Understanding and Managing Thyroid Disease

Understanding and Managing Thyroid Disease

Editor: Dakota Marshall

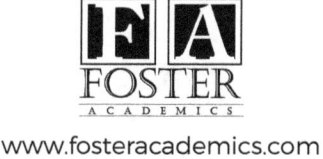

www.fosteracademics.com

www.fosteracademics.com

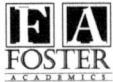

Cataloging-in-Publication Data

Understanding and managing thyroid disease / edited by Dakota Marshall.
    p. cm.
Includes bibliographical references and index.
ISBN 978-1-63242-947-6
1. Thyroid gland--Diseases. 2. Thyroid gland--Diseases--Diagnosis.
3. Thyroid gland--Diseases--Treatment. I. Marshall, Dakota.
RC655 .U53 2020
61644--dc23

Foster Academics,
118-35 Queens Blvd., Suite 400,
Forest Hills, NY 11375, USA

ISBN 978-1-63242-947-6 (Hardback)

Contents

Preface

This book has been a concerted effort by a group of academicians, researchers and scientists, who have contributed their research works for the realization of the book. This book has materialized in the wake of emerging advancements and innovations in this field. Therefore, the need of the hour was to compile all the required researches and disseminate the knowledge to a broad spectrum of people comprising of students, researchers and specialists of the field.

The thyroid is an endocrine gland consisting of two lobes which are connected by an isthmus. It produces various hormones that have determining roles in metabolic, cardiovascular, sexual and developmental processes. There are 20,000 protein coding genes of human cells, out of which 70% are expressed in the thyroid itself. The corresponding specific proteins are involved in hormone synthesis. When there is an excessive production of thyroid hormone, it results in a condition known as hyperthyroidism. It causes a number of non-specific syndromes, such as increased appetite, weight loss, tremor, decreased tolerance of heat, muscle weakness, etc. An underactive thyroid gland causes hypothyroidism characterized by symptoms such as abnormal weight gain, heavy menstruation, cold intolerance, hair loss, etc. Nodules in the thyroid gland can cause either cancerous or non-cancerous symptoms. Any of the functional disorders of the thyroid gland can cause the enlargement of the gland and cause goiter. This book is compiled in such a manner, that it will provide in-depth knowledge about thyroid disorders. The topics covered herein deal with the management and treatment of these disorders. The extensive content of this book provides the readers with a thorough understanding of the subject.

At the end of the preface, I would like to thank the authors for their brilliant chapters and the publisher for guiding us all-through the making of the book till its final stage. Also, I would like to thank my family for providing the support and encouragement throughout my academic career and research projects.

Editor

Why Can Insulin Resistance be a Natural Consequence of Thyroid Dysfunction?

Gabriela Brenta

Department of Endocrinology, Dr. César Milstein Hospital, La Rioja 951, C1221ACI, Buenos Aires, Argentina

Correspondence should be addressed to Gabriela Brenta, gbrenta@gmail.com

Academic Editor: Masanobu Yamada

Evidence for a relationship between T4 and T3 and glucose metabolism appeared over 100 years ago when the influence of thyroid hormone excess in the deterioration of glucose metabolism was first noticed. Since then, it has been known that hyperthyroidism is associated with insulin resistance. More recently, hypothyroidism has also been linked to decreased insulin sensitivity. The explanation to this apparent paradox may lie in the differential effects of thyroid hormones at the liver and peripheral tissues level. The purpose of this paper is to explore the effects of thyroid hormones in glucose metabolism and analyze the mechanisms whereby alterations of thyroid hormones lead to insulin resistance.

1. Introduction

The effects of T4 and T3 have a large impact on glucose homeostasis. This concept was acknowledged by Nobel Prize winner Dr. Bernardo Alberto Houssay in his lecture in 1947 *"The blood sugar and the production and consumption of glucose are kept within normal bounds, therefore there is an equilibrium between the glands of internal secretions which reduce the blood sugar (pancreas) and those which raise it (anterohypophysis, adrenals, thyroid, etc.)"*. Thyroid hormones exert both insulin agonistic and antagonistic actions in different organs. However, this occurs in a fine balance necessary for normal glucose metabolism. Deficit or excess of thyroid hormones can break this equilibrium leading to alterations of carbohydrate metabolism. Overt hyperthyroidism has been related to glucose intolerance and even ketoacidosis. With regards to hypothyroidism, cases of hypoglycemia have been reported in the literature despite the fact that peripheral insulin resistance may be present.

In the century that has elapsed, since the first observations of uncontrolled glucose metabolism in thyrotoxic diabetic patients [1], new pathways involved in the regulation of glucose homeostasis by thyroid hormones have been unveiled. Novel findings include the stimulation of hepatic glucose production by thyroid hormones acting via a sympathetic pathway from the hypothalamus [2] and

the discovery of transcriptional regulators of metabolic and mitochondrial genes that, influenced by intracellular T3 levels, may contribute to the development of insulin resistance [3]. The calorigenic-thermogenic activity of T3 long ascribed solely to uncoupling of mitochondrial oxidative phosphorylation has recently been related to T3-induced gating of mitochondrial permeability transition pore (PTP) of the inner mitochondrial membrane where the whole T3 transduction pathway integrates genomic and nongenomic activities of T3 in regulating mitochondrial energetics [4].

In this paper, we summarize the effects of thyroid hormones in glucose metabolism and its alterations when thyroid dysfunction is present.

2. Effects of Thyroid Hormones on Glucose Metabolism (Figure 1)

2.1. Direct Effects of Thyroid Hormones at the Liver Level (Table 1). Thyroid receptor-mediated effects on gene transcription and translation are key in the regulation of glucose metabolism. According to the results of studies with complementary DNA (cDNA) microarray analysis in mouse liver, this organ is a major target of thyroid hormones. Several genes involved in gluconeogenesis, glycogen metabolism, and insulin signaling that are regulated by thyroid hormones have been identified. In the study by Feng et al. [5], RNA

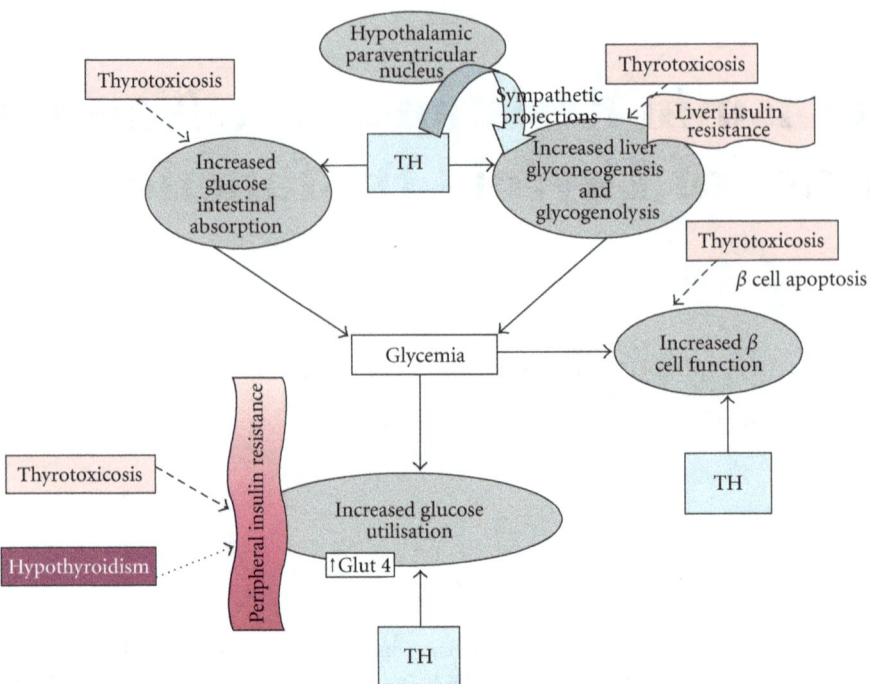

FIGURE 1: Effects of thyroid hormones on glucose metabolism in euthyroid (solid lines), hyperthyroid (rough-dashed lines), and hypothyroid conditions (fine-dashed lines). TH: thyroid hormones.

from hypothyroid mice treated with T3 was prepared, labeled with fluorescent dye, and hybridized with the cDNA microarray. An increase in glucose-6-phosphatase mRNA expression with T3 was reported. This enzyme hydrolyzes glucose-6-phosphate and completes the final step in gluconeogenesis and glycogenolysis, therefore playing an important role in the homeostatic regulation of blood glucose levels. Another finding was a decrease in mRNA expression of Akt2 (protein kinase B), a serine/threonine kinase that is an essential molecule in the insulin signaling pathway. Akt2 has been shown to promote glycogen synthesis in liver by inactivating glycogen synthase kinase 3. Thus, a decrease in Akt2 activity would decrease glycogen synthesis explaining the antagonistic insulin effect of thyroid hormones at the liver. Moreover, an induction of β2-adrenergic receptor mRNA and repression of inhibitory G protein (Gi) RNA of the adenylate cyclase cascade by T3 were also reported. All these results are in favour of a permissive influence of T3 in the glycogenolytic and gluconeogenic effects of epinephrine and glucagon. Other hepatic gluconeogenic enzymes that have been found to be positively regulated by thyroid hormones include phosphoenolpyruvate carboxykinase (PEPCK), the enzyme that catalyzes the rate-controlling step of gluconeogenesis [6] and pyruvate carboxylase, involved in the synthesis of oxaloacetate from pyruvate [7]. The catalytic activity of pyruvate carboxylase has been found increased approximately 2-fold in hyperthyroid rats compared with untreated or treated euthyroid controls.

Another mechanism, whereby thyroid hormones are known to increase hepatic glucose output, is through increased hepatic expression of the glucose transporter GLUT2

[8] as previously shown in a rat model where GLUT2 protein concentration in crude liver membranes was twice as high in chronically hyperthyroid versus hypothyroid animals.

It has been previously reported that, despite an expected resistance towards the insulin inhibitory effect on gluconeogenesis, the transcription of several enzymes involved in lipid synthesis or lipid metabolism is increased in hyperinsulinemic, insulin-resistant mice [9]. Furthermore, T3 induction of lipogenesis through the transcriptional activation of malic enzyme, involved in fatty acid synthesis, has been previously reported [10]. Therefore, it is possible that by the induction of lipogenic enzymes, T3 could be further aggravating the dysregulation of liver glucose and lipid metabolism characteristic of insulin resistance.

As a result of the long time quest for thyroid analogs that possess the favourable actions on metabolism without the unwanted thyroid cardiac effects, an indirect way of learning about T3 action in the different tissues has emerged [11]. The differential distribution of thyroid receptor (TR) isoforms in the tissues has been key for the development of these analogs. With regards to lipogenesis, carbohydrate-response element-binding protein (ChREBP) is a major transcription factor controlling the activation of glucose-induced lipogenesis in liver and is a direct target of thyroid hormones in liver and white adipose tissue (WAT), the two main lipogenic tissues in mice. ChREBP is shown to be specifically regulated by TRbeta but not by TRalpha in vivo, in liver where TRbeta represents 80% of the thyroid hormone bound TR, but also in WAT where both TR isoforms are expressed [12]. Although the area of thyroid analogs is beyond the scope of this paper, it is to be mentioned that

TABLE 1: Direct effects of T3 on genes that regulate glucose homeostasis at the liver and peripheral tissues (muscle, fat tissue, and fibroblasts).

Gene	Expression	Site	Net effect
glucose-6-phosphatase [5]	Increase	liver	Increase gluconeogenesis and glycogenolysis
protein kinase B (Akt2) [5]	decrease	liver	Decrease glycogen synthesis
β2-adrenergic receptor [5]	Increase	liver	Increase gluconeogenesis and glycogenolysis
inhibitory G protein (Gi) [5]	decrease	liver	Increase gluconeogenesis and glycogenolysis
phosphoenolpyruvate carboxykinase (PEPCK) [6]	Increase	liver	Increase gluconeogenesis
pyruvate carboxylase (PC) [7]	Increase	liver	Increase gluconeogenesis
GLUT2 [8]	Increase	liver	Increase glucose output
malic enzyme [10]	Increase	liver	lipogenesis
Carbohydrate-response element-binding protein (ChREBP) [12]	Increase	liver and fat tissue	lipogenesis
GLUT1 [14]	Increase	peripheral tissues	Increase glucose transport (basal)
GLUT4 [14]	Increase	peripheral tissues	Increase glucose transport (insulin-induced)
β2-adrenergic receptor [20]	Increase	Peripheral tissues	Increase lipolysis
phosphoglycerate kinase (PGK) [15]	Increase	peripheral tissues	Increase glycolysis
Hypoxia-inducible factor 1 (HIF-1α) [15]	Increase	peripheral tissues	Increase glycolysis
PPAR gamma coactivator-1 alpha (PGC-1 alpha) [27]	Increase	peripheral tissues	Increase mitochondrial biogenesis and function
uncoupling protein 3 (UCP3) [17]	Increase	peripheral tissues	Increase mitochondrial energy expenditure

some thyromimetic analogs, such as 3,5-l-diiodothyronine (T(2)), exert their beneficial action on metabolism, without inducing a thyrotoxic state, through a mechanism that does not involve binding to thyroid hormone receptors [13]. In rats fed a high-fat diet, the addition of T(2) to lipid-overloaded cells resulted in reduction in lipid content; downregulation of peroxisome proliferator-activated receptors (PPAR)α, PPARγ, and alternative oxidase (AOX) expression; increase in PPARδ expression; and stimulation of mitochondrial uncoupling thus preventing and reversing hepatic steatosis in this animal model. Surprisingly, in this study, these lipid-lowering actions not mediated by TR were also observed with T3.

To summarize, all these findings have helped to understand that thyroid hormones have insulin antagonistic effects at the liver that lead to an increased glucose hepatic output, via an enhanced rate of gluconeogenesis and glycogenolysis. With regards to lipid metabolism, both lipogenesis and lipolysis are stimulated by T3. However, in the context of insulin resistance, the conversion of glucose into fatty acids together with nonsuppressed gluconeogenesis is simply perpetuating the hyperinsulinemic state. Furthermore, nutritional influences, such as those of high-fat diets, should also be taken into consideration as modifiers of the effects of thyroid hormones on insulin sensitivity.

2.2. Direct Effects of Thyroid Hormones at the Peripheral Tissue Level (Table 1). Opposite to what occurs at the liver level, at peripheral tissues, thyroid hormones have been shown to exert some of their actions synergically with insulin. The upregulation of the expression of genes such as GLUT-4 [14] or phosphoglycerate kinase (PGK) [15], involved in

glucose transport and glycolysis respectively, is a good proof of concept.

In skeletal muscle, the main site of insulin-mediated glucose disposal, glucose transporter GLUT4, is induced by T3, revealing that it can increase basal and insulin-stimulated glucose transport in this tissue [14]. Another T3 target in skeletal muscle is mitochondrial uncoupling protein 3 (UCP3). Unveiling this association may be important since progressive reduction of UCP3 levels results in insulin resistance accompanied by decreased fatty acid oxidation and a less intense Akt/PKB and 5' adenosine monophosphate-activated protein kinase (AMPK) signaling [16]. Although discrepancies between the regulation by T3 of UCP3 expression in rats, humans, and mice have been observed, the rat model has shed some light into T3 actions in this tissue. T3 intravenous (i.v.) administration in hypothyroid rats showed a rise in serum fatty acid levels concomitant with a rapid increase in UCP3 expression in gastrocnemius muscle. These findings point to UCP as a possible molecular determinant of the action of T3 on energy metabolism [17].

Liver actions of the naturally occurring thyromimetic analog T2 have been discussed above. However, T2 actions have been also explored in skeletal muscle [18]. In a model of high-fat diet-induced insulin resistance in rat, the administration of T2, on the gastrocnemius muscle, induced remarkable changes on the metabolic/structural phenotype and insulin signaling. T2 increased insulin-stimulated Akt phosphorylation levels, the muscle contents of fast/glycolytic fibers and sarcolemmal GLUT4. Moreover, glycolytic enzymes and associated components were upregulated together with phosphofructokinase activity.

The result of cDNA microarray analysis on skeletal muscle of a group of healthy men receiving 75 μg/d of T3 for 14 days has shown that not only genes with agonistic insulin effects but several others with antagonistic insulin effects are upregulated by treatment with T3 [19], underlying the pleiotropic effect of thyroid hormone in energy metabolism. cDNA array data have also provided a molecular basis to the effect of T3 on adipose tissue. In human adipocytes, T3 increases the mRNA levels of the lipolytic β2-AR, favouring catecolamine-induced lipolysis and it also downregulates Sterol regulatory element binding protein (SREBP1c), involved in lipogenesis, which may constitute a link between hyperthyroidism and insulin resistance [20].

Skin fibroblasts have been also used to study thyroid hormone-responsive genes involved in metabolism in human cells. Although they are not as metabolically active as hepatic cells, they are easily obtained and also, thyroid hormone-responsive. In cultured human fibroblasts, Moeller et al. [15] observed that, opposite to a posttranscriptional regulation as reported for other growth factors and hormones, the mRNA of the transcription factor HIF-1α (Hypoxia-inducible factor 1), a key mediator of glycolysis, increased in response to T3. As the glucose transporter GLUT1, several enzymes of glycolysis, and the lactate exporter SLC16A3 were all also found induced by T3 and are target genes of the transcription factor HIF-1α, the authors postulated that the effect of thyroid hormones on the induction of these genes most probably was indirect and HIF-1α mediated. Furthermore, a new mechanism of thyroid action was unraveled by this group of researchers [21]. It was shown that T3 bound to TRbeta, *in lieu* of initiating gene transcription in the nucleus, activates the phosphatidylinositol 3-kinase (PI3K) signaling pathway in the cytosol in order to activate HIF-1α gene expression.

At the cellular level, thyroid hormones can also increase mitochondrial biogenesis, fatty acid oxidation, and TCA cycle activity [22]. These findings are quite relevant since the role of mitochondrial dysfunction, leading to cellular lipid excess and impaired oxidative metabolism, has been clearly demonstrated in the pathogenesis of type 2 diabetes [23–25]. Furthermore, it has been described that in skeletal muscle, the lack of thyroid hormones might dysregulate mitochondrial gene expression [26]. PPAR gamma coactivator-1 alpha (PGC-1 alpha), a key transcriptional regulator of mitochondrial content and function, fatty acid oxidation, and gluconeogenesis, has been involved in the process whereby thyroid hormones regulate mitochondrial function [3]. It has been shown that PGC-1 alpha gene expression is increased by T3, as much as 13-fold 6 hours after T3 treatment [27]. The regulation pattern of T3 on PGC-1 alpha is complex and may occur through nongenomic activation of kinases to induce the expression of PGC-1 alpha or through transcriptional upregulation via the presence of a thyroid responsive element (TRE) in the PGC-1 alpha promoter or by genomic upregulation of a transcription factor (via a TRE), which then binds to the PGC-1 alpha promoter and increases PGC-1 alpha transcription [28]. It is hypothesized that PGC-1 alpha can be dysregulated by reduced T3 levels [3], thus contributing to insulin resistance. Not only low circulating but also, intracellular T3 levels, could count for this matter. A lower expression and activity of type 2 iodothyronine-deiodinase (D2), the enzyme that is key for the conversion of T4 into T3 in muscle and thus, amplifies thyroid hormone signaling in individual cells, has been found linked to insulin resistance [29, 30]. If PGC-1 alpha effects on mitochondrial gene expression may indeed be regulated by thyroid hormone, normal activity of deiodinase type 2 is very relevant. Several factors, related to this enzymatic activity, are being currently studied. Bile acids are potent stimulators of the enzyme and may play an important role in the relationship between thyroid action and glucose metabolism [31]. On the other hand, the natural occurrence of polymorphisms of deiodinase type 2 such as Thr92Ala, with a lower activity, has also been implicated with increased risk for diabetes type 2 [29].

2.3. Indirect Effects of Thyroid Hormones to the Liver. It has been shown that the hypothalamus can modulate endogenous glucose production by using functionally reciprocal sympathetic and parasympathetic autonomic outputs to the liver [32]. Moreover, a sympathetic pathway from the hypothalamic paraventricular nucleus to the liver has been proposed as a central pathway for modulation of hepatic glucose metabolism by thyroid hormone [33]. Klieveric et al. [33] demonstrated that upon selective administration to the paraventricular nucleus (PVN), T3 increases endogenous glucose production and plasma glucose, and that these hypothalamic T3 effects are mediated via sympathetic projections to the liver. In order to arrive to such remarkable findings, the authors worked with euthyroid rats treated with methimazole and T4. First they administered an intracerebroventricular (i.c.v.) T3 or vehicle (Veh) infusion, and there was a significant increase in plasma glucose compared with Veh-treated rats. This meant that central T3 infusion could reproduce the characteristic increase in hepatic glucose output of thyrotoxicosis. To further identify the neuroanatomic region responsible for these changes, the authors infused T3 within the hypothalamus at the PVN. A similar response was obtained, that was independent of plasma T3, insulin, and corticosterone concentrations. They repeated the experiment in surgically hepatic sympathectomized animals (HSx) and sham-denervated animals. HSx animals showed a decrease of endogenous glucose output upon hypothalamic T3 infusion. The principal finding of this study is the description of a neural (autonomic) modulation of hepatic glucose metabolism by T3 at the hypothalamus that takes place independently of plasma glucoregulatory hormone concentrations.

3. Insulin Resistance as a Consequence of Hyperthyroidism

Thyrotoxic subjects frequently show impaired glucose tolerance. This is a result of increased glucose turnover with increased glucose absorption through the gastrointestinal tract, postabsorptive hyperglycemia, elevated hepatic glucose output, with elevated fasting and/or postprandial insulin and proinsulin levels, elevated free fatty acid concentrations and elevated peripheral glucose transport and utilization. The literature about this topic is vast and has been previously comprehensively reviewed by Dimitriadis and Raptis [34]. Thyrotoxic diabetic patients are more prone to ketosis [35]. Although ketoacidosis may result *per se* from the insulin resistance present in thyrotoxicosis, the stimulatory action of thyroid hormones in excess on lipolysis and free fatty acids availability can also contribute to increased ketogenesis [36].

3.1. Increased Hepatic Glucose Output in Hyperthyroidism.
Thyrotoxicosis has been reported to increase endogenous glucose production in the liver in the basal state and to decrease hepatic insulin sensitivity in humans [37]. The different mechanisms to explain this phenomenon include increased rates of gluconeogenesis and glycogenolysis [38] mainly explained by the above-mentioned effects on the liver by thyroid hormones. To summarize, these effects include thyroid receptor-mediated effects on liver gene transcription [5], increased sympathetic action in the liver mediated by hypothalamus [33], and increased concentrations of the GLUT2 glucose transporters in the liver plasma membrane that allows for glucose efflux [8, 39] together with increased concentration of free fatty acids in plasma [40].

3.2. Peripheral Tissues Glucose Metabolism in Hyperthyroidism.
The interpretation of the effects of hyperthyroidism on glucose utilization by peripheral tissues is by far the most complex issue on this topic. On one hand, the rates of glucose uptake in peripheral tissues have been found increased by thyroid hormones, suggesting that glucose utilization is highly increased, specially in skeletal muscle [34, 37, 41–44]. This increased utilization, as shown by indirect calorimetry during euglycemic hyperinsulinemic clamps, is mainly due to an increase in insulin-stimulated glucose oxidation rates [43, 45–48]. However, a decrease in insulin-stimulated nonoxidative glucose disposal, through reduced glycogenogenesis [43, 44, 49], takes place, with intracellular glucose being redirected towards glycolysis and lactate formation. The release of lactate from peripheral tissues back to the liver is a major contributor to the Cori cycle where more hepatic glucose is being produced [43, 49–51].

Although glucose intolerance in hyperthyroidism can be easily explained by hepatic insulin resistance without involvement of peripheral tissues, impaired insulin-stimulated peripheral glucose uptake has also been proven in some studies. By means of the arteriovenous difference technique in the forearm muscles of hyperthyroid subjects after the consumption of a mixed meal, it has been clearly demonstrated that muscle blood flow is increased, masking a defect in insulin-stimulated glucose uptake [52]. Moreover, in disagreement with previous reports [41, 45], Shen et al. [53] also described decreased peripheral insulin sensitivity in hyperthyroidism.

Alternative explanations for peripheral insulin resistance in hyperthyroidism include an increased secretion of bioactive mediators (adipokines) such as interleukin 6 (IL6) and tumour necrosis factor a (TNFα) from adipose tissue in hyperthyroidism [54]. These adipokines, that exert both proinflammatory and insulin resistant effects, have been found elevated in hyperthyroid women [54].

3.3. Insulin and Glucagon Secretion and Degradation in Hyperthyroidism.
In hyperthyroidism, decreased, normal, or even increased levels of plasma insulin have been reported [34]. However, a rather consistent finding has been the increased degradation of insulin in hyperthyroid subjects [43, 55]. It has been postulated that, in the long run, severe thyrotoxicosis can lead to irreversible pancreatic damage [56, 57].

With regards to glucagon, its secretion and metabolic clearance rates have been reported increased, explaining the normal fasting plasma levels described in hyperthyroidism [58].

3.4. Subclinical Hyperthyroidism and Insulin Resistance.
Subclinical hyperthyroidism has also been associated with insulin resistance [59–61] in some but not all studies [62]. The heterogenous nature of this condition can partly explain this controversy. Endogenous subclinical hyperthyroidism may have a larger impact on glucose metabolism due to its chronicity and higher T3 levels when compared to exogenous administration of T4 [61].

4. Hypothyroidism Can Also Lead to Insulin Resistance

Although seldom happening, hypothyroid patients can experience hypoglycaemia. This phenomenon can be interpreted in the light of reduced levels of gluconeogenesis leading to decreased liver glucose output [63, 64]. On the other hand, insulin resistance has been shown to be present in peripheral tissues in hypothyroid animal models [65, 66]. Hence, a poor utilization of glucose in hypothyroidism may be offset by a reduced release to circulation maintaining a balance of the glucose metabolism.

4.1. Animal Studies Showing Insulin Resistance in Hypothyroidism.
Studies performed in adipocytes and skeletal muscle of rats made hypothyroid have shown that these tissues are less responsive to insulin with regards to glucose metabolism [63, 65–69]. Czech et al. [65] studied insulin responsiveness in adipocytes and skeletal muscle of mature rats rendered hypothyroid by a low iodine diet and propylthiouracil. It was observed that glucose conversion to glycogen was partially inhibited while the glycolytic flux stimulation by insulin was totally frustrated. This decrease in insulin sensitivity occurred without an impaired membrane insulin effector system. Other authors [66, 67] showed decreased insulin-stimulated glucose transport and/or phosphorylation, as well as a lower rate of glycolysis in the isolated, incubated soleus muscle of the hypothyroid rat and also suggested that the effects of hypothyroidism in muscle were not mediated through an interference of insulin binding to its receptor. It was postulated that they rather occurred through a postreceptor mechanism that may include abnormal phosphorylation of insulin signaling proteins.

Insulin resistance was confirmed in another study of rats with mild hypothyroidism [69]. In this study, insulin responsiveness was measured by an insulin tolerance test and an euglycemic-hyperinsulinemic clamp followed by measurements of tissue-specific glucose utilization indices with the labelled 2-deoxy-D-[1-3H]glucose (2-DG) technique in muscles (red quadriceps) and white adipose tissue (epididymal fat). Several other parameters were also determined such as muscle triglyceride content, plasma leptin and nonesterified fatty acids (NEFA) levels, and mRNA expression of resistin in adipose tissue as well as adipose tissue and liver carnitine palmitoyl transferase 1α (CPT-1α), and muscle carnitine palmitoyl transferase 1β (CPT-1β) mRNA levels, explored by real-time quantitative PCR. Plasma leptin levels were lower and adipose tissue mRNA expression of resistin higher, in the hypothyroid state. Looking for a potential role of leptin in the metabolic consequences of hypothyroidism, leptin was infused, and it was found that glucose disposal was recovered. Increased expression of muscle and adipose tissue carnitine palmitoyl transferases, decreased plasma NEFA levels, and reduced muscle triglyceride content after leptin infusion were interpreted as the mediators of the recovery of the insulin resistant state. Therefore, one possible explanation to decreased insulin responsiveness in hypothyroidism, according to the authors of this study, includes a dysregulation of leptin action at the hypothalamus.

Adipocyte-myocyte crosstalk by adipokines has been reported to play a significant role in skeletal muscle insulin resistance and may partially explain insulin resistance present in hypothyroidism [70]. However, other factors associated with insulin resistance in hypothyroidism, such as altered blood flow, impaired GLUT4 translocation, decreased glycogen synthesis, and decreased muscle oxidative capacity have to be also considered [71].

4.2. Studies in Humans Demonstrating Insulin Resistance in Hypothyroidism. Compared to the number of reports about insulin resistance in hyperthyroid patients, there are relatively fewer studies in humans dealing with the effects of hypothyroidism on glucose metabolism. Rochon et al. [72] measured whole-body sensitivity of glucose disposal to insulin in hypothyroid patients using the euglycemic-hyperinsulinemic clamp technique. They demonstrated that hypothyroidism induced a decrease in the insulin-mediated glucose disposal that reverted upon treatment. Similar results were obtained by Stanická et al. [73]. By means of the same clamp technique and also measuring glucose tolerance and beta-cell activity with an oral glucose tolerance tests (OGTT), Handisurya et al. [74] confirmed these findings and added the knowledge that glucose-induced insulin secretion is diminished by thyroid replacement corresponding well with the observed improvement of insulin sensitivity.

Dimitriadis et al. [75] explored glucose uptake in muscle and adipose tissue of hypothyroid and control subjects by means of the arteriovenous difference technique in the anterior abdominal subcutaneous adipose tissue and the forearm muscles after the consumption of a mixed meal. A decreased net extraction of glucose and blood flow after the meal in hypothyroid muscle and adipose tissue was reported. This impairment in the ability of insulin to increase blood flow rate to the hypothyroid tissues is an alternative explanation to the mechanism whereby hypothyroidism

can induce lower glucose disposal. The short i.v. insulin tolerance test has been used to explore insulin sensitivity in acute overt hypothyroid patients. Compared to euthyroid controls, hypothyroid patients had a significantly lower glucose disposal [76].

Some negative results, however, in this field have been reported. A previous study in overt hypothyroid patients based on the homeostasis model assessment (HOMA-IR) [77] showed no association between hypothyroidism and insulin sensitivity. Moreover, Harris et al. [78] found unimpaired insulin-stimulated glucose disposal in the forearm of hypothyroid patients after treatment with levothyroxine.

4.3. Subclinical Hypothyroidism. With regards to subclinical hypothyroidism, insulin resistance has been demonstrated in some [60, 74, 79] but not all studies, where HOMA levels were found comparable to a control group [80–82]. However, in some of these negative studies [80, 81], hyperinsulinemia was reported in subclinical hypothyroid subjects and interpreted as an early sign of impairment of glucose metabolism.

5. Conclusions

Thyroid hormones have a large impact on glucose metabolism. A direct regulation on thyroid responsive genes at the target organ has been described and more recently an indirect effect involving hypothalamic pathways that regulate glucose metabolism via control of the sympathetic nervous system has been reported. Furthermore, thyroid hormone effects can be insulin agonistic, such as demonstrated in muscle or antagonistic such as observed in the liver. In hyperthyroidism, dysregulation of this balance may end in glucose intolerance mainly due to hepatic insulin resistance. In hypothyroidism the results are less evident. However, the available data suggest that insulin resistance is present mainly at the peripheral tissues. Possible explanations hypothesized to explain this phenomenon span from the dysregulation of mitochondrial oxidative metabolism to the reduction of blood flow in muscle and adipose tissue under hypothyroid conditions.

References

[1] G. L. Rohdenburg, "Thyroid diabetes," *Endocrinology*, vol. 4, p. 63, 1920.

[2] L. P. Klieverik, S. F. Janssen, A. Van Riel et al., "Thyroid hormone modulates glucose production via a sympathetic pathway from the hypothalamic paraventricular nucleus to the liver," *Proceedings of the National Academy of Sciences of the United States of America*, vol. 106, no. 14, pp. 5966–5971, 2009.

[3] S. Crunkhorn and M. E. Patti, "Links between thyroid hormone action, oxidative metabolism, and diabetes risk?" *Thyroid*, vol. 18, no. 2, pp. 227–237, 2008.

[4] E. Yehuda-Shnaidman, B. Kalderon, N. Azazmeh, and J. Bar-Tana, "Gating of the mitochondrial permeability transition pore by thyroid hormone," *Federation of American Societies for Experimental Biology Journal*, vol. 24, no. 1, pp. 93–104, 2010.

[5] X. Feng, Y. Jiang, P. Meltzer, and P. M. Yen, "Thyroid hormone regulation of hepatic genes in vivo detected by complementary

DNA microarray," *Molecular Endocrinology*, vol. 14, no. 7, pp. 947–955, 2000.

[6] E. A. Park, D. C. Jerden, and S. W. Bahouth, "Regulation of phosphoenolpyruvate carboxykinase gene transcription by thyroid hormone involves two distinct binding sites in the promoter," *Biochemical Journal*, vol. 309, no. 3, part 3, pp. 913–919, 1995.

[7] M. B. Weinberg and M. F. Utter, "Effect of thyroid hormone on the turnover of rat liver pyruvate carboxylase and pyruvate dehydrogenase," *Journal of Biological Chemistry*, vol. 254, no. 19, pp. 9492–9499, 1979.

[8] S. P. Weinstein, E. O'Boyle, M. Fisher, and R. S. Haber, "Regulation of GLUT2 glucose transporter expression in liver by thyroid hormone: evidence for hormonal regulation of the hepatic glucose transport system," *Endocrinology*, vol. 135, no. 2, pp. 649–654, 1994.

[9] W. Becker, R. Kluge, T. Kantner et al., "Differential hepatic gene expression in a polygenic mouse model with insulin resistance and hyperglycemia: evidence for a combined transcriptional dysregulation of gluconeogenesis and fatty acid synthesis," *Journal of Molecular Endocrinology*, vol. 32, no. 1, pp. 195–208, 2004.

[10] C. N. Mariash, C. R. McSwigan, H. C. Towle, H. L. Schwartz, and J. H. Oppenheimer, "Glucose and triiodothyronine both induce malic enzyme in the rat hepatocyte culture: evidence that triiodothyronine multiplies a primary glucose-generated signal," *Journal of Clinical Investigation*, vol. 68, no. 6, pp. 1485–1490, 1981.

[11] G. Brenta, S. Danzi, and I. Klein, "Potential therapeutic applications of thyroid hormone analogs," *Nature Clinical Practice Endocrinology & Metabolism*, vol. 3, pp. 632–664, 2007.

[12] K. Gauthier, C. Billon, M. Bissler et al., "Thyroid hormone receptor β(TRβ) and liver X receptor (LXR) regulate carbohydrate-response element-binding protein (ChREBP) expression in a tissue-selective manner," *Journal of Biological Chemistry*, vol. 285, no. 36, pp. 28156–28163, 2010.

[13] E. Grasselli, A. Voci, L. Canesi et al., "Non-receptor-mediated actions are responsible for the lipid-lowering effects of iodothyronines in FaO rat hepatoma cells," *Journal of Endocrinology*, vol. 210, no. 1, pp. 59–69, 2011.

[14] S. P. Weinstein, E. O'Boyle, and R. S. Haber, "Thyroid hormone increases basal and insulin-stimulated glucose transport in skeletal muscle. The role of GLUT4 glucose transporter expression," *Diabetes*, vol. 43, no. 10, pp. 1185–1189, 1994.

[15] L. C. Moeller, A. M. Dumitrescu, R. L. Walker, P. S. Meltzer, and S. Refetoff, "Thyroid hormone responsive genes in cultured human fibroblasts," *Journal of Clinical Endocrinology & Metabolism*, vol. 90, no. 2, pp. 936–943, 2005.

[16] R. Senese, V. Valli, M. Moreno et al., "Uncoupling protein 3 expression levels influence insulin sensitivity, fatty acid oxidation, and related signaling pathways," *Pflugers Archiv European Journal of Physiology*, vol. 461, no. 1, pp. 153–164, 2010.

[17] P. de Lange, A. Feola, M. Ragni et al., "Differential 3,5,3′-triiodothyronine-mediated regulation of uncoupling protein 3 transcription: role of fatty acids," *Endocrinology*, vol. 148, no. 8, pp. 4064–4072, 2007.

[18] M. Moreno, E. Silvestri, R. De Matteis et al., "3,5-Diiodo-L-thyronine prevents high-fat-diet-induced insulin resistance in rat skeletal muscle through metabolic and structural adaptations," *Journal of the Federation of American Societies for Experimental Biology*. In press.

[19] K. Clément, N. Viguerie, M. Diehn et al., "In vivo regulation of human skeletal muscle gene expression by thyroid hormone," *Genome Research*, vol. 12, no. 2, pp. 281–291, 2002.

[20] N. Viguerie, L. Millet, S. Avizou, H. Vidal, D. Larrouy, and D. Langin, "Regulation of human adipocyte gene expression by thyroid hormone," *Journal of Clinical Endocrinology & Metabolism*, vol. 87, no. 2, pp. 630–634, 2002.

[21] L. C. Moeller, X. Cao, A. M. Dumitrescu, H. Seo, and S. Refetoff, "Thyroid hormone mediated changes in gene expression can be initiated by cytosolic action of the thyroid hormone receptor beta through the phosphatidylinositol 3-kinase pathway," *Nuclear Receptor Signaling*, vol. 4, p. e020, 2006.

[22] F. Goglia, M. Moreno, and A. Lanni, "Action of thyroid hormones at the cellular level: the mitochondrial target," *Federation of the Societies of Biochemistry and Molecular Biology Letters*, vol. 452, no. 3, pp. 115–120, 1999.

[23] M. E. Patti, A. J. Butte, S. Crunkhorn et al., "Coordinated reduction of genes of oxidative metabolism in humans with insulin resistance and diabetes: potential role of PGC1 and NRF1," *Proceedings of the National Academy of Sciences of the United States of America*, vol. 100, no. 14, pp. 8466–8471, 2003.

[24] V. K. Mootha, C. M. Lindgren, K. F. Eriksson et al., "PGC-1α-responsive genes involved in oxidative phosphorylation are coordinately downregulated in human diabetes," *Nature Genetics*, vol. 34, no. 3, pp. 267–273, 2003.

[25] K. F. Petersen, D. Befroy, S. Dufour et al., "Mitochondrial dysfunction in the elderly: possible role in insulin resistance," *Science*, vol. 300, no. 5622, pp. 1140–1142, 2003.

[26] I. Irrcher, P. J. Adhihetty, T. Sheehan, A. M. Joseph, and D. A. Hood, "PPARγ coactivator-1α expression during thyroid hormone- and contractile activity-induced mitochondrial adaptations," *American Journal of Physiology—Cell Physiology*, vol. 284, no. 6, pp. 1669–1677, 2003.

[27] J. M. Weitzel, C. Radtke, and H. J. Seitz, "Two thyroid hormone-mediated gene expression patterns in vivo identified by cDNA expression arrays in rat," *Nucleic Acids Research*, vol. 29, no. 24, pp. 5148–5155, 2001.

[28] I. Irrcher, D. R. Walkinshaw, T. E. Sheehan, and D. A. Hood, "Thyroid hormone (T3) rapidly activates p38 and AMPK in skeletal muscle in vivo," *Journal of Applied Physiology*, vol. 104, no. 1, pp. 178–185, 2008.

[29] D. Mentuccia, L. Proietti-Pannunzi, K. Tanner et al., "Association between a novel variant of the human type 2 deiodinase gene Thr92Ala and insulin resistance: evidence of interaction with the Trp64Arg variant of the β-3-adrenergic receptor," *Diabetes*, vol. 51, no. 3, pp. 880–883, 2002.

[30] J. M. Dora, W. E. Machado, J. Rheinheimer, D. Crispim, and A. L. Maia, "Association of the type 2 deiodinase Thr92Ala polymorphism with type 2 diabetes: case-control study and meta-analysis," *European Journal of Endocrinology*, vol. 163, no. 3, pp. 427–434, 2010.

[31] M. Watanabe, S. M. Houten, C. Mataki et al., "Bile acids induce energy expenditure by promoting intracellular thyroid hormone activation," *Nature*, vol. 439, no. 7075, pp. 484–489, 2006.

[32] A. Kalsbeek, S. La Fleur, C. Van Heijningen, and R. M. Buijs, "Suprachiasmatic GABAergic inputs to the paraventricular nucleus control plasma glucose concentrations in the rat via sympathetic innervation of the liver," *Journal of Neuroscience*, vol. 24, no. 35, pp. 7604–7613, 2004.

[33] L. P. Klieverik, S. F. Janssen, A. Van Riel et al., "Thyroid hormone modulates glucose production via a sympathetic pathway from the hypothalamic paraventricular nucleus to the

liver," *Proceedings of the National Academy of Sciences of the United States of America*, vol. 106, no. 14, pp. 5966–5971, 2009.

[34] G. D. Dimitriadis and S. A. Raptis, "Thyroid hormone excess and glucose intolerance," *Experimental and Clinical Endocrinology and Diabetes*, vol. 109, no. 2, pp. S225–S239, 2001.

[35] M. Beylot, J. P. Riou, F. Bienvenu, and R. Mornex, "Increased ketonaemia in hyperthyroidism," *Diabetologia*, vol. 19, no. 6, pp. 505–510, 1980.

[36] M. Beylot, "Regulation of in vivo ketogenesis: role of free fatty acids and control by epinephrine, thyroid hormones, insulin and glucagon," *Diabetes and Metabolism*, vol. 22, no. 5, pp. 299–304, 1996.

[37] P. Cavallo-Perin, A. Bruno, L. Boine, M. Cassader, G. Lenti, and G. Pagano, "Insulin resistance in Graves' disease: a quantitative in-vivo evaluation," *European Journal of Clinical Investigation*, vol. 18, no. 6, pp. 607–613, 1988.

[38] L. Sestoft, P. D. Bartels, P. Flero, M. Folke, S. Gammeltoft, and L. O. Kristensen, "Influence of thyroid state on the effects of glycerol on gluconeogenesis and energy metabolism in perfused rat liver," *Biochimica et Biophysica Acta*, vol. 499, no. 1, pp. 119–130, 1977.

[39] T. Mokuno, K. Uchimura, R. Hayashi et al., "Glucose transporter 2 concentrations in hyper- and hypothyroid rat livers," *Journal of Endocrinology*, vol. 160, no. 2, pp. 285–289, 1999.

[40] J. Saunders, S. E. H. Hall, and P. H. Sonksen, "Glucose and free fatty acid turnover in thyrotoxicosis and hypothyroidism, before and after treatment," *Clinical Endocrinology*, vol. 13, no. 1, pp. 33–44, 1980.

[41] M. Laville, J. P. Rio, P. F. Bougneres, and R. Mornex, "Glucose metabolism in experimental hyperthyroidism: intact in vivo sensitivity to insulin with abnormal binding and increased glucose turnover," *Journal of Clinical Endocrinology & Metabolism*, vol. 58, no. 6, pp. 960–965, 1984.

[42] P. R. Bratusch-Marrain, S. Gasić, and W. K. Waldhäusl, "Triiodothyronine increases splanchnic release and peripheral uptake of glucose in healthy humans," *The American Journal of Physiology*, vol. 247, no. 5, part 1, pp. E681–E687, 1984.

[43] G. Dimitriadis, B. Baker, H. Marsh et al., "Effect of thyroid hormone excess on action, secretion, and metabolism of insulin in humans," *The American Journal of physiology*, vol. 248, no. 5, pp. E593–E601, 1985.

[44] J. Randin, B. Scarriga, F. Jequier, and J. Felber, "Studies of glucose and lipid metabolism and continues indirect calorimetry in Graves' disease: effect of an oral glucose load," *Journal of Clinical Endocrinology & Metabolism*, vol. 61, pp. 1165–1171, 1985.

[45] A. J. McCulloch, R. Nosadini, A. Pernet et al., "Glucose turnover and indices of recycling in thyrotoxicosis and primary thyroid failure," *Clinical Science*, vol. 64, no. 1, pp. 41–47, 1983.

[46] M. P. Sandler, R. P. Robinson, D. Rabin, W. W. Lacy, and N. N. Abumrad, "The effect of thyroid hormones on gluconeogenesis and forearm metabolism in man," *Clinical Endocrinology & Metabolism*, vol. 56, no. 3, pp. 479–485, 1983.

[47] F. Celsing, E. Blomstrand, J. Melichna et al., "Effect of hyperthyroidism on fibre-type composition, fibre area, glycogen content and enzyme activity in human skeletal muscle," *Clinical Physiology*, vol. 6, no. 2, pp. 171–181, 1986.

[48] M. C. Foss, G. M. G. F. Paccola, M. J. A. Saad, W. P. Pimenta, C. E. Piccinato, and N. Iazigi, "Peripheral glucose metabolism in human hyperthyroidism," *Journal of Clinical Endocrinology & Metabolism*, vol. 70, no. 4, pp. 1167–1172, 1990.

[49] G. D. Dimitriadis, B. Leighton, I. G. Vlachonikolis et al., "Effects of hyperthyroidism on the sensitivity of glycolysis and

[50] M. Parry-Billings, G. D. Dimitriadis, B. Leighton et al., "Effects of hyperthyroidism and hypothyroidism on glutamine metabolism by skeletal muscle of the rat," *Biochemical Journal*, vol. 272, no. 2, pp. 319–322, 1990.

[51] B. Leighton, G. D. Dimitriadis, M. Oarry-Billings, J. Bond, P. Kemp, and E. A. Newsholme, "Thyroid hormone analogue SKF L-94901: effects on amino acid and carbohydrate metabolism in rat skeletal muscle in vitro," *Biochemical Pharmacology*, vol. 40, no. 5, pp. 1161–1164, 1990.

[52] G. Dimitriadis, P. Mitrou, V. Lambadiari et al., "Insulin-stimulated rates of glucose uptake in muscle in hyperthyroidism: the importance of blood flow," *Journal of Clinical Endocrinology & Metabolism*, vol. 93, no. 6, pp. 2413–2415, 2008.

[53] D. C. Shen, M. B. Davidson, S. W. Kuo, and W. H. Sheu, "Peripheral and hepatic insulin antagonism in hyperthyroidism," *Journal of Clinical Endocrinology & Metabolism*, vol. 66, no. 3, pp. 565–569, 1988.

[54] P. Mitrou, E. Boutati, V. Lambadiari et al., "Insulin resistance in hyperthyroidism: the role of IL6 and TNFα," *European Journal of Endocrinology*, vol. 162, no. 1, pp. 121–126, 2010.

[55] J. P. Randin, L. Tappy, and B. Scazziga, "Insulin sensitivity and exogenous insulin clearance in Graves' disease. Measurement by the glucose clamp technique and continuous indirect calorimetry," *Diabetes*, vol. 35, no. 2, pp. 178–181, 1986.

[56] S. Lenzen and H. Kucking, "Inhibition of insulin secretion by L-thyroxine and thyroxine treatment in rats under the influence of drugs affecting the adrenergic nervous system," *Acta Endocrinologica*, vol. 100, no. 4, pp. 527–533, 1982.

[57] H. M. Ximenes, S. Lortz, A. Jörns, and S. Lenzen, "Triiodothyronine (T3)-mediated toxicity and induction of apoptosis in insulin-producing INS-1 cells," *Life Sciences*, vol. 80, no. 22, pp. 2045–2050, 2007.

[58] G. Dimitriadis, E. Hatziagelaki, P. Mitrou et al., "Effect of hyperthyroidism on clearance and secretion of glucagon in man," *Experimental and Clinical Endocrinology & Diabetes*, vol. 119, no. 4, pp. 214–217, 2011.

[59] D. G. Yavuz, M. Yüksel, O. Deyneli, Y. Ozen, H. Aydin, and S. Akalin, "Association of serum paraoxonase activity with insulin sensitivity and oxidative stress in hyperthyroid and TSH-suppressed nodular goitre patients," *Clinical Endocrinology*, vol. 61, no. 4, pp. 515–521, 2004.

[60] E. Maratou, D. J. Hadjidakis, M. Peppa et al., "Studies of insulin resistance in patients with clinical and subclinical hyperthyroidism," *European Journal of Endocrinology*, vol. 163, no. 4, pp. 625–630, 2010.

[61] J. Rezzonico, H. Niepomniszcze, M. Rezzonico, E. Pusiol, M. Alberto, and G. Brenta, "The association of insulin resistance with subclinical thyrotoxicosis," *Thyroid*, vol. 21, no. 9, pp. 945–949, 2011.

[62] K. A. Heemstra, J. W. Smit, C. F. Eustatia-Rutten et al., "Glucose tolerance and lipid profile in longterm exogenous subclinical hyperthyroidism and the effects of restoration of euthyroidism, a randomised controlled trial," *Clinical Endocrinology*, vol. 65, no. 6, pp. 737–744, 2006.

[63] A. J. McCulloch, D. G. Johnston, P. H. Baylis et al., "Evidence that thyroid hormones regulate gluconeogenesis from glycerol in man," *Clinical Endocrinology*, vol. 19, no. 1, pp. 67–76, 1983.

[64] F. Okajima and M. Ui, "Metabolism of glucose in hyper and hypothyroid rats in vivo. Glucose turnover values and futile cycle activities obtained with 14 C and 3H labelled glucose," *Biochemical Journal*, vol. 182, no. 2, pp. 565–575, 1979.

[65] M. P. Czech, C. C. Malbon, K. Kerman, W. Gitomer, and P. F. Pilch, "Effect of thyroid status on insulin action in rat adipocytes and skeletal muscle," *Journal of Clinical Investigation*, vol. 66, pp. 574–582, 1980.

[66] G. D. Dimitriadis, B. Leighton, M. Parry-Billings, D. West, and E. A. Newsholme, "Effects of hypothyroidism on the sensitivity of glycolysis and glycogen synthesis to insulin in the soleus muscle of the rat," *Biochemical Journal*, vol. 257, no. 2, pp. 369–373, 1989.

[67] G. Dimitriadis, M. Parry-Billings, S. Bevan et al., "The effects of insulin on transport and metabolism of glucose in skeletal muscle from hypothyroid rats," *European Journal of Clinical Investigation*, vol. 27, no. 6, pp. 475–483, 1997.

[68] A. Dubaniewicz, H. Kaciuba-Uscilko, K. Nazar, and L. Budohoski, "Sensitivity of the soleus muscle to insulin in resting and exercising rats with experimental hypo- and hyperthyroidism," *Biochemical Journal*, vol. 263, no. 1, pp. 243–247, 1989.

[69] P. Cettour-Rose, C. Theander-Carrillo, C. Asensio et al., "Hypothyroidism in rats decreases peripheral glucose utilization, a defect partially corrected by central leptin infusion," *Diabetologia*, vol. 48, no. 4, pp. 624–633, 2005.

[70] B. Havekes and H. P. Sauerwein, "Adipocyte-myocyte crosstalk in skeletal muscle insulin resistance; is there a role for thyroid hormone?" *Current Opinion in Clinical Nutrition and Metabolic Care*, vol. 13, no. 6, pp. 641–646, 2010.

[71] M. Peppa, C. Koliaki, P. Nikolopoulos, and S. A. Raptis, "Skeletal muscle insulin resistance in endocrine disease," *Journal of Biomedicine and Biotechnology*, vol. 2010, Article ID 527850, 2010.

[72] C. Rochon, I. Tauveron, C. Dejax et al., "Response of glucose disposal to hyperinsulinaemia in human hypothyroidism and hyperthyroidism," *Clinical Science*, vol. 104, no. 1, pp. 7–15, 2003.

[73] S. Stanická, K. Vondra, T. Pelikánová, P. Vlcek, M. Hill, and V. Zamrazil, "Insulin sensitivity and counter-regulatory hormones in hypothyroidism and during thyroid hormone replacement therapy," *Clinical Chemistry and Laboratory Medicine*, vol. 43, no. 7, pp. 715–720, 2005.

[74] A. Handisurya, G. Pacini, A. Tura, A. Gessl, and A. Kautzky-Willer, "Effects of thyroxine replacement therapy on glucose metabolism in subjects with subclinical and overt hypothyroidism," *Clinical Endocrinology*, vol. 69, no. 6, pp. 963–969, 2008.

[75] G. Dimitriadis, P. Mitrou, V. Lambadiari et al., "Insulin action in adipose tissue and muscle in hypothyroidism," *Journal of Clinical Endocrinology & Metabolism*, vol. 91, no. 12, pp. 4930–4937, 2006.

[76] G. Brenta, F. S. Celi, M. Pisarev, M. Schnitman, I. Sinay, and P. Arias, "Acute thyroid hormone withdrawal in athyreotic patients results in a state of insulin resistance," *Thyroid*, vol. 19, no. 6, pp. 665–669, 2009.

[77] M. Owecki, E. Nikisch, and J. Sowiński, "Hypothyroidism has no impact on insulin sensitivity assessed with HOMA-IR in totally thyroidectomized patients," *Acta Clinica Belgica*, vol. 61, no. 2, pp. 69–73, 2006.

[78] P. E. Harris, M. Walker, F. Clark, P. D. Home, and K. G. M. M. Alberti, "Forearm muscle metabolism in primary hypothyroidism," *European Journal of Clinical Investigation*, vol. 23, no. 9, pp. 585–588, 1993.

[79] P. H. Dessein, B. I. Joffe, and A. E. Stanwix, "Subclinical hypothyroidism is associated with insulin resistance in rheumatoid arthritis," *Thyroid*, vol. 14, no. 6, pp. 443–446, 2004.

[80] A. Tuzcu, M. Bahceci, D. Gokalp, Y. Tuzun, and K. Gunes, "Subclinical hypothyroidism may be associated with elevated high-sensitive C-reactive protein (low grade inflammation) and fasting hyperinsulinemia," *Endocrine Journal*, vol. 52, no. 1, pp. 89–94, 2005.

[81] A. Al Sayed, N. Al Ali, Y. Bo Abbas, and E. Alfadhli, "Subclinical hypothyroidism is associated with early insulin resistance in Kuwaiti women," *Endocrine Journal*, vol. 53, no. 5, pp. 653–657, 2006.

[82] G. Brenta, G. Berg, P. Arias et al., "Lipoprotein alterations, hepatic lipase activity, and insulin sensitivity in subclinical hypothyroidism: response to L-T4 treatment," *Thyroid*, vol. 17, no. 5, pp. 453–460, 2007.

2

Changes of TSH-Stimulation Blocking Antibody (TSBAb) and Thyroid Stimulating Antibody (TSAb) Over 10 Years in 34 TSBAb-Positive Patients with Hypothyroidism and in 98 TSAb-Positive Graves' Patients with Hyperthyroidism: Reevaluation of TSBAb and TSAb in TSH-Receptor-Antibody (TRAb)-Positive Patients

Nobuyuki Takasu and Mina Matsushita

Department of Endocrinology and Metabolism, Aizawa Hospital, 2-5-1 Honjo, Mtasumoto 390-8521, Japan

Correspondence should be addressed to Nobuyuki Takasu, takasunob@gmail.com

Academic Editor: Terry F. Davies

Two TRAbs: TSBAb and TSAb. TSBAb causes hypothyroidism. TSAb causes Graves' hyperthyroidism. TSBAb and TSAb block TSH-binding to cells as TRAb, measured as TSH-binding inhibitory immunoglobulin (TBII). We reevaluate TSBAb and TSAb. We studied TSBAb, TSAb, and TBII over 10 years in 34 TSBAb-positives with hypothyroidism and in 98 TSAb-positives with hyperthyroidism. Half of the 34 TSBAb-positives with hypothyroidism continued to have persistently positive TSBAb, continued to have hypothyroidism, and did not recover from hypothyroidism. Ten of the 98 TSAb-positives with hyperthyroidism continued to have positive TSAb and continued to have hyperthyroidism. TSBAb had disappeared in 15 of the 34 TSBAb-positives with hypothyroidism. With the disappearance of TSBAb, recovery from hypothyroidism was noted in 13 (87%) of the 15 patients. TSAb had disappeared in 73 of the 98 TSAb-positives with hyperthyroidism. With the disappearance of TSAb, remissions of hyperthyroidism were noted in 60 (82%) of the 73. Two of the 34 TSBAb-positives with hypothyroidism developed TSAb-positive Graves' hyperthyroidism. Two of the 98 TSAb-positive Graves' patients with hyperthyroidism developed TSBAb-positive hypothyroidism. TSBAb and TSAb are TRAbs. TSBAb-hypothyroidism and TSAb-hyperthyroidism may be two aspects of one disease (TRAb disease). Two forms of autoimmune thyroiditis: atrophic and goitrous. We followed 34 TSBAb-positive patients with hypothyroidism (24 atrophic and 10 goitrous) over 10 years. All of the 10 TSBAb-positive goitrous patients recovered from hypothyroidism and 19 (79%) of the 24 TSBAb-positive atrophic patients continued to have hypothyroidism.

1. Introduction

There are two types of TSH receptor antibodies (TRAbs): thyroid stimulating antibody (TSAb) [1, 2] and TSH-stimulation blocking antibody (TSBAb) [3]. TSAb stimulates the thyroid and causes Graves' hyperthyroidism. TSBAb blocks TSH-stimulation of the thyroid and causes hypothyroidism. Both TSAb and TSBAb block TSH-binding to thyroid cells as TSH-receptor antibody (TRAb), which has been measured as TSH-binding inhibitory immunoglobulin (TBII) [1–3]. TBII indicates the inhibition of TSH-binding to TSH receptor but does not indicate the function of TRAb. TRAb can be stimulatory or inhibitory. To know whether TRAb is stimulatory or inhibitory, TSAb and TSBAb have been measured [1–3]. TRAb has been measured by different assay methods and given various names. Among them, TBII [1, 4, 5] and TSAb [1, 2, 6–9] have been measured as TRAb to diagnose Graves' disease and to follow the patients. TBII is measured as a receptor assay. TSAb is measured as a stimulator assay, using porcine thyroid cells. TSAb indicates the stimulation activity of TRAb. TSBAb [3, 10–13] and TBII [3, 4, 10–13] have been measured as TRAb to diagnose TSBAb-positive hypothyroidism and to follow the patients. TSBAb has been measured as a TSH-stimulation blocking assay, using porcine thyroid cells [3, 10–13]. TSBAb indicates the inhibitory activity of TRAb. TSAb and TSBAb are TSH-receptor antibodies (TRAb). The former TRAb (TSAb) is a stimulating antibody [1, 2, 6–9], and the latter TRAb (TSBAb) is a blocking antibody [3, 10–13]. TSBAb blocks TSH-stimulation of the thyroid and causes hypothyroidism. TSBAb blocks TSH-binding to thyroid cells and is TRAb. TSBAb blocks TSH-stimulation of the thyroid and is measured as inhibition of TSH-stimulated cAMP synthesis of thyroid cells. TSBAb and TSAb are TRAb. TBII reflects TSBAb- and TSAb-activities.

TSAb stimulates the thyroid and causes Graves' hyperthyroidism. Treatment with antithyroid drugs (ATDs) decreases serum TSAb [14]. With the disappearance of TSAb, remissions of Graves' hyperthyroidism have been seen [14]. TSBAb blocks TSH-stimulation of the thyroid and causes hypothyroidism [3]. With the disappearance of TSBAb, recovery from hypothyroidism occurs [3].

It has been generally believed that Graves' patients have TSAb but do not have TSBAb, and that blocking antibody-(TSBAb-) positive patients with hypothyroidism have TSBAb but do not have TSAb. However, TSBAb-positive patients with hypothyroidism and TSAb-positive Graves' patients with hyperthyroidism could have both TSBAb and TSAb [13]. Some patients may have TSBAb and TSAb simultaneously or sequentially [13]. The balance of TSBAb and TSAb determines whether a patient has hypothyroidism or hyperthyroidism [13]. We have encountered TSBAb-positive patients with hypothyroidism, who developed TSAb-positive Graves' hyperthyroidism, and also TSAb-positive Graves' patients with hyperthyroidism, who developed TSBAb-positive hypothyroidism. Thyroid function can oscillate between hypothyroidism and hyperthyroidism as TSBAb or TSAb becomes dominant.

There are two forms of autoimmune thyroiditis: atrophic autoimmune thyroiditis and goitrous autoimmune thyroiditis [3]. It has become evident that hypothyroidism may occur as a result of the production of TSBAb. TSBAb has been said to cause hypothyroidism in the patients with atrophic autoimmune thyroiditis [3]. However, TSBAb has been found in patients with atrophic autoimmune thyroiditis, and also in patients with goitrous autoimmune thyroiditis [11]. TSBAb was detected in 25% of the patients with atrophic autoimmune thyroiditis and in 9% of those with goitrous autoimmune thyroiditis [3]. TSBAb causes hypothyroidism. With the disappearance of TSBAb, recovery from hypothyroidism has been reported [3]. Here, we followed 24 TSBAb-positive hypothyroid patients with atrophic autoimmune thyroiditis and 10 TSBAb-positive hypothyroid patients with goitrous autoimmune thyroiditis over 10 years. All of the 10 TSBAb-positive patients with goitrous autoimmune thyroiditis recovered from hypothyroidism and 19 (79%) of the 24 TSBAb-positive patients with atrophic autoimmune thyroiditis continued to have hypothyroidism.

We reevaluated TSBAb and TSAb in TRAb-positive patients. We studied serial changes of TSBAb and TSAb

over 10 years in 34 TSBAb-positive patients with hypothyroidism and in 98 TSAb-positive Graves' patients with hyperthyroidism. With persistently positive TSBAb, recovery from hypothyroidism was not observed. With persistently positive TSAb, remissions of Graves' hyperthyroidism were not obtained. With the disappearance of TSBAb, recovery from hypothyroidism was seen. With the disappearance of TSAb, remissions of Graves' hyperthyroidism were also seen. Two of the 34 TSBAb-positive patients with hypothyroidism developed TSAb-positive Graves' hyperthyroidism. Two of the 98 TSAb-positive Graves' patients with hyperthyroidism developed TSBAb-positive hypothyroidism. TSBAb-positive hypothyroidism and TSAb-positive hyperthyroidism may be two aspects of one disease (TRAb disease).

2. Subjects and Method

2.1. Subjects. We studied 34 TSBAb-positive patients with hypothyroidism and 98 TSAb-positive Graves' patients with hyperthyroidism (Table 1). The 34 TSBAb-positive patients with hypothyroidism were treated with thyroxine (T4) and the 98 TSAb-positive Graves' patients with hyperthyroidism were treated with antithyroid drugs (ATDs). Serial changes of TSBAb and TSAb over 10 years were studied in 34 TSBAb-positive patients with hypothyroidism (I) and in 98 TSAb-positive Graves' patients with hyperthyroidism (II). TSBAb-positive patients with hypothyroidism were diagnosed on the basis of the history, signs of hypothyroidism, and the laboratory findings, including positive TSBAb (>+40%) and decreased serum-free thyroxine (fT4) and free triiodothyronine (fT3) with high TSH [3, 13]. The diagnosis of goitrous autoimmune thyroiditis was based on the finding of palpable goiter and that of atrophic autoimmune thyroiditis on the absence of goiter [3]. The 34 TSBAb-positive patients with hypothyroidism were treated with thyroxine (T4). Thyroxine was discontinued at 3 months after the disappearance of TSBAb. After the discontinuation of T4, the patients had been seen every 1–3 months. When the patients continued to be in euthyroid states and to have negative TSBAb and negative TBII for more than 1 year after the T4-discontinuation, they were considered to have recovery from hypothyroidism; otherwise, they had recurrence [3]. When serum TSH became higher than 10 mIU/L, T4-administration was restarted [3]. TSAb-positive Graves' patients with hyperthyroidism were diagnosed on the basis of the history, signs of hyperthyroidism with diffuse goiter, and the laboratory findings, including positive TRAb (TSAb and/or TBII) and elevated fT4 and fT3 with low TSH [1, 2]. The 98 Graves' patients were treated with antithyroid drugs (ATDs). They had been treated with ATD over several years. ATD was discontinued at 6 months after the TSAb-disappearance. After the discontinuation of ATD, the patients had been seen every 1–3 months. When the patients continued to be in euthyroid states and to have negative TSAb and negative TBII for more than 1 year after the ATD-discontinuation, they were considered to be in remission; otherwise, they had recurrence [14]. When they had recurrence, ATD-treatment was restarted. We had followed these 34 TSBAb-positive patients with hypothyroidism and

TABLE 1: Changes of TSBAb (TSH-stimulation blocking antibody) and TSAb (thyroid stimulating antibody) over 10 years in 34 TSBAb-positive patients with hypothyroidism and in 98 TSAb-positive Graves' patients with hyperthyroidism.

	(I) 34 TSBAb-positive patients with hypothyroidism		34
Ia: Positive TSBAb persisted	Continued to have hypothyroidism	17	17
Ib: TSBAb disappeared	Ib1: Recovered from hypothyroidism	13	15
	Ib2: Continued to have hypothyroidism	2	
Ic: TSBAb → TSAb	TSBAb-positive hypo → Graves' hyper	2	2
	(II) 98 TSAb-positive Graves' patients with hyperthyroidism		98
IIa: Positive TSAb persisted	Continued to have Graves' hyperthyroidism	10	10
IIb: Complex changes of TSAb	IIb1: Remission	1	13
	IIb2: Recurrence	12	
IIc: TSAb disappeared	IIc1: Remission	60	73
	IIc2: Recurrence	13	
IId: TSAb → TSBAb	Graves' hyper → TSBAb-positive hypo	2	2

Numbers of the patients are shown.
Serial changes of TSBAb and TSAb over 10 years were studied in 34 TSBAb-positive patients with hypothyroidism (I) and in 98 TSAb-positive Graves' patients with hyperthyroidism (II). The 34 TSBAb-positive patients with hypothyroidism were treated with thyroxine (T4) and the 98 TSAb-positive Graves' patients with hyperthyroidism were treated with antithyroid drugs (ATDs). Half (17) (Ia) of the 34 TSBAb-positive patients with hypothyroidism (I) continued to have positive TSBAb and continued to have hypothyroidism. Ten (IIa) of the 98 TSAb-positive Graves' patients with hyperthyroidism (II) continued to have positive TSAb and continued to have Graves' hyperthyroidism. With the disappearance of TSBAb, recovery from hypothyroidism was noted in 13 (Ib1) (87%) of the 15 patients, in whom TSBAb had disappeared (Ib). With the disappearance of TSAb, remissions of Graves' hyperthyroidism were noted in 60 (IIc1) (82%) of the 73, in whom TSAb had disappeared (IIc). Two of the 34 TSBAb-positive patients with hypothyroidism developed TSBAb-positive Graves' hyperthyroidism (Ic), and two of the 98 TSAb-positive Graves' patients with hyperthyroidism developed TSBAb-positive hypothyroidism (IId).

98 TSAb-positive Graves' patients with hyperthyroidism over 10 years.

2.2. Porcine Thyroid Cell Cyclic AMP Production: TSBAb and TSAb. TSBAb and TSAb were measured as before [13, 14]. Cyclic AMP (cAMP) production was determined according to the instruction in commercial assay kit (Yamasa, Chosi, Chiba, Japan). Crude IgG, obtained as PEG (6000) 12.5% precipitated fraction- (final concentration) from 0.2 mL aliquot of test serum, was dissolved in modified Hanks' solution without NaCl. Porcine thyroid cells were incubated with test IgG in 0.25 mL Hanks' solution without NaCl, pH 7.5, containing 1.5% bovine serum albumin, 20 mM Hepes, and 0.5 mM 3-isobutyl-l-methylxanthine. Cyclic AMP production during 5 h incubation at 37°C was measured by radioimmunoassay (RIA), using a commercial kit (Yamasa). To measure TSBAb-activities, crude IgG was incubated with porcine thyroid cells in the presence of 25 μU bTSH (100 mU/L, final concentration), as before [3, 10–13, 15]. Cyclic AMP production during 5 h incubation was measured. TSBAb-activity was expressed as percentage inhibition of bTSH-stimulated cAMP production by test IgG. TSBAb-activity was calculated as follows: TSBAb (%) = $[1 - (c - b)/(a - b)] \times 100$ [3, 10–13, 15], where a: cAMP generated in the presence of normal IgG and bTSH, b: cAMP generated in the presence of normal IgG, and c: cAMP generated in the presence of test IgG and bTSH. Test IgG and normal IgG were the 12.5% PEG-precipitated fraction from test serum and normal human serum, respectively. TSBAb, described in this report, corresponds to TSBAb-A in the previous report [13]. TSBAb activities were studied in 95 normal subjects (normal values were less than +40%) [13]. TSBAb activities were more than +40% in all of the TSBAb-positive patients with hypothyroidism. TSAb activity was expressed as percentage

cAMP production compared with the mean values for 125 normal subjects (normal values were less than 180%) [1, 2, 14]: TSAb (%) = $[d/b] \times 100$, where b: cAMP generated in the presence of normal IgG, and d: cAMP generated in the presence of test IgG.

2.3. TSH-Binding Inhibitory Immunoglobulin (TBII). TBII was measured by radioreceptor assay with a commercial kit (R. S. R. Limited, Cardiff, UK). Assay results were expressed as the percentage inhibition of I^{125}-TSH-binding to thyroid plasma membrane as before [1, 2, 5, 14]. Normal values were obtained from 128 normal control subjects and were less than 10% [1, 2, 14].

2.4. Statistical Analysis and Others. All samples were tested in duplicate or triplicate. Statistical analysis was performed using Student's t-test or χ^2-test. P values less than 0.05 were considered to be statistically significant. Serum-free T3, -free T4, and TSH were determined by electrochemiluminescence immunoassays (ECLIAs) (Roche Diagnostics, Tokyo, Japan). Normal reference ranges are as follows: fT3 3.5–6.6 nmol/L, fT4 11.6–21.9 pmol/L, and TSH 0.4–4.20 mIU/L. The study plan was reviewed and approved by our institutional review committee. Written informed consent was obtained from the patient prior to publication of this paper.

3. Resuls

Serial changes of TSBAb and TSAb over 10 years were studied in 34 TSBAb-positive patients with hypothyroidism and in 98 Graves' patients with hyperthyroidism (Table 1). The 34 TSBAb-positive patients with hypothyroidism (I) were treated with thyroxine (T4) and the 98 TSAb-positive

TABLE 2: Characteristics of the 34 TSBAb-positive patients with hypothyroidism and the 98 TSAb-positive Graves' patients with hyperthyroidism.

	Number of patients	Gender Men/Women	Age (years)	Before treatment		
				TSBAb (%)	TSAb (%)	TBII (%)
(I) 34 TSBAb-positive patients with hypothyroidism						
Ia	17	5/12	42 ± 17	**94 ± 6**	146 ± 10	**95 ± 5**
Ib	15	4/11	45 ± 16	**90 ± 9**	136 ± 8	**92 ± 7**
Ic	2	1/1	38, 45	**98, 97**	100, 98	**96, 95**
Ia+Ib+Ic	34	10/24	43 ± 18	92 ± 7	140 ± 9	**94 ± 7**
(II) 98 TSAb-positive Graves' patients with hyperthyroidism						
IIa	10	3/7	40 ± 16	9 ± 8	**839 ± 421**	76 ± 15
IIb	13	3/10	42 ± 17	10 ± 11	**846 ± 195**	68 ± 16
IIc	73	18/55	44 ± 16	10 ± 10	**746 ± 390**	56 ± 18
IId	2	0/2	40, 48	2, 5	1625, 852	76, 58
IIa+IIb+IIc+IId	98	24/74	43 ± 17	10 ± 9	**775 ± 396**	57 ± 17

Values are means ± SD. I, Ia, Ib, Ic, II, IIa, IIb, IIc, and IId correspond to those in Table 1. No differences of gender and ages were noted among I, Ia, Ib, Ic, II, IIa, IIb, IIc, and IId. No differences of TSAb-, TSBAb-, and TBII-activities were noted among Ia, Ib, and Ic and among IIa, IIb, IIc, and IId.
All of the 34 TSBAb-positive patients with hypothyroidism had strongly positive TSBAb (85–103%, mean ± SD = 92 ± 7%) (Ia+Ib+Ic). Some of them had weakly positive TSAb. Their TSAb activity ranged from 92% to 240%. The TSAb activities were 180–240% in 7 (21%) of the 34 TSBAb-positive patients with hypothyroidism and were less than 180% in the other 27 patients (79%). Seven (21%) of the 34 TSBAb-positive patients with hypothyroidism had positive TSAb. TSBAb-positive patients with hypothyroidism had narrow distribution of TSBAb (82–104%, 92 ± 7%) and TSAb (92–240%, 140 ± 9%). All of the 98 Graves' patients with hyperthyroidism had positive TSAb (250–1795%, 775 ± 396%) (IIa+IIb+IIc+IId). Some of them had TSBAb. The TSBAb activities were +40–+52% in 11 (11%) and were less than +40% in the other 87 patients (89%). Graves' patients with hyperthyroidism had wide distributions of TSAb (250–1795%, 775 ± 396%) and TSBAb (−28–+52%, 10 ± 9%).

Graves' patients with hyperthyroidism (II) were treated with antithyroid drugs (ATDs). Among the 34 TSBAb-positive patients with hypothyroidism (I), 17 patients (Ia) continued to have persistently positive TSBAb and continued to have hypothyroidism. Half (17) (Ia) of the 34 TSBAb-positive patients continued to have persistently positive TSBAb, continued to have hypothyroidism, and did not recover from hypothyroidism. TSBAb disappeared in 15 (Ib) of the 34 TSBAb-positive patients with hypothyroidism. With the disappearance of TSBAb, recovery from hypothyroidism was seen in 13 (Ib1) (87%) of the 15 patients, in whom TSBAb had disappeared (Ib). Among the 98 TSAb-positive Graves' patients with hyperthyroidism (II), 10 patients (IIa) continued to have persistently positive TSAb and continued to have hyperthyroidism. Ten of the 98 TSAb-positive Graves' patients with hyperthyroidism continued to have persistently positive TSAb. They continued to have hyperthyroidism and did not get remissions of Graves' hyperthyroidism. They continued to take ATD. Complex changes of TSAb were noted in 13 TSAb-positive patients (IIb). One (IIb1) of the 13 patients with complex changes of TSAb got remissions, but the other 12 patients (IIb2) did not. TSAb disappeared in 73 (IIc) (74%) of the 98 TSAb-positive Graves' patients with hyperthyroidism. With the disappearance of TSAb, 60 (IIc1) (82%) of the 73 patients, in whom TSAb had disappeared (IIc), got remissions of Graves' hyperthyroidism. Two TSBAb-positive patients with hypothyroidism developed TSAb-positive Graves' hyperthyroidism (Ic). Two TSAb-positive Graves' patients with hyperthyroidism developed TSBAb-positive hypothyroidism (IId).

Table 2 shows characteristics of the 34 TSBAb-positive patients with hypothyroidism (I) and the 98 TSAb-positive Graves' patients with hyperthyroidism (II). I, Ia, Ib, Ic, II, IIa, IIb, IIc, and IId correspond to those in Table 1. No differences of gender and ages were noted among I, Ia, Ib, Ic, II, IIa, IIb, IIc, and IId. No differences of TSAb-, TSBAb-, and TBII-activities were noted among Ia, Ib, and Ic and among IIa, IIb, IIc, and IId. All of the 34 TSBAb-positive patients with hypothyroidism had strongly positive TSBAb (85–103%, mean ± SD = 92 ± 7%) (Table 2, Ia+Ib+Ic). Some of them had weakly positive TSAb. Their TSAb activity ranged from 92% to 240%. The TSAb activities were 180–240% in 7 (21%) of the 34 TSBAb-positive patients with hypothyroidism and were less than 180% in the other 27 patients (79%). Seven (21%) of the 34 TSBAb-positive patients with hypothyroidism had positive TSAb. TSBAb-positive patients with hypothyroidism had narrow distribution of TSBAb (82–104%, 92 ± 7%) and TSAb (92–240%, 140 ± 9%). All of the 98 Graves' patients with hyperthyroidism had positive TSAb (250–1795%, 775 ± 396%) (Table 2, IIa+IIb+IIc+IId). Some of them had TSBAb. The TSBAb activities were +40–+ 52% in 11 (11%) and were less than +40% in the other 87 patients (89%). Graves' patients with hyperthyroidism had wide distributions of TSAb (250–1795%, 775 ± 396%) and TSBAb (−28–+52%, 10 ± 9%).

3.1. 34 TSBAb-Positive Patients with Hypothyroidism (I) (Tables 1 and 2, I). All of the 34 TSBAb-positive patients with hypothyroidism had strongly positive TSBAb. Some of them had weakly positive TSAb. TSBAb-positive patients with hypothyroidism had narrow distributions of TSBAb (82–104%, 92 ± 7%) and TSAb (92–240%, 140 ± 9%) (Table 2, Ia+b+c). Figure 1 shows the changes of TSBAb

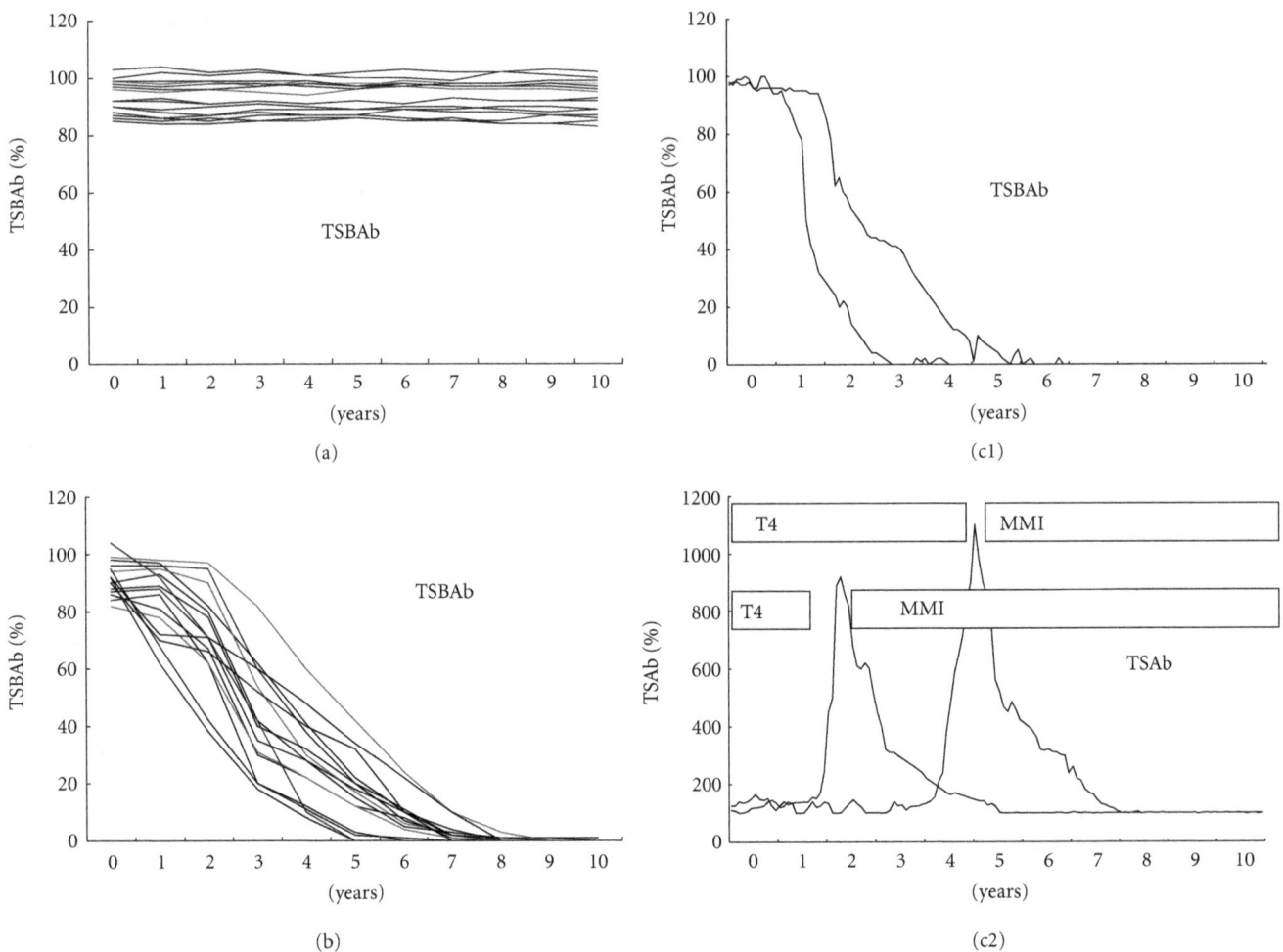

FIGURE 1: The changes of TSBAb in 34 TSBAb-positive patients with hypothyroidism (Table 1, I). Among the 34 TSBAb-positive patients with hypothyroidism, 17 patients continued to have persistently positive TSBAb and continued to have hypothyroidism (Table 1, Ia) (a). Half of the 34 TSBAb-positive patients continued to have persistently positive TSBAb, continued to have hypothyroidism, and did not recover from hypothyroidism. They continued to take thyroxine (T4). TSBAb disappeared in 15 of the 34 TSBAb-positive patients with hypothyroidism (Table 1, Ib) (b). Recovery from hypothyroidism was noted with the disappearance of TSBAb in 13 (87%) of the 15 patients, in whom TSBAb had disappeared. (c1, c2) show the changes of TSBAb and TSAb, respectively, in the 2 patients with TSBAb-positive hypothyroidism, who developed TSAb-positive Graves' hyperthyroidism (Table 1, Ic). In these 2 patients, TSBAb was dominant initially (c1), and then TSAb became dominant (c2); 2 patients with TSBAb-positive hypothyroidism developed TSAb-positive Graves' hyperthyroidism. Hypothyroidism was treated with thyroxine (T4). Graves' hyperthyroidism was treated with 1-methyl 2-mercapto imidazole (MMI). TSBAb: TSH-stimulation blocking antibody; TSAb: thyroid stimulating antibody.

in the 34 TSBAb-positive patients with hypothyroidism (Table 1, I). Among the 34 TSBAb-positive patients with hypothyroidism (I), 17 (Ia) (Table 1, Ia, Figure 1(a)) continued to have persistently positive TSBAb and continued to have hypothyroidism. Half (17) (Ia) of the 34 TSBAb-positive patients (I) continued to have persistently positive TSBAb, continued to have hypothyroidism, and did not recover from hypothyroidism. They continued to take T4. TSBAb disappeared in 15 (Ib) (Table 1, Ib, Figure 1(b)) of the 34 TSBAb-positive patients (I) with hypothyroidism. With the disappearance of TSBAb, recovery from hypothyroidism was noted in 13 (Ib1) (87%) of the 15 patients, in whom TSBAb had disappeared (Ib).

Figures 1(c1) and 1(c2) show the changes of TSBAb and TSAb, respectively, in the 2 patients with TSBAb-positive hypothyroidism, who developed TSAb-positive Graves' hyperthyroidism (Table 1, Ic). In these 2 patients, TSBAb was dominant initially (Figure 1(c1)), and then TSAb became dominant (Figure 1(c2)). These 2 TSBAb-positive patients had hypothyroidism and then developed TSAb-positive Graves' hyperthyroidism. They were treated with T4 and then treated with 1-methyl 2-mercapto imidazole (MMI). Figure 2 demonstrates the clinical course of one of these 2 patients with TSBAb-positive hypothyroidism, who developed TSAb-positive Graves' hyperthyroidism (Table 1, Ic). A 45-year-old woman with TSBAb-positive hypothyroidism developed TSAb-positive Graves' hyperthyroidism. TSBAb was dominant initially (Figure 2(a)), and then TSAb became dominant (Figure 2(b)). She had TSBAb-positive hypothyroidism with

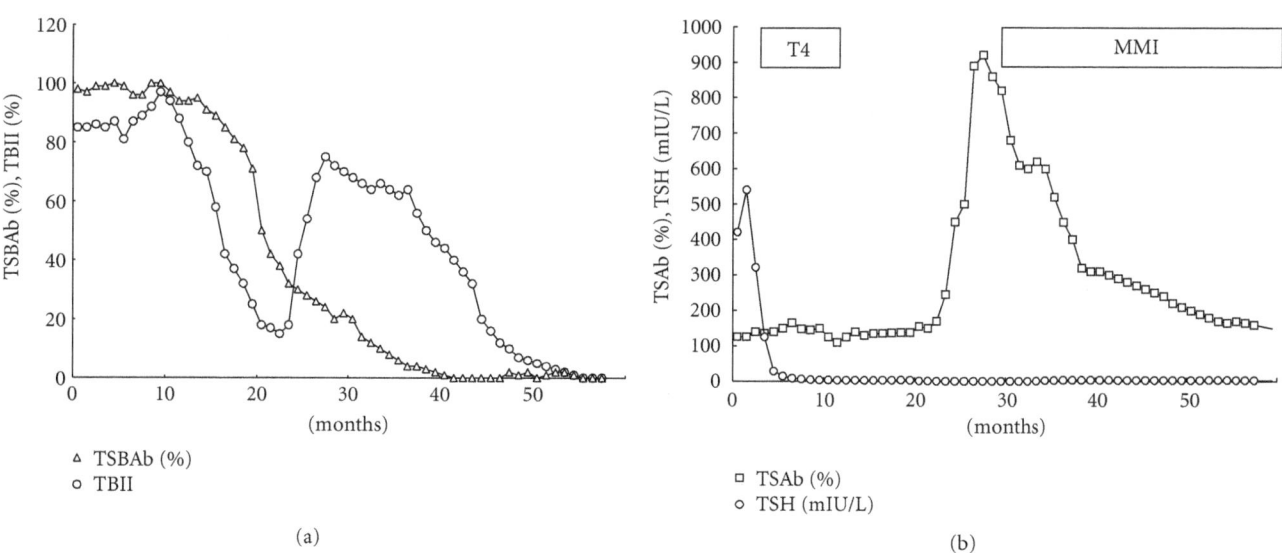

FIGURE 2: The clinical course of one of the 2 patients, who initially had TSBAb-positive hypothyroidism and then developed TSAb-positive Graves' hyperthyroidism (Table 1, Ic). A 45-year-old woman with TSBAb-positive hypothyroidism developed TSAb-positive Graves' hyperthyroidism. She had TSBAb-positive hypothyroidism ((a), △) with high serum TSH ((b), ○) and then developed TSAb-positive Graves' hyperthyroidism ((b), □) with undetectable serum TSH ((b), ○). TSBAb was dominant initially ((a), △), and then TSAb became dominant ((b), □). TBII (TSH-binding inhibitory immunoglobulin) ((a), ○) reflects TSBAb- and TSAb-activity. A patient with TSBAb-positive hypothyroidism developed TSAb-positive Graves' hyperthyroidism. She was treated with T4 and then with MMI.

high serum TSH and then developed TSAb-positive Graves' hyperthyroidism with undetectable serum TSH. She was treated with T4 and then treated with MMI. She had a goiter initially and had goitrous autoimmune thyroiditis.

Among the 34 TSBAb-positive patients with hypothyroidism (Table 1, I), 24 had atrophic autoimmune thyroiditis and 10 had goitrous autoimmune thyroiditis (Table 3(a)). The 34 TSBAb-positive patients with hypothyroidism consisted of 17 patients (a: positive TSBAb persisited), 15 patients (b: TSBAb disappeared), and 2 patients (c: TSBAb → TSAb) (Table 3(a)). All of the 17 (a) patients continued to have positive TSBAb and continued to have hypothyroidism. All of the 17 (a) patients had atrophic autoimmune thyroiditis and none of them had goitrous autoimmune thyroiditis. TSBAb disappeared in the 15 (b) patients: 13 (b1) (87%) of the 15 (b) patients recovered from hypothyroidism and 2 (b2) (13%) of the 15 (b) patients continued to have hypothyroidism. Of the 13 (b1) patients, who recovered from hypothyroidism, 5 had atrophic autoimmune thyroiditis and 8 had goitrous autoimmune thyroiditis. The 2 (b2) patients, who continued to have hypothyroidism, had atrophic autoimmune thyroiditis. Of the 15 (b) patients, in whom TSBAb had disappeared, 7 [5 (b1) + 2 (b2)] had atrophic autoimmune thyroiditis and 8 [8 (b1)] had goitrous autoimmune thyroiditis. Two (c) patients of the 34 TSBAb-positive patients with hypothyroidism developed TSAb-positive Graves' hyperthyroidism had goitrous autoimmune thyroiditis.

Table 3(b) demonstrates recovery from hypothyroidism in the 34 TSBAb-positive patients with hypothyroidism (24 patients with atrophic autoimmune thyroiditis and 10 patients with goitrous autoimmune thyroiditis). Among

the 34 TSBAb-positive patients with hypothyroidism, 19 [(17 (a) + 2 (b2)) in Table 3(a)] continued to have hypothyroidism over 10 years and 15 [13 (b1) + 2 (c)] recovered from hypothyroidism (13 (b1) recovered from hypothyroidism and had remissions and 2 (c) recovered from hypothyroidism and developed hyperthyroidism). All of the 19 TSBAb-positive patients with hypothyroidism, who continued to have hypothyroidism [17 (a) + 2 (b2)], had atrophic autoimmune thyroiditis, and none of them had goitrous autoimmune thyroiditis. Fifteen [13 (b1) + 2 (c)] of the 34 TSBAb-positive patients with hypothyroidism recovered from hypothyroidism. Five [5 (b1)] of the 15 patients, who recovered from hypothyroidism, had atrophic autoimmune thyroiditis and the other 10 [8 (b1) + 2 (c)] had goitrous autoimmune thyroiditis. Nineteen (79%) of the 24 TSBAb-positive hypothyroid patients with atrophic autoimmune thyroiditis continued to have hypothyroidism and the other 5 (21%) recovered from hypothyroidism. All (100%) of the 10 TSBAb-positive hypothyroid patients with goitrous autoimmune thyroiditis [8 (b1) + 2 (c)] recovered from hypothyroidism. Significant differences of recovery from hypothyroidism were noted between the patients with goitrous autoimmune thyroiditis and those with atrophic autoimmune thyroiditis ($\chi^2 = 17.9$, P value < 0.05). All of the 10 TSBAb-positive patients with goitrous autoimmune thyroiditis recovered from hypothyroidism and 19 (79%) of the 24 patients with atrophic autoimmune thyroiditis continued to have hypothyroidism.

3.2. 98 TSAb-Positive Graves' Patients with Hyperthyroidism (II) (Tables 1 and 2, II). All of the 98 Graves' patients

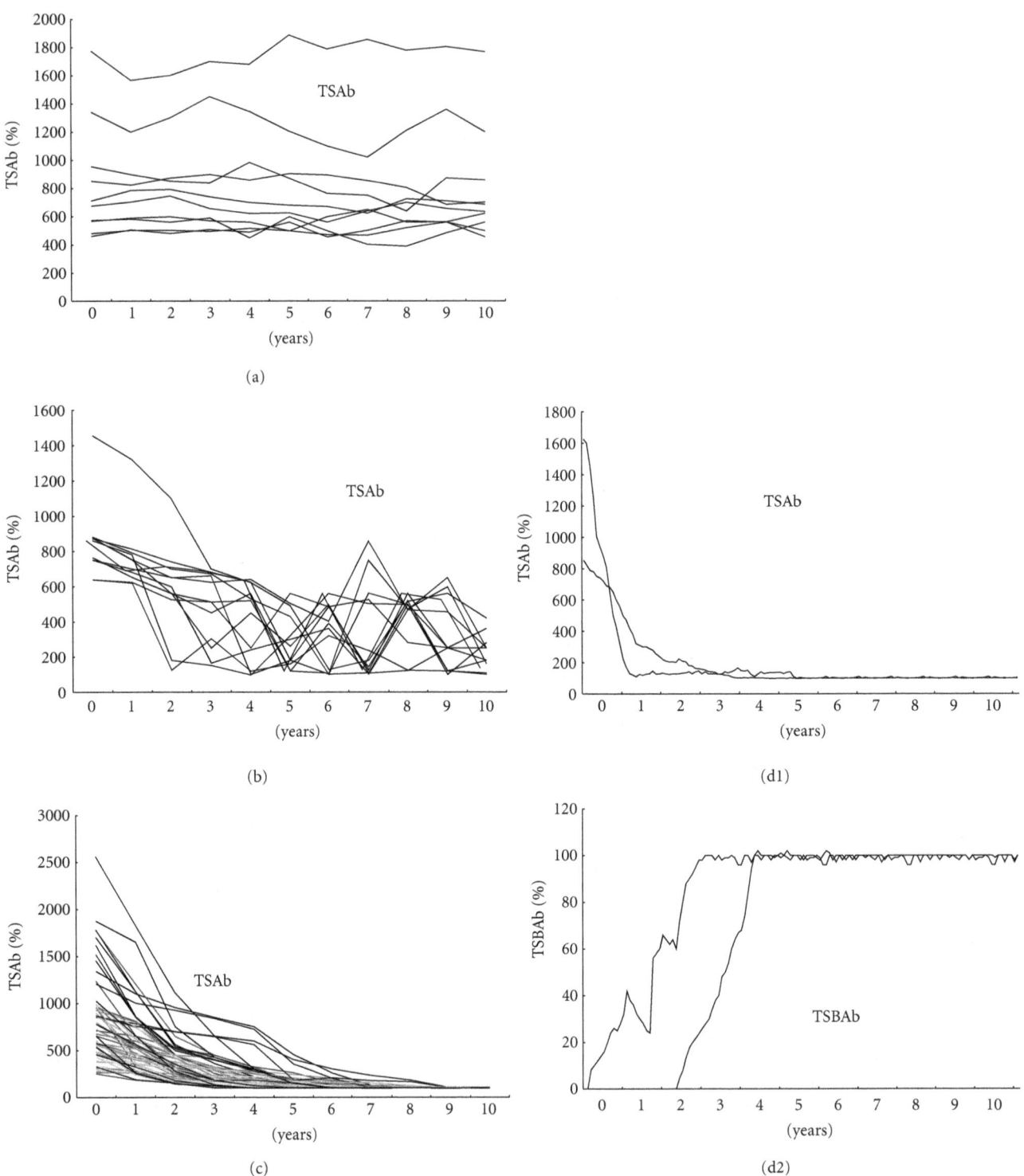

FIGURE 3: The changes of TSAb in 98 Graves' patients with hyperthyroidism (II) (Table 1, II). Among the 98 Graves' patients with hyperthyroidism, 10 patients continued to have persistently positive TSAb and continued to have hyperthyroidism (Table 1, IIa) (a). Ten of the 98 TSAb-positive Graves' patients with hyperthyroidism continued to have persistently positive TSAb. They continued to have hyperthyroidism and did not get remissions of Graves' hyperthyroidism. They continued to take MMI. Complex changes of TSAb were noted in 13 TSAb-positive patients (Table 1, IIb) (b). One of the 13 patients with complex changes of TSAb got remissions, but the other 12 patients did not get remissions. TSAb disappeared in 73 (74%) of the 98 TSAb-positive Graves' patients with hyperthyroidism (Table 1, IIc) (c). With the disappearance of TSAb, 60 (82%) of the 73 patients, in whom TSAb had disappeared, got remissions of Graves' hyperthyroidism. (d1, d2) show the changes of TSAb and TSBAb, respectively, in the 2 patients with TSAb-positive Graves' hyperthyroidism, who developed TSBAb-positive hypothyroidism (Table 1, IId). In these 2 patients, TSAb was dominant initially (d1), and then TSBAb became dominant (d2). Two patients with TSAb-positive Graves' hyperthyroidism developed TSBAb-positive hypothyroidism. Graves' hyperthyroidism was treated with MMI, and hypothyroidism was treated with T4.

TABLE 3: Atrophic autoimmune thyroiditis or goitrous autoimmune thyroiditis in the 34 TSBAb (TSH-stimulation-blocking-antibody)-positive patients with hypothyroidism (a) and recovery from hypothyroidism (b).

(a) Atrophic autoimmune thyroiditis (atrophic) or goitrous autoimmune thyroiditis (goitrous) in the 34 TSBAb-positive patients with hypothyroidism

34 TSBAb-positive patients with hypothyroidism (I in Table 1)[†]			34	
			Atrophic (24)	Goitrous (10)
a: Positive TSBAb persisted (Ia)		17	17	0
b: TSBAb disappeared (Ib) 15	b1: recovered (Ib1)	13	5	8
	b2: hypothyroid (Ib2)	2	2	0
c: TSBAb → TSAb (Ic)		2	0	2

Numbers of the patients are shown. (I in Table 1)[†] correspond to those in Table 1
Among the 34 TSBAb-positive patients with hypothyroidism (Table 1, I), 24 had atrophic autoimmune thyroiditis and 10 had goitrous autoimmune thyroiditis. The 34 TSBAb-positive patients with hypothyroidism consisted of 17 patients (a: positive TSBAb persisited), 15 patients (b: TSBAb disappeared), and 2 patients (c: TSBAb → TSAb). All of the 17 (a) patients continued to have positive TSBAb and continued to have hypothyroidism. All of the 17 (a) patients had atrophic autoimmune thyroiditis and none of them had goitrous autoimmune thyroiditis. TSBAb disappeared in the 15 (b) patients: 13 (b1) (87%) of the 15 (b) patients recovered from hypothyroidism and 2 (b2) (13%) of the 15 (b) patients continued to have hypothyroidism. Of the 13 (b1) patients, who recovered from hypothyroidism, 5 had atrophic autoimmune thyroiditis and 8 had goitrous autoimmune thyroiditis. The 2 (b2) patients, who continued to have hypothyroidism, had atrophic autoimmune thyroiditis. Of the 15 (b) patients, in whom TSBAb had disappeared, 7 [5 (b1) + 2 (b2)] had atrophic autoimmune thyroiditis and 8 [8 (b1)] had goitrous autoimmune thyroiditis. Two (c) patients of the 34 TSBAb-positive patients with hypothyroidism who developed TSAb-positive Graves' hyperthyroidism who had goitrous autoimmune thyroiditis.

(b) Recovery from hypothyroidism in the patients with atrophic autoimmune thyroiditis (atrophic) and in those with goitrous autoimmune thyroiditis (goitrous)

	Atrophic (24)	Goitrous (10)		
Continued to have hypothyroidism	19 (79%) [17 (a) + 2 (b2)]*	0 (0%)	19	
Recovered from hypothyroidism	5 (21%) [5 (b1)]*	10 (100%) [8 (b1) + 2 (c)]*	15	$\chi^2 = 17.9$ P value < 0.05
	24 (100%)	10 (100%)	34	

Numbers (%) of the patients are shown. [ ]* corresponds to Table 3(a).
Among the 34 TSBAb-positive patients with hypothyroidism (Table 1, I), 24 had atrophic autoimmune thyroiditis and 10 had goitrous autoimmune thyroiditis. Among the 34 TSBAb-positive patients with hypothyroidism, 19 [(17 (a) + 2 (b2)] (Table 3(a)) continued to have hypothyroidism over 10 years and 15 [13 (b1) + 2 (c)] recovered from hypothyroidism [13 (b1) recovered from hypothyroidism and had remissions and 2 (c) recovered from hypothyroidism and developed hyperthyroidism]. All of the 19 TSBAb-positive patients with hypothyroidism, who continued to have hypothyroidism [17 (a) + 2 (b2)], had atrophic autoimmune thyroiditis, and none of them had goitrous autoimmune thyroiditis. Fifteen [13 (b1) + 2 (c)] of the 34 TSBAb-positive patients with hypothyroidism recovered from hypothyroidism. Five [5 (b1)] of the 15 patients, who recovered from hypothyroidism, had atrophic autoimmune thyroiditis and the other 10 [8 (b1) + 2 (c)] had goitrous autoimmune thyroiditis. Nineteen (79%) of the 24 TSBAb-positive hypothyroid patients with atrophic autoimmune thyroiditis continued to have hypothyroidism and the other 5 (21%) of them recovered from hypothyroidism. All of the 10 TSBAb-positive hypothyroid patients with goitrous autoimmune thyroiditis [8 (b1) + 2 (c)] recovered from hypothyroidism. Significant differences of recovery from hypothyroidism were noted between the patients with goitrous autoimmune thyroiditis and those with atrophic autoimmune thyroiditis ($\chi^2 = 17.9$, P value < 0.05). All (100%) of the 10 TSBAb-positive patients with goitrous autoimmune thyroiditis recovered from hypothyroidism and 19 (79%) of the 24 patients with atrophic autoimmune thyroiditis continued to have hypothyroidism.

with hyperthyroidism had positive TSAb. Some of them had positive TSBAb. Graves' patients with hyperthyroidism had wide distributions of TSAb and TSBAb. Some of the Graves' patients had both positive TSAb and TSBAb. Figure 3 shows the changes of TSAb in 98 Graves' patients with hyperthyroidism (II) (Table 1, II). Among the 98 Graves' patients with hyperthyroidism, 10 patients continued to have persistently positive TSAb and continued to have hyperthyroidism (IIa) (Figure 3(a)). Ten of the 98 TSAb-positive Graves' patients with hyperthyroidism continued to have positive TSAb and continued to have Graves' hyperthyroidism. They did not get remissions of Graves' hyperthyroidism and continued to take ATD. Complex changes of TSAb were noted in 13 TSAb-positive patients (IIb) (Figure 3(b)). One (IIb1) of the 13 patients with complex changes of TSAb got remissions, but the other 12 patients (IIb2) did not get remissions. TSAb disappeared in 73 (IIc) (74%) of the 98 TSAb-positive

Graves' patients with hyperthyroidism (IIc) (Figure 3(c)). With the disappearance of TSAb, 60 (IIc1) (82%) of the 73 patients, in whom TSAb had disappeared (IIc), got remissions of Graves' hyperthyroidism. Figures 3d1 and 3d2 show the changes of TSAb and TSBAb, respectively, in the 2 patients with TSAb-positive Graves' hyperthyroidism, who developed TSBAb-positive hypothyroidism (IId) (Table 1, IId). In these 2 patients, TSAb was dominant initially (Figure 3(d1)), and then TSBAb became dominant (Figure 3(d2)). The 2 patients had TSAb-positive Graves' hyperthyroidism and then developed TSBAb-positive hypothyroidism. They were treated with MMI, and then treated with T4. Figure 4 demonstrates the clinical course of one of these 2 patients with TSAb-positive Graves' hyperthyroidism, who developed TSBAb-positive hypothyroidism (Table 1, IId). A 40-year-old woman with TSAb-positive Graves' hyperthyroidism developed TSBAb-positive

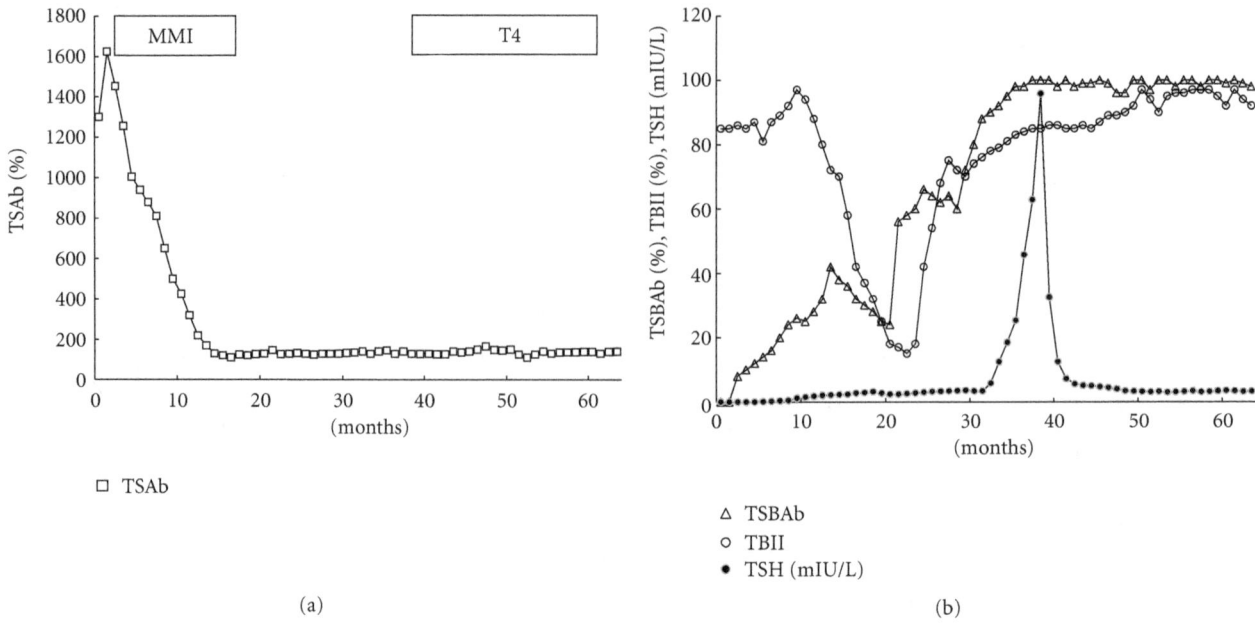

(a)

(b)

FIGURE 4: Clinical course of one of the 2 patients, who had TSAb-positive Graves' hyperthyroidism and then developed TSBAb-positive hypothyroidism (Table 1, IId). A 40-year-old woman with TSAb-positive Graves' hyperthyroidism developed TSBAb-positive hypothyroidism. She had TSAb-positive Graves' hyperthyroidism ((a), □) with undetectable serum TSH ((b), •) and then developed TSBAb-positive hypothyroidism ((b), △) with high serum TSH ((b), •). TSAb was dominant initially ((a), □), and then TSBAb became dominant ((b), △). TBII ((b), ○) reflects TSBAb- and TSAb-activity. A patient with TSAb-positive Graves' hyperthyroidism developed TSBAb-positive hypothyroidism. She was treated with MMI and then with T4.

4. Discussion

hypothyroidism. TSAb was dominant initially (Figure 4(a)), and then TSBAb became dominant (Figure 4(b)). She had TSAb-positive Graves' hyperthyroidism with undetectable serum TSH and then developed TSBAb-positive hypothyroidism with high TSH. She was treated with MMI and then treated with T4. She had a goiter over 10 years.

4. Discussion

We have reevaluated TSBAb and TSAb in 34 TSBAb-positive patients with hypothyroidism and in 98 TSAb-positive Graves' patients with hyperthyroidism. Half of the 34 TSBAb-positive patients continued to have persistently positive TSBAb, continued to have hypothyroidism and did not recover from hypothyroidism. Ten of the 98 Graves' patients continued to have positive TSAb. They continued to have hyperthyroidism, and did not get remissions of Graves' hyperthyroidism. TSBAb had disappeared in 15 of the 34 TSBAb-positive patients with hypothyroidism. With the disappearance of TSBAb, recovery from hypothyroidism was noted in 13 (87%) of the 15 TSBAb-positive patients. TSAb had disappeared in 73 of the 98 TSAb-positive Graves' patients with hyperthyroidism. With the disappearance of TSAb, 60 (82%) of the 73 TSAb-positive patients got remissions. Two of the 34 TSBAb-positive patients with hypothyroidism developed TSAb-positive Graves' hyperthyroidism. Two of the 98 TSAb-positive Graves' patients with hyperthyroidism developed TSBAb-positive hypothyroidism. TSBAb causes hypothyroidism. TSAb causes Graves' hyperthyroidism. TSBAb and TSAb are TRAb. TSBAb-

positive hypothyroidism and TSAb-positive hyperthyroidism may be two aspects of one disease (TRAb disease).

TSBAb blocks TSH-stimulation of the thyroid and causes hypothyroidism. TSAb stimulates the thyroid and causes Graves' hyperthyroidism. Both TSBAb and TSAb block TSH-binding to thyroid cells as TSH receptor antibodies (TRAbs), which have been measured as TSH-binding inhibitory immunoglobulin (TBII) [1–3, 13]. TBII reflects TSBAb- and TSAb-activities. TBII measures the binding of antibody to TSH receptor by competition with radiolabeled TSH and does not distinguish between TSBAb and TSAb. TSBAb is measured as a TSH-stimulation blocking assay and TSAb as a stimulator assay. TSBAb is a blocking antibody [3, 13] and TSAb is a stimulating antibody [1, 2, 13].

TSBAb-activities were expressed as percentage inhibition of TSH-stimulated cAMP production by test IgG [3, 10–13, 15–20]. Two formulas (TSBAb-A and TSBAb-B) have been proposed to calculate TSBAb [3, 10–13]. TSBAb-A was used in the earlier reports [3, 10–13], and TSBAb-B in the later report [13]. TSBAb-A ignores TSAb activity in serum and might give low TSBAb activity. TSBAb-B considers TSAb activity in serum and might give high TSBAb activity. All of the TSBAb-positive patients with hypothyroidism had strongly positive TSBAb-A and TSBAb-B. Both TSBAb-A and TSBAb-B could be used to estimate TSBAb activities [13]. The details were discussed in the previous paper [13]. TSBAb, described in this paper, corresponds to TSBAb-A in the previous paper [13]. TSBAb-A [13] is used as TSBAb in this report.

All of the 34 TSBAb-positive patients with hypothyroidism and all of the 98 TSAb-positive Graves' patients had positive TBII (TRAb). TSBAb and TSAb are TSH-receptor antibodies (TRAbs), which have been measured as TBII. TBII does not distinguish between TSBAb and TSAb. TBII reflects TSBAb- and TSAb-activities [1–3, 13]. All of the 34 TSBAb-positive patients with hypothyroidism had strongly positive TSBAb. Some of them had positive TSAb [13]. All of the 98 Graves' patients had positive TSAb. Some of them had positive TSBAb [13]. TSBAb-positve patients with hypothyroidism had narrow distributions of TSBAb and TSAb, and Graves' patients with hyperthyroidism had wide distributions of TSBAb and TSAb [13]. TSBAb-positive patients with hypothyroidism have strongly positive TSBAb.

TBII reflects TSBAb- and TSAb-activities [1–3, 13]. Some of the TBII-positive patients have hypothyroidism, and the other TBII-positive patients have hyperthyroidism. The former TBII is TSBAb, and the latter TBII is TSAb. The numbers of the former TSBAb-positive patients with hypothyroidism are less than those of the latter TSAb-positive Graves' patients with hyperthyroidism. All of the TSBAb-positive patients with hypothyroidism have high titers of TBII, which is TSBAb [3]. Almost all of the untreated Graves' patients with hyperthyroidism have TBII, which is TSAb [1, 2]. TSBAb- (TRAb-) positive hypothyroidism and TSAb- (TRAb-) positive Graves' hyperthyroidism may be two aspects of one disease (TRAb disease).

Hypothyroidism may result from the production of TSBAb [3]. In 1992, we followed 21 TSBAb-positive patients with hypothyroidism over 10 years and found that with the disappearance of TSBAb, recovery from hypothyroidism was noted in 6 (40%) of the 15 TSBAb-positive patients [3]. Here, we followed 34 TSBAb-positive patients with hypothyroidism over 10 years and found that with the disappearance of TSBAb, recovery from hypothyroidism was noted in 13 (87%) of the 15 patients. The frequency of recovery from hypothyroidism with the disappearance of TSBAb in this paper is much higher than that in the previous one [3]. With the disappearance of TSBAb, recovery from hypothyroidism is observed. The production of TSBAb may subside, producing remissions of hypothyroidism.

It is important to know whether a patient with Graves' disease gets remission or not during ATD treatment. Disappearance of TSAb predicted the remissions of Graves' hyperthyroidism [14]. With the disappearance of TSAb, 36 (82%) of the 44 patients were reported to get remissions in the previous paper [14] and 60 (82%) of the 73 patients are reported to get remissions in this paper. Disappearance of TSAb predicts the remissions of Graves' hyperthyroidism.

Two of the 34 TSBAb-positive patients with hypothyroidism developed TSAb-positive Graves' hyperthyroidism (Ic). Two of the 98 TSAb-positive Graves' patients with hyperthyroidism developed TSBAb-positive hypothyroidism (IId). In the former, TSBAb was dominant initially and then TSAb became dominant. In the latter, TSAb was dominant initially and then TSBAb became dominant. Thyroid function can oscillate between hypothyroidism and hyperthyroidism as TSBAb or TSAb becomes dominant. TSAb and TSBAb can be used to document the functions of TRAb

[13]. TBII-positive patients with strongly positive TSBAb have hypothyroidism. TBII-positive patients with positive TSAb have hyperthyroidism. TSBAb-positive patients with hypothyroidism and TSAb-positive Graves' patients with hyperthyroidism may have both TSBAb and TSAb [1, 2, 13, 21–26]. TSBAb-positive patients with hypothyroidism may develop TSAb-positive hyperthyroidism. TSAb-positive Graves' patients with hyperthyroidism may develop TSBAb-positive hypothyroidism. TSBAb and TSAb are TRAb. TSBAb- (TRAb-) positive hypothyroidism and TSAb- (TRAb-) positive hyperthyroidism may be two aspects of one disease (TRAb disease).

In Japan, TRAb has been measured as TBII and TSAb [14]. TSAb is a bioassay, using porcine thyroid cells. We usually measure TSAb, using a commercially available kit [14]. In Japan, TSAb-assay kit is available, but TSBAb-assay kit is not. When a patient has hypothyroidism with elevated TSH and positive TBII, this TBII is thought to be TSBAb. We usually do not measure TSBAb. Practically, when a patient with hypothyroidism has positive TBII, this TBII may be TSBAb. When a patient with hyperthyroidism has positive TBII, this TBII may be TSAb. TSAb and TSBAb can be used to document TRAb-function. TBII, measuring the antibody-binding to the receptor by competition with radio-labeled TSH, does not distinguish between TSAb and TSBAb. A positive TBII result in a patient with hypothyroidism is evidence for the presence of TSBAb. A positive TBII result in a patient with hyperthyroidism is evidence for the presence of TSAb. These bioassays (TSAb and TSBAb) are useful to detect transient neonatal hyperthyroidism and hypothyroidism [10] and are also important to confirm the causes of hyperthyroidism and hypothyroidism [13]. TBII-positive patients may have TSBAb or TSAb. Thyroid function can oscillate between hypothyroidism and hyperthyroidism as TSBAb or TSAb becomes dominant. TSAb and TSBAb can be used to document TRAb-function [13].

There are two forms of autoimmune thyroiditis: atrophic autoimmune thyroiditis and goitrous autoimmune thyroiditis [3]. We followed 34 TSBAb-positive patients with hypothyroidism (24 patients with atrophic autoimmune thyroiditis and 10 with goitrous autoimmune thyroiditis) over 10 years. TSBAb has been found in patients with atrophic autoimmune thyroiditis, and also in patients with goitrous autoimmune thyroiditis [11]. All of the 10 TSBAb-positive patients with goitrous autoimmune thyroiditis recovered from hypothyroidism and 19 (79%) of the 24 with atrophic autoimmune thyroiditis continued to have hypothyroidism. With the disappearance of TSBAb, recovery from hypothyroidism has been seen. TSBAb-positive hypothyroid patients with goitrous autoimmune thyroiditis may recover from hypothyroidism, and those with atrophic autoimmune thyroiditis may continue to have hypothyroidism.

References

[1] N. Takasu, C. Oshiro, H. Akamine et al., "Thyroid-stimulating antibody and TSH-binding inhibitor immunoglobulin in 277 Graves' patients and in 686 normal subjects," *Journal of Endocrinological Investigation*, vol. 20, no. 8, pp. 452–461, 1997.

[2] N. Takasu, K. Kamijo, Y. Sato et al., "Sensitive thyroid-stimulating antibody assay with high concentrations of polyethylene glycol for the diagnosis of Graves' disease," *Clinical and Experimental Pharmacology and Physiology*, vol. 31, no. 5-6, pp. 314–319, 2004.

[3] N. Takasu, T. Yamada, M. Takasu et al., "Disappearance of thyrotropin-blocking antibodies and spontaneous recovery from hypothyroidism in autoimmune thyroiditis," *The New England Journal of Medicine*, vol. 326, no. 8, pp. 513–518, 1992.

[4] K. Endo, K. Kasagi, J. Konishi et al., "Detection and properties of TSH-binding inhibitor immunoglobulins in patients with Graves' disease and Hashimoto's thyroiditis," *Journal of Clinical Endocrinology and Metabolism*, vol. 46, no. 5, pp. 734–739, 1978.

[5] B. R. Smith and R. Hall, "Measurement of thyrotropin receptor antibodies," *Methods in Enzymology*, vol. 74, pp. 405–420, 1981.

[6] K. Kasagi, J. Konishi, and Y. Iida, "A new in vitro assay for human thyroid stimulator using cultured thyroid cells: effect of sodium chloride on adenosine 3',5'-monophosphate increase," *Journal of Clinical Endocrinology and Metabolism*, vol. 54, no. 1, pp. 108–114, 1982.

[7] T. F. Davies, M. Platzer, A. Schwartz et al., "Functionality of thyroid-stimulating antibodies assessed by cryopreserved human thyroid cell bioassay," *Journal of Clinical Endocrinology and Metabolism*, vol. 57, no. 5, pp. 1021–1027, 1983.

[8] B. Rapoport, F. S. Greenspan, S. Filetti et al., "Clinical experience with a human thyroid cell bioassay for thyroid-stimulating immunoglobulin," *Journal of Clinical Endocrinology and Metabolism*, vol. 58, no. 2, pp. 332–338, 1984.

[9] M. Ludgate, J. Perret, M. Parmentier et al., "Use of the recombinant human thyrotropin receptor (TSH-R) expressed in mammalian cell lines to assay TSH-R autoantibodies," *Molecular and Cellular Endocrinology*, vol. 73, no. 1, pp. R13–R18, 1990.

[10] N. Takasu, T. Mori, Y. Koizumi et al., "Transient neonatal hypothyroidism due to maternal immunoglobulins that inhibit thyrotropin-binding and post-receptor processes," *Journal of Clinical Endocrinology and Metabolism*, vol. 59, no. 1, pp. 142–146, 1984.

[11] N. Takasu, T. Yamada, M. Katakura et al., "Evidence for thyrotropin (TSH)-blocking activity in goitrous Hashimoto's thyroiditis with assays measuring inhibition of TSH receptor binding and TSH-stimulated thyroid adenosine 3',5'-monophosphate responses/cell growth by immunoglobulins," *Journal of Clinical Endocrinology and Metabolism*, vol. 64, no. 2, pp. 239–245, 1987.

[12] N. Takasu, T. Yamada, A. Sato et al., "Graves' disease following hypothyroidism due to Hashimoto's disease: studies of eight cases," *Clinical Endocrinology*, vol. 33, no. 6, pp. 687–698, 1990.

[13] N. Takasu, K. Yamashiro, Y. Ochi et al., "TSBAb (TSH-stimulation blocking antibody) and TSAb (Thyroid stimulating antibody) in TSBAb-positive patients with hypothyroidism and graves' patients with hyperthyroidism," *Hormone and Metabolic Research*, vol. 33, no. 4, pp. 232–237, 2001.

[14] N. Takasu, K. Yamashiro, I. Komiya et al., "Remission of graves' hyperthyroidism predicted by smooth decreases of thyroid-stimulating antibody and thyrotropin-binding inhibitor immunoglobulin during antithyroid drug treatment," *Thyroid*, vol. 10, no. 10, pp. 891–896, 2000.

[15] T. Kouki, T. Inui, K. Yamashiro et al., "Demonstration of fragments with thyroid stimulating activity from Thyroid stimulation blocking antibodies-IgG molecules by papain digestion," *Clinical Endocrinology*, vol. 47, no. 6, pp. 693–698, 1997.

[16] J. Konishi, Y. Iida, K. Endo et al., "Inhibition of thyrotropin-induced adenosine 3'5'-monophosphate increase by immunoglobulins from patients with primary myxedema," *Journal of Clinical Endocrinology and Metabolism*, vol. 57, no. 3, pp. 544–549, 1983.

[17] H. Inomata, N. Sasaki, and K. Tamaru, "Relationship between potency of blocking type thyrotropin-binding inhibitor immunoglobulin in three women with primary myxedema and thyroid function of their neonates," *Endocrinologia Japonica*, vol. 33, no. 3, pp. 353–359, 1986.

[18] N. Yokoyama, M. Izumi, S. Katamine et al., "Heterogeneity of Graves immunoglobulin G: comparison of thyrotropin receptor antibodies in serum and in culture supernatants of lymphocytes transformed by Epstein-Barr virus infection," *Journal of Clinical Endocrinology and Metabolism*, vol. 64, no. 2, pp. 215–218, 1987.

[19] I. Matsui, S. Sakata, T. Ogawa et al., "Biological activities of rat antisera raised against synthetic peptides of human thyrotropin receptor," *Endocrine Journal*, vol. 40, no. 5, pp. 607–612, 1993.

[20] Y. Hidaka, V. Guimaraes, M. Soliman et al., "Production of thyroid-stimulating antibodies in mice by immunization with T-cell epitopes of human thyrotropin receptor," *Endocrinology*, vol. 136, no. 4, pp. 1642–1647, 1995.

[21] E. Macchia, R. Concetti, G. Carone et al., "Demonstration of blocking immunoglobulins G, having a heterogeneous behaviour, in sera of patients with Graves' disease: possible coexistence of different autoantibodies directed to the TSH receptor," *Clinical Endocrinology*, vol. 28, no. 2, pp. 147–156, 1988.

[22] A. Miyauchi, N. Amino, H. Tamaki et al., "Coexistence of thyroid-stimulating and thyroid-blocking antibodies in a patient with Graves' disease who had transient hypothyroidism," *The American Journal of Medicine*, vol. 85, no. 3, pp. 418–420, 1988.

[23] H. Tamai, K. Kasagi, Y. Takaichi et al., "Development of spontaneous hypothyroidism in patients with Graves' disease treated with antithyroidal drugs: clinical, immunological, and histological findings in 26 patients," *Journal of Clinical Endocrinology and Metabolism*, vol. 69, no. 1, pp. 49–53, 1989.

[24] K. Kasagi, A. Hidaka, K. Endo et al., "Fluctuating thyroid function depending on the balance between stimulating and blocking types of TSH receptor antibodies: a case report," *Thyroid*, vol. 3, no. 4, pp. 315–318, 1993.

[25] K. Takeda, J. Takamatsu, K. Kasagi et al., "Development of hyperthyroidism following primary hypothyroidism: a case report with changes in thyroid-related antibodies," *Clinical Endocrinology*, vol. 28, no. 4, pp. 341–344, 1988.

[26] V. P. Michelangeli, C. Poon, D. J. Topliss et al., "Specific effects of radioiodine treatment on TSAb and TBAb levels in patients with Graves' disease," *Thyroid*, vol. 5, no. 3, pp. 171–176, 1995.

Suspected Spontaneous Reports of Birth Defects in the UK Associated with the use of Carbimazole and Propylthiouracil in Pregnancy

Pamela Bowman[1, 2] and Bijay Vaidya[3]

[1] Department of Paediatrics, Royal Devon and Exeter Hospital, Exeter, Devon EX25DW, UK
[2] Department of Endocrinology, Royal Devon and Exeter Hospital, Exeter, Devon EX25DW, UK
[3] Peninsula NIHR Clinical Research Facility, Level 2, Peninsula Medical School, University of Exeter, Barrack Road, Exeter, Devon EX25DW, UK

Correspondence should be addressed to Pamela Bowman, pamelabowman@nhs.net

Academic Editor: Kris Gustave Poppe

The concept of a carbimazole embryopathy underlies current Endocrine Society advice to avoid this drug in early pregnancy, favouring propylthiouracil as an alternative for the treatment of maternal hyperthyroidism. We aimed to establish whether suspected spontaneous reporting of adverse drug reactions in the UK via the Yellow Card Scheme supports a carbimazole embryopathy and the lack of association between propylthiouracil and congenital anomalies. All birth defects related to maternal treatment with carbimazole or propylthiouracil reported over a 47-year period via the Yellow Card Scheme were analysed. 57 cases with 97 anomalies were reported following in utero exposure to carbimazole. These anomalies included aplasia cutis, choanal atresia, tracheo-oesophageal fistula, and patent vitellointestinal duct, which have previously been reported in association with carbimazole/methimazole exposure in utero. Only 6 cases with 11 anomalies were reported for propylthiouracil, all within the last 15 years. Therefore, these findings may support a carbimazole embryopathy. There are few birth defects associated with propylthiouracil, but this should be interpreted in the context of higher historical prescription rates for carbimazole.

1. Introduction

Hyperthyroidism, primarily caused by Graves' disease, affects about 1 in 500 pregnancies. Although not common, it is important to recognise and treat maternal hyperthyroidism, because failing to do so can have detrimental effects. In the mother, untreated hyperthyroidism can cause spontaneous miscarriage, pregnancy induced hypertension, preterm labour, congestive cardiac failure, and thyroid storm; for the fetus this could mean still birth, intrauterine growth restriction, or low birth-weight [1]. Further, hyperthyroid states in the mother have been associated with congenital anomalies including oesophageal atresia, tracheo-oesophageal fistula, and biliary tree atresia [2, 3].

There is also an association between the antithyroid drugs used to treat maternal hyperthyroidism and congenital anomalies. This association is most widely reported for carbi-mazole and its active metabolite, methimazole, such that the concept of a carbimazole embryopathy is being increasingly acknowledged amongst prescribing clinicians [4–9]. There has been no convincing link between the alternative thion-amide drug propylthiouracil and birth defects [10] despite the rate of placental transfer of the drug being the same as that of carbimazole [11]. Both drugs are equally efficacious at controlling maternal hyperthyroidism [12]. This has led to the Endocrine Society's current advice to use propy-lthiouracil as a first-line drug during pregnancy, if available, especially during first trimester organogenesis [13]. Carbimazole or methimazole should be used only if propy-lthiouracil is not available or if the patient cannot tolerate or has an adverse response to it [13].

Recognition of serious adverse effects of anti-thyroid drugs in pregnancy is dependent upon reporting of such effects by prescribing clinicians. Since 1964, the Yellow Card

Scheme has allowed healthcare professionals involved in prescribing in the UK to report suspected serious adverse drug reactions (ADRs) to the Commission on Human Medicines (CHM)/Medicines and Healthcare Products Regulatory Agency (MHRA). The professional reporting the suspected ADR submits a Yellow Card found at the back of the British National Formulary, or electronically via the MHRA website, giving brief clinical details supporting their suspicions that the drug is responsible for the adverse outcome(s) seen. In addition, pharmaceutical companies are legally required to report suspected serious ADRs of their products. Since October 2005, patients have also been able to report suspected ADRs through the Yellow Card Scheme.

In this paper, we aimed to establish whether spontaneous reporting via the Yellow Card Scheme in the UK lends support to an association between congenital anomalies and the use of carbimazole or propylthiouracil in pregnancy.

2. Methods

Data on all birth defects reported via the Yellow Card Scheme in association with treatment with carbimazole or propylthiouracil between July 1963 and September 2010 was obtained in "Drug Analysis Prints" from the MHRA [14]. Drug Analysis Prints give a complete listing of all UK spontaneous suspected ADRs reported through the Yellow Card Scheme by healthcare professionals, patients, and the pharmaceutical industry to the MHRA and CHM. They do not present a complete overview of the risks associated with specific medicines, and conclusions on the safety and risks of medicines cannot be made on the information contained in Drug Analysis Prints alone.

3. Results

The Drug Analysis Print from the MHRA included 64 reports of birth defects following exposure to antithyroid drugs, reported between 1963 and 2010. Of these, 54 reports came from healthcare professionals, 9 from pharmaceutical companies, and one from a patient. On review, one of the reports was found not to comprise birth defect and was excluded from further analysis.

Figure 1 shows the total numbers of birth defects reported following exposure to carbimazole and propylthiouracil by decade. For carbimazole, there have been 57 cases with a total of 97 congenital anomalies. Three (5%) of these cases (with tracheo-oesophageal fistula, anencephaly, and unspecified congenital heart disease, respectively) have been reported as fatal. For propylthiouracil, only 6 cases with 11 congenital anomalies have been reported, but these have all been within the last 15 years. None of the six cases has been reported as fatal.

Table 1 describes the type of birth defects reported for carbimazole and propylthiouracil exposure in utero and the number of defects seen in conjunction with other anomalies in the same individual. Two-thirds of the cases with birth defects associated with both carbimazole and propylthiouracil exposure had multiple anomalies in the same individuals. Birth defects associated with carbimazole exposure in-

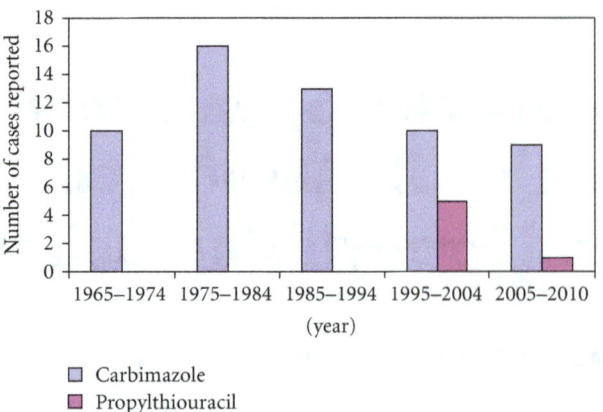

FIGURE 1: Bar graph showing number of cases with congenital malformations reported following exposure to carbimazole or propylthiouracil by decade from 1965 until 2010.

cluded aplasia cutis, choanal atresia, tracheo-oesophageal fistula, patent vitellointestinal duct, and dysmorphic facies, which have been previously reported as components of carbimazole embryopathy [9]. The doses of carbimazole used were known for 34 out of 57 cases (60%), and ranged between 5 mg and 60 mg daily (median 15 mg). Similarly, the dose of propylthiouracil, known for 5 out of 6 cases (83%), ranged widely from 50 mg to 350 mg daily (median 50 mg).

4. Discussion

Our results support an association between exposure to carbimazole in utero and birth defects. There have been far fewer reports via the Yellow Card Scheme of birth defects related to propylthiouracil exposure, but all the reports related to this drug have been within the last 15 years; this may reflect the fact that historically carbimazole has been the more widely prescribed drug in the UK [15], rather than it its rate of teratogenicity being significantly higher. There has been a 3.5-fold increase in PTU prescription relative to carbimazole since 1981 in the UK [15], which may have unmasked adverse effects that had previously gone unnoticed. Changes in prescribing trends are also reflected by data from the USA, where between 2002 and 2008, propylthiouracil use increased in women of childbearing age [16].

The teratogenicity of anti-thyroid drugs remains a source of controversy [17]. Two previous studies comparing carbimazole with propylthiouracil showed no difference in the number of major congenital anomalies seen in babies exposed to these drugs in utero [12, 18]. However, both studies were relatively small. A study from Sweden found 4 reports between 1995–2000 of infants born with oesophageal atresia and omphalocele or choanal atresia, 3 of whom had been exposed to methimazole in the first trimester; there was no association between these anomalies and propylthiouracil [19]. A recent larger case control study which included over 18,000 cases with congenital malformations, 127 of whom were exposed to antithyroid drugs in the first trimester, showed a significant association between exposure to carbimazole/methimazole and choanal atresia or omphalocele [20]. For

TABLE 1: Suspected adverse drug reactions of congenital anomalies associated with carbimazole and propylthiouracil received via the UK Yellow Card Scheme.

System	Congenital anomalies*	Carbimazole			Propylthiouracil		
		Number of anomalies (total)	Number with single anomaly	Number with other anomalies	Number of anomalies (total)	Number with single anomaly	Number with other anomalies
Skin	Aplasia cutis	6	2	4	0	0	0
	Other (skin disorder, ulcer)	2	0	2	0	0	0
Respiratory	Choanal atresia	5	2	3	0	0	0
	Tracheo-oesophageal fistula	2	2	0	0	0	0
	Other (neonatal respiratory distress syndrome, respiratory disorder)	2	0	2	0	0	0
Gastrointestinal	Cleft palate	5	3	2	1	1	0
	Omphalocele/umbilical abnormalities	4	2	2	2	0	2
	Patent vitellointestinal duct	1	0	1	0	0	0
	Duodenal atresia	1	1	0	0	0	0
	Anal atresia	1	0	1	0	0	0
	Other (neonatal jaundice and abnormal liver function tests)	2	0	2	0	0	0
	Not specified	3	2	1	0	0	0
Cardiovascular	Septal defects	3	1	2	0	0	0
	Other (Fallot's tetralogy and coarctation of aorta)	2	2	0	0	0	0
	Not specified	1	0	1	0	0	0
Musculoskeletal	Limb/hand/foot malformation	4	1	3	3	1	2
	Not specified	4	3	1	0	0	0
Neurological	Spina bifida	3	1	2	0	0	0
	Hydrocephalus	5	1	4	0	0	0
	Anencephaly	4	4	0	1	0	1
	Hypotonia	2	0	2	0	0	0
	Other (spine malformation and holoprosencephaly)	1	0	1	1	0	1
Renal/urinary tract	Renal aplasia	1	0	1	0	0	0
	Other (urinary tract malformation, epispadias)	1	0	1	1	1	0
Endocrine	Thyroid disorder	1	0	1	0	0	0
	Hypogonadism	1	0	1	0	0	0
Craniofacial	Dysmorphic facies	2	0	2	1	0	1
	Skull malformation	4	1	3	0	0	0
	Ear malformation	3	1	2	0	0	0
	Deafness	4	2	2	0	0	0
	Eye malformation	4	1	3	0	0	0
	Other (nose malformation and teeth malformation)	2	0	2	0	0	0
Others	Nipple/breast anomalies (athelia and hypoplastic nipples)	2	0	2	0	0	0
	Developmental delay	2	0	2	0	0	0
	Autism	0	0	0	1	0	1
	Not specified	7	1	6	0	0	0
Total		97	33	64	11	3	8

*One Yellow Card report may contain more than one reaction term. Therefore, the total number of reactions is greater than the total number of reports.

propylthiouracil, there was a tentative suggestion of an association with situs inversus, renal agenesis, or dysgenesis and cardiac outflow tract malformations although these were not as strong as the associations reported for carbimazole [20]. Consistent with these observations, we found five cases of choanal atresia and four cases of umbilical anomalies associated with carbimazole exposure in our study (Table 1). There were no reports of situs inversus, renal agenesis, or cardiac malformations associated with propylthiouracil exposure (Table 1).

The nature of congenital malformations seen in our cases is wide ranging, keeping with previous reports of birth defects related to these drugs (Table 1). Several of the congenital malformations associated with carbimazole exposure observed in this study, including aplasia cutis, choanal atresia, tracheo-oesophageal fistula, omphalocele, patent vitellointestinal duct, nipple abnormalities, and dysmorphic facies, have previously been reported in association with carbimazole/methimazole exposure in utero [9]. Furthermore, two-thirds of the anomalies associated with carbimazole exposure occurred with other defects in the same cases, lending further support to an embryopathy as opposed to a single malformation which might have occurred spontaneously irrespective of exposure to teratogens or not. It should be noted that most of the anomalies seen following propylthiouracil exposure also did not occur in isolation, but given the small numbers for propylthiouracil, this should be interpreted with caution.

We acknowledge that there are several limitations to our study. Firstly, true prevalence of birth defects related to carbimazole and propylthiouracil cannot be calculated from the information we have collated. We do not know the total number of births to mothers with Graves' disease over the study period, and we do not have data relating to the types of anti-thyroid drugs prescribed to pregnant women over the study period. In addition, Yellow Card data cannot be used as a reliable indicator of the frequency of suspected ADRs to medicines. The number of reports received via the Yellow Card Scheme does not directly equate to the number of people who suffer adverse reactions to drugs. It is recognised that this scheme is associated with an unknown and variable level of underreporting. The level of ADR reporting may fluctuate between given years due to a variety of reasons, for example, a medicine being new, stimulated interest/publicity, and variations in exposure to the medicine. In this case, there is potential for bias in that prescribers may be more likely to make an association between a congenital anomaly and carbimazole given previous reports of an embryopathy related to the drug which is not the case for propylthiouracil. Similarly, carbimazole and propylthiouracil were introduced to the market at different times, and therefore, reporting bias means that they should not be directly compared.

Secondly, causality cannot be proven. It is important to note that a report of an ADR does not necessarily mean that it was caused by the drug. Many factors have to be taken into account in assessing causal relationships including temporal association, the possible contribution of concomitant medication, and the underlying disease. We do not have information on maternal thyroid function for our cases; this is important, because maternal hyperthyroidism itself is associated with congenital anomalies [2, 3]. Furthermore, in a cohort study of infants of mothers with Graves' disease, the incidence of congenital malformations was significantly higher in infants whose mothers were hyperthyroid in the first trimester compared to those who were euthyroid, with a reported prevalence of 6% and 0.3% in the two groups, respectively [21].

Thirdly, we do not have a complete data on the doses and durations of the carbimazole or propylthiouracil exposure in our cases. We only know doses used for 60% of patients treated with carbimazole and 83% of patients treated with propylthiouracil.

Nevertheless, the multiple characteristic congenital anomalies we have reported in this study lend support to the teratogenicity of thionamide drugs, in particular carbimazole. This has important clinical implications, and prescribing physicians should be aware of the potential association with congenital anomalies whilst balancing this risk with that of uncontrolled maternal hyperthyroidism in pregnancy.

5. Conclusion

The evidence we have described in this study may support a carbimazole embryopathy. There are few birth defects associated with propylthiouracil, but this should be interpreted in the context of higher historical prescription rates for carbimazole.

Acknowledgments

The authors are grateful to staff at the Medicines and Healthcare Products Regulatory Agency (MHRA), UK, for extracting the data from the Yellow Cards, and providing helpful comments on our manuscript. Work of BV was partly supported by the National Institute for Health Research (NIHR). The views expressed in this publication are those of the authors and not necessarily those of the National Health Service, the NIHR or the Department of Health, United Kingdom.

References

[1] G. E. Krassas, K. Poppe, and D. Glinoer, "Thyroid function and human reproductive health," *Endocrine Reviews*, vol. 31, no. 5, pp. 702–755, 2010.

[2] P. Barbero, R. Valdez, H. Rodríguez et al., "Choanal atresia associated with maternal hyperthyroidism treated with methimazole: a case-control study," *American Journal of Medical Genetics Part A*, vol. 146, no. 18, pp. 2390–2395, 2008.

[3] M. Seoud, A. Nassar, I. Usta, M. Mansour, I. Salti, and K. Younes, "Gastrointestinal malformations in two infants born to women with hyperthyroidism untreated in the first trimester," *American Journal of Perinatology*, vol. 20, no. 2, pp. 59–62, 2003.

[4] N. Foulds, I. Walpole, F. Elmslie, and S. Mansour, "Carbimazole embryopathy: an emerging phenotype," *American Journal of Medical Genetics*, vol. 132, no. 2, pp. 130–135, 2005.

[5] A. K. Myers and W. Reardon, "Choanal atresia—a recurrent feature of foetal carbimazole syndrome," *Clinical Otolaryngology*, vol. 30, pp. 364–383, 2005.

[6] D. Wolf, N. Foulds, and H. Daya, "Antenatal carbimazole and choanal atresia: a new embryopathy," *Archives of Otolaryngology—Head and Neck Surgery*, vol. 132, no. 9, pp. 1009–1011, 2006.

[7] L. Kannan, S. Mishra, R. Agarwal, V. Kartikeyan, N. Gupta, and M. Kabra, "Carbimazole embryopathy-bilateral choanal atresia and patent vitello-intestinal duct: a case report and review of literature," *Birth Defects Research Part A*, vol. 82, no. 9, pp. 649–651, 2008.

[8] D. Koenig, A. Spreux, S. Hiéronimus et al., "Birth defects observed with maternal carbimazole treatment: six cases reported to Nice's Pharmacovigilance Center," *Annales d'Endocrinologie*, vol. 71, no. 6, pp. 535–542, 2010.

[9] P. Bowman, N. J. Osborne, R. Sturley, and B. Vaidya, "Carbimazole Embryopathy: implications for the choice of antithyroid drugs in pregnancy," *QJM*. In press.

[10] O. Diav-Citrin and A. Ornoy, "Teratogen update: antithyroid drugs—methimazole, carbimazole, and propylthiouracil," *Teratology*, vol. 65, no. 1, pp. 38–44, 2002.

[11] R. H. Mortimer, G. R. Cannell, R. S. Addison, L. P. Johnson, M. S. Roberts, and I. Bernus, "Methimazole and propylthiouracil equally cross the perfused human term placental lobule," *Journal of Clinical Endocrinology and Metabolism*, vol. 82, no. 9, pp. 3099–3102, 1997.

[12] D. A. Wing, L. K. Millar, P. P. Koonings, M. N. Montoro, and J. H. Mestman, "A comparison of propylthiouracil versus methimazole in the treatment of hyperthyroidism in pregnancy," *American Journal of Obstetrics and Gynecology*, vol. 170, no. 1, pp. 90–95, 1994.

[13] M. Abalovich, N. Amino, L. A. Barbour et al., "Management of thyroid dysfunction during pregnancy and postpartum: an endocrine society clinical practice guideline," *Journal of Clinical Endocrinology and Metabolism*, vol. 92, no. 8, pp. S1–S47, 2007.

[14] Medicines and Healthcare Products Regulatory Agency/Commission on Human Medicines, United Kingdom, http://www.mhra.gov.uk/.

[15] S. H. S. Pearce, "Spontaneous reporting of adverse reactions to carbimazole and propylthiouracil in the UK," *Clinical Endocrinology*, vol. 61, no. 5, pp. 589–594, 2004.

[16] A. B. Emiliano, L. Governale, M. Parks, and D. S. Cooper, "Shifts in propylthiouracil and methimazole prescribing practices: antithyroid drug use in the United States from 1991 to 2008," *Journal of Clinical Endocrinology and Metabolism*, vol. 95, no. 5, pp. 2227–2233, 2010.

[17] F. Azizi and A. Amouzegar, "Management of hyperthyroidism during pregnancy and lactation," *European Journal of Endocrinology*, vol. 164, no. 6, pp. 871–876, 2011.

[18] H. Rosenfeld, A. Ornoy, S. Shechtman, and O. Diav-Citrin, "Pregnancy outcome, thyroid dysfunction and fetal goitre after in utero exposure to propylthiouracil: a controlled cohort study," *British Journal of Clinical Pharmacology*, vol. 68, no. 4, pp. 609–617, 2009.

[19] F. A. Karlsson, O. Axelsson, and H. Melhus, "Severe embryopathy and exposure to methimazole in early preganancy," *Journal of Clinical Endocrinology and Metabolism*, vol. 87, no. 2, pp. 947–948, 2002.

[20] M. Clementi, E. Di Gianantonio, M. Cassina et al., "Treatment of hyperthyroidism in pregnancy and birth defects," *Journal of Clinical Endocrinology and Metabolism*, vol. 95, no. 11, pp. E337–E341, 2010.

[21] N. Momotani, K. Ito, N. Hamada, Y. Ban, Y. Nishikawa, and T. Mimura, "Maternal hyperthyroidism and congenital malformation in the offspring," *Clinical Endocrinology*, vol. 20, no. 6, pp. 695–700, 1984.

4

Subclassification of the "Grey Zone" of Thyroid Cytology; A Retrospective Descriptive Study with Clinical, Cytological, and Histological Correlation

Mariella Bonzanini,[1] **Pierluigi Amadori,**[2] **Luca Morelli,**[1] **Silvia Fasanella,**[1]
Riccardo Pertile,[3] **Angela Mattiuzzi,**[4] **Giorgio Marini,**[4]
Mauro Niccolini,[5] **Giuseppe Tirone,**[6] **Marco Rigamonti,**[7] **and Paolo Dalla Palma**[1]

[1] Department of Surgical Pathology, S. Chiara Hospital, 38100 Trento, Italy
[2] Outpatient Endocrine Surgery, Local Public Health Service, 38100 Trento, Italy
[3] Epidemiological Survey, Local Public Health Service, Trento, Italy
[4] Department of Radiology, S. Chiara Hospital, 38100 Trento, Italy
[5] Department of Radiology, Villa Bianca Hospital, 38100 Trento, Italy
[6] Department of Surgery, S. Chiara Hospital, 38100 Trento, Italy
[7] Department of Surgery, Cles Hospital, 38100 Trento, Italy

Correspondence should be addressed to Mariella Bonzanini, mariella.bonzanini@apss.tn.it

Academic Editor: Nelson Wohllk

Undetermined thyroid cytology precludes any definitive distinction between malignant and benign lesions. Recently several classifications have been proposed to split this category into two or more cytological subcategories related to different malignancy risk rates. The current study was performed retrospectively to investigate the results obtained separating "undetermined" cytologic reports into two categories: "follicular lesion" (FL) and "atypia of undetermined significance" (AUS). Biochemical, clinical, and echographic features of each category were also retrospectively analyzed. Altogether, 316 undetermined fine-needle aspirated cytologies (FNACs) were reclassified as 74 FL and 242 AUS. Histological control leads to a diagnosis of carcinomas, adenomas, and nonneoplastic lesions, respectively, in 42.2%, 20%, and 37.8% of AUS and in 8.3%, 69.4%, and 22.2% of FL. Among biochemical, clinical, cytological, and echographic outcomes, altered thyroid autoantibodies, multiple versus single nodule, AUS versus FL, and presence of intranodular vascular flow were statistically significant to differentiate adenoma from carcinoma and from nonneoplastic lesions, whereas no significant differences were found between carcinomas and nonneoplastic lesions for these parameters. The results of this retrospective study show that undetermined FNAC category can further be subclassified in AUS and FL, the former showing higher malignancy rate. Further prospective studies are needed to confirm our results.

1. Introduction

Fine-needle aspiration cytology (FNAC) has become the dominant method in the evaluation of thyroid nodules, being fast, reliable, safe, minimally invasive, cost-effective, and reaching high sensitivity and specificity [1].

FNAC has allowed a dramatic decrease in surgical treatment of patients with thyroid nodular disease [2], enhancing the percentage of malignant operated nodules over 50% [3].

However, even in adequate cellular specimens, the method shows certain limitations and leads to an "undetermined" result in 4–15% of all cases [4, 5], precluding any definitive distinction between malignant and benign lesions.

To assess terminology, description, and interpretation of cytological appearances and transmit them to the clinicians in a clear and reproducible way, several classifications for thyroid cytology report have been proposed [6–10].

All are based on a risk of malignancy scale for adequate specimens."Undetermined" results are mostly composed of atypia of undetermined significance (AUS) and follicular patterned lesions (FL).

According to the recent Bethesda System for Reporting Thyroid Cytopathology (BSRTC), "atypia of undetermined significance/follicular lesion of undetermined significance" (AUS/FLUS) is a heterogeneous category that includes cases with ambiguous cytological findings that appear to be greater than what would be expected of a nonneoplastic process, yet the degree of cellular or architectural atypia is insufficient for an interpretation of "follicular neoplasm" or "suspicious for malignancy" [8].

Therefore, undetermined cytology is a sort of "grey zone" also for the clinicians, whose main goal is a correct therapeutic approach to thyroid lesions, that is, surgery, with its extension, or medical followup. Practically, most of these lesions are surgically removed, in total or subtotal thyroidectomy, although only a minority of them are malignant.

However, true malignancy incidence in undetermined lesions is not definitely known, because not all of them are histologically checked, and the literature reports largely heterogeneous data.

In AUS, malignancy is reported in 25% of operated patients, but it is thought to be closer to 5–10% of the total [8]. Papillary carcinoma is by far the commonest tumour [3, 11, 12].

Malignancy incidence in FL is even more variously reported than in AUS.

Cancer ratio in all FL lesions (operated and nonoperated) is about 20% in several surveys [3, 11–13], but other authors reported much lesser incidences of 0–7% [14–16].

In this study we have retrospectively split "undetermined" thyroid FNAC into two categories: "follicular lesion" (FL) and "atypia of undetermined significance" (AUS) in order to evaluate

(i) the relative incidences of AUS and FL in thyroid FNA specimens in our district,

(ii) the incidence of malignant lesions in AUS and FL,

(iii) the presence of biochemical, clinical, and echographic features possibly predictive of malignancy related to AUS and FL.

2. Materials and Methods

We reviewed the thyroid FNAC data of our institution from June 2004 to December 2007.

For each FNAC, a specific module was performed, including patient data, clinical and biochemical thyroid status (hypo-, hyper, or euthyroidism), thyroid autoantibodies, and thyroid medication. Moreover, detailed ultrasound features such as size, echogenicity, microcalcifications, boundaries, and color Doppler vascular flow pattern (intra/perinodular) were described for each nodule.

FNACs were mainly performed by four radiologists and one endocrinologist with ultrasound guide, using 25 or 27 gauge needles.

Two-three samplings were performed for each nodule. Papanicolaou and May-Grünwald-Giemsa stains were both used for FNA smears preparations.

2.1. Cytological Classification Criteria. Cytological specimens were evaluated by 3 pathologists, and careful cytological description was reported for each case.

Original cytologic reports were reclassified into 5 categories: inadequate, benign, undetermined, suspicious, and malignant, not knowing the followup.

The undetermined results were divided into two further categories.

(1) FL for samples suggesting follicular neoplasms. In this category were included FNACs with high to moderate cellularity, predominantly or partially microfollicular pattern, scanty or absent colloid, and mild or absent nuclear atypia. Samples consisting almost exclusively/exclusively of Hurthle cells were also included here.

Follicular patterned lesions or Hurthle cells lesions with overt cytological architectural or nuclear atypical features (that is irregular or variably sized follicle, crowding of cells, many single cells, pleomorphic, enlarged nuclei, nuclear grooves, coarse and irregular chromatin, prominent and multiple nucleoli, atypical or numerous mitosis) [17] were reported as suspicious and were not included in this study.

(2) AUS for samples exhibiting cytological atypia or other features raising the possibility of neoplasia, but which were insufficient to enable confident placing into any other category.

This is intended as a broad category encompassing focal features suggestive of papillary carcinoma, cellular atypia hindered by sample preparation artifact, cellular atypia engendered by cystic alteration, repair, and therapy. Atypical lymphoid infiltrate was included [8, 10].

2.2. Histological, Cytological, and Clinical Followup. Corresponding histologic and clinical-cytological followup was reviewed.

The histological diagnosis was made according to the World Health Organization guidelines [18].

The patients who did not undergo thyroid surgery, with benign repeated FNAC, were followed by clinical and periodic thyroid sonographic evaluation, at least once within 2 years from the last FNA. If the thyroid nodule did not undergo any modifications it was considered "bona fide" benign.

2.3. Statistical Analysis. The descriptive analyses included the observed frequencies calculation with the respective percentages for each categorical variable, while median and range were computed for patients' age and diameter of nodules (continuous variables).

Multivariate stepwise logistic regression analysis was performed in order to identify clinical, echographic, and cytological categories associated with the lesion type (carcinomas versus adenomas, carcinomas versus nonneoplastic lesions, adenomas versus nonneoplastic lesions). In stepwise selection analysis, any significant variables (P value $\leq$ .05) are inserted in the model as covariates, but an attempt is made to remove any insignificant variables from the model before adding a new significant variable to the model. Each addition or deletion of a variable to or from a model is listed as a separate step and at each step, a new model is fitted. In this study only the final model is presented. Results are given in terms of odds ratio (OR).

Multivariate analyses were performed with SAS software, version 9.1.3 (SAS Institute Inc., SAS 9.1.3, Cary, NC, USA, 2003).

3. Results

Between June 2004 and December 2007, 2422 FNAs were performed in 1883 patients with thyroid nodule(s). There were 348 men and 1535 women, aged 13–88 years (median 54 years).

Reclassification of the cytological reports yielded 397 (16.4%) nondiagnostic samples, 1554 (64.2%) benign cytology, 84 (3.5%) diagnoses of suspect malignant neoplasia, 71 (2.9%) diagnoses of malignant cytology, and 316 (13%) undetermined cytologic reports. 74 (3%) reports corresponding to follicular lesion were reclassified as FL, and 242 (10%) reports were reclassified as AUS (Figure 1).

3.1. Histological Followup. The histological diagnosis was available for 81 nodules of the undetermined category: 36 of 74 (48.6%) nodules classified as FL, and 45 of 242 (18.6%) nodules classified as AUS.

There were 22 malignant tumors, 34 follicular adenomas, and 25 nonneoplastic lesions.

Among malignant tumors, 19 were PTC, 15 classic and 4 follicular variant, and 3 were follicular carcinomas.

Follicular adenomas were Hurtle cells type in 13 cases and follicular in 21 cases.

Nonneoplastic lesions have been shown to be nodular hyperplasia in 18 cases, Hashimoto's thyroiditis in 5, granulomatous thyroiditis in 1, and spindled, probably reactive, lesion in 1. Among histologically proven carcinomas, 19 (42.2%) were observed in nodules with preoperative AUS reclassification, whereas 3 (8.3%) were observed in nodules with preoperative FL reclassification.

Adenomas were observed in 25 (69.4%) nodules classified as FL and in 9 (20%) classified as AUS.

Seventeen benign lesions (nodular hyperplasia and thyroiditis) corresponded to cytological reclassification of AUS (37.8%) and 8 to FL (22.2%) (Table 1).

3.2. Clinical Followup. Repetition of FNAC was performed in 73 AUS lesions. Nine resulted inadequate, 46 benign, 10 AUS, 1 FL, 5 suspicious, and 2 malignant.

Repetition of FNAC was performed in 8 FL. In 5 cases the same cytological category was confirmed, whereas in 3 cases the cytological diagnosis was benign.

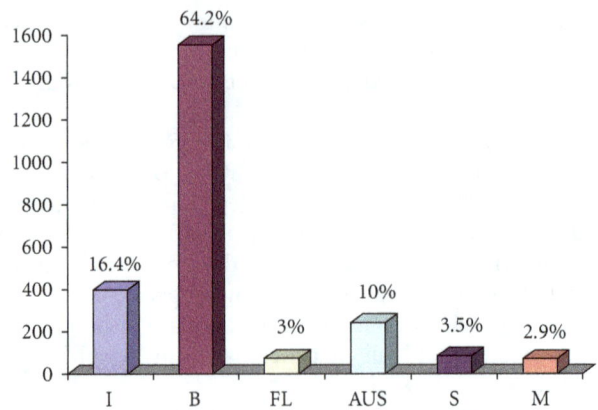

FIGURE 1: I: inadequate; B: benign; FL: follicular lesion; AUS: atypia of undetermined significance; S: suspicious for malignant neoplasia; M: malignant neoplasia. Distribution of cytological categories after reclassification.

For 49 lesions with repeated benign FNA (46 AUS and 3 FL), in which the patients did not undergo thyroid surgery, clinical and echographic followup supported the benign nature of the lesion.

3.3. Clinical and Echographic Features. Clinical, echographic features and cytological diagnosis of histologically proven carcinomas and adenomas and of nonneoplastic lesions with histological or clinical followup are reported in Table 2.

No significant statistical differences were found according to age, gender, and thyroid function between carcinomas, adenomas, and nonneoplastic lesions. Moreover, there were no significant differences for clinical, echographic, and cytological reclassification between carcinomas and nonneoplastic lesions. However, altered autoantibodies, multiple nodules versus single nodule, and AUS versus FL cytological category showed a statistically significant difference between carcinomas and adenomas (Table 3). In detail, after conditioning on the other variables entered in the model, the probability of observing a carcinoma was more than 15 times higher when thyroid autoantibodies were altered (OR = 15.43 with a P value = .046), multiple nodules increased the probability of identifying a carcinoma by almost 79 times (OR = 78.94 with a P value = .003), and the presence of AUS cytological category increased the probability of recognizing a carcinoma by more than 21 times (OR = 21.49 with a P value = .023). Total variance explained by these three variables entered in the final model is 56% (R^2 = 0.56) and concordance percentage is 92.9% which means that 93 of every 100 nodules will be well classified using alteration in thyroid autoantibodies, multiple/single nodules, and cytological category as predictors.

Concerning the comparison between nonneoplastic lesions and adenomas, single nodule (versus multiple nodules), follicular lesion (versus AUS), higher diameter, and no vascular flow are all statistically significant features in adenomas compared to nonneoplastic lesions (Table 4). Keeping the other variables constant in the model, the

TABLE 1: Histologic followup of cases.

	AUS (242 cases)		FL (74 cases)	
	45	18.6%	36	48.6%
Benign	26	57.8%	33	91.6%
Follicular adenoma	5	19.2%	16	48.5%
Hurtle cell adenoma	4	15.4%	9	27.3%
Nodular hyperplasia	11	43.3%	7	21.2%
Hashimoto thyroiditis	4	15.4%	1	3%
De Quervain thyroiditis	1	3.8%	—	—
Reactive nodule	1	3.8%	—	—
Malignant	19	42.2%	3	8,4%
Papillary carcinoma classic type	14	73.7%	1	33.3%
Follicular variant of papillary carcinoma	3	15.8%	1	33.3%
Follicular carcinoma	2	10.5%	1	33.3%

AUS: atypia of undetermined significance; FL: follicular lesion.

TABLE 2: Clinical, biochemical, and echographic features of 130 thyroid nodules with histological (81 cases) or benign repeated cytology with clinical-echographic followup (49 cases).

	Carcinoma		Adenoma		Nodular hyperplasia/thyroiditis	
	22	16.9%	33	25.4%	75	57.7%
Clinical and biochemical features						
Age (years)	Range 25–75		Range 18–81		Range 27–72	
	Median 53		Median 49		Median 51	
Female	18	80.8%	26	78.8%	68	90.7%
Male	4	19.2%	7	21.2%	7	9.3%
AbHTG and/or AbTPO	7	31.8%	4	12.1%	27	36.0%
Hypothyroidism	1	4.5%	—	—	3	4.0%
Hyperthyroidism	1	4.5%	1	3.0%	2	2.7%
Single nodule	8	36.4%	25	75.8%	24	32.0%
Unknown	—		1	3.0%	3	4.0%
Diameter (mm)	Range 6–48		Range 7–54		Range 8–50	
	Median 18		Median 23		Median 15	
Palpable	14	63.6%	22	66.7%	35	46.7%
Echographic features						
Solid	20	90.9%	26	78.8%	54	72.0%
Hypoechoic	14	70.0%	20	76.9%	37	68.5%
Hyperechoic	2	10%	1	3.8%	10	18.5%
Isoechoic	4	20%	5	19.2%	7	13.0%
Microcalcifications	5	25%	5	19.2%	3	5.6%
Vascular flow	4	20%	14	53.8	11	20.4%
Irregular margins	3	15%	2	7.7%	3	5.6%
Unknown	—		2	6.1%	3	4.0%
Mixed	2	9.1%	5	15.1%	16	21.3%
Cystic	—	—	—	—	2	2.7%
Cytologic category						
AUS	19	86.4%	9	27.3%	65	86.7%
FL	3	13.6%	24	72.7%	10	13.3%

AUS: atypia of undetermined significance; FL: follicular lesion.

TABLE 3: Multivariate logistic analysis of the probability of identifying a carcinoma versus an adenoma by clinical, echographic features and cytologic category.

	Parameters entered in the model	OR	P value	Concordance percentage	R2
All nodules (n = 54)	Ab altered (yes versus no)	15.43	.046	92.9%	0.56
	Multiple versus single nodule	78.94	.003		
	Cytologic Category (AUS versus FL)	21.49	.023		
Only solid nodules (n = 45)	Multiple versus single nodule	29.53	.005	85.9%	0.48
	Cytologic Category (AUS versus FL)	12.50	.044		

AUS: atypia of undetermined significance; FL: follicular lesion.

TABLE 4: Multivariate logistic analysis of the probability of identifying a benign nodule (NH and thyroiditis) versus an adenoma by clinical, echographic features and cytologic category.

	Parameters entered in the model	OR	P value	Concordance percentage	R^2
All nodules (n = 108)	Multiple versus single nodule	14.47	.002	81.3%	0.38
	Cytologic Category (AUS versus FL)	11.96	.000		
	Diameter (mm)	0.94	.043		
Only solid nodules (n = 80)	Multiple versus single nodule	10.93	.006	80.8%	0.37
	Cytologic Category (AUS versus FL)	8.48	.005		
	Vascular flow (yes versus No)	0.14	.035		

AUS: atypia of undetermined significance; FL: follicular lesion.

probability of identifying a benign lesion increased by 14.5 times in case of multiple nodules (OR = 14.47 with a P value = .002) and by 12 times with an AUS cytological category (OR = 11.96 with a P value ≤ .0001). Finally, for each mm. of increase in the nodule diameter, the logistic regression model predicted a 6% decrease in the probability of observing a nonneoplastic lesion rather than an adenoma (OR = 0.94 and P value = .043). Concordance percentage of the model is 81.3% and R^2 is 0.38.

Taking into account only solid nodules (n = 80), the diameter was no more statistically significant, but another variable entered in the model, that is, vascular flow: the presence of vascular flow decreased the probability of observing a nonneoplastic lesion by 86% (OR = 0.14 and P value = .035).

4. Conclusions

Although FNAC has been used with success in the diagnosis of papillary, medullary, and anaplastic thyroid carcinomas, it is difficult to assess its value in follicular lesions. The main problem is the distinction between benign lesions, such as follicular adenoma or nodular adenomatous goiter, and follicular carcinoma or follicular variant of papillary carcinoma (FVPTC).

Therefore, histological evaluation is necessary to demonstrate capsular/vascular invasion for follicular carcinoma and the subtle nuclear aspects in FVPTC [11].

Classifications, practically overlapping as for benign and malignant definitions, show some substantial differences managing undetermined lesions.

Follicular lesions are managed in two main different ways depending on the classification.

The Bethesda System distinguishes 3 subcategories: "follicular neoplasm or suspicious for a follicular neoplasm" refers to a cellular aspirate comprised of follicular cells, most of which are arranged in an altered architectural pattern characterized by significant cell crowding and/or microfollicle formation; "follicular neoplasm, Hurthle cell type/suspicious for follicular neoplasm, Hurthle cell type" refers to a cellular aspirate consisting exclusively (or nearly exclusively) of Hurthle cells.

Follicular patterned aspirates that do not otherwise fulfil the aforementioned criteria are set together with AUS (AUS/FLUS).

However, a significant difference in malignancy incidence seems not to appear from the document [8].

The recently published "Guidance on the reporting of thyroid cytology specimens" of English Royal College of Pathologist (RCP) names "neoplasm possible" (Thy3) the undetermined category and separates samples suggesting follicular neoplasms (Thy3f-f for follicular) from samples which exhibit cytological atypia or other features which raise the possibility of neoplasia but which are insufficient to enable confident placing into any other category (Thy3a-a for atypia).

Operative indications emerging from BSRTC recommend FNAC repetition for AUS/FLUS (with subsequent surgery if AUS/FLUS, or worse category, are found) [8], whereas RCP recommends an individualized and multidisciplinary assessment for each patient [10].

As for AUS, its incidence among thyroid cytological specimens is variably reported, ranging from 2% to 6%, although some heterogeneity in its definition makes it difficult to draw consistent conclusions [3, 5, 11, 12]. The Bethesda System for Reporting Thyroid Cytopathology recommends to use this category as a last resort and limit its use to approximately 7% [8].

In our institution, thyroid FNAC classification similar to that of The Royal College of Pathologists [9, 10] has been actually chosen, where the presence/absence of nuclear atypia is the key of the undetermined lesions subclassification in AUS and FL.

In the present study, data obtained on this basis indicate that AUS is associated with higher malignancy rates than FL.

Low malignancy incidence in FL emerging from our study contradicts the usually accepted rates of about 20% reported by some studies [3, 5, 13, 14, 19, 20] but it is in agreement with others.

Two Italian studies found no cancers in all operated nodules with cytological diagnosis of FL [15, 21].

DeMay, at histological examination, found only 2 cancers (none follicular) among 138 FL [16].

Such a discrepancy may reflect inconsistent patterns in cytological criteria of classification.

One of the heaviest factors influencing this discrepancy is cellular atypia, particularly its definition and association with follicular patterned lesions.

The role of atypia as an independent risk factor for malignancy has been matter of interest and debate. Although some authors report no correlation between atypia and malignancy [5, 22, 23], other studies show, conversely, that atypia alone or in association with a follicular patterned FNAC can be linked to a higher risk of malignancy [12, 14, 16, 20, 24, 25].

Interestingly, most literature showing high malignancy rates in FL, actually reports substantial reduction when lesions with atypia are excluded [12, 14, 19].

Moreover, among the malignancies histologically proven in FL, FVPTC appears to be the commonest one, whereas follicular carcinoma and Hurthle cell carcinomas seem to be much rarer than usually reported both in FL and, generally, among all thyroid cancers [13–16].

It is well known that the cytological diagnosis of FVPTC is challenging, due to a paucity or lack of well-defined nuclear features of papillary carcinoma, leading, in samples containing few cellular groups, to a diagnosis of AUS or FL [13].

However, an accurate evaluation of focal cytological features and the architectural pattern has been shown to allow a correct diagnosis of malignancy or suspect for malignancy [26, 27], but adequate smears and skilled pathologists are necessary, and this could play some role in outcome differences.

Multivariate analysis of our data allows to draw some other relevant conclusions.

Among the cytological undetermined lesions of thyroid, adenomas seem to be the more correctly classifiable on the basis of cytological, immunological, and ultrasound data.

Firstly, most of FL specimens lead to a histological diagnosis of adenoma.

Secondly, thyroid autoantibodies appear to be more common in non-neoplastic lesions and in carcinomas than in adenomas. As for carcinomas, this is not surprising. Coexistence of chronic lymphocytic thyroiditis and PTC has

been reported, at variable frequencies, although it remains unclear whether these two thyroid disorders share a common aetiology or thyroiditis represents a host tumor immune response [28–30].

Moreover, Kim et al. recently reported positive serum antithyroglobulin antibodies as an independent predictor for thyroid malignancy in thyroid nodules, regardless of the presence of autoimmune thyroiditis [31].

Our results, although limited to thyroid cancers discovered in undetermined cytology, seem to be in agreement with this observation.

Conversely, the overlapping incidences of thyroid autoantibodies in carcinomas and in non-neoplastic lesions in the present study could almost partially be due to the fact that, in the latter, both autoimmune thyroiditis and nodular hyperplasia were enclosed.

In conclusion, our outcomes suggest higher malignancy risk in cytological undetermined thyroid lesions with atypia than without atypia.

The very low incidence of thyroid cancer found in FL refers to the same perplexity about an unavoidable surgical treatment, arisen by other authors with similar results [15, 16, 21].

Although all patients with FL should be considered for surgical resection, they should be also informed about the low malignancy risk of their condition and other aspects, such as underlying medical conditions and age of the patients, presence/absence of thyroid autoantibodies, growth rate of the nodule, which could be taken in account for the decision.

Conversely, a more relevant indication to surgery could be advisable for AUS.

In this lesion, FNAC repetition seems also appropriate. Our data confirm that about half of these aspirates are reclassified as benign, as already reported in the literature [3, 12].

Being based on the review of previous cytological data, our study shares the same limitations of the retrospective studies, not allowing a prospective, two-arm followup of operated versus nonoperated cases. Therefore our findings should be evaluated in this light. Anyway, we clearly documented clinical and cytological findings in subclassified undetermined cytologic category in 81 nodules histologically checked and in 49 nodules with repeated FNAC and clinical and echographic followup.

Two years ago our results led to the employment, in our department, of a cytological classification similar to that of the RCP. A larger, prospective study design has been planned for the risk assessment in each cytological category.

In recent years, molecular tests have been shown to be useful in the diagnosis of thyroid neoplasms. Point mutations in BRAF and RAS genes and gene rearrangements involving PAX8/PPARγ and RET/PTC have been found in approximately 70% of thyroid neoplasia [32].

The B-RAF V600E mutation has been shown as diagnostic marker for PTC, and there have been many reports on its diagnostic usefulness in refining the cytological diagnosis of this tumor [33–37]. But, unfortunately BRAF analysis is of limited value in preoperative diagnosis of FVPTC [38].

Moreover, several studies indicate that molecular testing of thyroid nodules for a panel of mutations can enhance the accuracy of undetermined FNAC [39, 40], but at present no single marker seems to be accurate enough to distinguish thyroid carcinoma from its benign mimics to be introduced in the routine [41].

Finally, our results support the indication to distinguish undetermined thyroid cytological samples with follicular patterned feature without atypia from the undetermined samples with atypical cells and to relate the FNAC results with clinical and echographic findings.

References

[1] M. W. Ashcraft and A. J. Van Herle, "Management of thyroid nodules. I: history and physical examination, blood tests, X-ray tests, and ultrasonography," *Head and Neck Surgery*, vol. 3, no. 3, pp. 216–230, 1981.

[2] H. Gharib and J. R. Goellner, "Fine-needle aspiration biopsy of the thyroid: an appraisal," *Annals of Internal Medicine*, vol. 118, no. 4, pp. 282–289, 1993.

[3] L. Yassa, E. S. Cibas, C. B. Benson et al., "Long-term assessment of a multidisciplinary approach to thyroid nodule diagnostic evaluation," *Cancer*, vol. 111, no. 6, pp. 508–516, 2007.

[4] Z. W. Baloch, M. J. Sack, G. H. Hu, V. A. Livolsi, and P. K. Gupta, "Fine-needle aspiration of thyroid: an institutional experience," *Thyroid*, vol. 8, no. 7, pp. 565–569, 1998.

[5] J. Yang, V. Schnadig, R. Logrono, and P. G. Wasserman, "Fine-needle aspiration of thyroid nodules: a study of 4703 patients with histologic and clinical correlations," *Cancer*, vol. 111, no. 5, pp. 306–315, 2007.

[6] H. H. Wang, "Reporting thyroid fine-needle aspiration: literature review and a proposal," *Diagnostic Cytopathology*, vol. 34, no. 1, pp. 67–76, 2006.

[7] "Papanicolau Society of cytopathology recommandetionsfor thyroid fine-needle aspiration," 2010, http://www.pathology.org/guidelines.html.

[8] S. Z. Ali and E. S. Cibas, *The Bethesda System for Reporting Thyroid Cytopathology. Definitions, Criteria and Explanatory Notes*, Springer, New York, NY, USA, 2010.

[9] British Thyroid Association Royal College of Physicians, "Guidelines for the management of thyroid cancer," in *Report of the Thyroid Cancer Guidelines Update Group*, P. Perros, Ed., Royal College of Physicians, London, UK, 2nd edition, 2007.

[10] The Royal College of Pathologists, "Guidance on the reporting of thyroid cytology specimens," London: RCP 2009, http://www.rcpath.org/resources/pdf/g089guidanceonthere-portingofthyroidcytologyfinal.pdf.

[11] Y. Shi, X. Ding, M. Klein et al., "Thyroid fine-needle aspiration with atypia of undetermined significance: a necessary or optional category?" *Cancer Cytopathology*, vol. 117, no. 5, pp. 298–304, 2009.

[12] R. E. Goldstein, J. L. Netterville, B. Burkey, and J. E. Johnson, "Implications of follicular neoplasms, atypia, and lesions suspicious for malignancy diagnosed by fine-needle aspiration of thyroid nodules," *Annals of Surgery*, vol. 235, no. 5, pp. 656–664, 2002.

[13] W. C. Faquin and Z. W. Baloch, "Fine-Needle aspiration of follicular patterned lesions of the thyroid: diagnosis, management, and follow-up according to National Cancer Institute (NCI) recommendations," *Diagnostic Cytopathology*, vol. 38, pp. 731–739, 2010.

[14] N. Dabelić, N. Matesa, D. Matesa-Anić, and Z. Kusić, "Malignancy risk assessment in adenomatoid nodules and suspicious follicular lesions of the thyroid obtained by fine needle aspiration cytology," *Collegium Antropologicum*, vol. 34, pp. 349–354, 2010.

[15] L. Foppiani, M. Tancredi, G. L. Ansaldo et al., "Absence of histological malignancy in a patient cohort with follicular lesions on fine-needle aspiration," *Journal of Endocrinological Investigation*, vol. 26, no. 1, pp. 29–34, 2003.

[16] R. M. DeMay, "Follicular lesions of the thyroid: W(h)ither follicular carcinoma?" *American Journal of Clinical Pathology*, vol. 114, no. 5, pp. 681–683, 2000.

[17] R. M. De May, "Thyroid," in *The Art and Science of Cytopathology*, pp. 724–729, ASCP Press, Chigago, Ill, USA, 1996.

[18] C. Hedinger, *Histological Typing of Thyroid Tumours*, Springer, Berlin, Germany, 2nd edition, 1988.

[19] R. Mihai, A. J. C. Parker, D. Roskell, and G. P. Sadler, "One in four patients with follicular thyroid cytology (THY3) has a thyroid carcinoma," *Thyroid*, vol. 19, no. 1, pp. 33–37, 2009.

[20] G. Bahar, D. Braslavsky, T. Shpitzer et al., "The cytological and clinical value of the thyroid "follicular lesion"," *American Journal of Otolaryngology*, vol. 24, no. 4, pp. 217–220, 2003.

[21] D. Piromalli, G. Martelli, I. Del Prato, P. Collini, and S. Pilotti, "The role of fine needle aspiration in the diagnosis of thyroid nodules: analysis of 795 consecutive cases," *Journal of Surgical Oncology*, vol. 50, no. 4, pp. 247–250, 1992.

[22] T. S. Greaves, M. Olvera, B. D. Florentine et al., "Follicular lesions of thyroid: a 5-year fine-needle aspiration experience," *Cancer*, vol. 90, no. 6, pp. 335–341, 2000.

[23] C. R. McHenry, S. R. Thomas, S. J. Slusarczyk, and A. Khiyami, "Follicular or Hurthle cell neoplasm of the thyroid: can clinical factors be used to predict carcinoma and determine extent of thyroidectomy?" *Surgery*, vol. 126, no. 4, pp. 798–804, 1999.

[24] A. Carpi, E. Ferrari, M. G. Toni, A. Sagripanti, A. Nicolini, and G. Di Coscio, "Needle aspiration techniques in preoperative selection of patients with thyroid nodules: a long-term study," *Journal of Clinical Oncology*, vol. 14, no. 5, pp. 1704–1712, 1996.

[25] A. S. Kelman, A. Rathan, J. Leibowitz, D. E. Burstein, and R. S. Haber, "Thyroid cytology and the risk of malignancy in thyroid nodules: importance of nuclear atypia in indeterminate specimens," *Thyroid*, vol. 11, no. 3, pp. 271–277, 2001.

[26] S. Logani, P. K. Gupta, V. A. LiVolsi, S. Mandel, and Z. W. Baloch, "Thyroid nodules with FNA cytology suspicious for follicular variant of papillary thyroid carcinoma: follow-up and management," *Diagnostic Cytopathology*, vol. 23, no. 6, pp. 380–385, 2000.

[27] I. A. El Hag and S. M. Kollur, "Benign follicular thyroid lesions versus follicular variant of papillary carcinoma: differentiation by architectural pattern," *Cytopathology*, vol. 15, no. 4, pp. 200–205, 2004.

[28] K. C. Loh, F. S. Greenspan, F. Dong, T. R. Miller, and P. P. B. Yeo, "Influence of lymphocytic thyroiditis on the prognostic outcome of patients with papillary thyroid carcinoma," *Journal of Clinical Endocrinology and Metabolism*, vol. 84, no. 2, pp. 458–463, 1999.

[29] E. Kebebew, P. A. Treseler, P. H. G. Ituarte, and O. H. Clark, "Coexisting chronic lymphocytic thyroiditis and papillary thyroid cancer revisited," *World Journal of Surgery*, vol. 25, no. 5, pp. 632–637, 2001.

[30] S. Arif, A. Blanes, and S. J. Diaz-Cano, "Hashimoto's thyroiditis shares features with early papillary thyroid carcinoma," *Histopathology*, vol. 41, no. 4, pp. 357–362, 2002.

[31] E. S. Kim, D. J. Lim, K. H. Baek et al., "Thyroglobulin antibody is associated with increased cancer risk in thyroid nodules," *Thyroid*, vol. 20, pp. 885–891, 2010.

[32] Y. E. Nikiforov, "Thyroid carcinoma: molecular pathways and therapeutic targets," *Modern Pathology*, vol. 21, supplement 2, pp. S37–S43, 2008.

[33] G. Salvatore, R. Giannini, P. Faviana et al., "Analysis of BRAF point mutation and RET/PTC rearrangement refines the fine-needle aspiration diagnosis of papillary thyroid carcinoma," *Journal of Clinical Endocrinology and Metabolism*, vol. 89, no. 10, pp. 5175–5180, 2004.

[34] K. W. Chung, S. K. Yang, G. K. Lee et al., "Detection of BRAF mutation on fine needle aspiration specimens of thyroid nodule refines cyto-pathology diagnosis, especially in BRAF mutation-prevalent area," *Clinical Endocrinology*, vol. 65, no. 5, pp. 660–666, 2006.

[35] M. R. Sapio, D. Posca, A. Raggioli et al., "Detection of RET/PTC, TRK and BRAF mutations in preoperative diagnosis of thyroid nodules with indeterminate cytological findings," *Clinical Endocrinology*, vol. 66, no. 5, pp. 678–683, 2007.

[36] G. Troncone, I. Cozzolino, M. Fedele, U. Malapelle, and L. Palombini, "Preparation of thyroid FNA material for routine cytology and BRAF testing: a validation study," *Diagnostic Cytopathology*, vol. 38, no. 3, pp. 172–176, 2010.

[37] S. Girlando, L. V. Cuorvo, M. Bonzanini et al., "High prevalence of B-RAF mutation in papillary carcinoma of the thyroid in North-East Italy," *International Journal of Surgical Pathology*, vol. 18, no. 3, pp. 173–176, 2010.

[38] A. Proietti, R. Giannini, C. Ugolini et al., "BRAF status of follicular variant of papillary thyroid carcinoma and its relationship to its clinical and cytological features," *Thyroid*, vol. 20, pp. 1263–1270, 2010.

[39] Y. E. Nikiforov, D. L. Steward, T. M. Robinson-Smith et al., "Molecular testing for mutations in improving the fine-needle aspiration diagnosis of thyroid nodules," *Journal of Clinical Endocrinology and Metabolism*, vol. 94, no. 6, pp. 2092–2098, 2009.

[40] N. P. Ohori, M. N. Nikiforova, K. E. Schoedel et al., "Contribution of molecular testing to thyroid fine-needle aspiration cytology of "follicular lesion of undetermined significance/atypia of undetermined significance"," *Cancer Cytopathology*, vol. 118, no. 1, pp. 17–23, 2010.

[41] B. C. G. Freitas and J. M. Cerutti, "Genetic markers differentiating follicular thyroid carcinoma from benign lesions," *Molecular and Cellular Endocrinology*, vol. 321, no. 1, pp. 77–85, 2010.

5

Incremental Healthcare Expenditures Associated with Thyroid Disorders among Individuals with Diabetes

Amit D. Raval and Usha Sambamoorthi

Department of Pharmaceutical Systems and Policy, School of Pharmacy, West Virginia University, P.O. Box 9510, Morgantown, WV-26505, USA

Correspondence should be addressed to Amit D. Raval, adraval@hsc.wvu.edu

Academic Editor: C. Marcocci

Objective. To estimate incremental healthcare expenditures associated with thyroid disorders among individuals with diabetes. *Research Design and Methods.* Cross-sectional study design with data on adults over 20 years of age with diabetes ($N = 4,490$) from two years (2007 and 2009) of the Medical Expenditure Panel Survey (MEPS) was used. Ordinary least square regressions on log-transformed total expenditures and type of healthcare expenditures (inpatient, emergency room, outpatient, prescription drug, and other) were performed to estimate the incremental expenditures associated with thyroid disorders after controlling for demographic, socioeconomic, health status, lifestyle risk factors, macrovascular comorbid conditions (MCCs), and chronic conditions (CCs). *Results.* Among individuals with diabetes, those with thyroid disorders had significantly greater average annual total healthcare expenditures ($15,182) than those without thyroid disorders ($11,093). Individuals with thyroid disorders had 34.3% greater total healthcare expenditures compared to those without thyroid disorders, after controlling for demographic, socio-economic, and perceived health status. Furthermore, controlling for CCs and MCCs, this increase in expenditures was reduced to 21.4%. *Conclusions.* Among individuals with diabetes, thyroid disorders were associated with greater healthcare expenditures; such excess expenditures may be due to CCs and MCCs. Comanagement of CCs and reducing MCCs may be a pathway to reduce high healthcare expenditures.

1. Introduction

In 2011, approximately 20 million Americans were affected by thyroid disorders [1]. Individuals with diabetes are at greater risk for developing thyroid disorders and have a higher prevalence of thyroid disorders compared to the general population. Prevalence of thyroid disorders among individuals with diabetes ranges from 13%–32% compared to 5%–8% in the general population [2–5]. Although hypothyroidism is a common disorder among individuals with diabetes [2–5], hyperthyroidism is also prevalent and is estimated to be around 12% [6].

As thyroid hormones affect glucose metabolism [7–10], individuals with diabetes and hypothyroidism may suffer from frequent recurrent hypoglycemic episodes [11] and insulin resistance [12, 13]. Thyroid hormones also affect body weight, placing individuals with thyroid disorders at increased risk of obesity and negative consequences related to obesity [8, 12, 13]. Individuals with diabetes and hyperthyroidism may suffer from hyperglycemia possibly due to increased metabolism of insulin, increase in glucose absorption from gut, increase in endogenous glucose production, lipolysis resulted in hepatic gluconeogenesis, increase in growth hormones, glucagon and catecholamine levels [7, 9, 14–18].

Elevated risk of microvascular complications such as retinopathy and nephropathy among individuals with diabetes and subclinical hypothyroidism compared to individuals with diabetes and without subclinical hypothyroidism has been documented [19–22]. In addition, thyroid disorders may lead to macrovascular complications. In a recent study, subclinical hypothyroidism was associated with increased risk of cardiovascular mortality and morbidity specifically increased incidence of atrial fibrillation [23]. In addition, thyroid disorders cooccur with many common chronic conditions, for example, depression, arthritis, and asthma [24–28] which can further complicate the management of both diabetes and thyroid disorders.

The negative consequences of abnormally high or low levels of thyroid hormones on glycemic control, micro- and macrovascular complications can lead to greater economic burden as well. Among individuals with diabetes, macrovascular conditions are reported to be a major driver of healthcare expenditures [29–31]. However, studies that examine the excess economic burden measured by direct healthcare expenditures associated with thyroid disorders among individuals with diabetes are scarce. There is a need for studies in this area to better understand the drivers of greater healthcare expenditures among individuals with diabetes and thyroid disorders and develop strategies and programs to reduce the economic burden in this group. Therefore, the primary objective of the study is to provide cross-sectional estimates of additional healthcare expenditures associated with thyroid disorders among adults with diabetes by comparing them to those with diabetes and without thyroid disorders, using a nationally representative survey of households and families.

2. Methods

2.1. Study Design.
This study utilized a cross-sectional design and compared healthcare expenditures among individuals with thyroid disorders and diabetes to individuals with diabetes without thyroid disorders.

2.1.1. Data Source.
The Medical Expenditure Panel Survey (MEPS) data for the years 2007 and 2009 were used for this study. The MEPS is a set of large-scale surveys of families and individuals, their medical providers (doctors, hospitals, pharmacies, etc.), and employers across the United States of America (USA). The MEPS is cosponsored by the Agency for Healthcare Research and Quality (AHRQ) and the National Center for Health Statistics. The survey provides nationally representative estimates of healthcare use, expenditures, payment sources, health insurance coverage, health status, health conditions, and treatment for the civilian noninstitutionalized population of USA.

For the current study, we used household and medical conditions files of the MEPS. The household component collects person-level data on demographic characteristics, health conditions, health status, use of medical services, charges and payments, access to care, employment, health insurance coverage, and income for a period of two years. Medical conditions file provides information on medical conditions that were reported by the households. The medical conditions and procedures reported by the household component respondent are usually recorded by the interviewer as verbatim text, which is then coded by professional coders to fully specifiedInternational Classification of Diseases, Ninth Revision, Clinical Modification (ICD-9-CM) codes, including medical condition and V codes [32, 33]. However, to preserve confidentiality, the MEPS

data provide nearly all of the diagnosis condition codes only 3-digit ICD-9 CM codes. In addition, the MEPS data provide clinical classification codes, which are aggregated ICD-9-CM codes into clinically meaningful categories that group similar conditions. For the purpose of this study, we used both ICD-9 CM as well as clinical classification codes to identify the medical condition appropriately (see details of ICD-9CM and CCS crosswalk on: http://meps.ahrq.gov/mepsweb/data_stats/download_data/pufs/h128/h128_icd9codes.shtml).

We included data for the years 2007 and 2009 to gain sufficient sample size. As individuals are followed for two years, to avoid including repeated observations from the same individual, we selected alternate years.

2.2. Study Sample.
The study sample included adults, aged 21 years or older, and reported diabetes during the calendar years and alive during the calendar years. Diabetes was identified from clinical classification codes 49 and 50 (Table 5). Detailed information on the crosswalk between ICD-9-CM codes and clinical classification codes is available elsewhere [32, 33]. The final study sample consisted of 4,490 individuals with diabetes, of whom 545 reported having thyroid disorders.

2.3. Measures

2.3.1. Dependent Variables

Healthcare Expenditures: Total and Type of Expenditures. Within MEPS, healthcare services, which were paid by third-party payers and/or individuals themselves are defined as health expenditures and reported for each year. Expenditures are also distinguished by the type of expenditures, and aggregated by inpatient care; ambulatory care, provided in offices and hospital outpatient departments; care provided in emergency departments; prescribed medications, vision, dental, home health care, and others. Sources include direct payments from individuals, private insurance, Medicare, Medicaid, Veteran Affairs, other public insurance, workers' compensation, and other sources [32, 33]. In current study, we classified the types of expenditures into: (1) inpatient; (2) emergency room; (3) outpatient; (4) prescription drugs; (5) other. Other expenditures included home health care, vision, dental, durable medical equipment, and ambulance services, orthopedic items, hearing devices, prostheses, bathroom aids, medical equipment, disposable supplies, alterations/modifications, and other miscellaneous items or services that were obtained, purchased, or rented during the year [32, 33]. Expenditures in 2007 were converted to 2009 dollars using the annual consumer price index for medical care services available from the bureau of labor statistics [34]. As expenditures data were skewed to the right, we transformed expenditures to natural logarithmic scale and we used logged expenditures as dependent variables in regression analysis.

Key Independent Variable: Presence of Thyroid Disorders.
Thyroid disorders were identified using clinical classification code of 48, which represented all thyroid disorders such as acquired hypothyroidism (ICD-9-CM code −244), thyrotoxicosis (ICD-9-CM code −242), thyroiditis (ICD-9-CM code −245), and other disorders of thyroid (ICD-9-CM code −246) [35]. We created a dummy variable for presence of thyroid disorder for the purpose of analysis.

2.3.2. Other Independent Variables. Demographic variables included gender (women, men), categories of age in years (21–49, 50–64, and 65 and +), race/ethnicity (White, African American, Latino, and other), marital status (married, widowed, separated/divorced, and never married), and area of residence (metro and nonmetro). Socioeconomic characteristics were categorized by education (less than high school, high school, and above high school) and poverty status. The poverty status variable was defined poor (less than 100% federal poverty line), near poor (100% to less than 200%), middle income (200% to less than 400%), and high income (greater than or equal to 400%) available from MEPS represented family income in relation to the federal poverty line (based on family size and composition).

Health status was measured with widely used standard scales of perceived physical and mental health. Perceived physical and mental health status were categorized into excellent/very good, good, and fair/poor. Body mass index categories (BMI—normal or underweight, overweight, and obese), current smoking (yes/no), and vigorous physical activity at least 3 times/week (yes/no) represented lifestyle risk factors. Healthcare expenditures are often influenced by the presence of chronic physical conditions such as arthritis, chronic obstructive pulmonary disease (COPD), gastroesophageal reflux disease (GERD), other endocrine disease, and osteoporosis and mental health conditions such as depression and anxiety [31, 36–38]. Therefore, we also included the total number of cooccurring chronic conditions as one of the independent variables. For details of conditions and codes, please see Table 5.

Macrovascular Comorbid Conditions. To understand the association between diabetes complications and expenditures, we included macrovascular comorbid conditions as defined by Fu and colleagues [31] as one of the independent variables. The macrovascular comorbid conditions were defined using clinical classification codes and appropriate ICD-9 CM 3-digit codes, which included codes for cardiovascular disease (ischemic heart disease, congestive heart failure, aortic/visceral/peripheral aneurysms, visceral atherosclerosis, and peripheral vascular disease) and cerebrovascular disease (strokes and transient ischemic attacks).

2.4. Statistical Techniques. To test unadjusted differences in logged expenditures, ordinary least square regressions were used to estimate the incremental expenditures associated with thyroid disorders among individuals with diabetes. Effect estimates for continuous independent variables on the

log of annual expenditures can be interpreted as percentage change for each unit of change in the independent variable. The effect of categorical variables in terms of percentage of expenditures can be estimated by exponentiating the regression coefficients of dummy variables and subtracting one (i.e., percent change = $e^\beta − 1$) [39]. Therefore, in tables, we also present percent change in expenditures in addition to parameter estimates.

To understand the association between thyroid disorders expenditures among individuals with diabetes, we conducted four different regression models in which independent variables were entered in blocks. In Model 1, we controlled for age, gender and race/ethnicity. In Model 2, we adjusted for other demographic, socioeconomic, and life-style factors in addition to variables used in Model 1. In Model 3, in addition to the variables used in Model 2, we included number of cooccurring chronic conditions. In Model 4, we controlled for the presence of macrovascular comorbid conditions, in addition to all other variables included in Model 3. All analyses account for complex survey design of the MEPS and statistical testing was carried out with survey procedures in SAS 9.2.

3. Results

3.1. Description of the Study Sample. In our study sample, 12% (N = 545) individuals reported having cooccurring thyroid disorders. The demographics and socio-economic characteristics, access to care, health status, and personal health practices of individuals with diabetes with or without thyroid disorders are presented in Table 1.

Among individuals with diabetes, gender, age, race/ethnicity, marital status, poverty status, health insurance, BMI, smoking status, and physical activity were significantly different between individuals with and without thyroid disorders. For example, a significantly higher proportion of women (20%) than men (7%) reported having thyroid disorders. Similarly, a significantly higher proportion of elderly who were 65 years or older (17.8%) reported having thyroid disorders compared to young adults in the age group 21–50 years (10.1%). Compared to African Americans (8.6%), a significantly higher proportion of Whites reported having thyroid disorders (16.3%). Regarding lifestyle risk factors, a lower proportion of smokers (10.5%) reported having thyroid disorders compared to nonsmokers (15%). Individuals who performed moderate-to-vigorous physical activity at least three times a week had lower rates of thyroid disorders (12.3%) compared to individuals who did not perform moderate-to-vigorous physical activity at least three times a week (15%).

We examined the prevalence of cooccurring chronic and macrovascular comorbid conditions (Table 2). Among individuals with diabetes, those with thyroid disorders reported significantly higher rates of cooccurring chronic conditions and macrovascular comorbid conditions compared to their counterparts without thyroid disorders. For example, 39.5% of those with thyroid disorders reported the presence of any macrovascular comorbid conditions compared to 30.6%

TABLE 1: Description of sample characteristics of individuals with diabetes by the presence of thyroid disorders from the Medical Expenditure Panel Survey, 2007 and 2009.

	Total sample		No thyroid		Thyroid		Sig.
	N	wt%	N	Row wt%	N	Row wt%	
All	4,490	100.0%	3,945	87.8%	545	12.1%	
Sex							
Female	2,519	55.0	2,090	79.7	429	20.3	* * *
Male	1,971	45.0	1,855	93.0	116	7.0	
Age							
21–50 years	1,001	20.5	924	89.9	77	10.1	
51–64 years	1,741	38.2	1,548	88.2	193	11.8	* * *
65 years or older	1,748	41.2	1,473	82.2	275	17.8	
Race/ethnicity							
White	2,079	66.1	1,739	83.7	340	16.3	
African American	1,037	14.4	956	91.4	81	8.6	* * *
Latino	1,023	12.7	927	89.4	96	10.6	
Other	351	6.7	323	91.4	28	8.6	
Marital status							
Married	2,550	59.4	2,280	87.5	270	12.5	
Widowed	696	14.9	567	79.0	129	21.0	* * *
Separated/divorced	799	16.9	703	87.5	96	12.5	
Never married	445	8.8	395	86.0	50	14.0	
Metro							
Metro	3,627	80.4	3,192	86.1	435	13.9	
Nonmetro	863	19.6	753	86.1	110	13.9	
Education							
Less than high school	1,465	24.3	1,288	85.4	177	14.6	
High school	1,418	34.2	1,241	85.6	177	14.4	
Above high school	1,565	41.5	1,379	86.9	186	13.1	
Poverty status							
Poor	875	13.9	782	89.1	93	10.9	
Near poor	1,121	21.5	976	82.8	145	17.2	* *
Middle income	1,321	30.2	1,145	84.7	176	15.3	
High income	1,173	34.4	1,042	88.1	131	11.9	
Health insurance							
Private	2,346	60.6	2,066	86.8	280	13.2	
Public	1,706	32.1	1,472	83.4	234	16.6	* *
Uninsured	438	7.3	407	92.0	31	8.0	
Body mass index categories							
Under/normal weight	721	15.4	647	87.8	74	12.2	
Overweight	1,342	28.4	1,203	87.4	139	12.6	
Obese	2,321	54.2	2,004	84.8	317	15.2	
Missing	106	2.1	91	86.9	15	13.1	
Perceived health							
Excellent/very good	1,033	25.3	922	87.8	111	12.2	
Good	1,674	39.4	1,480	86.2	194	13.8	
Fair/poor	1,783	35.2	1,543	84.7	240	15.3	
Mental health							
Excellent/very good	2,113	49.8	1,867	86.7	246	13.3	
Good	1,607	34.9	1,423	86.0	184	14.0	
Fair/poor	770	15.3	655	84.3	115	15.7	

TABLE 1: Continued.

	Total sample		No thyroid		Thyroid		Sig.
	N	wt%	N	Row wt%	N	Row wt%	
All	4,490	100.0%	3,945	87.8%	545	12.1%	
Current smoker							
Yes	666	14.8	601	89.5	65	10.5	
Other	3,528	78.9	3,076	85.0	452	15.0	**
Missing	296	6.2	268	91.2	28	8.8	
Exercise							
≥3 times a week	1,800	41.1	1,618	87.7	182	12.3	
No exercise	2,656	58.9	2,298	85.0	358	15.0	*
Missing	296	6.2	268	91.2	28	8.8	

Based on 4,490 individuals with diabetes, aged 21 years or older and were alive during the calendar years 2007 and 2009.

Asterisks represent significant group differences by the presence of thyroid disorders based on chi-square tests.

***$P < .001$; **$.001 \leq P < .01$; *$.01 \leq P < .05$.

Please note that the percentages cannot be calculated by dividing the unweighted number by total sample size because the percentages are derived after accounting for the complex survey design of the MEPS.

TABLE 2: Prevalence of co-occurring chronic conditions by the presence of thyroid disorders among individuals with diabetes from the Medical Expenditure Panel Survey, 2007 and 2009.

	No thyroid disorders		Thyroid disorders		Sig.
	N	Col. wt%	N	Col. wt%	
All	3,945	100.0	545	100.0	
Any macrovascular comorbid conditions	**1,181**	**30.6**	**213**	**39.5**	***
Heart disease	1,061	28.0	193	35.8	**
Stroke	225	5.2	41	8.0	*
Peripheral vascular disease	36	1.0	6	0.8	
Any cooccurring physical chronic conditions	**2233**	**58.5**	**414**	**78.9**	***
Arthritis	1635	41.4	313	55.9	***
Cancer	398	11.8	91	21.4	***
Chronic obstructive pulmonary disease	621	16.3	120	20.5	*
Gastroesophageal reflux disease	497	13.1	100	17.9	*
Asthma	380	9.3	77	12.6	*
Anemia	140	3.1	34	5.9	**
Osteoporosis	103	2.8	33	5.5	**
Endocrine disorders	54	1.6	16	3.0	
Any cooccurring mental health conditions	**929**	**24.9**	**192**	**34.2**	***
Depression	623	17.2	137	25.1	***
Anxiety	406	10.6	91	15.7	***
Schizophrenia	22	0.5	7	0.8	

Based on 4,490 individuals with diabetes, aged 21 years or older and were alive during the calendar years 2007 and 2009.

Asterisks represent significant group differences by the presence of thyroid disorders based on chi-square tests.

***$P < .001$; **$.001 \leq P < .01$; *$.01 \leq P < .05$.

Please note that the percentages cannot be calculated by dividing the unweighted number by total sample size because the percentages are derived after accounting for the complex survey design of the MEPS.

of individuals with diabetes and without thyroid disorders. Similarly, 35.8% of those with thyroid disorders reported heart disease compared to 28% among those with diabetes and without thyroid disorders.

In terms of number chronic conditions, 14.6% of those with thyroid disorders reported 5 or more conditions compared to 6.7% among those with diabetes and without thyroid disorders (data not shown in tabular form). In addition, individuals with thyroid disorders had significantly greater number of chronic physical and mental conditions compared to individuals without thyroid disorders.

3.2. Healthcare Expenditures. Among individuals with diabetes, comparisons of average total, inpatient, emergency room, outpatient, prescription drug, and other expenditures for those with and without thyroid disorders are presented in Table 3. Significant group differences in expenditures were tested using log-transformed expenditures using an OLS

TABLE 3: Average total and type of expenditures (2009$) by the presence and absence of thyroid disorders individuals with diabetes from the Medical Expenditure Panel Survey, 2007 and 2009.

	No thyroid disorders		Thyroid disorders		Unadjusted OLS regression on logged dollars			
	Mean ($)	SE	Mean ($)	SE	Beta	SE	% Change	Sig.
Total	**$11,093**	**$382**	**$15,182**	**$1,055**	**0.50**	**0.006**	**64.4**	∗∗∗
Inpatient	3,560	250	4,743	808	0.49	0.020	63.1	∗∗∗
Outpatient	3,118	188	4,403	487	0.61	0.012	84.2	∗∗∗
Prescription	3,214	87	4,157	239	0.50	0.005	64.7	∗∗∗
Emergency room	298	26	328	74	0.17	0.006	18.6	∗∗∗
Other	903	52	1552	220	0.99	0.024	170.7	∗∗∗

Based on 4,490 individuals with diabetes, aged 21 years or older and were alive during the calendar years 2007 and 2009.
Asterisks represent significant group differences by the presence of thyroid using ordinary least squares regression log transformed expenditures. Other expenditures included dental, vision, durable medical equipment use, and others.
Percentage expenditures associated with thyroid disorders were estimated by exponentiating the regression coefficients of dummy variables and subtracting one (i.e., percent change = $e^\beta - 1$)
SE: standard error.
$∗∗∗P < .001; ∗∗.001 \leq P < .01; ∗.01 \leq P < .05$.

regression in which the presence of thyroid disorders was the independent variable. Individuals with diabetes and thyroid disorders had significantly greater total healthcare expenditures than those without thyroid disorders ($15,182 versus $11,093, $P < 0.001$). Using OLS on logged dollars, with only the presence of thyroid disorders as the independent variable, we found that among individuals with diabetes, presence of thyroid disorders was associated with 64.4% greater total expenditures compared to those without thyroid disorders.

With respect to types of expenditures, similar patterns were observed for outpatient, prescription drug, and other expenditures with presence of thyroid disorders among individuals with diabetes. However, the percent increase associated with thyroid disorders varied from as high as 170.7% for other expenditures to as low as 18.6% for emergency room expenditures.

Table 4 summarizes the parameter estimates, standard errors and P values of parameter estimates from separate OLS regressions on logged values of total and types of expenditures among individuals with diabetes with and without thyroid disorders. We also present percent change in expenditures associated with presence of thyroid disorders (last column of Table 4). In the first model, in addition to presence/absence of thyroid disorders, we also included demographic (sex, age, and race/ethnicity). After controlling for these variables, the association between presence of between thyroid disorders and total healthcare expenditures remained significant. However, presence of thyroid disorders was associated with 43.8% greater total expenditures compared to those without thyroid disorders. When additional demographic factors (marital status, area of residence), economic factors (education, family poverty status), access to care factors (health insurance), lifestyle risk factors (smoking, physical activity), and health status factors (perceived mental and physical health) were controlled in Model 2, those with thyroid disorders had 34.3% greater total expenditures compared to those without thyroid disorders.

When cooccurring chronic conditions were entered into the model, those with thyroid disorders had 23.7%

greater total expenditures compared to those without thyroid disorders. In the final model, when macrovascular comorbid conditions were included, the association between presence of thyroid disorders and total expenditures remained highly significant (beta = 0.19 which translated to 21.4% change in expenditures, $P < .001$).

When examined by type of expenditures, however, for emergency-room-related expenditures, the presence of thyroid disorders was non-significant with the addition of chronic cooccurring conditions in Model 3. In the addition, the presence of thyroid disorders was inversely associated with emergency room expenditures with addition of macrovascular comorbid conditions in Model 4.

4. Discussion

The current paper estimated incremental healthcare expenditures associated with thyroid disorders among individuals with diabetes. Individuals with diabetes and thyroid disorders had greater healthcare expenditures compared to individuals with diabetes without thyroid disorders, even after adjusting for demographic, economic, lifestyle risk factors, health status, number of cooccurring chronic conditions, and macrovascular comorbid conditions. Our estimates can be considered as an underestimate of the true economic burden because we did not include productivity lost due to missed work days and disability days due to thyroid disorders. Our exploratory analysis suggested that employed individuals with diabetes and thyroid disorders had greater number of work-loss days compared to employed individuals without thyroid disorders and diabetes. These findings indicate that the economic burden among individuals with thyroid disorders may even be greater than suggested by our estimates.

There are plausible reasons as to why direct healthcare expenditures may be greater for those with thyroid disorders and diabetes compared to individuals with no thyroid disorders and diabetes. For example, different types of thyroid

TABLE 4: Intercept and parameter estimates for the presence of thyroid disorders from ordinary least squares regression on logged healthcare expenditures individuals with diabetes from the Medical Expenditure Panel Survey, 2007 and 2009.

Thyroid disease	Beta	SE	% Change (exp(beta) − 1)	Significance
Total				
Model 1	0.363	0.005	43.8	* * *
Model 2	0.295	0.004	34.3	* * *
Model 3	0.213	0.005	23.7	* * *
Model 4	0.194	0.006	21.4	* * *
Inpatient				
Model 1	0.389	0.02	47.6	* * *
Model 2	0.299	0.016	34.9	* * *
Model 3	0.2	0.017	22.1	* * *
Model 4	0.152	0.02	16.4	* * *
Emergency room				
Model 1	0.124	0.006	13.2	* * *
Model 2	0.089	0.007	9.3	* * *
Model 3	0.01	0.006	1.0	
Model 4	−0.02	0.005	−2.0	* * *
Outpatient				
Model 1	0.393	0.011	48.1	* * *
Model 2	0.299	0.016	34.9	* * *
Model 3	0.208	0.008	23.1	* * *
Model 4	0.196	0.009	21.7	* * *
Prescription drug				
Model 1	0.348	0.009	41.6	* * *
Model 2	0.282	0.009	32.6	* * *
Model 3	0.193	0.01	21.3	* * *
Model 4	0.179	0.01	19.6	* * *
Other				
Model 1	0.752	0.03	112.1	* * *
Model 2	0.727	0.03	106.9	* * *
Model 3	0.646	0.03	90.8	* * *
Model 4	0.630	0.03	87.8	* * *

Based on 4,490 adults with diabetes, aged 21 years or older and were alive during the calendar year 2007 and 2009. Asterisks represent significant group differences by the presence of thyroid disorders using t-tests.
Model 1, included age, gender, and race/ethnicity as independent variables. In Model 2, in addition to the variables used in Model 1, other demographic (marital status and metro status), socioeconomic (education, poverty status, and health insurance) health status (perceived physical and mental health) and lifestyle factors (body mass index categories and smoking status) were included. We controlled for number of cooccurring chronic conditions as an additional variable in Model 3., Finally, in Model 4, we also additionally entered presence of any macrovascular comorbid conditions.
$*P < .001$; $**.001 \leq P < .01$; $*.01 \leq P < .05$.

TABLE 5: CCS codes used to identify cooccurring and macrovascular comorbid conditions from the Medical Expenditure Panel Survey, 2007 and 2009.

Disease category	Clinical classification code(s)
Diabetes	49, 50
Thyroid disorders	48
Any macrovascular comorbid conditions	
Heart disease	96, 97, 100 through 108
Stroke*	342, 430, 431, 432, 434, 435, 436, 437, 438
Peripheral vascular disease	114, 248
Any cooccurring physical chronic conditions	
Arthritis	201, 202, 203, 204
Cancer	11 through 44
Chronic obstructive pulmonary disease	127
Gastro esophageal reflux disease	138
Asthma	128
Anemia*	280 thru 285
Osteoporosis*	206
Endocrine disorders	51
Any cooccurring mental health conditions	
Depression	657
Anxiety	651
Schizophrenia	659

*Indicates used on ICD-9, 3-digit codes instead of CCS codes in defining those conditions.
Details of codes and crosswalk of ICD-9 codes and CCS codes are available on html: http://meps.ahrq.gov/mepsweb/data_stats/download_data/pufs/h128/h128_icd9codes.shtml.

diseases and management of thyroid disorders (i.e., thyroidectomy or radioiodine or medical therapy) may increase the direct healthcare expenditures because these procedures can be very resource-intensive [40]. Future research needs to examine the contribution of specific procedures in thyroid management to the economic burden of individuals with thyroid disorders and diabetes.

A closer examination of factors explaining the incremental direct healthcare expenditures associated with thyroid disorders revealed that nonmodifiable risk factors such as age, gender, and race/ethnicity explained 29.7% the incremental expenditures. After adjustment of other demographic and socioeconomic characteristics, access to care, lifestyle risk factors, perceived physical health, and perceived mental health, the presence of thyroid disorders was associated with nearly one-fifth (18.7%) greater total expenditures. These findings suggest that lifestyle risk factors such as smoking, obesity, and physical activity can be modified to reduce economic burden of thyroid disorders among individuals with diabetes.

Approximately one-fifth of incremental (21.6%) expenditures were explained by cooccurring chronic conditions. This is not surprising given that three-quarters of individuals with diabetes and thyroid disorders reported cooccurring conditions such as arthritis, depression cancer, and others compared to approximately one-half individuals with diabetes without thyroid disorders. Our findings suggest high comorbidity burden among individuals with thyroid disorders and diabetes. In addition, these findings highlight the need for providers to focus on comanagement of thyroid disorders, diabetes, and other cooccurring chronic conditions to reduce the economic burden of these individuals.

In terms of types of expenditures, it is interesting to note that there was no significant association between thyroid disorders and emergency room expenditures when controlled for chronic cooccurring condition. When macrovascular comorbid conditions were additionally entered into the model, the association was negative. Individuals with thyroid disorders had 2% lower expenditures compared to those without thyroid disorders. These findings suggest that excess emergency room expenditures due to thyroid disorders may be driven by cooccurring chronic conditions macrovascular comorbid conditions. It is also well documented that emergency room visits are associated with a greater number of chronic conditions and/or macrovascular comorbid conditions [41–43].

Our study findings have implications for healthcare management strategies for individuals with diabetes. With the growing economic burden of diabetes, healthcare management needs to focus on reducing excess economic burden associated with thyroid disorders among individuals with diabetes. These steps may include early detection and treatment of thyroid disorders. However, there is no systematic approach to screening for thyroid disorders among individuals with type 2 diabetes. Although ADA suggests for screening for thyroid disease at the time of diagnosis of type 2 diabetes [44], screening practices vary widely and pragmatic guidelines are lacking [45]. Our findings highlight the need for developing guidelines in terms of frequency and target population such as women and the elderly for thyroid screening among individuals with diabetes [44]. Furthermore, future studies need to evaluate cost effectiveness of routine thyroid screening among individuals with diabetes.

Our study had many strengths and some limitation. The strengths of our study include nationally representative study of adults with diabetes, large sample size, comprehensive list of variables that can influence expenditures such as cooccurring chronic conditions, health status, and capturing health care expenditures from a variety of sources. There are some limitations also. In MEPS, data on medical conditions and utilization are self-reported and may not be accurate. However, validation of chronic conditions against provider reports suggested that households tended to be accurate for conditions that affect daily life (e.g., diabetes, sensitivity 92.1%; thyroid disorders, sensitivity 85%) [46]. It has been reported that MEPS household respondents accurately reported inpatient hospitalizations but underreport emergency room and outpatient visits. However, such underreporting did not affect behavioral analyses [47]. Severity and duration information for diabetes, thyroid disorders, surgical procedures for thyroid disorders, and other conditions was not available; these may have further narrowed the incremental expenditures associated with thyroid disorders. However, the current study controlled for perceived health status and perceived mental health status. Although steps were taken by the MEPS designers to minimize recall bias (diaries and extensive probes to enhance recall), many variables were self-reported and subject to recall bias. In addition, information of microvascular complications may provide insight nto initial economic burden associated with those conditions in individuals with thyroid disorders. Finally, as our study used a cross-sectional design, therefore, we cannot establish causality.

5. Conclusion

In conclusion, our study may be the first study to use a nationally representative survey to report that thyroid disorders were associated with higher healthcare expenditures among individuals with diabetes. Presence of cooccurring chronic conditions was one of the drivers of economic burden in these individuals. Our findings highlight the importance of comanagement of diabetes, thyroid disorders, and other chronic conditions. Future research need to focus on feasibility and cost effectiveness of routine thyroid screening among individuals with diabetes.

Disclaimer

The views expressed in this academic research paper are those of the authors and do not reflect the official policy or position of West Virginia University (WVU) or any other affiliated organizations.

Acknowledgments

The authors would also like to thank Mrs. Parul Agarwal for her support and suggestions. U. Sambamoorthi was partially supported for infrastructure from the West Virginia Collaborative Health Outcomes Research of Therapies and Services (WV CoHORTS) Center.

References

[1] "Prevalence and impact of thyroid disease," 2012, http://www.thyroid.org/thyroid-events-education-media/about-hypothyroidism/.

[2] J. J. Díez, P. Sánchez, and P. Iglesias, "Prevalence of thyroid dysfunction in patients with type 2 diabetes," *Experimental and Clinical Endocrinology and Diabetes*, vol. 119, no. 4, pp. 201–207, 2011.

[3] P. Perros, R. J. McCrimmon, G. Shaw, and B. M. Frier, "Frequency of thyroid dysfunction in diabetic patients: value of annual screening," *Diabetic Medicine*, vol. 12, no. 7, pp. 622–627, 1995.

[4] A. Papazafiropoulou, A. Sotiropoulos, A. Kokolaki, M. Kardara, P. Stamataki, and S. Pappas, "Prevalence of thyroid dysfunction among greek type 2 diabetic patients attending an outpatient clinic," *Journal of Clinical Medicine and Research*, vol. 2, no. 2, pp. 75–78, 2010.

[5] D. H. Akbar, M. M. Ahmed, and J. Al-Mughales, "Thyroid dysfunction and thyroid autoimmunity in Saudi type 2 diabetics," *Acta Diabetologica*, vol. 43, no. 1, pp. 14–18, 2006.

[6] P. Wu, "Thyroid disease and diabetes," *Clinical Diabetes*, vol. 18, pp. 38–39, 2000.

[7] G. Dimitriadis, B. Baker, H. Marsh et al., "Effect of thyroid hormone excess on action, secretion, and metabolism of insulin in humans," *The American Journal of Physiology*, vol. 248, no. 5, part 1, pp. E593–E601, 1985.

[8] G. Dimitriadis, P. Mitrou, V. Lambadiari et al., "Insulin action in adipose tissue and muscle in hypothyroidism," *Journal of Clinical Endocrinology and Metabolism*, vol. 91, no. 12, pp. 4930–4937, 2006.

[9] N. M. O'Meara, J. D. Blackman, J. Sturis, and K. S. Polonsky, "Alterations in the kinetics of C-peptide and insulin secretion in hyperthyroidism," *Journal of Clinical Endocrinology and Metabolism*, vol. 76, no. 1, pp. 79–84, 1993.

[10] F. Okajima and M. Ui, "Metabolism of glucose in hyper- and hypo-thyroid rats in vivo. Relation of catecholamine actions to thyroid activity in controlling glucose turnover," *Biochemical Journal*, vol. 182, no. 2, pp. 585–592, 1979.

[11] K. S. Leong, M. Wallymahmed, J. Wilding, and I. MacFarlane, "Clinical presentation of thyroid dysfunction and Addison's disease in young adults with type 1 diabetes," *Postgraduate Medical Journal*, vol. 75, no. 886, pp. 467–470, 1999.

[12] P. Cettour-Rose, C. Theander-Carrillo, C. Asensio et al., "Hypothyroidism in rats decreases peripheral glucose utilisation, a defect partially corrected by central leptin infusion," *Diabetologia*, vol. 48, no. 4, pp. 624–633, 2005.

[13] E. Maratou, D. J. Hadjidakis, A. Kollias et al., "Studies of insulin resistance in patients with clinical and subclinical hypothyroidism," *European Journal of Endocrinology*, vol. 160, no. 5, pp. 785–790, 2009.

[14] R. J. Levin and D. H. Smyth, "The effect of the thyroid gland on intestinal absorption of hexoses," *The Journal of physiology*, vol. 169, pp. 755–769, 1963.

[15] A. J. Matty and B. Seshadri, "Effect of thyroxine on the isolated rat intestine," *Gut*, vol. 6, pp. 200–202, 1965.

[16] H. F. Kemp, H. S. Hundal, and P. M. Taylor, "Glucose transport correlates with GLUT2 abundance in rat liver during altered thyroid status," *Molecular and Cellular Endocrinology*, vol. 128, no. 1-2, pp. 97–102, 1997.

[17] T. Mokuno, K. Uchimura, R. Hayashi et al., "Glucose transporter 2 concentrations in hyper- and hypothyroid rat livers," *Journal of Endocrinology*, vol. 160, no. 2, pp. 285–289, 1999.

[18] M. Vaughan, "An in vitro effect of triiodothyronine on rat adipose tissue," *Journal of Clinical Investigation*, vol. 46, no. 9, pp. 1482–1491, 1967.

[19] H. S. Chen, T. E. J. Wu, T. S. Jap et al., "Subclinical hypothyroidism is a risk factor for nephropathy and cardiovascular diseases in Type 2 diabetic patients," *Diabetic Medicine*, vol. 24, no. 12, pp. 1336–1344, 2007.

[20] M. A. Singer, "Of mice and men and elephants: metabolic rate sets glomerular filtration rate," *American Journal of Kidney Diseases*, vol. 37, no. 1, pp. 164–178, 2001.

[21] J. G. Den Hollander, R. W. Wulkan, M. J. Mantel, and A. Berghout, "Correlation between severity of thyroid dysfunction and renal function," *Clinical Endocrinology*, vol. 62, no. 4, pp. 423–427, 2005.

[22] G. R. Yang, J. K. Yang, L. Zhang, Y. H. An, and J. K. Lu, "Association between subclinical hypothyroidism and proliferative diabetic retinopathy in type 2 diabetic patients: a case-control study," *Tohoku Journal of Experimental Medicine*, vol. 222, no. 4, pp. 303–310, 2010.

[23] T.-H. Collet, J. Gussekloo, D. C. Bauer et al., "Subclinical hyperthyroidism and the risk of coronary heart disease and mortality," *Archives of Internal Medicine*, vol. 172, no. 10, pp. 799–809, 2012.

[24] R. Bunevičius and A. J. Prange, "Thyroid disease and mental disorders: cause and effect or only comorbidity?" *Current Opinion in Psychiatry*, vol. 23, no. 4, pp. 363–368, 2010.

[25] L. T. Dilas, T. Icin, J. N. Paro, and I. Bajkin, "Autoimmune thyroid disease and other non-endocrine autoimmune diseases," *Medicinski Pregled*, vol. 64, pp. 3183–3147, 2011.

[26] T. C. Robazzi and F. F. Adan, "Autoimmune thyroid disease in patients with rheumatic diseases," *Revista Brasileira de Reumatologia*, vol. 52, no. 3, pp. 423–430, 2012.

[27] M. D. Williams, R. Harris, C. M. Dayan, J. Evans, J. Gallacher, and Y. Ben-Shlomo, "Thyroid function and the natural history of depression: findings from the Caerphilly Prospective Study (CaPS) and a meta-analysis," *Clinical Endocrinology*, vol. 70, no. 3, pp. 484–492, 2009.

[28] P. Mitrou, S. A. Raptis, and G. Dimitriadis, "Thyroid disease in older people," *Maturitas*, vol. 70, no. 1, pp. 5–9, 2011.

[29] T. P. Gilmer, P. J. O'Connor, W. A. Rush et al., "Predictors of health care costs in adults with diabetes," *Diabetes Care*, vol. 28, no. 1, pp. 59–64, 2005.

[30] J. G. Trogdon and T. Hylands, "Nationally representative medical costs of diabetes by time since diagnosis," *Diabetes Care*, vol. 31, no. 12, pp. 2307–2311, 2008.

[31] A. Z. Fu, Y. Qiu, L. Radican, and B. J. Wells, "Health care and productivity costs associated with diabetic patients with macrovascular comorbid conditions," *Diabetes Care*, vol. 32, no. 12, pp. 2187–2192, 2009.

[32] Agency for Healthcare Research and Quality, "The medical expenditure panel survey: household component full year files, MEPS HC-129 2009 full year consolidated data file," 2012, http://meps.ahrq.gov/mepsweb/data_stats/download_data/pufs/h129/h129doc.pdf.

[33] Agency for Healthcare Research and Quality, "The medical expenditure panel survey: MEPS HC-123: 2009 full year population characteristics," 2012, http://meps.ahrq.gov/mepsweb/data_stats/download_data/pufs/h123/h123doc.pdf.

[34] "Bureau of labor statistics: consumer price index," 2012, http://www.bls.gov/cpi/#tables.

[35] Medical Expenditure Panel Survey, "use and expenditures related to thyroid disease among women age 18 and older, U.S. noninstitutionalized population," Statistical Report no. 348, 2008, http://meps.ahrq.gov/mepsweb/data_files/publications/st348/stat348.pdf.

[36] J. L. Rosenzweig, K. Weinger, L. Poirier-Solomon, and M. Rushton, "Use of a disease severity index for evaluation of healthcare costs and management of comorbidities of patients with diabetes mellitus," *American Journal of Managed Care*, vol. 8, no. 11, pp. 950–958, 2002.

[37] E. N. Pearce, "In people with subclinical hypothyroidism, TSH level >10 mIU/l may predict increased risk of coronary heart disease and related mortality," *Evidence-Based Medicine*, vol. 16, no. 1, pp. 31–32, 2011.

[38] American Diabetes Association, "Economic costs of diabetes in the U.S. in 2007," *Diabetes Care*, vol. 31, no. 3, pp. 596–615.

[39] R. Halvorsen and R. Palmquist, "The interpretation of dummy variables in semilogarithmic equations," *American Economic Review*, vol. 70, no. 3, pp. 474–475, 1980.

[40] K. Zanocco, M. Heller, D. Elaraj, and C. Sturgeon, "Is subtotal thyroidectomy a cost-effective treatment for Graves disease? A cost-effectiveness analysis of the medical and surgical treatment options," *Surgery*, vol. 152, no. 2, pp. 164–172, 2012.

[41] "Hospital stays for patients with diabetes, 2008," 2012, http://www.hcup-us.ahrq.gov/reports/statbriefs/sb93.pdf.

[42] V. C. Woo, M. Carter, M. Bialy, and J. Rehman, "Emergency room visits: comparison of individuals with type 1

and type 2 diabetes," 2012, http://professional.diabetes.org/Abstracts_Display.aspx?TYP=1&CID=55894.

[43] L. E. Egede, "Patterns and correlates of emergency department use by individuals with diabetes," *Diabetes Care*, vol. 27, no. 7, pp. 1748–1750, 2004.

[44] American Diabetes Association, "Standards of medical care in diabetes—2012," *Diabetes Care*, vol. 35, supplement 1, pp. S11–S63, 2012.

[45] R. Kadiyala, R. Peter, and O. E. Okosieme, "Thyroid dysfunction in patients with diabetes: clinical implications and screening strategies," *International Journal of Clinical Practice*, vol. 64, no. 8, pp. 1130–1139, 2010.

[46] S. MacHlin, J. Cohen, A. Elixhauser, K. Beauregard, and C. Steiner, "Sensitivity of household reported medical conditions in the medical expenditure panel survey," *Medical Care*, vol. 47, no. 6, pp. 618–625, 2009.

[47] S. H. Zuvekas and G. L. Olin, "Validating household reports of health care use in the medical expenditure panel survey," *Health Services Research*, vol. 44, no. 5, pp. 1679–1700, 2009.

6

Maternal Thyroid Function during the Second Half of Pregnancy and Child Neurodevelopment at 6, 12, 24, and 60 Months of Age

Jonathan Chevrier, Kim G. Harley, Katherine Kogut, Nina Holland, Caroline Johnson, and Brenda Eskenazi

Center for Environmental Research and Children's Health (CERCH), School of Public Health, University of California, Berkeley, CA 94704-7392, USA

Correspondence should be addressed to Jonathan Chevrier, chevrier@berkeley.edu

Academic Editor: Joanne Rovet

Although evidence suggests that maternal hypothyroidism and mild hypothyroxinemia during the first half of pregnancy alters fetal neurodevelopment among euthyroid offspring, little data are available from later in gestation. In this study, we measured free T4 using direct equilibrium dialysis, as well as total T4 and TSH in 287 pregnant women at 27 weeks' gestation. We also assessed cognition, memory, language, motor functioning, and behavior in their children at 6, 12, 24, and 60 months of age. Increasing maternal TSH was related to better performance on tests of cognition and language at 12 months but not at later ages. At 60 months, there was inconsistent evidence that higher TSH was related to improved attention. We found no convincing evidence that maternal TH during the second half of pregnancy was related to impaired child neurodevelopment.

1. Introduction

The profound deleterious neurodevelopmental effect of maternal and fetal hypothyroidism caused by iodine deficiency has been recognized for more than a century [1]. More recent evidence from experimental and observational studies suggests that even among euthyroid offspring, maternal hypothyroidism and hypothyroxinemia (low thyroxine (T4) with normal thyroid-stimulating hormone (TSH) levels) during early pregnancy may be associated with impaired brain development. Man and colleagues, for instance, reported associations between maternal hypothyroxinemia in early pregnancy and lower scores on neurodevelopmental scales at 8 months, 4 years, and 7 years of age [2–4]. A more recent study by Haddow et al. found reduced scores on tests of intelligence, attention, and visual-motor performance at 8 years of age among children of 48 mothers with untreated clinical hypothyroidism (defined as TSH levels >99.7th percentile or TSH between the 98th and the 99.6th percentile and total T4 < 7.75 μg/dL) at the 17th week of gestation

relative to 124 controls [5]. A Chinese study ($n = 1,268$) also found that children of 19 women with hypothyroxinemia (defined as total T4 below the reference range but normal TSH and free T4) and 18 women with subclinical hypothyroidism (high TSH and normal free and total T4) in the first half of pregnancy scored 7.6–10.0 point lower than controls on the mental (MDI) and psychomotor (PDI) development indices of the Bayley Scales of Infant Development [6].

Studies have reported reduced scores on cognitive, motor, and language scales even among children of mothers with mild hypothyroxinemia. For instance, in a large population-based cohort study conducted in The Netherlands ($n = 3,659$), Henrichs et al. found 80% increased odds of expressive language delays at 18 and 30 months of age among children whose mother had free T4 levels <10th percentile at 13 weeks' gestation [7]. Pop and colleagues also reported lower scores on the orientation cluster of the Neonatal Behavioral Assessment Scale three weeks after birth ($n = 204$) [8] and a 7.4 point decrease on the PDI at 10 months of age ($n = 220$) [9] in children of mothers with lower free T4 at 12 weeks' gestation. They also found 8–10 point reductions on the MDI and the PDI at 12 and 24 months of age in children of 57 mothers with low-normal free T4 relative to 50 controls [10]. The one study to contradict the above findings did not measure free T4 [11]. Thus, the bulk of the literature points to an association between adverse neurodevelopmental outcomes in offspring and maternal hypothyroidism, hypothroxinemia, and low-normal free T4 levels during the first half of pregnancy.

Evidence suggests that TH of maternal origin may also play a role in fetal development later in pregnancy. This hypothesis was supported by early studies which demonstrated that transfer of radiolabeled T4 and T3 through the placenta continues to occur after the onset of fetal thyroid function [12]. Maternal T4 appears to reach the fetus in significant amounts up until birth, as evidenced by a study conducted by Vulsma et al. [13]. In that study, T4 was detected in the cord blood of 25 neonates with a complete iodide organification defect, a genetic condition that prevents the iodination of tyrosine and therefore inhibits T4 synthesis. T4 measured in cord blood reached concentrations equivalent to 30–60% of the mean values found in full-term fetuses without this condition [14]. Given that a substantial proportion of thyroid hormone reaching the fetus is of maternal origin in the latter part of gestation, it is conceivable that maternal thyroid hormone may continue to affect fetal neurodevelopment during this period. To date, only the studies by Pop and colleagues examined this question in humans and found no relationship between low-normal maternal free T4 (<10th percentile) measured at 24 and 32 weeks' gestation and child neurodevelopment [8–10]. To our knowledge, these results have not been replicated by other groups.

Most studies investigating the association of maternal thyroid function during pregnancy and child cognitive development have focused on hypothyroidism/hypothyroxinemia, perhaps because this condition is more common than hyperthyroidism. Maternal hyperthyroidism is nevertheless a significant condition that affects 0.05–0.2% of pregnancies in the form of Graves' disease; an additional 2-3% of pregnant women are also believed to experience gestational transient thyrotoxicosis [15]. In rats, fetal/neonatal hyperthyroidism causes decreased brain and cerebellar weight as well as abnormal brain development, including an acceleration of neuronal differentiation, a delay in glial cell differentiation and early termination of cell proliferation, resulting in a smaller number of granular and basket cells [16]. In humans, maternal hyperthyroidism during pregnancy has been linked to preeclampsia, fetal loss, premature births, growth restriction, and low birth weight [17–21]. Subclinical hyperthyroidism (defined as TSH values below the reference range with normal free T4 levels [22]), on the other hand, was not found to be associated with low birth weight, major malformations, or fetal, neonatal, or perinatal mortality in infants of 433 women with TSH levels ≤2.5th percentile and normal free T4 (≤1.75 ng/dL) relative to 23,124 women with normal TSH levels [23]. However, we are aware of no studies that investigated associations between

high-normal T4 or subclinical hyperthyroidism and neurodevelopment.

The current study thus aims to examine whether maternal TH levels in the second half of pregnancy are associated with child neurodevelopment at 6, 12, 24, and 60 months of age. Prior studies used immunoassays to determine free T4 levels, but these measurements are influenced by T4-bound protein concentrations which increase during pregnancy [24]. In the present study, we used direct equilibrium dialysis to measure free T4 [25], a method that yields valid results in samples with normal or elevated T4-bound protein levels [26].

2. Methods

2.1. Participants. Pregnant women were recruited through the Center for the Health Assessment of Mothers and Children of Salinas (CHAMACOS), a birth cohort study of primarily Latino children born in the Salinas Valley, California. Women were eligible for inclusion in the study if they were ≥18 years old, had completed <20 weeks' gestation, spoke English or Spanish, were Medi-Cal eligible (state-sponsored health care for low-income families), were planning to deliver at the Monterey county hospital (Natividad Medical Center), and received prenatal care in this hospital or at one of five clinics of Clinica de Salud del Valle de Salinas. Screening and enrollment occurred between October 1999 and October 2000. We obtained informed consent from the 601 women who agreed to participate. Out of the 526 singleton live births (there were 20 miscarriages, 3 stillbirths, 2 neonatal deaths, 5 twin births, and 45 women were lost to follow-up), we excluded children with conditions that may impact scores on neurodevelopmental tests such as hydrocephaly ($n = 1$), autism ($n = 1$), and a history of seizures ($n = 7$). Children whose neurodevelopment was never assessed ($n = 139$) or whose mother's banked serum volume was insufficient for TH analysis ($n = 91$) were also excluded, leaving a final sample of 287 mother-child pairs. A total of 271 children were included at 6 months, 258 at 12 months, 240 at 24 months, and 207 at 60 months of age.

Women who were excluded or who dropped out at one or more time-point were more likely to be employed, to have been born in the US, to be depressed, and had lived longer in the US compared to those who were included in analyses. Excluded children were more likely to be firstborns and to have had lower birth weights compared to those who were included in the analyses. This study was approved by the University of California, Berkeley Committee for the Protection of Human Subjects.

2.2. Interviews. Women were interviewed in English or Spanish by bilingual, bicultural staff during pregnancy (at 13 and 27 weeks' gestation on average), at delivery, and when their children were 6, 12, 24, and 60 months of age. We obtained information about sociodemographic and lifestyle characteristics at each interview, including smoking, alcohol consumption, drug use, and diet during pregnancy; and on childcare, breastfeeding, number of children in the home, and housing density (number of people per room) after birth. The Peabody Picture Vocabulary Test (PPVT; at the 6 month visit) [27] and the Center for Epidemiologic Studies Depression Scale (CES-D; at the 12 month visits) [28] were also administered to mothers. In addition, the Infant-Toddler Home Observation for Measurement of the Environment (HOME) [29] was completed at 6 and 12 months; some subscales of the HOME were completed at 24 months. We also administered the Kotelchuck Adequacy of Prenatal Care Utilization Index [30], the Duke-UNC Functional Social Support Questionnaire [31], and the Diet Quality Index proposed by Bodnar and Siega-Riz [32] and modified by Harley and Eskenazi [33]. Mothers' (during pregnancy) and children's (up to age 24 months) medical records were abstracted by a registered nurse. We obtained data on delivery complications including vacuum extraction, placental abruption, amnionitis, and hemorrhage, or other bleeding; and on neonatal TSH levels (see below).

2.3. Neurodevelopmental Evaluations. Children were evaluated at the ages of 6, 12, 24, and 60 months. We selected for analyses those tests that assessed the same constructs examined in previous studies of maternal thyroid hormone and child neurodevelopment [2–7, 9–11]. Children were assessed at 6, 12, and 24 months of age on the Mental Development Index (MDI) and Psychomotor Development Index (PDI) of the Bayley Scales of Infant Development-Second Edition [34], and at 6 and 12 months on the auditory and expressive comprehension subscales of the Preschool Language Scale (PLS). At 60 months of age, the Performance Intellectual Quotient (IQ) was evaluated using the Wechsler Preschool and Primary Scale of Intelligence 3rd edition (WPPSI-III) [35]. We also administered the Vocabulary subtest of the WPPSI-III. Motor and language development, memory, attention, and school readiness were assessed using the McCarthy Scales of Children's Abilities (Digit Span Forward and Backward, Words and Sentences, Draw-a-Child, and Gross Motor Leg and Arm) [36], the Woodcock-Johnson Test of Cognitive Ability (Letter-Word and Applied Problems) and its Spanish-validated version (the Woodcock-Muñoz Test [37, 38]), the Pegboard subtest of the Wide Range Assessment of Visual-Motor Abilities (WRAVMA) for both dominant and non-dominant hands [39], the Conner's Kiddie Continuous Performance Test (KCPT) [40], and the PPVT [27]. The mother was queried about her child's behavior using the Child Behavior Checklist (CBCL). The Bayley Scales, the WPPSI performance IQ, the WRAVMA, the Woodcock-Johnson/Muñoz test, and the PPVT are age-standardized to a mean of 100 and a standard deviation of 15. Standardized scores on the McCarthy Scales are only available for full subscales but not for individual subtests. Raw scores were thus used for gross motor subtests. Scores on other McCarthy subtests were determined by subtracting children's chronological age from their developmental age (in months), as determined using methods published by Kaufman and Kaufman [41]. Positive scores show accelerated development while negative scores represent a delay. Finally, raw scores were used for the CBCL following recommendations from the test manual [42].

Neurodevelopmental evaluations were conducted in Spanish and/or English by psychometricians blind to mothers' TH levels in the study office or in a recreational vehicle (RV) modified for this purpose. Psychometricians were trained and supervised by a child neuropsychologist (CJ) and were videotaped and evaluated on a regular basis to ensure consistency across psychometricians and over time. All tests were reviewed by graduate students trained by the child neuropsychologist to ensure accurate scoring.

2.4. Thyroid Hormone Measurements. We measured TSH, free T4 and total T4 in serum collected by venipuncture from pregnant women at the time of the second interview (Mean ± SD = 26.9 ± 3.4 weeks' gestation). Samples were processed immediately at Natividad Medical Center and stored at −80°C at the UC Berkeley School of Public Health Biorepository until shipment to Quest Diagnostic's Nichols Institute (San Juan Capistrano, CA) where they were analyzed on a Bayer ADVIA Centaur system (Siemens Healthcare Diagnostics, Deerfield, IL). A pilot experiment revealed that every freeze-thaw cycle was associated with a 0.1 ng/dL increase in free T4 levels ($P < 0.001$); this variable accounted for 33% of the variance (unpublished results). Samples were thus thawed only once for aliquoting, shipped refrigerated, and analyzed within 48 hours. TSH was measured by ultrasensitive third generation immunochemiluminometric assay (ICMA; functional sensitivity (FS): 0.01 mIU/L, intra-assay coefficients of variation (CV) = 2.3–6.0%); total T4 was determined by solid-phase ICMA (FS: 0.1 μg/dL, CV: 4.5–5.7%); free T4 was analyzed by direct equilibrium dialysis (ED) followed by radioimmunoassay (RIA; FS: 0.1 ng/dL, CV: 2.4–6.2%) [25]. Serum protein-bound T4 levels usually increase during pregnancy [15], which may bias results obtained by immunoassays not preceded by ED [24]. ED uses a semipermeable membrane to physically separate the bound hormone from the free portion, which is then measured using a highly sensitive RIA. This method measures free T4 accurately in samples with normal or elevated protein-bound T4 levels [26]. Previous studies used butanol-extractable iodine [2–4], which estimates T4 levels by measuring protein-bound iodine [43] or immunoassays [5–10]. Trimester-specific reference ranges for TH levels were provided by the analytical laboratory. Neonatal TSH was also measured in dried blood spots by the Genetics Disease Branch of the California Department of Health Services as part of the State's Newborn Screening Program. Hospital staff collected blood spots by heel stick on average 24.8 hours after birth (SD = 15.5); samples were analyzed by solid-phase, time-resolved sandwich fluoroimmunoassay (AutoDELPHIA; PerkinElmer, Wellesley, MA).

2.5. Statistical Analyses. Multiple linear regression models were used to evaluate associations between TH and neurodevelopmental outcomes. Models were first run with TH expressed continuously. We also ran models with TSH categorized as low ($n = 43$) versus normal based on trimester-specific reference ranges provided by the analytical laboratory. There were however not enough women with high

Table 1: Demographic characteristics of study participants ($n = 287$).

	No. (%)
Mothers	
Age (years)	
18–24	130 (45.3)
25–29	95 (33.1)
30–34	42 (14.6)
35–45	20 (7.0)
Race/Ethnicity	
White	5 (1.7)
Latino	278 (96.9)
Other	4 (1.4)
Education	
≤6th grade	121 (42.2)
7–12th grade	105 (36.6)
≥High School	61 (21.3)
Income (% poverty)	
<100	171 (59.6)
100–200	105 (36.6)
>200	11 (3.8)
Country of birth	
United States	32 (11.1)
Mexico	251 (87.5)
Other	4 (1.4)
Time in the USA (years)	
≤5	156 (54.4)
6–10	69 (24.0)
≥11	62 (21.6)
Parity	
0	91 (31.7)
≥1	196 (68.3)
Smoking during pregnancy	
No	271 (94.4)
Yes	16 (5.6)
Alcohol during pregnancy (≥one serving)	
No	282 (98.3)
Yes	5 (1.7)
Children	
Sex	
Boy	140 (48.8)
Girl	147 (51.2)
Birthweight (g)	
<2500 g	10 (3.5)
2500–3500 g	149 (51.9)
>3500 g	128 (44.6)
Gestational duration (weeks)	
<37	21 (7.3)
37–42	266 (92.7)
>42	0 (0.0)

TSH or with other TH measurements outside of the reference range to conduct such analyses. Therefore, to obtain sufficient sample size and to replicate methods used in prior studies [7–10], we dichotomized TH at the 10th and the 90th percentile based on distributions in our sample and at 0.8 ng/dL. Neurodevelopmental scores were expressed continuously. We used generalized additive models with a 3-degrees-of-freedom cubic spline function to evaluate the shape of the relationship between continuously expressed TH and scores on neurodevelopmental assessments and to test for linearity [44]. Since altered neurodevelopment was hypothesized to occur at both ends of the distribution of TH values (i.e., following an inverse U-shaped association), scores with P values for digression from linearity <0.10 were fit using a quadratic term while scores with a P value ≥0.10 were fit linearly in multiple regression models. Conclusions were similar when using quadratic or linear terms. We therefore only present results using linear terms.

We removed outliers as identified by the Generalized Extreme Studentized Deviates Many-Outlier procedure at an $\alpha = 0.01$ [45]. Covariates considered for inclusion in models were identified based on prior reports suggesting that they influenced neurodevelopment (see Appendix A for a complete list). They included (categorized as shown in Table 1 or as indicated below): maternal age at enrollment (continuously), race, education, income, parity (continuously), depression (yes versus no), maternal PPVT score (continuously), Diet Quality Index (continuously), Kotelchuck Adequacy of Prenatal Care Utilization Index (adequate plus, adequate, inadequate), Composite Social Support Index (continuously), employment status at the time of and prior to assessments (yes versus no), smoking (yes versus no), alcohol (yes versus no) and illegal drug (yes versus no) consumption during pregnancy, delivery type (natural versus cesarean section), pregnancy complications (any versus none), infant sex, premature birth (yes versus no), months of breastfeeding (continuously), HOME score at the time of and prior to assessments, and psychometrician administering assessments.

To ensure that neurodevelopment was not affected by neonatal hypothyroidism, we also considered neonatal TSH levels as a covariate. In addition, we considered the potential confounding effect of some known neurotoxicants. Lead was measured in maternal and cord blood samples using graphite furnace atomic absorption spectrophotometry. As exposure to organophosphate insecticides has been associated with altered neurodevelopment in this cohort of farmworker families [46, 47], this variable was also considered. Organophosphate insecticide exposure was assessed by measuring dialkyl phosphate metabolites in maternal urine collected at approximately 13 and 26 weeks' gestation by highresolution gas chromatography-tandem mass spectrometry (HRGC/MS-MS) with isotope dilution quantification [48]. Measurements at the two time points were averaged and log10-transformed. For each time point, covariates were included in final models if they were associated with any of the TH measurements at $P < 0.10$ based on analysis of variance (ANOVA) or Pearson's correlations.

In order to control for potential selection bias due to exclusion from analyses and/or loss to followup, we ran all models with and without weights determined as the inverse

TABLE 2: Mean scores on neurodevelopmental scales at 6, 12, and 24 months of age.

| | 6 Months | | 12 Months | | 24 Months | |
	N	Mean (SD)	N	Mean (SD)	N	Mean (SD)
Bayley						
Mental development index	271	95.0 (7.9)	258	101.3 (9.1)	240	86.4 (11.7)
Psychomotor development index	271	96.2 (11.1)	257	107.0 (12.8)	240	98.2 (10.4)
Preschool language scale						
Auditory comprehension	270	104.6 (12.9)	257	99.1 (12.9)		
Expressive comprehension	270	91.1 (13.5)	257	94.5 (13.8)		
Total score	270	97.7 (11.3)	257	96.6 (13.5)		

TABLE 3: Mean scores on neurodevelopmental scales at 5 years of age.

	N	Mean (SD)
Intelligence		
WPPSI[1]		
Performance IQ	207	94.7 (14.7)
Motor		
WRAVMA[2]		
Pegboard-Dominant	205	110.7 (17.4)
Pegboard-Nondominant	204	110.3 (17.2)
McCarthy		
Draw-a-Child	206	3.9 (16.1)
Gross Motor-Leg	194	11.0 (2.2)
Gross Motor-Arm	202	4.1 (2.4)
Language Development		
WPPSI[1] Vocabulary	207	8.8 (2.6)
PPVT[3]	205	94.8 (17.5)
Memory		
McCarthy		
Words and Sentences	205	−4.5 (16.6)
Digit Span Forward	204	−15.2 (13.0)
Digit Span Backward	199	−15.3 (10.6)
School Readiness		
Woodcock-Johnson/Muñoz		
Letter-Word	199	92.4 (12.1)
Applied Problems	206	87.0 (15.8)
Attention		
CBCL[4]		
ADHD[5]	200	4.7 (2.8)
KCPT[6]		
ADHD Confidence Index[5]	188	45.7 (17.5)

[1] Weschler Preschool and Primary Scale of Intelligence.
[2] Wide Range Assessment of Visual Motor Ability.
[3] Peabody Picture Vocabulary Test.
[4] Child Behavior Checklist.
[5] Attention Deficit Hyperactivity Disorder.
[6] Kiddie Continuous Performance Test.
Note: We report differences between chronological and developmental ages for the McCarthy Draw-a-Child, Words and Sentences, and Digit Span Forward and Backward subtests (in months). Raw scores are reported for the gross motor tasks of the McCarthy scales (no developmental ages are available for these subtests) and for the CBCL as recommended by the test manual [42]. Standardized scores are used for other tests.

probability of inclusion in our samples at each time-point [49]. Probability of inclusion was determined based on

multiple logistic regression models using covariates listed in the Statistical Analyses section as potential predictors. Model selection was performed using a Deletion-Substitution-Addition (DSA) algorithm, which finds the combination of variables (including interactions and polynomials) that minimizes cross-validated risk [50]. Results were similar with and without this adjustment; we present results without the adjustment. Missing covariates were imputed. In addition, two free T4 and two TSH values below the limit of detection (LOD) (0.1 ng/dL and 0.01 mIU/L, resp.) were imputed as half the LOD. Statistical significance was defined as $P < 0.05$ on two-tailed tests. TSH values were $\log_2$-transformed for all statistical analyses. Analyses were performed using Intercooled STATA, version 10.0 (StataCorp, College Station, TX) and R, version 2.6.1 (R Foundation for Statistical Computing, Vienna, Austria).

3. Results

Mothers were mostly low-income, Mexican-born, Spanish-speaking Latinas with a low level of education, and many were recent immigrants to the United States (Table 1). A large proportion of women (73.7%) lived in farmworker families. During pregnancy, smoking was rare in this population (5.2%), and only 2.6% of women had ≥1 serving of alcohol per week. Mothers' mean PPVT score was 88.0 (SD = 21.2).

Mean free and total T4 levels were 0.8 ng/dL (SD = 0.2) and 10.5 μg/dL (SD = 1.5), respectively; the geometric mean for TSH was 1.2 mIU/L (GSD = 1.7). Nine (2.7%) women had low free T4 (<0.5 ng/dL) and 13 (3.9%) had low total T4 (<8.0 μg/dL) levels. None of the women were hypothyroidic based on the reference range for TSH provided by the analytical laboratory (TSH > 5.2 mIU/L), but 16 were hypothyroidic using the criteria proposed by the National Academy of Clinical Biochemistry (TSH > 2.5 mIU/L) [51, 52]. Five women had high free T4 (>1.6 ng/dL), none had elevated total T4 (>17.8 and >20.1 μg/dL in the second and third trimesters, resp.), and 43 had low TSH (<0.5 and <0.8 mIU/L in the second and third trimesters, resp.). All children had normal TSH levels at birth (<25 mIU/L).

Scores on neurodevelopmental scales when children were aged 6, 12, 24, and 60 months are shown in Tables 2 and 3. Except for a low MDI score at 24 months (mean = 86.1; SD = 12.0), Bayley and PLS scores were close to the expected mean (i.e., 100) at all time points. At 60 months of age, children performed well on fine motor tests but scored relatively low

TABLE 4: Associations between maternal thyroid hormone levels during pregnancy (27 weeks' gestation) and child neurodevelopment at 6, 12 and 24 months of age.

			Bayley scales		Preschool language scale		
			Mental development index	Psychomotor development index	Auditory comprehension	Expressive comprehension	Total score
6 Months[1]	Free T4	β	−3.14	−3.27	−2.03	1.65	−0.10
		(95% CI)	(−7.65, 1.36)	(−9.36, 2.82)	(−9.80, 5.75)	(−5.48, 8.79)	(−6.45, 6.25)
	Total T4	β	0.03	−0.06	−0.24	0.58	0.19
		(95% CI)	(−0.57, 0.62)	(−0.86, 0.74)	(−1.28, 0.80)	(−0.37, 1.53)	(−0.66, 1.05)
	TSH	β	0.85	1.46	1.51	0.24	1.06
		(95% CI)	(−0.49, 2.18)	(−0.33, 3.26)	(−0.81, 3.84)	(−1.91, 2.38)	(−0.87, 2.98)
12 Months[2]	Free T4	β	−0.48	−6.40	4.39	1.26	3.45
		(95% CI)	(−6.22, 5.26)	(−13.89, 1.08)	(−3.56, 12.34)	(−7.20, 9.72)	(−4.76, 11.67)
	Total T4	β	−0.12	−0.45	0.33	−0.15	0.12
		(95% CI)	(−0.92, 0.68)	(−1.53, 0.63)	(−0.79, 1.46)	(−1.34, 1.04)	(−1.05, 1.28)
	TSH	β	1.71	0.10	2.92	0.46	1.91
		(95% CI)	(0.05, 3.37)*	(−2.16, 2.35)	(0.59, 5.25)*	(−2.04, 2.95)	(−0.51, 4.33)
24 Months[3]	Free T4	β	−4.29	−2.67			
		(95% CI)	(−11.60, 3.02)	(−8.95, 3.62)			
	Total T4	β	−0.17	0.43			
		(95% CI)	(−1.20, 0.85)	(−0.43, 1.30)			
	TSH	β	0.33	−1.31			
		(95% CI)	(−1.97, 2.63)	(−3.25, 0.63)			

*$P < 0.05$.

[1] Models adjusted for maternal age, employment status at enrollment and at the 6-months visit, country of birth, time lived in the US, Diet Quality Index, blood lead levels and delivery complications; child hospitalization before 6 months, season of assessment and psychometrician.

[2] Models adjusted for maternal age, employment status at enrollment and at the 6 months visit, country of birth, time lived in the US, Diet Quality Index, Kotelchuck Adequacy of Prenatal Care Utilization Index, blood lead levels, delivery complications and PPVT score; child age, preterm birth, hospitalization at 6 months and 1 year, family structure at 1 year; season, and language spoken at the time of assessment.

[3] Models adjusted for maternal age, income, employment status at enrollment, 6 months and 1 year, country of birth, Diet Quality Index, Kotelchuck Adequacy of Prenatal Care Utilization Index, blood lead levels, delivery complications, PPVT score; child hospitalization at 1 year; number of children in the home at 6 months, home density at 2 years, family structure at 1 year; season, psychometrician and language of assessment.

[4] Since TSH was expressed on a $\log_2$ basis, β are equal to the change in neurodevelopmental outcomes for a doubling in TSH levels.

on cognitive (verbal and nonverbal), language, and memory tests.

Table 4 shows associations between maternal thyroid hormone levels and child scores on the Bayley and Preschool Language scales at 6, 12, and 24 months of age. Associations between maternal free T4 and scores on the Bayley scales were consistently negative but none were statistically significant either in unadjusted (results not shown) or adjusted models. Associations between Bayley scores and total T4 were also generally negative but not statistically significant. Increasing maternal TSH was related to better performance on the Bayley MDI and on the auditory comprehension subscale of the PLS at 12 months but maternal thyroid hormone was not related to these constructs at later points. Maternal free and total T4 levels were not significantly associated with scores on the PLS.

Maternal free T4, total T4, and TSH were not associated with performance on any tests of neurodevelopment in 60-month-old children (Table 5) with one exception: every doubling in TSH levels was associated with a 0.65 point decrease (95%CI = −1.26, −0.04) on the Attention Deficit Hyperactivity Disorder (ADHD) subscale of the CBCL, although

there was no significant association between maternal TH levels and CBCL Attention Problems and Pervasive Developmental Problems scales nor on child's performance on the KCPT (results not shown). Categorizing each measure of TH at the 10th or 90th percentiles yielded no significant association; subclinical hyperthyroidism was also not related with outcomes.

4. Discussion

We found little evidence that TH levels measured around the 27th week of gestation in mothers of euthyroid infants living in an iodine-sufficient area [53] were associated with child neurodevelopment. Although increasing maternal TSH levels were associated with better performance on the Bayley MDI at 12 months, these results did not persist at 24 months. Similarly, a reduction in ADHD symptoms, as reported by mothers in 60-month-old children, was not supported by other measures of hyperactivity and/or inattention at this age (i.e., maternal report on the Attention Problems scale of the CBCL or child performance on the KCPT). Better Auditory

TABLE 5: Associations between maternal thyroid hormone levels during pregnancy (27 weeks' gestation) and child neurodevelopment at 5 years of age.[1]

	Free T4		Total T4		TSH[2]	
	β	(95% CI)	β	(95% CI)	β	(95% CI)
Performance IQ						
WPPSI[3]	−4.12	(−13.73, 5.49)	0.03	(−1.35, 1.41)	−2.26	(−5.27, 0.74)
Motor Development						
WRAVMA[4]						
Pegboard-Dominant	−3.76	(−15.45, 7.93)	−0.97	(−2.64, 0.70)	0.51	(−3.12, 4.15)
Pegboard-Nondominant	−4.21	(−16.03, 7.61)	−1.55	(−3.23, 0.13)	0.02	(−3.65, 3.68)
McCarthy						
Draw-a-Child	−5.98	(−16.74, 4.77)	0.10	(−1.44, 1.63)	0.06	(−3.27, 3.39)
Gross Motor-Leg	−0.14	(−1.60, 1.32)	0.00	(−0.22, 0.22)	0.16	(−0.31, 0.63)
Gross Motor-Arm	0.08	(−1.51, 1.66)	−0.04	(−0.27, 0.19)	0.04	(−0.45, 0.53)
Language Development						
WPPSI[3] Vocabulary	−0.21	(−1.98, 1.57)	−0.22	(−0.47, 0.03)	−0.37	(−0.92, 0.19)
PPVT[5]	−2.71	(−14.18, 8.77)	−0.89	(−2.54, 0.76)	−1.05	(−4.66, 2.57)
Memory						
McCarthy						
Words and Sentences	0.10	(−11.32, 11.52)	−0.55	(−2.17, 1.07)	−1.44	(−4.97, 2.09)
Digit Span Forward	4.06	(−4.72, 12.83)	0.77	(−0.46, 2.00)	−1.83	(−4.51, 0.86)
Digit Span Backward	4.43	(−2.55, 11.42)	−0.10	(−1.13, 0.94)	−0.38	(−2.63, 1.87)
School Readiness						
Woodcock-Johnson/Muñoz						
Letter-Word	−1.86	(−9.33, 5.60)	0.21	(−0.88, 1.31)	1.43	(−0.94, 3.80)
Applied Problems	−3.82	(−14.06, 6.42)	−0.51	(−2.01, 1.00)	−1.48	(−4.74, 1.78)
Attention						
CBCL[6]						
ADHD[7]	−0.10	(−2.03, 1.82)	0.00	(−0.28, 0.27)	−0.65	(−1.26, −0.04)*
KCPT[8]						
ADHD[7] Confidence Index	7.52	(−4.86, 19.91)	0.09	(−1.70, 1.87)	−0.75	(−4.61, 3.12)

*$P < 0.05$.
[1] Models adjusted for maternal age, income, employment status at 6 months, country of birth, Diet Quality Index, delivery complications, PPVT score; child 5-minute APGAR, hospitalization at 1 year; number of children in home at 1 and 2 years, home density at 2 years, family structure at 1 year; season of assessment.
[2] Since TSH was expressed on a $\log_2$ basis, β are equal to the change in neurodevelopmental outcomes for a doubling in TSH levels.
[3] Weschler Preschool and Primary Scale of Intelligence.
[4] Wide Range Assessment of Visual Motor Ability.
[5] Peabody Picture Vocabulary Test.
[6] Child Behavior Checklist.
[7] Attention Deficit Hyperactivity Disorder.
[8] Kiddie Continuous Performance Test.

Comprehension also was noted at 12 months but not on other tests of language (WPPSI Vocabulary and PPVT) at 60 months.

Our results are in agreement with those reported by Pop and colleagues, the only other group that examined associations between maternal TH levels during the second half of gestation and child neurodevelopment [8–10]. In these studies, authors reported no associations between free T4 levels measured at 24 and 32 weeks' gestation and infant and toddler development, but did find relations with maternal thyroid hormone measured earlier in pregnancy. Other studies that measured TH during the first half of pregnancy have also reported associations with child neurodevelopment [2–10]

with a notable exception in the study by Oken et al., which found no association between maternal TSH and total T4 at 10 weeks' gestation and child cognition at 6 months and 3 years of age in a large study of 500 mothers and children dyads [11]. TH of maternal origin may thus be of particular importance to brain development before the onset of fetal thyroid function, which occurs around midgestation [54]. Evidence for the potential role of maternal TH before the onset of fetal thyroid function includes the detection of T4 in coelomic fluid as early as 6 weeks' gestation [55], the fact that nuclear T3 receptors were identified in the brain of 10 week old fetuses [56], and that T3 binding to these receptors was detected between 9 and 13 weeks' gestation [57].

This study has some limitations. Women who were excluded from analyses were more likely to be depressed and to give birth to children of lower birth weight. This may have introduced bias since these variables are related to both thyroid hormone levels and neurodevelopment. However, our results were not substantially altered after applying inverse probability of inclusion weights, suggesting that this potential bias may not explain our null finding. In addition, in our study, as well as in those of Pop and colleagues [8–10], most women were euthyroid. Hence, our findings do not preclude the possibility that more extreme maternal thyroid hormone levels in the latter half of pregnancy may influence fetal neurodevelopment.

This study has a number of strengths. We examined a wide range of domains of behavior and neurodevelopment at multiple ages and examined maternal thyroid hormone using direct equilibrium dialysis, which is currently considered the gold standard method to measure free T4. Prior studies exclusively used immunoassays, which, according to the National Academy of Clinical Biochemistry, may only be considered as free T4 "estimates" [52]. Another strength of the present study is that we were able to consider, and control for, a large number of potential confounders, including exposure to neurotoxicants such as lead, cigarette smoke, and organophosphate insecticides [58]. In addition, our population is demographically homogenous, further reducing the potential for confounding. Finally, Zoeller and Rovet proposed that maternal hypothyroxinemia and hypothyroidism at the beginning of the third trimester (when we determined thyroid function in CHAMACOS women) primarily affects gross and fine motor skills, memory, and visuospatial skills [59]. In this study, we evaluated these constructs using well-validated and widely used instruments and yet found no clear evidence of a relationship between maternal thyroid hormone levels and child neurodevelopment.

In summary, this is the first study of maternal thyroid hormone and child neurodevelopment to use direct equilibrium dialysis to measure free T4. Although prior studies did report associations between maternal clinical hypothyroidism and mild hypothyroxinemia during the first half of pregnancy and cognitive impairments in children, we find no convincing evidence that TH measured during later gestation is associated with neurodevelopment in euthyroid children living in an iodine-sufficient area.

Appendices

A. Maternal Covariates

Baseline visit	
Age at enrollment (years), No. (%)	
18–24	130 (45.3)
25–29	95 (33.1)
30–34	42 (14.6)
34–45	20 (7.0)
Age at enrollment (years), Mean (SD)	25.8 (5.0)
Race, No. (%)	
White	5 (1.7)
Latino	278 (96.9)
Other	4 (1.4)
Education, No. (%)	
≤6th grade	121 (42.2)
7–12th grade	105 (36.6)
≥High School	61 (21.3)
Income (% poverty), No. (%)	
<100	171 (59.6)
100–200	105 (36.6)
>200	11 (3.8)
Average income per person per month ($), Mean (SD)	413.8 (255.7)
Employment status, No. (%)	
No	209 (72.8)
Yes	78 (27.2)
Country of birth, No. (%)	
United States	32 (11.1)
Mexico	251 (87.5)
Other	4 (1.4)
Time in the USA (years), No. (%)	
≤5	156 (54.4)
6 to 10	69 (24.0)
≥11	62 (21.6)
Parity, Mean (SD)	1.3 (1.2)
Smoking during pregnancy, No. (%)	
No	271 (94.4)
Yes	16 (5.6)
Smokers in household during pregnancy, No. (%)	
No	258 (89.9)
Yes	29 (10.1)
Any second-hand smoke exposure during pregnancy, No. (%)	
No	179 (62.4)
Yes	108 (37.6)
More than one alcoholic drink per week during pregnancy, No. (%)	
No	282 (98.3)
Yes	5 (1.7)
Any drug consumption during pregnancy, No. (%)	
No	282 (98.3)
Yes	5 (1.7)
Kotelchuck Adequacy of Prenatal Care Utilization Index, No. (%)	
Inadequate	62 (21.6)
Adequate	93 (32.4)
Adequate Plus	132 (46.0)
Diet Quality Index during pregnancy, Mean (SD)	45.3 (9.7)
Composite Social Support Index, Mean (SD)	3.7 (0.9)
Urinary DAP[1] metabolites during pregnancy (nmol/L), Mean (SD)	2.1 (0.4)

Lead levels during pregnancy (ug/dL), Mean (SD)	1.5 (2.1)
6-Month Visit	
Income (% poverty), No. (%)	
<100	199 (69.3)
100–200	86 (30.0)
>200	2 (0.7)
Employment status, No. (%)	
No	199 (69.3)
Yes	88 (30.7)
PPVT[2] score, Mean (SD)	88.2 (21.1)
WAIS[3] score, Mean (SD)	6.3 (2.6)
12-Month Visit	
Income (% poverty), No. (%)	
<100	179 (62.4)
100–200	99 (34.5)
>200	9 (3.1)
Employment status, No. (%)	
No	198 (69.0)
Yes	89 (31.0)
Composite Social Support Index, Mean (SD)	3.8 (1.0)
Depression, No. (%)	
No	140 (48.8)
Yes	147 (51.2)
24-Month Visit	
Income (% poverty), No. (%)	
<100	167 (58.2)
100–200	107 (37.3)
>200	13 (4.5)
Employment status, No. (%)	
No	174 (60.6)
Yes	113 (39.4)
Composite Social Support Index, Mean (SD)	3.9 (1.0)
Three-Year Visit	
Income (% poverty), No. (%)	
<100	178 (62.0)
100–200	103 (35.9)
>200	6 (2.1)
Employment status, No. (%)	
No	175 (61.0)
Yes	112 (39.0)
Depression, No. (%)	
No	161 (56.1)
Yes	126 (43.9)
60-Month visit	
Income (% poverty), No. (%)	
<100	182 (63.4)
100–200	93 (32.4)
>200	12 (4.2)
Employment status, No. (%)	
No	158 (55.1)
Yes	129 (44.9)

Composite Social Support Index, Mean (SD)	3.9 (1.0)

[1]Dialkyl phosphates (DAPs) measured in maternal urine (organophosphate pesticide metabolites).
[2]Peabody Picture Vocabulary Test (PPVT).
[3]Wechsler Adult Intelligence Scale (WAIS).

B. Child Covariates

Baseline visit	
Sex, No. (%)	
Boy	140 (48.8)
Girl	147 (51.2)
Birthweight (g), Mean (%)	
<2500	10 (3.5)
2500–3500	149 (51.9)
>3500	128 (44.6)
Gestational duration (weeks), No. (%)	
≥37	266 (92.7)
<37	21 (7.3)
Cesarean section, No. (%)	
No	220 (76.7)
Yes	67 (23.3)
Pregnancy complications, No. (%)	
No	284 (99.0)
Yes	3 (1.0)
5-minute APGAR score, Mean (SD)	8.9 (0.4)
Months child breastfed, Mean (SD)	8.6 (8.2)
Neonatal TSH (mIU/L), Mean (SD)	6.5 (3.5)
6-Month Visit	
Number of children in household, Mean (SD)	2.1 (0.4)
Housing density (people per room), No. (%)	
≤0.5	4 (1.4)
0.51–1.00	52 (18.1)
1.01–1.50	93 (32.4)
≥1.51	138 (48.1)
Lived with father, No. (%)	
All the time	242 (84.3)
Most of the time	11 (3.8)
Some of the time	14 (4.9)
Not at all	20 (7.0)
HOME[1] score, Mean (SD)	32.0 (4.1)
Hospitalized overnight, No. (%)	
No	253 (88.2)
Yes	34 (11.8)
Age at assessment (months), Mean (SD)	6.6 (1.1)
Medication/herbal intake within 24 hours of assessment, No. (%)	
No	279 (97.2)
Yes	8 (2.8)

Location assessment performed, No. (%)

Office	187 (65.2)
Other	100 (34.8)

Season assessment performed, No. (%)

January–March	68 (23.7)
April–June	71 (24.7)
July–September	77 (26.8)
October–December	71 (24.7)

Psychometrician at assessment, No. (%)

01	117 (40.8)
07	32 (11.1)
13	42 (14.6)
16	4 (1.4)
23	92 (32.1)

12-Month Visit

Number of children in household, Mean (SD)	2.0 (1.7)

Housing density (people per room), No. (%)

≤0.5	1 (0.3)
0.51–1.00	55 (19.2)
1.01–1.50	105 (36.6)
≥1.51	126 (43.9)

Lived with father, No. (%)

All the time	239 (83.3)
Most of the time	11 (3.8)
Some of the time	13 (4.5)
Not at all	24 (8.4)
HOME[1] score, Mean (SD)	35.9 (3.1)

Hospitalized overnight, No. (%)

No	276 (96.2)
Yes	11 (3.8)
Age at assessment (months), Mean (SD)	12.7 (1.3)

Medication/herbal intake within 24 hours of assessment, No. (%)

No	255 (88.9)
Yes	32 (11.1)

Location assessment performed, No. (%)

Office	190 (66.2)
Other	97 (33.8)

Season assessment performed, No. (%)

January–March	73 (25.4)
April–June	67 (23.3)
July–September	74 (25.8)
October–December	73 (25.4)

Psychometrician at assessment, No. (%)

01	109 (38.0)
07	83 (28.9)
23	95 (33.1)

24-Month visit

Number of children in household, Mean (SD)	1.8 (1.5)

Housing density (people per room), No. (%)

≤0.5	2 (0.7)
0.51–1.00	51 (17.8)
1.01–1.50	94 (32.8)
≥1.51	140 (48.8)

Lived with father, No. (%)

All the time	236 (82.2)
Most of the time	23 (8.0)
Some of the time	5 (1.7)
Not at all	23 (8.0)
HOME[1] score, Mean (SD)	26.1 (2.5)

Hospitalized overnight, No. (%)

No	275 (95.8)
Yes	12 (4.2)
Age at assessment (months), Mean (SD)	24.7 (1.2)

Medication/herbal intake within 24 hours of assessment, No. (%)

No	205 (71.4)
Yes	82 (28.6)

Location assessment performed, No. (%)

Office	194 (67.6)
Other	93 (32.4)

Season assessment performed, No. (%)

January–March	73 (25.4)
April–June	85 (29.6)
July–September	71 (24.7)
October–December	58 (20.2)

Psychometrician at assessment, No. (%)

01	122 (42.5)
07	31 (10.8)
23	134 (46.7)

60-Month visit

Number of children in household, Mean (SD)	1.9 (1.3)

Housing density (people per room), No. (%)

≤0.5	1 (0.3)
0.51–1.00	87 (30.3)
1.01–1.50	126 (43.9)
≥1.51	73 (25.4)

Lived with father, No. (%)

All the time	221 (77.0)
Most of the time	16 (5.6)
Some of the time	11 (3.8)
Not at all	39 (13.6)

Hospitalized overnight, No. (%)

No	279 (97.2)
Yes	8 (2.8)

Attended preschool, No. (%)	
No	124 (43.2)
Yes	163 (56.8)
Attended kindergarten, No. (%)	
No	68 (23.7)
Yes	219 (76.3)
Age at assessment (months), Mean (SD)	60.7 (2.2)
Medication/herbal intake within 24 hours of assessment, No. (%)	
No	240 (83.6)
Yes	47 (16.4)
Location assessment performed, No. (%)	
Office	245 (85.4)
Other	42 (14.6)
Season assessment performed, No. (%)	
January–March	76 (26.5)
April–June	72 (25.1)
July–September	86 (30.0)
October–December	53 (18.5)
Psychometrician at assessment, No. (%)	
01	117 (40.8)
21	23 (8.0)
23	32 (11.1)
43	115 (40.1)

[1]Home Observation for Measurement of the Environment (H.O.M.E).

Acknowledgments

This publication was supported by grant numbers: RD 83171001 from the US Environmental Protection Agency and P01 ES009605 from the National Institute for Environmental Health Sciences. Additional funding was provided by the University of California Institute for Mexico and the United States (UC MEXUS), the Fonds de la Recherche en Santé du Québec and the Canadian Institutes for Health Research. The contents of this publication are solely the responsibility of the authors and do not necessarily represent funders' official views. The authors gratefully acknowledge study participants as well as Jon Nakamoto, MD, Ph.D., Michelle Vedar, MPH and Kristin M. Tyler, BA, for their invaluable contributions. Authors declare that they have no competing financial interests.

References

[1] J. T. Dunn, "Iodine supplementation and the prevention of cretinism," *Annals of the New York Academy of Sciences*, vol. 678, pp. 158–168, 1993.

[2] E. B. Man, R. H. Holden, and W. S. Jones, "Thyroid function in human pregnancy. VII. Development and retardation of 4-year-old progeny of euthyroid and of hypothyroxinemic women," *American Journal of Obstetrics and Gynecology*, vol. 109, no. 1, pp. 12–19, 1971.

[3] E. B. Man and W. S. Jones, "Thyroid function in human pregnancy. V. Incidence of maternal serum low butanol-extractable iodines and of normal gestational TBG and TBPA capacities; Retardation of 8-month-old infants," *American Journal of Obstetrics and Gynecology*, vol. 104, no. 6, pp. 898–908, 1969.

[4] E. B. Man and S. A. Serunian, "Thyroid function in human pregnancy. IX. Development or retardation of 7 year old progeny of hypothyroxinemic women," *American Journal of Obstetrics and Gynecology*, vol. 125, no. 7, pp. 949–957, 1976.

[5] J. E. Haddow, G. E. Palomaki, W. C. Allan et al., "Maternal thyroid deficiency during pregnancy and subsequent neuropsychological development of the child," *The New England Journal of Medicine*, vol. 341, no. 8, pp. 549–555, 1999.

[6] Y. Li, Z. Shan, W. Teng et al., "Abnormalities of maternal thyroid function during pregnancy affect neuropsychological development of their children at 25-30 months," *Clinical Endocrinology*, vol. 72, no. 6, pp. 825–829, 2010.

[7] J. Henrichs, J. J. Bongers-Schokking, J. J. Schenk et al., "Maternal thyroid function during early pregnancy and cognitive functioning in early childhood: the generation R study," *Journal of Clinical Endocrinology and Metabolism*, vol. 95, no. 9, pp. 4227–4234, 2010.

[8] L. Kooistra, S. Crawford, A. L. Van Baar, E. P. Brouwers, and V. J. Pop, "Neonatal effects of maternal hypothyroxinemia during early pregnancy," *Pediatrics*, vol. 117, no. 1, pp. 161–167, 2006.

[9] V. J. Pop, J. L. Kuijpens, A. L. Van Baar et al., "Low maternal free thyroxine concentrations during early pregnancy are associated with impaired psychomotor development in infancy," *Clinical Endocrinology*, vol. 50, no. 2, pp. 147–155, 1999.

[10] V. J. Pop, E. P. Brouwers, H. L. Vader, T. Vulsma, A. L. Van Baar, and J. J. De Vijlder, "Maternal hypothyroxinaemia during early pregnancy and subsequent child development: a 3-year follow-up study," *Clinical Endocrinology*, vol. 59, no. 3, pp. 282–288, 2003.

[11] E. Oken, L. E. Braverman, D. Platek, M. L. Mitchell, S. L. Lee, and E. N. Pearce, "Neonatal thyroxine, maternal thyroid function, and child cognition," *Journal of Clinical Endocrinology and Metabolism*, vol. 94, no. 2, pp. 497–503, 2009.

[12] N. B. Myant, "Passage of thyroxine and tri-iodol-thyronine from mother to foetus in pregnant women," *Clinical Science*, vol. 17, no. 1, pp. 75–79, 1958.

[13] T. Vulsma, M. H. Gons, and J. J. M. De Vijlder, "Maternal-fetal transfer of thyroxine in congenital hypothyroidism due to a total organification defect or thyroid agenesis," *The New England Journal of Medicine*, vol. 321, no. 1, pp. 13–16, 1989.

[14] J. G. Thorpe-Beeston, K. H. Nicolaides, C. V. Feelton, J. Butler, and A. M. McGregor, "Maturation of the secretion of thyroid hormone and thyroid-stimulating hormone in the fetus," *The New England Journal of Medicine*, vol. 324, no. 8, pp. 532–536, 1991.

[15] D. Glinoer, "The regulation of thyroid function in pregnancy: pathways of endocrine adaptation from physiology to pathology," *Endocrine Reviews*, vol. 18, no. 3, pp. 404–433, 1997.

[16] I. M. Evans, M. R. Pickard, A. K. Sinha, A. J. Leonard, D. C. Sampson, and R. P. Ekins, "Influence of maternal hyperthyroidism in the rat on the expression of neuronal and astrocytic cytoskeletal proteins in fetal brain," *Journal of Endocrinology*, vol. 175, no. 3, pp. 597–604, 2002.

[17] J. Anselmo, D. Cao, T. Karrison, R. E. Weiss, and S. Refetoff, "Fetal loss associated with excess thyroid hormone exposure," *Journal of the American Medical Association*, vol. 292, no. 6, pp. 691–695, 2004.

[18] M. Phoojaroenchanachai, S. Sriussadaporn, T. Peerapatdit et al., "Effect of maternal hyperthyroidism during late pregnancy on the risk of neonatal low birth weight," *Clinical Endocrinology*, vol. 54, no. 3, pp. 365–370, 2001.

[19] L. K. Millar, D. A. Wing, A. S. Leung, P. P. Koonings, M. N. Montoro, and J. H. Mestman, "Low birth weight and preeclampsia in pregnancies complicated by hyperthyroidism," *Obstetrics and Gynecology*, vol. 84, no. 6, pp. 946–949, 1994.

[20] J. H. Lazarus, "Thyroid disease in pregnancy and childhood," *Minerva Endocrinologica*, vol. 30, no. 2, pp. 71–87, 2005.

[21] S. Luewan, P. Chakkabut, and T. Tongsong, "Outcomes of pregnancy complicated with hyperthyroidism: a cohort study.," *Archives of Gynecology and Obstetrics*, vol. 283, no. 2, pp. 243–247, 2011.

[22] M. I. Surks, E. Ortiz, G. H. Daniels et al., "Subclinical thyroid disease: scientific review and guidelines for diagnosis and management," *Journal of the American Medical Association*, vol. 291, no. 2, pp. 228–238, 2004.

[23] B. M. Casey, J. S. Dashe, C. E. Wells, D. D. McIntire, K. J. Leveno, and F. G. Cunningham, "Subclinical hyperthyroidism and pregnancy outcomes," *Obstetrics and Gynecology*, vol. 107, no. 2 I, pp. 337–341, 2006.

[24] R. Wang, J. C. Nelson, R. M. Weiss, and R. B. Wilcox, "Accuracy of free thyroxine measurements across natural ranges of thyroxine binding to serum proteins," *Thyroid*, vol. 10, no. 1, pp. 31–39, 2000.

[25] J. C. Nelson and R. T. Tomei, "Direct determination of free thyroxin in undiluted serum by equilibrium dialysis/radioimmunoassay," *Clinical Chemistry*, vol. 34, no. 9, pp. 1737–1744, 1988.

[26] J. C. Nelson, R. M. Weiss, and R. B. Wilcox, "Underestimates of serum free thyroxine (T4) concentrations by free T4 immunoassays," *Journal of Clinical Endocrinology and Metabolism*, vol. 79, no. 1, pp. 76–79, 1994.

[27] L. Dunn and L. Dunn, *Peabody Picture Vocabulary Test*, American Guidance Service, Circle Pines, Minn, USA, 1981.

[28] L. S. Radloff, "The CES-D scale: a self-report depression scale for research in the general population," *Applied Psychological Measurement*, vol. 1, no. 3, pp. 385–401, 1977.

[29] B. Caldwell and R. Bradley, *Home Observation for Measurement of the Environment*, University of Arkansas, Little Rock, Ark, USA, 1984.

[30] M. Kotelchuck, "An evaluation of the Kessner Adequacy of Prenatal Care Index and a proposed Adequacy of Prenatal Care Utilization Index," *American Journal of Public Health*, vol. 84, no. 9, pp. 1414–1420, 1994.

[31] W. E. Broadhead, S. H. Gehlbach, F. V. de Gruy, and B. H. Kaplan, "The Duke-UNC Functional Social Support Questionnaire. Measurement of social support in family medicine patients," *Medical Care*, vol. 26, no. 7, pp. 709–723, 1988.

[32] L. M. Bodnar and A. M. Siega-Riz, "A diet quality index for pregnancy detects variation in diet and differences by sociodemographic factors," *Public Health Nutrition*, vol. 5, no. 6, pp. 801–809, 2002.

[33] K. Harley and B. Eskenazi, "Time in the United States, social support and health behaviors during pregnancy among women of Mexican descent," *Social Science and Medicine*, vol. 62, no. 12, pp. 3048–3061, 2006.

[34] N. Bayley, *Bayley Scales of Infant Development*, The Psychological Corporation, San Antonio, Tex, USA, 2nd edition, 1993.

[35] D. Wechsler, *WPPSI-III Administration and Scoring Manual*, The Psychological Corporation, San Antonio, Tex, USA, 2002.

[36] D. McCarthy, *Manual for the McCarthy Scales of Children's Abilities*, The Psychological Corporation, New York, NY, USA, 1972.

[37] R. W. Woodcock and A. F. Munoz-Sandoval, *Bateria Woodcock-Munoz: Pruebas de Habilidad Cognitiva-Revisada*, The Riverside Publishing Company, Itasca, Ill, USA, 1996.

[38] R. W. Woodcock and M. B. Johnson, *Woodcock-Johnson Tests of Cognitive Ability*, The Riverside Publishing Company, Itasca, Ill, USA, 1990.

[39] W. Adams and D. Sheslow, *WRAVMA: Wide Range Assessment of Visual Motor Abilities*, Wide Range, Wilmington, Del, USA, 1995.

[40] C. K. Conners, *Conners' K-CPT: Kiddie Continuous Performance Test*, Multi-Health Systems, North Tonawanda, NY, USA, 2001.

[41] A. S. Kaufman and N. L. Kaufman, *Clinical Evaluation of Young Children with the McCarthy Scales*, Grune & Stratton, New York, NY, USA, 1977.

[42] T. M. Achenbach and L. A. Rescorla, *Manual for the ASEBA Preschool Forms & Profiles*, University of Vermont, Research Center for Children, Youth & Families, Burlington, Vt, USA, 2000.

[43] E. B. Man, D. M. Kudd, and J. P. Peters, "Butanol-extractable iodine of serum," *The Journal of Clinical Investigation*, vol. 30, no. 5, pp. 531–538, 1951.

[44] T. Hastie and R. Tibshirani, "Generalized additive models for medical research," *Statistical Methods in Medical Research*, vol. 4, no. 3, pp. 187–196, 1995.

[45] B. Rosner, "Percentage points for a generalized ESD many-outlier procedure," *Technometrics*, vol. 25, no. 2, pp. 165–172, 1983.

[46] J. G. Young, B. Eskenazi, E. A. Gladstone et al., "Association between in utero organophosphate pesticide exposure and abnormal reflexes in neonates," *NeuroToxicology*, vol. 26, no. 2, pp. 199–209, 2005.

[47] B. Eskenazi, A. R. Marks, A. Bradman et al., "Organophosphate pesticide exposure and neurodevelopment in young Mexican-American children," *Environmental Health Perspectives*, vol. 115, no. 5, pp. 792–798, 2007.

[48] R. Bravo, L. M. Caltabiano, G. Weerasekera et al., "Measurement of dialkyl phosphate metabolites of organophosphorus pesticides in human urine using lyophilization with gas chromatography-tandem mass spectrometry and isotope dilution quantification," *Journal of Exposure Analysis and Environmental Epidemiology*, vol. 14, no. 3, pp. 249–259, 2004.

[49] J. W. Hogan, J. Roy, and C. Korkontzelou, "Tutorial in biostatistics. Handling drop-out in longitudinal studies," *Statistics in Medicine*, vol. 23, no. 9, pp. 1455–1497, 2004.

[50] S. E. Sinisi and M. J. van der Laan, "Loss-based cross-validated deletion/substitution/addition algorithms in estimation," UC Berkeley Division of Biostatistics Working Paper Series, Working Paper 143, 2004, http://www.bepress.com/ucbbiostat/paper143.

[51] S. J. Mandel, C. A. Spencer, and J. G. Hollowell, "Are detection and treatment of thyroid insufficiency in pregnancy feasible?" *Thyroid*, vol. 15, no. 1, pp. 44–53, 2005.

[52] National Academy of Clinical Biochemistry, "Laboratory support for the diagnosis of thyroid disease," in *Laboratory Medicine Practice Guidelines*, L. M. Demers and C. A. Spencer, Eds., NACB, Washington, DC, USA, 2002.

[53] K. L. Caldwell, G. A. Miller, R. Y. Wang, R. B. Jain, and R. L. Jones, "Iodine status of the U.S. population, National Health and Nutrition Examination Survey 2003-2004," *Thyroid*, vol. 18, no. 11, pp. 1207–1214, 2008.

[54] G. Morreale De Escobar, M. J. Obregon, and F. Escobar Del Rey, "Clinical perspective: is neuropsychological development related to maternal hypothyroidism or to maternal hypothyroxinemia?" *Journal of Clinical Endocrinology and Metabolism*, vol. 85, no. 11, pp. 3975–3987, 2000.

[55] B. Contempre, E. Jauniaux, R. Calvo, D. Jurkovic, S. Campbell, and G. M. De Escobar, "Detection of thyroid hormones in human embryonic cavities during the first trimester of pregnancy," *Journal of Clinical Endocrinology and Metabolism*, vol. 77, no. 6, pp. 1719–1722, 1993.

[56] J. Bernal and F. Pekonen, "Ontogenesis of the nuclear 3,5,3'-triiodothyronine receptor in the human fetal brain," *Endocrinology*, vol. 114, no. 2, pp. 677–679, 1984.

[57] B. Ferreiro, J. Bernal, C. G. Goodyer, and C. L. Branchard, "Estimation of nuclear thyroid hormone receptor saturation in human fetal brain and lung during early gestation," *Journal of Clinical Endocrinology and Metabolism*, vol. 67, no. 4, pp. 853–856, 1988.

[58] J. Chevrier, B. Eskenazi, A. Bradman, L. Fenster, and D. B. Barr, "Associations between prenatal exposure to polychlorinated biphenyls and neonatal thyroid-stimulating hormone levels in a Mexican-American population, Salinas Valley, California," *Environmental Health Perspectives*, vol. 115, no. 10, pp. 1490–1496, 2007.

[59] R. T. Zoeller and J. Rovet, "Timing of thyroid hormone action in the developing brain: clinical observations and experimental findings," *Journal of Neuroendocrinology*, vol. 16, no. 10, pp. 809–818, 2004.

7

Mechanisms of L-Triiodothyronine-Induced Inhibition of Synaptosomal Na$^+$-K$^+$-ATPase Activity in Young Adult Rat Brain Cerebral Cortex

Pradip K. Sarkar,[1,2,3] Avijit Biswas,[2] Arun K. Ray,[3] and Joseph V. Martin[2]

[1] *Department of Basic Sciences, Parker University, 2500 Walnut Hill Lane, Dallas, TX 75229, USA*
[2] *Center for Computational & Integrative Biology, Rutgers University, 315 Penn Street, Camden, NJ 08102, USA*
[3] *Department of Molecular Medicine, Bose Institute, P-1/12, CIT, Scheme VII-M, Calcutta 700054, India*

Correspondence should be addressed to Pradip K. Sarkar; psarkar@parker.edu

Academic Editor: Noriyuki Koibuchi

The role of thyroid hormones (TH) in the normal functioning of adult mammalian brain is unclear. Our studies have identified synaptosomal Na$^+$-K$^+$-ATPase as a TH-responsive physiological parameter in adult rat cerebral cortex. L-triiodothyronine (T$_3$) and L-thyroxine (T$_4$) both inhibited Na$^+$-K$^+$-ATPase activity (but not Mg^{2+}-ATPase activity) in similar dose-dependent fashions, while other metabolites of TH were less effective. Although both T$_3$ and the β-adrenergic agonist isoproterenol inhibited Na$^+$-K$^+$-ATPase activity in cerebrocortical synaptosomes in similar ways, the β-adrenergic receptor blocker propranolol did not counteract the effect of T$_3$. Instead, propranolol further inhibited Na$^+$-K$^+$-ATPase activity in a dose-dependent manner, suggesting that the effect of T$_3$ on synaptosomal Na$^+$-K$^+$-ATPase activity was independent of β-adrenergic receptor activation. The effect of T$_3$ on synaptosomal Na$^+$-K$^+$-ATPase activity was inhibited by the α_2-adrenergic agonist clonidine and by glutamate. Notably, both clonidine and glutamate activate G$_i$-proteins of the membrane second messenger system, suggesting a potential mechanism for the inhibition of the effects of TH. In this paper, we provide support for a nongenomic mechanism of action of TH in a neuronal membrane-related energy-linked process for signal transduction in the adult condition.

1. Introduction

Thyroid hormones (TH) exert major influences on the growth and development of the mammalian brain through specific nuclear receptor-mediated gene expression. Although several different isoforms of nuclear receptors for TH have been described in adult mammalian brain, their physiological function is quite unclear [1–4]. Still, adult onset of dysthyroidism develops a number of functional, neurological and psychological manifestations in humans [5–7]. In contrast to the developing brain, most of the changes resulting from hormone variations in the adult condition are reversible with the proper adjustment of circulatory TH [5–7].

Recent evidence has demonstrated that L-triiodothyronine (T$_3$) is distributed, concentrated, and metabolized in the synaptosomal fraction of adult rat cerebral cortex [5, 8, 9].

Specific T$_3$-binding sites have also been described in cerebrocortical synaptosomes [10, 11] and a graded binding of T$_3$ to its synaptosomal receptor binding sites has been correlated with the corresponding inhibition of the Na$^+$-K$^+$-ATPase activities in adult rat brain [11]. TH rapidly alters *in vitro* phosphorylation of synaptosomal proteins in a dose-dependent fashion [12]. TH levels are also altered in adult rat brain in different thyroid conditions [9]. TH enhances calcium entry in adult rat brain synaptosomes [13–15], in hypothyroid mouse brain [16], and in single rat myocytes [17].

However, there is a lack of clear understanding of the mechanism(s) of action of TH in the regulation of synaptic functions in adult neurons. The present study investigates the pathways of T$_3$-mediated signaling from its binding to the synaptosomal membrane receptors to the subsequent activation of second messenger system components that ultimately affect the further downstream effector molecule, the Na^+-K^+-ATPase. In this paper, we hypothesize a nongenomic mechanism of action of TH in neuronal membrane-related energy-linked process(es) for signal transduction in adult condition. We have used α- and β-adrenoceptor agonists and antagonists for modulation of the activity of G_s- and G_i-proteins of the membrane adenylate cyclase system. Portions of this work have appeared elsewhere in a preliminary form [18, 19].

2. Materials and Methods

2.1. Materials. The following compounds were purchased from Sigma Chemical Company, USA: bovine serum albumin (BSA), clonidine hydrochloride (CLO), disodium-ATP, isoproterenol hydrochloride (ISO), 2-mercaptoethanol, ouabain octahydrate, prazosin hydrochloride (PRA), phenylephrine hydrochloride (PHE), propranolol hydrochloride (PROP), sodium glutamate, 3,5,3'-L-triiodothyronine (T_3), L-thyroxine (T_4), 3,3',5'-L-triiodothyronine (reverse T_3 or r-T_3), 3,5-L-diiodothyronine (T_2), Tris-ATP, yohimbine hydrochloride (YOH), dibutyryl 3',5'-cyclic adenosine monophosphate sodium salt (DB cAMP), and sodium orthovanadate.

2.2. Treatment of Animals. Adult male Charles Foster rats (3 months old) were housed at $25 \pm 1°C$ in 12 h dark-12 h light conditions and fed *ad libitum* with standard rat diet and water. The animals were sacrificed by quick decapitation and the brains were removed into ice-cold 250 mM sucrose solution. The cerebral cortices were dissected out for synaptosomal fraction preparation.

2.3. Preparation of Synaptosomes. The synaptosomes from thecerebral cortex were prepared as described previously [20]. Briefly, the cerebral cortex was homogenized (10% weight/volume) in 0.32 M sucrose and centrifuged at 1000 g for 10 minutes to remove cell debris and nuclei. The supernatant was collected and recentrifuged at 1000 g for another 10 min. The resulting pellet was discarded and the supernatant was layered over 1.2 M sucrose and centrifuged at 34,000 g for 50 min at 4°C. The fraction collected between the 0.32 M and 1.2 M sucrose layer was diluted at 1 : 1.5 with ice-cold bidistilled water, further layered on 0.8 M sucrose, and again centrifuged at 34,000 g for 30 min. The pellet thus obtained was washed and repelleted at 20,000 g for 20 min. Synaptosomal pellets were lysed by suspending in ice-cold bidistilled water to release the occluded Na^+-K^+-ATPase activity.

2.4. Assay of Synaptosomal Na^+-K^+-ATPase Activity. Synaptosomal Na^+-K^+-ATPase activity was assayed as ouabain-sensitive ATP hydrolysis in reaction mixtures of (i) 30 mM imidazole-HCl, 130 mM NaCl, 20 mM KCl, and 4 mM $MgCl_2$ and (ii) 30 mM imidazole-HCl, 4 mM $MgCl_2$, and 1 mM ouabain, at pH 7.4. Both the reaction media (i) and (ii) were first preincubated *in vitro* with or without simultaneous addition of various concentrations of thyroid hormones (T_3, T_4) and TH-analogue (T_2) (0.001 nM to 1 μM), adrenergic drugs (1 nM for ISO, PRA, PHE and YOH; 1 nM–100 nM for CLO and PROP), glutamate (100 μM), DB cAMP (1 μM–5 mM), and sodium orthovanadate (10 nM–2 mM) followed by addition of the synaptosomal lysates, each containing 20–50 μg synaptosomal protein, at 0°C for 60 minutes in dark. To get a steady-state ouabain binding, both the assay media (i) and (ii), with and without ouabain, respectively, as described above, were preincubated for 60 min at 0°C in the dark, followed by a 5-min incubation at 37°C to equilibrate the temperature. The reaction was started by adding 4 mM Tris-ATP and incubated at 37°C for 10 min. An aliquot of 100 μL of 10% sodium dodecylsulfate was added to stop the enzymatic reaction. The inorganic phosphate (P_i) formed was determined in the reaction mixture [21]. Na^+-K^+-ATPase activity was calculated as difference in the P_i content between media (i) and (ii) and expressed as μmols P_i/h/mg protein [22]. The ouabain-sensitive portion of the total ATPase (Na^+-K^+-Mg^{2+}-ATPase) was determined from the P_i released in the medium (i) minus that in medium (ii). The P_i released from the reaction medium (ii) was used for determination of the synaptosomal Mg^{2+}-ATPase activity. Synaptosomal Mg^{2+}-ATPase activity, therefore, was assayed as the ouabain-insensitive ATP hydrolysis.

2.5. Measurement of Protein. Synaptosomal protein content was measured using bovine serum albumin as a standard [23].

2.6. Statistical Analysis. Results are expressed as the mean $\pm$ SEM of 3-4 separate experiments or as mentioned. Each experiment was made from six rats. The statistical analysis of the data was performed by Student's t-test, considering $P < 0.05$ as the significance level. The data for multiple groups were also analyzed by one-way ANOVA followed by Student Newman-Keuls post-hoc comparisons using Sigmastat software. Nonlinear regression analysis was performed using GraphPad Prism software.

3. Results

3.1. Effects of T_3 and Metabolites on Na^+-K^+-ATPase Activity. *In vitro* addition of various doses of T_3 to the synaptosomal fraction (which is devoid of cell nuclei) confirmed our previous observation [11] and showed nearly the same trend of a dose-dependent inhibition ($IC_{50} = 166.4 \pm 55.0$ pM; maximal inhibition = $63.2 \pm 3.4\%$ at 95% confidence levels) of Na^+-K^+-ATPase activity. No significant effect of T_3 was noticed on the Mg^{2+}-ATPase specific activity (Figure 1). T_4 had a similar inhibitory effect as T_3 on Na^+-K^+-ATPase activity ($IC_{50} = 77.2 \pm 31.8$ pM; maximal inhibition = $66.5 \pm 7.2\%$), while T_2 had minimal effects (Figure 2). Furthermore, the same range of doses (10^{-12}–10^{-8} M) of r-T_3 did not inhibit either Na^+-K^+-ATPase or Mg^{+2}-ATPase activities (data not shown).

3.2. Effect of T_3 and β-Adrenergic Agonists/Antagonists on Na^+-K^+-ATPase Activity. Equimolar doses (1 nM) of T_3 and

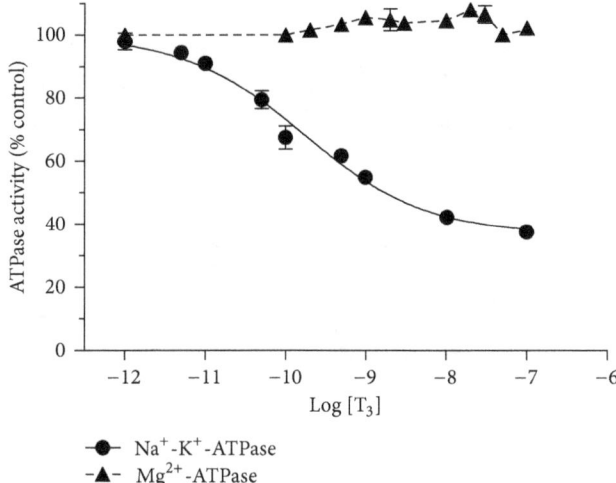

FIGURE 1: Inhibitory effect of various doses (0.001 nM–100 nM) of T_3 on synaptosomal Na^+-K^+-ATPase or Mg^{2+}-ATPase activity, *in vitro*. The data are represented as mean ± SEM of ten separate experiments, taking six animals in each group. The vertical lines denote SEM. Filled circles indicate Na^+-K^+-ATPase while filled triangles indicate Mg^{2+}-ATPase activity.

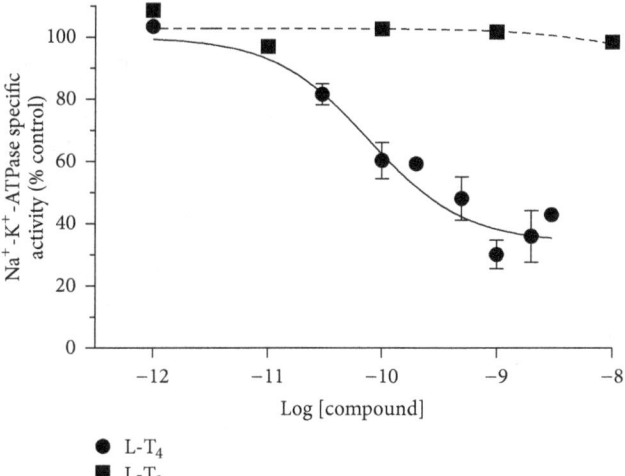

FIGURE 2: Inhibitory effect of various doses (0.001 nM–10 nM) of T_4 or T_2 on synaptosomal Na^+-K^+-ATPase activity, *in vitro*. The data are represented as mean ± SEM of four separate experiments, taking six animals in each group. The vertical lines denote SEM. Filled circles indicate effects of T_4 on Na^+-K^+-ATPase activity while filled squares indicate effects of T_2.

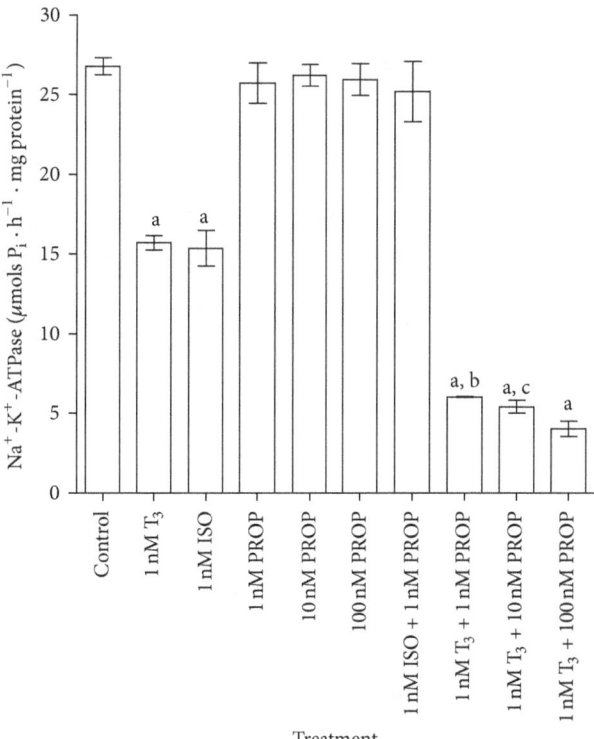

FIGURE 3: Effect of T_3 on synaptosomal Na^+-K^+-ATPase activity and its modulation by a β-adrenergic receptor agonist (ISO) and a β-adrenergic receptor antagonist (PROP) *in vitro*. A half-maximally effective dose of T_3 (1 nM) was chosen from the dose-response curve for T_3 in Figure 1. The data are represented as mean ± SEM of five separate experiments taking six animals in each group. [a]$P < 0.001$, compared to the control group. [b]$P < 0.001$ and [c]$P < 0.05$, compared to T_3 (1 nM) + PROP (100 nM) group (one-way ANOVA followed by Newman-Keuls test). The vertical lines denote SEM.

the nonselective β-adrenergic agonist ISO were added separately *in vitro*, inhibited the Na^+-K^+-ATPase enzyme activity by 41.3% and 42.6%, respectively (Figure 3). The nonselective β-adrenergic antagonist PROP alone did not alter the enzyme activity at different doses (1 nM, 10 nM, and 100 nM). The inhibitory action of ISO (1 nM) on the Na^+-K^+-ATPase activity was counteracted by PROP (1 nM), whereas PROP could not block T_3-mediated inhibition of the enzyme activity. Instead PROP potentiated the T_3-mediated inhibition of the enzyme activity in a dose-dependent manner. Significant

differences in the potentiation of the T_3 effect (1 nM) by PROP on Na^+-K^+-ATPase activity were noticed between 1 nM and 100 nM ($P < 0.001$) and between 10 nM and 100 nM ($P < 0.05$) doses (Figure 3).

3.3. Effects of T_3 and α-Adrenergic Agonists/Antagonists on Na^+-K^+-ATPase Activity.

The effects of *in vitro* addition of 1 nM doses of PHE (selective α_1-adrenergic receptor agonist) and PRA (α_1-adrenergic receptor antagonist) on synaptosomal Na^+-K^+-ATPase activity or Mg^{2+}-ATPase activity were minimal (Figure 4). Furthermore, 1 nM doses of PHE or PRA did not alter the inhibitory effect of 1 nM T_3 on Na^+-K^+-ATPase activity, nor did it change the Mg^{2+}-ATPase activity, *in vitro* (Figure 4).

Similarly, *in vitro* addition of CLO (α_2-adrenergic agonist) at different doses did not elicit significant changes in the synaptosomal Na^+-K^+-ATPase activity (Figure 5). However, when CLO was added in the presence of an equimolar dose of T_3, the inhibitory effect of T_3 on the Na^+-K^+-ATPase activity was completely counteracted. The effect of T_3 on the enzyme activity remained prominent at a 100 nM dose of T_3 (100 nM T_3: 10.29 ± 0.2 μmols P_i/h/mg protein;

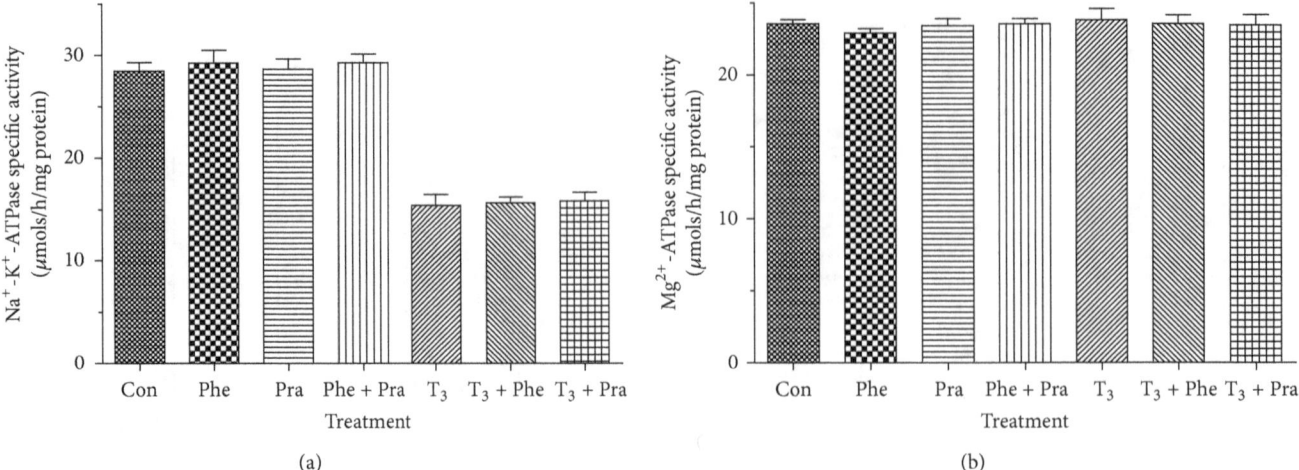

(a)   (b)

FIGURE 4: Modulation of the T_3 action on synaptosomal Na^+-K^+-ATPase activity by a selective α_1-adrenergic agonist (PHE) and a selective α_1-antagonist (PRA) *in vitro*. A half-maximally effective dose of T_3 (1 nM) was chosen from the dose-response curve for T_3 in Figure 1. The doses for PHE and PRA used for the *in vitro* experiment were 1 nM in each case. The data are represented as mean ± SEM of five separate experiments, taking six animals in each group. The vertical lines denote SEM.

Control: 26.22 ± 0.2 μmols P_i/h/mg protein) along with 1 nM CLO (100 nM T_3 + 1 nM CLO: 15.23 ± 0.4 μmols P_i/h/mg protein); however, 1 nM CLO attenuated the effect of T_3 (100 nM) by 32% more towards the control value (data not shown graphically). The α_2-adrenergic receptor antagonist YOH also inhibited synaptosomal Na^+-K^+-ATPase activity (Figure 5). Inhibition of the enzyme activity in the presence of both 1 nM T_3 and 1 nM YOH was found to be intermediate between the levels of inhibition by either compound alone, although there were no significant differences between these groups (Figure 5).

3.4. Effect of T_3 and Glutamate on Na^+-K^+-ATPase Activity. In vitro addition of 100 μM glutamate alone did not alter the synaptosomal Na^+-K^+-ATPase activity compared to control values, whereas, addition of 100 μM glutamate showed complete attenuation of T_3 (10 nM)-mediated inhibition of synaptosomal Na^+-K^+-ATPase activity in adult rat cerebral cortex (Figure 6). A higher dose of T_3 (10 nM) was chosen, in order to test the effect of glutamate against a greater inhibitory action on the Na^+-K^+-ATPase activity.

3.5. Effect of DB cAMP and T_3 on Na^+-K^+-ATPase Activity. To study the effect of DB cAMP on modulation of Na^+-K^+-ATPase activity by T_3, first a dose response experiment with various concentrations of DB cAMP (0.001 mM to 5 mM) was performed. *In vitro* addition of DB cAMP showed a typical sigmoidal curve with gradual decrease in the Na^+-K^+-ATPase activity to a maximal inhibition at 0.2 mM (Figure 7(a)). From this standardization, we chose to use a 0.2 mM final concentration of DB cAMP for further experiments. *In vitro* addition of DB cAMP (0.2 mM) with and without various doses of T_3 (0.001 nM–10 nM) was examined for effects on Na^+-K^+-ATPase activity (Figure 7(b)). T_3-induced inhibition of synaptosomal Na^+-K^+-ATPase activity was further

depressed in the presence of 0.2 mM DB cAMP. However, the two curves appeared to converge at the highest doses of T_3.

3.6. Influence of Sodium Orthovanadate on Modulation of Na^+-K^+-ATPase Activity by T_3. The *in vitro* effect of sodium orthovanadate, a protein tyrosine phosphatase inhibitor, was examined in cerebrocortical synaptosomes. The cerebrocortical synaptosomes were treated with a fixed dose of T_3 (10 nM) with or without different doses of sodium o-vanadate (Figure 8). A higher dose of T_3 (10 nM) was chosen from the T_3 dose-response curve, considering its greater inhibitory action on the Na^+-K^+-ATPase activity. T_3 caused an inhibition of Na^+-K^+-ATPase specific activity, and this effect was enhanced by sodium orthovanadate in a dose-dependent way. In general, the effects of sodium orthovanadate and T_3 appeared to be additive until the Na^+-K^+-ATPase specific activity was completely inhibited.

4. Discussion

The objective of the present investigation was to search for possible mechanisms for the inhibition by TH of synaptosomal Na^+-K^+-ATPase activity in adult rat cerebral cortex.

Initial studies examined the specificity of the effect according to the pattern of iodination of the hormone derivatives (Figures 1 and 2). *In vitro* inhibitory effect of T_3 on synaptosomal Na^+-K^+-ATPase activity supported our previous observation and showed nearly the same trend of a dose-dependent inhibition of Na^+-K^+-ATPase activity [11]. In addition to our earlier report, the current study showed an insignificant effect of T_3 on the synaptosomal Mg^{2+}-ATPase specific activity (Figure 1). *In vitro* addition of T_4 also indicated similar pattern of inhibitory influence on the synaptosomal Na^+-K^+-ATPase activity, like the effect of T_3, with no significant changes on the Mg^{2+}-ATPase activity. The effects of TH on Na^+-K^+-ATPase activity seemed to be

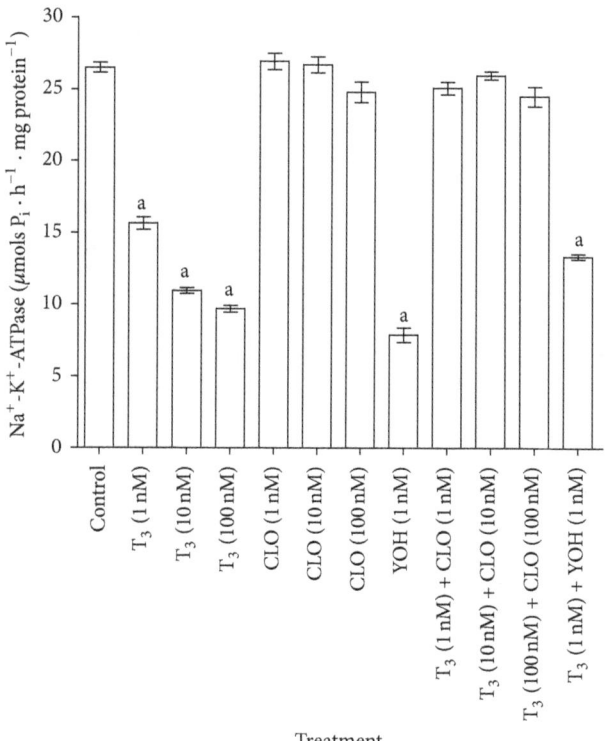

FIGURE 5: Modulation of the T_3 action on synaptosomal Na^+-K^+-ATPase activity by an α_2-adrenergic agonist (CLO) and an α_2-adrenergic antagonist (YOH) *in vitro*. The data are represented as mean ± SEM of six separate experiments taking six animals in each group. [a]$P < 0.001$, compared to the control group (one-way ANOVA followed by Newman-Keuls test). The vertical lines denote SEM.

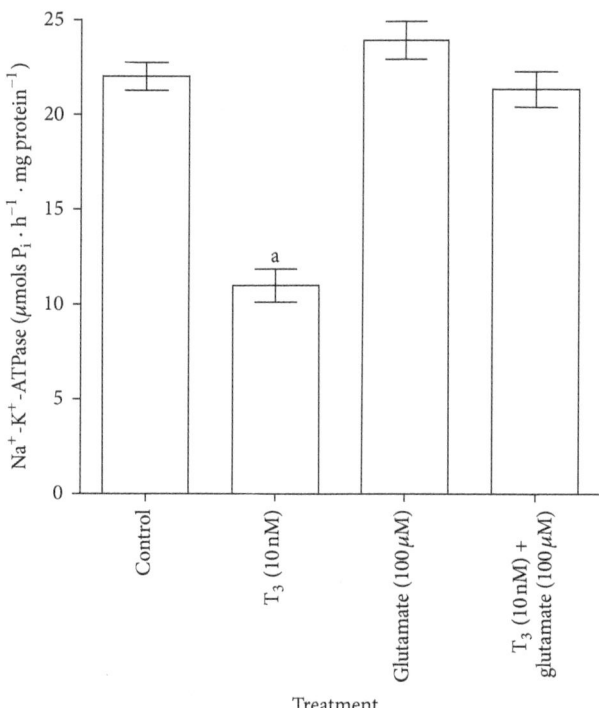

FIGURE 6: Modulatory effect of glutamate on T_3-induced inhibition of synaptosomal Na^+-K^+-ATPase activity in cerebral cortex, *in vitro*. A higher dose of T_3 (10 nM) was chosen from the T_3 dose-response curve, considering its greater inhibitory action on the Na^+-K^+-ATPase activity and to observe the effect of 100 μM glutamate on this T_3-induced inhibition. The data are represented as mean ± SEM of four separate experiments taking six animals in each group. [a]$P < 0.001$, compared to the control group (one-way ANOVA followed by Newman-Keuls test).

specific for compounds with 2 iodine atoms on the inner ring, as T_2 and r-T_3 were without activity in the current studies. T_3 was less potent than T_4. It is consistent with reports of the relative affinities of the two compounds for a cell surface receptor, integrin $\alpha_v\beta_3$ known to mediate a variety of nongenomic effects of THs [24].

Binding of T_4 to integrin $\alpha_v\beta_3$ causes internalization of the receptor and nongenomically promotes phosphorylation of mitogen-activated protein kinase/extracellular regulated kinase 1 and 2 (MAPK/ERK$_{1/2}$) in the CV-1 line of monkey fibroblasts [24]. A similar mechanism seems likely in chick chorioallantoic membrane [25]. Following the internalization of the integrin $\alpha_v\beta_3$, the α_v monomer is translocated to the nucleus, where it may transcriptionally regulate expression of protein [26]. TH causes lungs to rapidly (within hours) increase alveolar fluid clearance [27] and to express increased Na^+-K^+-ATPase protein by a MAPK/ERK$_{1/2}$-dependent pathway [28]. Note, however, that the current finding of an immediate effect to decrease Na^+-K^+-ATPase activity could not be due to a mechanism involving transcriptional regulation, since the synaptosomal preparation is devoid of cell nuclei. It is also suggested that some of the effects of T_3 stimulation of the integrin $\alpha_v\beta_3$ could be more direct than the nuclear interaction [29].

A potential mechanism for the inhibitory effects of TH in the present study might be the regulation of phosphorylation of Na^+-K^+-ATPase or a modulatory molecule. It is well known that catecholamine-mediated phosphorylation of Na^+-K^+-ATPase inhibits enzymatic activity in Chinese hamster ovary (CHO) cells, but not through a process of internalization of the enzyme [30–32]. Intriguingly in this respect, one of the proteins found to be phosphorylated at the tyrosyl residue in synaptosomes treated for 5 s with TH had a molecular weight of 95 kD [12], matching the size of α-subunit of Na^+-K^+-ATPase [33].

The significant inhibition of the synaptosomal Na^+-K^+-ATPase activity *in vitro* by T_3 confirmed our previous *in vivo* observations [22]. In order to characterize this inhibitory influence of THs on the synaptosomal membrane, we intended to study the effect of adrenergic receptor agonists and antagonists which regulate guanine nucleotide binding proteins (G-proteins) via their activating and inhibitory actions. Both T_3 and ISO (β-adrenergic receptor agonist) showed an analogous but independent (parallel) inhibitory effect on the enzyme activity (Figure 3). ISO-induced inhibition of Na^+-K^+-ATPase activity was blocked by PROP (β-adrenergic receptor blocker) indicating that the synaptosomal membrane interaction with ISO was likely

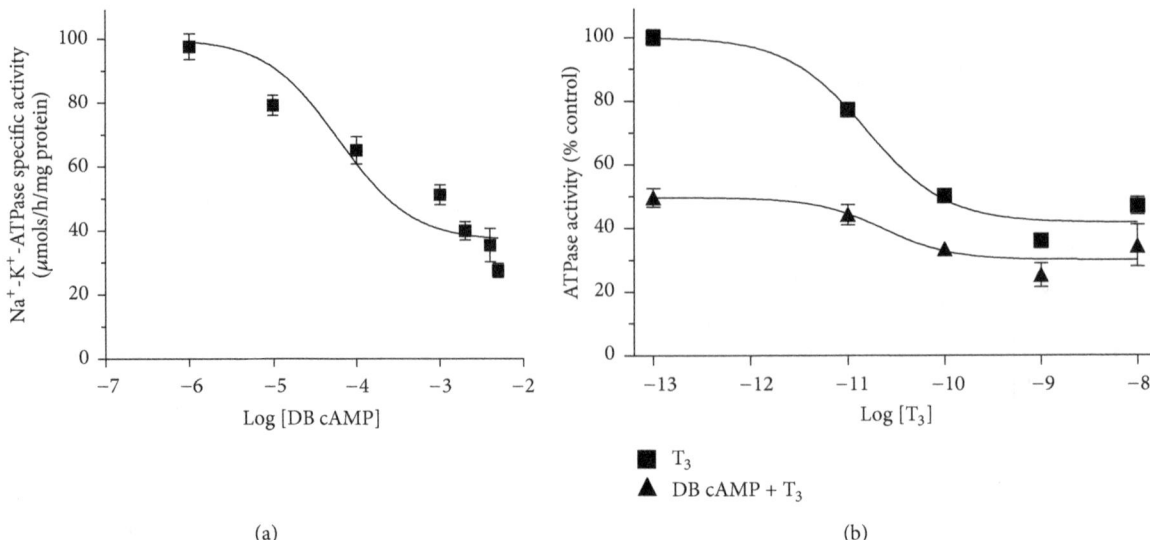

FIGURE 7: Influence of DB cAMP and T_3 on synaptosomal Na^+-K^+-ATPase activity, *in vitro*. (a) Inhibitory effect of various doses of DB cAMP on synaptosomal Na^+-K^+-ATPase activity, *in vitro*. The data are represented as mean ± SEM of four separate experiments, taking six animals in each group. The vertical bars denote SEM. (b) Interaction of the effects of of DB cAMP and T_3 on synaptosomal Na^+-K^+-ATPase activity, *in vitro*. Filled squares indicate effects of graded doses of T_3 (0.001 nM–10 nM) alone on Na^+-K^+-ATPase activity while filled triangles indicate effects of the 0.2 mM dose of DB cAMP with graded doses of T_3 (0.1 pM–1 μM).

a β-adrenoceptor-mediated event, potentially coupled to G_s-protein. However, PROP was completely unable to block T_3-mediated inhibition of synaptosomal Na^+-K^+-ATPase activity. This clearly indicated that T_3-mediated inhibition of the enzyme activity was not coupled to β-adrenoceptor, but rather, may have had a similar effect through another kind of receptor. The augmentation of the T_3 effect by PROP appeared to be a type of synergistic action, the mechanism of which remains unclear at present. Increased activity of adenylate cyclase caused by THs, independent of propranolol blockade, has been shown in cultured cerebral cells from embryonic mice, suggesting that the effect of T_3 was not mediated through a β-adrenergic-dependent system [34]. The T_3-induced increase in sodium current in neonatal rat myocytes also could not be blocked by PROP, whereas it was antagonized by amiodarone, a nonspecific blocker of β-adrenoceptor, suggesting that the effects were not mediated through β-adrenergic signaling pathways [35]. However, β-adrenoceptor blockade by chronic subcutaneous delivery of PROP for 14 days has been shown to downregulate levels of TH receptor TR α_1-mRNA and β_1-mRNA in mouse heart, which may influence the genomic effect of the hormone [36].

Next, we wanted to check for the role of an α_1-adrenergic receptor agonist and antagonist. Agonists for the α_1-adrenergic receptor mediate their actions through G_q protein followed by activation of phospholipase C and subsequent production of the second messengers inositol triphosphate and diacylglycerol, an activator of protein kinase C [37]. Neither PHE (selective α_1 agonist) nor PRA (α_1 antagonist) had an influence on Na^+-K^+-ATPase activity. Furthermore, neither compound interacted with the effects of T_3. Mg^{2+}-ATPase activity remained unaltered when treated with either of these α_1-adrenergic drugs (agonist and antagonist)

and T_3, alone or in combination (Figure 4). These results suggest that the effects of T_3 on Na^+-K^+-ATPase activity do not share common mechanisms with α_1-receptors.

On the other hand, CLO, an α_2-adrenergic receptor agonist (Figure 5), and glutamate (Figure 6), possibly acting via a metabotropic glutamate receptor (mGluR), blocked T_3-induced inhibition of Na^+-K^+-ATPase activity. Neither CLO nor glutamate showed any significant effect on the Na^+-K^+-ATPase activity in rat hippocampus and frontal cortex homogenates [38]. One possibility would be that the counteraction of the effect of T_3 on synaptosomal Na^+-K^+-ATPase by CLO and glutamate might be mediated through the inhibition of adenylate cyclase activity with the activation of inhibitory G-protein (G_i) followed by the inhibition of cAMP synthesis and the protein phosphorylation cascade mechanism. It is well known that α_2-adrenergic agonists act through stimulation of G_i-protein [18, 19, 39, 40].

Association of the glutamate transporter with Na^+-K^+-ATPase in synaptosomes has been implicated by their correlated regulation via protein kinases [41]. Glutamate also has been reported to inhibit adenylate cyclase activity in rat hippocampal synaptosomes [39, 40, 42, 43], as well as in striatal and cerebrocortical neurons, both in intact cells and membranes [40] via metabotropic glutamate receptors (mGluRs), which are coupled to effector systems through GTP binding proteins. In fact, in the nucleus tractus solitarius of adult brain, it was shown that an antibody to the G_i inhibited the effects of mGluRs [44]. $mGluR_1$ and $mGluR_5$ subtypes are coupled to phosphatidyl inositol hydrolysis/Ca^{2+}-signal transduction. $mGluR_1$ has also been shown to stimulate release of arachidonic acid and to increase cAMP formation. The $mGluR_2$, $mGluR_3$, $mGluR_4$, and $mGluR_5$ subtypes appear to be coupled to inhibition

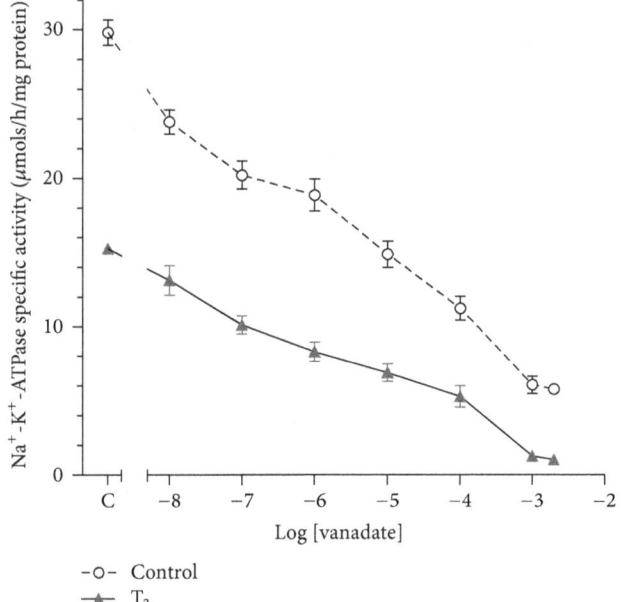

FIGURE 8: Modulation of the T_3 action on synaptosomal Na^+-K^+-ATPase activity by sodium orthovanadate. A higher dose of T_3 (10 nM) was chosen from the T_3 dose-response curve considering its greater inhibitory action on the Na^+-K^+-ATPase activity and to observe the effect of graded doses (1 nM–2 mM) of sodium orthovanadate on this T_3-induced inhibition. The data are represented as mean ± SEM of four separate experiments, taking six animals in each group. The vertical bars denote SEM. Open circles indicate mean values for a set of control incubations without T_3. Filled triangles indicate the results of a set of incubations with 10 nM T_3.

of cAMP synthesis, but differ in their agonist selectivity. mGluR$_2$ and mGluR$_3$ mRNAs are highly expressed in the cerebral cortex [40, 42, 43]. Activation of mGluR has been shown to counteract β-adrenoceptor-mediated inhibition of afterhyperpolarization in hippocampal neurons of the CA1 area. This has been suggested to be by mGluR-mediated activation of protein kinase C, which inhibited adenylate cyclase pathways [42, 43]. The physiological functions of these mGluRs are still being clarified. Thus, T_3 action in adult rat synaptosomal membrane, ultimately to inhibit the effector molecule Na^+-K^+-ATPase, might be mediated through G_s stimulation. mGlu receptors may then have some regulatory roles in counteracting T_3-induced action.

Our observation showed that DB cAMP (a nonhydrolyzable form of cAMP and activator of cAMP-dependent protein kinases) had a T_3-like effect on Na^+-K^+-ATPase activity (Figure 7). Furthermore, the *in vitro* addition of increased doses of T_3 lowered the slope of the dose-response curve for DB cAMP. Such a finding might be consistent with a related mechanism for the effects of DB cAMP and T_3, and would not represent merely additive effects of two distinct mechanisms. Our previous observations suggested that the phosphorylation status of certain synaptosomal proteins could be mediated via cAMP- and/or Ca^{2+}-dependent pathways [12, 45]. A differential stoichiometry of phosphorylation of the α-subunit of the Na^+-K^+-ATPase by protein kinase A

and protein kinase C has been shown to inhibit this enzymatic activity in shark rectal gland, rat renal cortex, and basolateral membrane vesicles from rat renal cortex [46].

The effect of the protein tyrosine phosphatase inhibitor sodium orthovanadate [47] appeared to be additive to the effect of T_3, implying that there could be a separate mechanism of action of the two compounds (Figure 8). Since vanadate is a blocker of tyrosine phosphatase activity, it also could be speculated that T_3-induced inhibition of Na^+-K^+-ATPase activity is further suppressed by synergistic action by vanadate via keeping the enzyme in its phosphorylated form, causing inhibition of its activity. A point to note here is that the α-subunit is the catalytic subunit and its phosphorylation causes inhibition of this enzyme [46]. T_3 appears not to have the inhibitory effect on Na^+-K^+-ATPase activity by an influence on phosphatase activity.

5. Conclusion

Our results regarding T_3 action in relation to the inhibition of synaptosomal Na^+-K^+-ATPase are consistent with a T_3-synaptosomal membrane component binding site interaction sensitive to the activation of G_i-protein. Such a membrane binding component might interact with a G_s-protein, resulting in increased synthesis of cAMP. The membrane Na^+-K^+-ATPase is involved in several aspects of physiological processes. In the neuron, its inhibition is linked with neurotransmitter release [46]. Hence, the present study provides further evidence of a nongenomic membrane-related action of T_3 in the mature mammalian synaptosome. Understanding of the mechanism of action of TH in adult mammalian brain has major implications in the higher mental functions and in the regulation of several neuropsychiatric disorders developed in thyroid dysfunctions in adult humans.

Acknowledgments

Financial support was from the Council of Scientific & Industrial Research, India, and the Department of Science & Technology, Government of India, to Pradip K. Sarkar, and NSF grant IBN-0110961 to Pradip K. Sarkar and Joseph V. Martin.

References

[1] J. H. Dussault and J. Ruel, "Thyroid hormones and brain development," *Annual Review of Physiology*, vol. 49, pp. 321–334, 1987.

[2] J. Puymirat, "Thyroid receptors in the rat brain," *Progress in Neurobiology*, vol. 39, no. 3, pp. 281–294, 1992.

[3] J. H. Oppenheimer, "Evolving concepts of thyroid hormone action," *Biochimie*, vol. 81, no. 5, pp. 539–543, 1999.

[4] J. Zhang and M. A. Lazar, "The mechanism of action of thyroid hormones," *Annual Review of Physiology*, vol. 62, pp. 439–466, 2000.

[5] M. B. Dratman and J. T. Gordon, "Thyroid hormones as neurotransmitters," *Thyroid*, vol. 6, no. 6, pp. 639–647, 1996.

[6] W. N. Henley and T. J. Koehnle, "Thyroid hormones and the treatment of depression: an examination of basic hormonal

actions in the mature mammalian brain," *Synapse*, vol. 27, pp. 36–44, 1997.

[7] R. Bunevicius and A. J. Prange, "Mental improvement after replacement therapy with thyroxine plus triiodothyronine: relationship to cause of hypothyroidism," *International Journal of Neuropsychopharmacology*, vol. 3, no. 2, pp. 167–174, 2000.

[8] G. A. Mason, C. H. Walker, and A. J. Prange, "L-triiodothyronine: is this peripheral hormone a central neurotransmitter?" *Neuropsychopharmacology*, vol. 8, no. 3, pp. 253–258, 1993.

[9] P. K. Sarkar and A. K. Ray, "Synaptosomal T_3 content in cerebral cortex of adult rat in different thyroidal states," *Neuropsychopharmacology*, vol. 11, no. 3, pp. 151–155, 1994.

[10] Y. Mashio, M. Inada, and K. Tanaka, "Synaptosomal T_3 binding sites in rat brain: their localization on synaptic membrane and regional distribution," *Acta Endocrinologica*, vol. 104, no. 2, pp. 134–138, 1983.

[11] P. K. Sarkar and A. K. Ray, "Specific binding of L-triiodothyronine modulates Na^+-K^+-ATPase activity in adult rat cerebrocortical synaptosomes," *NeuroReport*, vol. 9, no. 6, pp. 1149–1152, 1998.

[12] P. K. Sarkar, N. D. Durga, J. J. Morris, and J. V. Martin, "In vitro thyroid hormone rapidly modulates protein phosphorylation in cerebrocortical synaptosomes from adult rat brain," *Neuroscience*, vol. 137, no. 1, pp. 125–132, 2006.

[13] P. K. Sarkar and A. K. Ray, "Calcium mobilization within hypothyroid adult rat brain synaptosomes," *Hormone and Metabolic Research*, vol. 35, no. 9, pp. 562–564, 2003.

[14] G. A. Mason, C. H. Walker, and A. J. Prange Jr., "Depolarization-dependent ^{45}Ca uptake by synaptosomes of rat cerebral cortex is enhanced by L-triiodothyronine," *Neuropsychopharmacology*, vol. 3, no. 4, pp. 291–295, 1990.

[15] N. Chakrabarti and A. K. Ray, "Rise of intrasynaptosomal Ca^{2+} level and activation of nitric oxide synthase in adult rat cerebral cortex pretreated with 3-5-3′-L-triiodothyronine," *Neuropsychopharmacology*, vol. 22, no. 1, pp. 36–41, 2000.

[16] Z. Iqbal, H. Koenig, and J. J. Trout, "Triiodothyronine (T3) stimulates calcium influx and membrane trasport processes in nerve cells and terminals of hypothyroid mouse cortex," *Federation proceedings*, vol. 43, p. 735, 2002.

[17] R. B. Lomax, P. H. Cobbold, A. P. Allshire, K. S. R. Cuthbertson, and W. R. Robertson, "Tri-iodothyronine increases intracellular calcium levels in single rat myocytes," *Journal of Molecular Endocrinology*, vol. 7, no. 1, pp. 77–79, 1991.

[18] P. K. Sarkar and A. K. Ray, "Thyroid hormone and membrane-related processes in synaptosomes," in *Proceedings of the 60th Annual Meeting of Society of Biological Chemists (India)*, Section Endocrinology & Reproductive Biology, Abstract 147, 1991.

[19] P. K. Sarkar, *Thyroid hormone action in synaptosome of adult rat brain [Ph.D. thesis]*, University of Calcutta, Calcutta, India, 1995.

[20] P. K. Sarkar and A. K. Ray, "A simple biochemical approach to differentiate synaptosomes and non-synaptic mitochondria from rat brain," *Methods and Findings in Experimental and Clinical Pharmacology*, vol. 14, no. 7, pp. 493–497, 1992.

[21] P. K. Sarkar, "A quick assay for Na^+-K^+-ATPase specific activity," *Zeitschrift fur Naturforschung C*, vol. 57, no. 5-6, pp. 562–564, 2002.

[22] P. K. Sarkar and A. K. Ray, "Synaptosomal action of thyroid hormone: changes in Na^+-K^+-ATPase activity in adult rat cerebral cortex," *Hormone and Metabolic Research*, vol. 25, no. 1, pp. 1–3, 1993.

[23] J. C. Vera, "Measurement of microgram quantities of protein by a generally applicable turbidimetric procedure," *Analytical Biochemistry*, vol. 174, no. 1, pp. 187–196, 1988.

[24] J. J. Bergh, H. Lin, L. Lansing et al., "Integrin $\alpha V \beta 3$ contains a cell surface receptor site for thyroid hormone that is linked to activation of mitogen-activated protein kinase and induction of angiogenesis," *Endocrinology*, vol. 146, no. 7, pp. 2864–2871, 2005.

[25] F. B. Davis, S. A. Mousa, L. O'Connor et al., "Proangiogenic action of thyroid hormone is fibroblast growth factor-dependent and is initiated at the cell surface," *Circulation Research*, vol. 94, no. 11, pp. 1500–1506, 2004.

[26] A. B. Glinskii, G. V. Glinsky, H. Lin et al., "Modification of survival pathway gene expression in human breast cancer cells by tetraiodothyroacetic acid (tetrac)," *Cell Cycle*, vol. 8, no. 21, pp. 3554–3562, 2009.

[27] M. Bhargava, M. R. Runyon, D. Smirnov et al., "Triiodo-L-thyronine rapidly stimulates alveolar fluid clearance in normal and hyperoxia-injured lungs," *American Journal of Respiratory and Critical Care Medicine*, vol. 178, no. 5, pp. 506–512, 2008.

[28] J. Lei, C. N. Mariash, M. Bhargava, E. V. Wattenberg, and D. H. Ingbar, "T_3 increases Na-K-ATPase activity via a MAPK/ERK1/2-dependent pathway in rat adult alveolar epithelial cells," *American Journal of Physiology—Lung Cellular and Molecular Physiology*, vol. 294, no. 4, pp. L749–L754, 2008.

[29] H. Y. Lin, H. Y. Tang, F. B. Davis et al., "Nongenomic regulation by thyroid hormone of plasma membrane ion and small molecule pumps," *Discovery Medicine*, vol. 14, pp. 199–206, 2012.

[30] X. Cheng, J. Höög, A. C. Nairn, P. Greengard, and A. Aperia, "Regulation of rat Na^+-K^+-ATPase activity by PKC is modulated by state of phosphorylation of Ser-943 by PKA," *American Journal of Physiology—Cell Physiology*, vol. 273, no. 6, pp. C1981–C1986, 1997.

[31] X. Cheng, G. Fisone, O. Aizman et al., "PKA-mediated phosphorylation and inhibition of Na^+-K^+-ATPase in response to β-adrenergic hormone," *American Journal of Physiology—Cell Physiology*, vol. 273, no. 3, pp. C893–C901, 1997.

[32] R. M. Andersson, S. X. J. Cheng, and A. Aperia, "Forskolin-induced down-regulation of Na^+, K^+-ATPase activity is not associated with internalization of the enzyme," *Acta Physiologica Scandinavica*, vol. 164, no. 1, pp. 39–46, 1998.

[33] W. L. Stahl and R. W. Albers, "The Na,K-ATPase of nervous tissue," *Neurochemistry International*, vol. 8, no. 4, pp. 449–476, 1986.

[34] S. G. Amur, G. Shanker, and R. A. Pieringer, "β-adrenergic stimulation of protein (arginine) methyltransferase activity in cultured cerebral cells from embryonic mice," *Journal of Neuroscience Research*, vol. 16, no. 2, pp. 377–386, 1986.

[35] C. Huang, H. M. Geller, W. L. Green, and W. Craelius, "Acute effects of thyroid hormone analogs on sodium currents in neonatal rat myocytes," *Journal of Molecular and Cellular Cardiology*, vol. 31, no. 4, pp. 881–893, 1999.

[36] S. Shahrara, C. Sylven, and V. Drvota, "Subtype specific down-regulation of thyroid hormone receptor mRNA by β-adrenoreceptor blockade in the myocardium," *Biological and Pharmaceutical Bulletin*, vol. 23, no. 11, pp. 1303–1306, 2000.

[37] R. M. Graham, D. M. Perez, J. Hwa, and M. T. Piascik, "Alpha 1-adrenergic receptor subtypes. Molecular structure, function, and signaling," *Circulation Research*, vol. 78, no. 5, pp. 737–749, 1996.

[38] M. B. Conto and M. A. Venditti, "In vitro studies of the influence of glutamatergic agonists on the Na$^+$, K$^+$-ATPase and K$^+$-p-nitrophenylphosphatase activities in the hippocampus and frontal cortex of rats," *Journal of Negative Results in BioMedicine*, vol. 11, p. 12, 2012.

[39] W. L. Stahl and W. E. Harris, "Na$^+$,K$^+$-ATPase: structure, function, and interactions with drugs," *Advances in Neurology*, vol. 44, pp. 681–693, 1986.

[40] A. Levitzki, "Signal transduction in hormone-dependent adenylate cyclase," *Cell Biophysics*, vol. 12, pp. 133–143, 1988.

[41] E. M. Rose, J. C. P. Koo, J. E. Antflick, S. M. Ahmed, S. Angers, and D. R. Hampson, "Glutamate transporter coupling to Na,K-ATPase," *The Journal of Neuroscience*, vol. 29, no. 25, pp. 8143–8155, 2009.

[42] M. A. Musgrave, M. A. Madigan, B. M. Bennett, and J. W. Goh, "Stimulation of postsynaptic and inhibition of presynaptic adenylyl cyclase activity by metabotropic glutamate receptor activation," *Journal of Neurochemistry*, vol. 62, no. 6, pp. 2316–2324, 1994.

[43] R. Nouranifar, R. D. Blitzer, T. Wong, and E. Landau, "Metabotropic glutamate receptors limit adenylyl cyclase-mediated effects in rat hippocampus via protein kinase C," *Neuroscience Letters*, vol. 244, no. 2, pp. 101–105, 1998.

[44] T. Endoh, "Characterization of modulatory effects of postsynaptic metabotropic glutamate receptors on calcium currents in rat nucleus tractus solitarius," *Brain Research*, vol. 1024, no. 1-2, pp. 212–224, 2004.

[45] P. K. Sarkar, "l-Triiodothyronine differentially and nongenomically regulates synaptosomal protein phosphorylation in adult rat brain cerebral cortex: role of calcium and calmodulin," *Life Sciences*, vol. 82, no. 17-18, pp. 920–927, 2008.

[46] A. M. Bertorello, A. Aperia, S. I. Walaas, A. C. Nairn, and P. Greengard, "Phosphorylation of the catalytic subunit of Na$^+$,K$^+$-ATPase inhibits the activity of the enzyme," *Proceedings of the National Academy of Sciences of the United States of America*, vol. 88, no. 24, pp. 11359–11362, 1991.

[47] J. A. Gordon, "Use of vanadate as protein-phosphotyrosine phosphatase inhibitor," *Methods in Enzymology*, vol. 201, pp. 477–482, 1991.

8

Thyroid and Aging or the Aging Thyroid? An Evidence-Based Analysis

Naveen Aggarwal[1] and Salman Razvi[1,2]

[1] Department of Endocrinology, Gateshead Health NHS Foundation NHS Trust, UK
[2] Institute of Genetic Medicine, Newcastle University, UK

Correspondence should be addressed to Salman Razvi; salman.razvi@ncl.ac.uk

Academic Editor: Glenn D. Braunstein

Thyroid hormone production, metabolism, and action change with aging. The reference ranges for serum thyrotropin and thyroid hormones are derived mainly from younger populations. Thus, the prevalence of subclinical thyroid dysfunction is increased greatly in the elderly. However, it is unclear whether mild thyroid dysfunction in the elderly is associated with adverse outcomes. In this review, we discuss current evidence-based literature on thyroid function in the elderly and whether subclinical thyroid dysfunction in the elderly should be treated.

1. Introduction

As a result of declining fertility and increasing longevity, the populations of a growing number of countries are aging rapidly. Between 2005 and 2050, half of the increase in the world population will be accounted for by a rise in the population aged 60 years or over, whereas the number of children (persons under age 15) will decline slightly. Furthermore, in the more developed regions, the population aged 60 or over is expected to nearly double (from 245 million in 2005 to 406 million in 2050), whereas that of persons under age 60 will probably decline (from 971 million in 2005 to 839 million in 2050) [1].

As one ages, changes occur in all body systems including the endocrine system. These changes may be due to the amount of hormones secreted or the sensitivity of target organs. In some cases, the changes in amount of hormones secreted may be secondary to changes in target organs (e.g., LH and FSH). In addition, there may also be some change in the rate of metabolism of other hormones (e.g., increased peripheral degradation of thyroid hormones) [2].

There has been increasing interest in thyroid function in the elderly because of association of thyroid status with disability, cognitive function, cardiovascular disease risk, and longevity. The effects of overt thyroid dysfunction are well documented in all age groups. The effects of subclinical thyroid disease in elderly population are still unclear, mainly due to lack of randomized control trials (RCTs). In this paper, we evaluate the evidence about association of subclinical thyroid disease in the elderly with adverse outcomes and the evidence regarding intervention in this particular age group.

2. What Is "Normal Thyroid Function" in the Elderly?

There has been long standing controversy about the thyroid function test results in the elderly [3]. Serum TSH, free T4, and free T3 concentrations change with aging [4–13]. The first Whickham survey, published in 1977, showed that TSH levels did not vary with age in males but increased markedly in females after the age of 45 years. The rise of TSH with age in females was virtually abolished when persons with thyroid antibodies were excluded from the sample [14]. However, in this landmark study, the number of individuals aged 75 or more was quite small, thus limiting the ability to detect a significant increase in TSH in this age group. The 20-year follow-up Whickham survey showed that with increasing age, the incidence of positive antithyroid antibodies and hypothyroidism also increased [15]. This follow-up study, though, was unable to assess longitudinal change in serum TSH and thyroid hormones as more sensitive assays had been utilized, thus making any meaningful comparisons difficult. The larger and more recent NHANESIII survey showed that serum TSH concentrations as well as serum thyroid peroxidase (TPOAb) and thyroglobulin (TgAb) antibodies rise with age in both men and women [16]. In this study, the median TSH increased and T4 decreased after age 20 in all ethnic groups, even after excluding thyroid antibody status and other risk factors. In a subsequent further analysis, Surks and Hollowell examined the NHANESIII data which showed a progressive increase in mean, median, and 97.5 centile for TSH concentration with age in the disease-free and reference populations. This analysis suggested that the 97.5 centile is about 3.6 mIU/litre in people who are 20–39 yr of age and 5.9 and 7.5 mIU/litre in those who are 70–79 and 80 yr old and older, respectively [17]. They also demonstrated that about 70% of older patients who would be classified as subclinical hypothyroidism with TSH greater than 4.5 mIU/litre were within their age-specific reference range. Consequently, the authors have suggested that age-based reference ranges for TSH should be considered [18].

Moreover, a recent longitudinal study from Western Australia (Busselton survey), for the first time, showed that serum TSH increases (mean increase of 0.32 mU/L over 13 years) with no significant change in free T4 concentrations with aging [19]. Similarly, another longitudinal thyroid function evaluation in a very elderly subgroup (mean age 85 years) of the Cardiovascular Health Study (All Stars Study) found that serum TSH increased by 13% over an average of 13 years of follow-up associated with a 1.7% increase in FT4 and a 13% reduction in total T3 levels [20].

All the above studies (Whickham, NHANESIII, Busselton, and CVHS All Stars Surveys) have been conducted in iodine sufficient areas. Contrary to these findings, a cross-sectional study performed in an area of borderline sufficient iodine intake showed that serum TSH concentrations decreased gradually with age throughout life, whereas FT4 levels increased only in participants older than 60 years [21]. The authors hypothesized that this finding could be a result of development of thyroid autonomy after longstanding iodine insufficiency although iodine status itself was not measured in this cohort. An earlier study performed in a previously iodine deficient area in Germany showed a lower reference range (0.25 to 2.12 mIU/litre) for serum TSH in people without thyroid disease [22].

Moreover, there are studies which show that subclinical hypothyroidism and subclinical hyperthyroidism may correct spontaneously over time. A study by Parle et al. showed that over 1 year follow-up, TSH returned to normal spontaneously in 5% of people aged 60 years or more with subclinical hypothyroidism and in 76% of patients with low but detectable TSH [23]. In another similar and larger study, albeit in adults across all age groups, over a 5-year period, TSH normalized without any intervention in more than 50% of patients with elevated or decreased serum TSH level [24].

Setting an upper limit for the normal value of TSH for a population has implications for the diagnosis of subclinical hypothyroidism as well as related issues such as screening, association with comorbidities, especially cardiovascular risks, and treatment. Thus, the current data support the view that serum TSH rises slightly with aging, but the data on free T4 is conflicting. Prospective large studies are required to confirm whether age-specific reference ranges should be utilized when reporting thyroid parameters.

3. Thyroid Status and Cardiovascular Risks

A number of studies have shown an association between hypothyroidism and atherosclerosis; one of the early ones being the study by Vanhaelst et al. in 1967, which showed a greater prevalence and severity of coronary atherosclerosis in the hypothyroid patients as compared to controls [25].

Subclinical hypothyroidism (SCH) is associated with impaired left ventricular diastolic function at rest, systolic dysfunction on effort, and enhanced risk for atherosclerosis and myocardial infarction [26]. SCH has been shown to be associated with adverse lipid profile [27–29], increased carotid intimal thickness [28], and endothelial dysfunction [29, 30], with all these parameters reversing with levothyroxine replacement.

A fundamental issue to consider is the effect of age on the association between SCH and ischemic heart disease (IHD). The Cardiovascular Health Study cohort showed that in people above age of 65, SCH is not associated with increased risk of cardiovascular disease, mortality, or heart failure, although the latter was significantly higher in those with serum TSH > 10 mIU/litre [31, 32]. A similar result was obtained in an analysis from the Health, Aging, and Body Composition Study of individuals aged 70–79 years [33]. In a meta-analysis performed by one of the authors of this review, subjects were divided into those below and those above the age of 65 years [34]. Interestingly, the incidence and prevalence of IHD and cardiovascular mortality was higher in the younger age group but not in the group above 65 years of age. Another recent study has shown no association between persistent or transient subclinical hypothyroidism and incident IHD, heart failure, or cardiovascular death [35]. In this study, the authors used 2 models to define persistent SCH: in one model, there were two readings of TSH in SCH range in samples taken 2 years apart, and in the second model, there were 4 readings in similar range over a period of up to 8 years. In both of these models, the findings were similar: not showing any association between SCH and cardiovascular disease. Furthermore, an observational study of *real life* practice performed from data obtained from the United Kingdom General Practitioners Research Database (GPRD) showed that treatment of SCH with levothyroxine was associated with fewer IHD events in younger individuals (40–70 years), but this was not evident in older people (>70 years) [36]. The Leiden 85+ study in which 599 people were followed from age of 85 years through age 89 years (mean follow up 3.7 years) showed that increasing levels of TSH and decreasing levels of free thyroxine, both representing lower thyroid function, were associated with a survival benefit mainly due to reduced IHD events [37].

There have been a number of observational studies reporting an association of subclinical hyperthyroidism with IHD [38, 39], atrial fibrillation [31, 39–41], and cardiac dysfunction [32, 42]. A recent large study by Collet et al. [43] pooled individual data from 10 prospective cohort studies and concluded that endogenous subclinical hyperthyroidism is associated with increased risks of total and IHD mortality, and incident AF, with highest risks of IHD mortality and AF when TSH level is lower than 0.10 mIU/litre.

These results indicate that a higher TSH in the elderly may not have any adverse effects on the cardiovascular system and may even be protective. On the other hand, a low TSH is associated with adverse vascular outcomes. Large adequately designed trials are required to confirm that the association between serum TSH levels and adverse vascular outcomes in the elderly is causal. At this juncture, one European study has commenced recruitment investigating whether levothyroxine treatment improves outcomes in SCH patients aged 65 years or older [44].

4. Thyroid Status and Cognitive Function

Overt hypothyroidism is associated with cognitive impairment and depression [45–48]. There are few studies that have explored the relationship between thyroid function in euthyroid elderly people and cognition [37, 49–53]. All studies have shown a relationship between thyroid function and cognition, but the results are conflicting regarding the most sensitive marker (TSH, T4, or T3). Furthermore, there is variation regarding the particular domain of cognition affected by changes in thyroid hormone concentrations.

A number of studies have shown the adverse effect of SCH on cognition in younger age groups [54–56]. However, in the elderly population, the studies give conflicting results. One study in individuals with mean age of 74 years showed that people with SCH had worse performance on verbal recall and MMSE, but working memory and processing speed were unaffected [57]. The PAQUID survey of individuals aged 65 yr or more showed that increased TSH levels were significantly linked with the presence of symptoms of depression but not with impairment of cognitive function [58]. There have been other studies which also do not support any association between SCH and cognitive impairment [59–62].

There have been few RCTs investigating improvement in cognition with levothyroxine replacement in SCH. Three small RCTs in middle aged individuals showed improvement in cognitive function with levothyroxine replacement therapy in people with SCH [63–65]. Two larger RCTs with longer followup have not shown any benefit in cognition with levothyroxine replacement [66, 67]; the latter study was specifically in the elderly population aged 65 years or over.

A recent systematic review has considered the association of subclinical hyperthyroidism with dementia [68]. It concluded that there is a substantial body of evidence to support the association between subclinical hyperthyroidism and cognitive impairment. It also concluded that at present, there is lack of evidence to suggest that antithyroid treatment might ameliorate dementia.

5. Thyroid Status, Depression, and Disability

Some studies have shown an association of subclinical thyroid disease with depression [57, 65]. In the Leiden 85+ study which studied individuals > 85 years in age, no consistent association between thyroid status and disability or depressive symptoms was detected [37]. Another observational study also showed that SCH is not associated with metabolic derangement, cognitive impairment, depression, or poor quality of life (QoL) in elderly subjects [61]. A recent study too did not support deleterious effects of subclinical thyroid disorders on physical or cognitive function, depression, or mortality in an older population [62]. Analysis of individuals aged 70–79 years from the Health, Aging, and Body Composition Study showed that higher TSH may be associated with a slight functional mobility advantage [69]. The RCT by Jorde et al. concluded that in SCH where the serum TSH level is in the 3.5–10.0 mIU/litre range, there is no neuropsychological dysfunction or increased symptoms of hypothyroidism compared those in with healthy controls [66].

6. Thyroid Status and Longevity

There have been few studies exploring the effect of thyroid disease on mortality and longevity in the elderly population. It is important to point out that these results differ from studies in younger population, and they should not be extrapolated to them.

As mentioned earlier, the Leiden 85+ study showed that higher TSH concentrations and lower free thyroxine levels were associated with a survival benefit [37]. In this study, participants with low levels of TSH at baseline had highest mortality rate, and participants with high TSH levels and low FT4 levels had the lowest mortality rate. The authors speculated that lower thyroid function may lead to lower metabolic rate which in turn could cause caloric restriction. Lower metabolic rate and caloric restriction have both been shown to be associated with improved survival in several animal studies [70–72].

Atzmon et al. conducted their study in elderly Ashkenazi Jews with the median age of study population being 98 years [73]. They demonstrated that centenarians have significantly higher median serum TSH concentrations compared with younger Ashkenazi controls (median age 72 years) and in a population of thyroid disease-free individuals (median age 68 yr) from the US National Health and Nutrition Examination Survey 1998–2002. Similar results were noted in the study by van den Beld et al. who showed that low serum free T4 was associated with a better 4-year survival in men aged 73 to 94 years [74]. The study by de Jongh et al. showed no difference in mortality in elderly population with subclinical thyroid disorders [62]. Another recent study in men aged > 65 years concluded that there was no beneficial or detrimental effect of subclinical thyroid dysfunction in older men [75]. On the other hand, various studies have shown subclinical hyperthyroidism to be associated with higher mortality or no association with mortality. The studies by van den Beld et al. [74] and de Jongh et al. [62] have not shown any change in mortality in their subjects with subclinical hyperthyroidism. Previously, Parle et al. showed that a single measurement of low serum thyrotropin in individuals aged 60 years or older is associated with increased mortality from all causes, and in particular mortality due to circulatory and cardiovascular diseases [38]. Similar results were found by Collet et al. [43] that endogenous subclinical hyperthyroidism is associated with increased risks of total as well as IHD mortality, with highest risks of CHD mortality and AF when TSH level is lower than 0.10 mIU/litre.

These results are not entirely unexpected as similar results have been shown in animal studies. It has been reported that rats in which hyperthyroidism was induced had a shorter life span [76, 77]. Wistar rats with induced hypothyroidism had a longer life span than euthyroid rats [78]. Ames and Snell dwarf mice have low levels of prolactin, growth hormone, and thyroid hormones and have both reduced body core temperature and metabolic rates consistent with hypothyroidism and live 40–70% longer than euthyroid mice [79].

There have been few recent studies exploring the longevity with raised TSH and familial/genetic basis for this phenomenon. Rozing et al. in Leiden Longevity Study showed that when compared with their partners, the group of offspring of nonagenarian siblings showed a trend toward higher serum TSH levels in conjunction with lower free T4 levels and lower free T3 levels [80]. In their extension to this study, they found that lower mortality in the parents of nonagenarian siblings was associated with higher serum TSH levels, lower free serum T4 levels, and lower free T3 levels in the nonagenarian siblings [81]. In the study of Ashkenazi Jews, a heritable phenotype characterized by raised serum TSH which is associated with human longevity was identified. Carriers of rs12050077 and rs10149689 single nucleotide polymorphism in the TSH receptor gene had higher serum TSH, possibly contributing to decreased thyroid function and longevity [82].

7. Thyroid Status and Bone Health

In 1891, von Recklinghausen reported a "worm eaten" appearance of the long bones in a young woman who died from hyperthyroidism [83]. Thyroid hormone affects bone calcium metabolism by direct action on osteoclasts or by acting on osteoblasts which in turn mediate osteoclastic bone resorption [84]. TSH may also have a direct effect on bone formation and bone resorption, mediated via the TSH receptor on osteoblast and osteoclast precursors [85]. Various studies have examined the association of thyroid function with bone mineral density (BMD) and/or fracture risk. In the Tromsø study, the subjects with serum TSH below the 2.5 centile had significantly lower BMD as compared to that of controls with serum TSH in the normal range. Conversely, the postmenopausal women with serum TSH above the 97.5 centile had significantly higher BMD at the femoral neck than women with serum TSH in the normal range [86].

A study from Japan, using quantitative ultrasound, demonstrated that subclinical hypothyroidism does not affect bone turnover but has an impact on bone structure [87].

In the Study of Osteoporotic Fractures in women > 65 years, low TSH was not associated with BMD or accelerated bone loss in older ambulatory women [88]. However, the study group, analysing data from the same cohort, also showed that low serum TSH levels were associated with increased risk for new hip and vertebral fractures [89]. Another study in men > 65 years showed that patients with subclinical hyperthyroidism or hypothyroidism were at increased risk of hip fracture [90]. The recent MrOS study concluded that although neither TSH nor FT4 are associated with bone loss, lower serum TSH may be associated with an increased risk of hip fractures in older men [91]. There has been two meta-analyses on the effects of long-term thyroxine replacement [92, 93]. Both of these showed that levothyroxine therapy leading to suppressed TSH was associated with significant bone loss in postmenopausal women but not those that were premenopausal.

8. Conclusions and Recommendations

There is increasing wealth of data suggesting that serum TSH levels increase with age, particularly after 70 years. This might reflect reduced end organ sensitivity, reduced turnover, and clearance, a genetic trait conferring a survival benefit or a combination of factors. In addition, no clear benefit is seen in treating a high TSH on a multitude of outcomes in the elderly. In fact, there is a possibility that treatment of SCH in the very elderly may lead to adverse outcomes. On the other hand, a low TSH has been associated with worse outcomes in the older age group. However, to confirm these findings, large scale intervention trials assessing mortality, cardiovascular events, mood, disability, fractures, and cognition are required. This could then lead to the use of age-specific TSH reference ranges.

9. Summary of Recommendations— For Elderly Population Only

(i) Thyroid function results in the elderly (>70 years) should be interpreted with caution as the "normal" range may be different from that in younger population.

(ii) A single abnormal TSH result should be monitored over time as a substantial number of people with subclinical thyroid disease will normalise spontaneously.

(iii) Subclinical hypothyroidism may be associated with adverse cardiac outcome if TSH is > 10 mU/litre, but there is no evidence that it has any adverse cardiac effect in people with TSH < 10 mU/litre.

(iv) Subclinical hyperthyroidism is associated with increased incidence of heart failure, AF, IHD, and mortality, especially if TSH is < 0.1 mU/litre.

(v) There is conflicting evidence linking subclinical hypothyroidism with cognitive impairment, but more recent larger studies are against any association or benefit with intervention.

(vi) Subclinical hyperthyroidism is associated with higher incidence of cognitive impairment, but at present, there is no evidence to support use of antithyroid drugs for dementia.

(vii) There appears to be no association of subclinical thyroid disease with depression and physical disability.

(viii) Subclinical hypothyroidism appears to lead to a survival benefit in the elderly population.

(ix) Subclinical hyperthyroidism appears to be associated with higher mortality.

(x) Subclinical hypothyroidism in elderly people should not be treated routinely if TSH is < 10 mU/litre and if the patient is otherwise well.

(xi) Subclinical hyperthyroidism on the other hand should be evaluated further especially regarding other cardiovascular risk factors and comorbidities, and then a decision should be made regarding treatment, especially in people with TSH < 0.1 mU/litre.

References

[1] "World Population Prospects. The 2006 Revision. Executive Summary," United Nations, Department of Economic and Social Affairs, Population Division, 2006.

[2] S. Mariotti, C. Franceschi, A. Cossarizza, and A. Pinchera, "The aging thyroid," *Endocrine Reviews*, vol. 16, no. 6, pp. 686–715, 1995.

[3] K. A. Woeber, "Aging and the thyroid," *The Western Journal of Medicine*, vol. 143, no. 5, pp. 668–669, 1985.

[4] R. D. Hesch, J. Gatz, and J. Pape, "Total and free triiodothyronine and thyroid binding globulin concentration in elderly human persons," *European Journal of Clinical Investigation*, vol. 6, no. 2, pp. 139–145, 1976.

[5] J. Herrmann, H. J. Rusche, H. J. Kröll, P. Hilger, and H. L. Krüskemper, "Free triiodothyronine T3 and thyroxine T4 serum levels in old age," *Hormone and Metabolic Research*, vol. 6, no. 3, pp. 239–240, 1974.

[6] R. D. Hesch, J. Gatz, H. Jueppner, and P. Stubbe, "TBG dependency of age related variations of thyroxine and triiodothyronine," *Hormone and Metabolic Research*, vol. 9, no. 2, pp. 141–146, 1977.

[7] T. Pawlikowski, I. Owczarczyk, J. K. Komorowski andWisniewska Roszkowska, and W. Roszkowska, "Blood serum thyroxine and triiodothyronine in men over 60," *Endokrynologia Polska*, vol. 26, no. 6, pp. 593–601, 1975.

[8] U. Westgren, A. Burger, and S. Ingemansson, "Blood levels of 3,5,3′ triiodothyronine and thyroxine: differences between children, adults, and elderly subjects," *Acta Medica Scandinavica*, vol. 200, no. 6, pp. 493–495, 1976.

[9] H. A. Rubenstein, V. P. Butler Jr., and S. C. Werner, "Progressive decrease in serum triiodothyronine concentrations with human aging: radioimmunoassay following extraction of serum," *Journal of Clinical Endocrinology and Metabolism*, vol. 37, no. 2, pp. 247–253, 1973.

[10] W. Jeske and M. Thorner, "Serum T3 T4 and TSH in the elderly," *Endokrynologia Polska*, vol. 28, no. 2, pp. 117–123, 1977.

[11] J. Herrmann, H. J. Rusche, H. J. Kroll, K. H. Rudorff, and H. L. Krüskemper, "Trijodthyronin: abnahme der serumkonzentration mit zunehmendem alter," *Deutsche Medizinische Wochenschrif*, vol. 99, no. 42, pp. 2122–2124, 1974.

[12] J. M. Hansen, L. Skovsted, and K. Siersbaek Nielsen, "Age dependent changes in iodine metabolism and thyroid function," *Acta Endocrinologica*, vol. 79, no. 1, pp. 60–65, 1975.

[13] A. Lipson, E. L. Nickoloff, and T. H. Hsu, "A study of age-dependent changes in thyroid function tests in adults," *Journal of Nuclear Medicine*, vol. 20, no. 11, pp. 1124–1130, 1979.

[14] W. M. G. Tunbridge, D. C. Evered, and R. Hall, "The spectrum of thyroid disease in a community: the Whickham survey," *Clinical Endocrinology*, vol. 7, no. 6, pp. 481–493, 1977.

[15] M. P. J. Vanderpump, W. M. G. Tunbridge, J. M. French et al., "The incidence of thyroid disorders in the community: a twenty-year follow-up of the Whickham Survey," *Clinical Endocrinology*, vol. 43, no. 1, pp. 55–68, 1995.

[16] J. G. Hollowell, N. W. Staehling, W. Dana Flanders et al., "Serum TSH, T4, and thyroid antibodies in the United States population (1988 to 1994): national Health and Nutrition Examination Survey (NHANES III)," *Journal of Clinical Endocrinology and Metabolism*, vol. 87, no. 2, pp. 489–499, 2002.

[17] M. I. Surks and J. G. Hollowell, "Age-specific distribution of serum thyrotropin and antithyroid antibodies in the U.S. population: implications for the prevalence of subclinical hypothyroidism," *Journal of Clinical Endocrinology and Metabolism*, vol. 92, no. 12, pp. 4575–4582, 2007.

[18] M. I. Surks and L. Boucai, "Age- and race-based serum thyrotropin reference limits," *Journal of Clinical Endocrinology and Metabolism*, vol. 95, no. 2, pp. 496–502, 2010.

[19] A. P. Bremner, P. Feddema, P. J. Leedman et al., "Age-related changes in thyroid function: a longitudinal study of a community-based cohort," *Journal of Clinical Endocrinology & Metabolism*, vol. 97, pp. 1554–1562, 2012.

[20] A. C. Waring, A. M. Arnold, A. B. Newman, P. Bùzková, C. Hirsch, and A. R. Cappola, "Longitudinal changes in thyroid function in the oldest old and survival: the cardiovascular health study all-stars study," *Journal of Clinical Endocrinology & Metabolism*, vol. 97, no. 11, pp. 3944–3950, 2012.

[21] E. H. Hoogendoorn, A. R. Hermus, F. de Vegt et al., "Thyroid function and prevalence of anti-thyroperoxidase antibodies in a population with borderline sufficient iodine intake: influences of age and sex," *Clinical Chemistry*, vol. 52, no. 1, pp. 104–111, 2006.

[22] H. Völzke, D. Alte, T. Kohlmann et al., "Reference intervals of serum thyroid function tests in a previously iodine-deficient area," *Thyroid*, vol. 15, no. 3, pp. 279–285, 2005.

[23] J. V. Parle, J. A. Franklyn, K. W. Cross, S. C. Jones, and M. C. Sheppard, "Prevalence and follow-up of abnormal thyrotrophin (TSH) concentrations in the elderly in the United Kingdom," *Clinical Endocrinology*, vol. 34, no. 1, pp. 77–83, 1991.

[24] J. Meyerovitch, P. Rotman-Pikielny, M. Sherf, E. Battat, Y. Levy, and M. I. Surks, "Serum thyrotropin measurements in the community: five-year follow-up in a large network of primary care physicians," *Archives of Internal Medicine*, vol. 167, no. 14, pp. 1533–1538, 2007.

[25] L. Vanhaelst, P. Neve, P. Chailly, and P. A. Bastenie, "Coronary-artery disease in hypothyroidism. Observations in clinical myxoedema," *Lancet*, vol. 2, no. 7520, pp. 800–802, 1967.

[26] B. Biondi, E. A. Palmieri, G. Lombardi, and S. Fazio, "Effects of subclinical thyroid dysfunction on the heart," *Annals of Internal Medicine*, vol. 137, no. 11, pp. 904–914, 2002.

Thyroid and Aging or the Aging Thyroid? An Evidence-Based Analysis

71

[27] N. Caraccio, E. Ferrannini, and F. Monzani, "Lipoprotein profile in subclinical hypothyroidism: response to levothyroxine replacement, a randomized placebo-controlled study," *Journal of Clinical Endocrinology and Metabolism*, vol. 87, no. 4, pp. 1533–1538, 2002.

[28] F. Monzani, N. Caraccio, M. Kozàkowà et al., "Effect of levothyroxine replacement on lipid profile and intima-media thickness in subclinical hypothyroidism: a double-blind, placebo-controlled study," *Journal of Clinical Endocrinology and Metabolism*, vol. 89, no. 5, pp. 2099–2106, 2004.

[29] S. Razvi, L. Ingoe, G. Keeka, C. Oates, C. McMillan, and J. U. Weaver, "The beneficial effect of L-thyroxine on cardiovascular risk factors, endothelial function, and quality of life in subclinical hypothyroidism: randomized, crossover trial," *Journal of Clinical Endocrinology and Metabolism*, vol. 92, no. 5, pp. 1715–1723, 2007.

[30] S. Taddei, N. Caraccio, A. Virdis et al., "Impaired endothelium-dependent vasodilatation in subclinical hypothyroidism: beneficial effect of levothyroxine therapy," *Journal of Clinical Endocrinology and Metabolism*, vol. 88, no. 8, pp. 3731–3737, 2003.

[31] A. R. Cappola, L. P. Fried, A. M. Arnold et al., "Thyroid status, cardiovascular risk, and mortality in older adults," *Journal of the American Medical Association*, vol. 295, no. 9, pp. 1033–1041, 2006.

[32] N. Rodondi, D. C. Bauer, A. R. Cappola et al., "Subclinical thyroid dysfunction, cardiac function, and the risk of heart failure: the cardiovascular health study," *Journal of the American College of Cardiology*, vol. 52, no. 14, pp. 1152–1159, 2008.

[33] N. Rodondi, A. B. Newman, E. Vittinghoff et al., "Subclinical hypothyroidism and the risk of heart failure, other cardiovascular events, and death," *Archives of Internal Medicine*, vol. 165, no. 21, pp. 2460–2466, 2005.

[34] S. Razvi, A. Shakoor, M. Vanderpump, J. U. Weaver, and S. H. S. Pearce, "The influence of age on the relationship between subclinical hypothyroidism and ischemic heart disease: a meta-analysis," *Journal of Clinical Endocrinology and Metabolism*, vol. 93, no. 8, pp. 2998–3007, 2008.

[35] K. A. Hyland, A. M. Arnold, J. S. Lee, and A. R. Cappola, "Persistent subclinical hypothyroidism and cardiovascular risk in the elderly: the cardiovascular health study," *Journal of Clinical Endocrinology & Metabolism*, vol. 98, no. 2, pp. 533–540, 2013 2013.

[36] S. Razvi, J. U. Weaver, T. J. Butler, and S. H. Pearce, "Levothyroxine treatment of subclinical hypothyroidism, fatal and nonfatal cardiovascular events, and mortality," *Archives of Internal Medicine*, vol. 172, no. 10, pp. 811–817, 2012.

[37] J. Gussekloo, E. van Exel, A. J. M. de Craen, A. E. Meinders, M. Frölich, and R. G. J. Westendorp, "Thyroid status, disability and cognitive function, and survival in old age," *Journal of the American Medical Association*, vol. 292, no. 21, pp. 2591–2599, 2004.

[38] J. V. Parle, P. Maisonneuve, M. C. Sheppard, P. Boyle, and J. A. Franklyn, "Prediction of all-cause and cardiovascular mortality in elderly people from one low serum thyrotropin result: a 10-year cohort study," *Lancet*, vol. 358, no. 9285, pp. 861–865, 2001.

[39] G. Iervasi, S. Molinaro, P. Landi et al., "Association between increased mortality and mild thyroid dysfunction in cardiac patients," *Archives of Internal Medicine*, vol. 167, no. 14, pp. 1526–1532, 2007.

[40] C. T. Sawin, A. Geller, P. A. Wolf et al., "Low serum thyrotropin concentrations as a risk factor for atrial fibrillation in older persons," *New England Journal of Medicine*, vol. 331, no. 19, pp. 1249–1252, 1994.

[41] J. Auer, P. Scheibner, T. Mische, W. Langsteger, O. Eber, and B. Eber, "Subclinical hyperthyroidism as a risk factor for atrial fibrillation," *American Heart Journal*, vol. 142, no. 5, pp. 838–842, 2001.

[42] B. Biondi, E. A. Palmieri, S. Fazio et al., "Endogenous subclinical hyperthyroidism affects quality of life and cardiac morphology and function in young and middle-aged patients," *Journal of Clinical Endocrinology and Metabolism*, vol. 85, no. 12, pp. 4701–4705, 2000.

[43] T. Collet, J. Gussekloo, D. C. Bauer et al., "Subclinical hyperthyroidism and the risk of coronary heart disease and mortality," *Archives of Internal Medicine*, vol. 172, no. 10, pp. 799–809, 2012.

[44] Thyroid Hormone Replacement for Subclinical Hypo-Thyroidism Trial (TRUST), http://www.trustthyroidtrial.com.

[45] J. D. Davis and G. Tremont, "Neuropsychiatric aspects of hypothyroidism and treatment reversibility," *Minerva Endocrinologica*, vol. 32, no. 1, pp. 49–65, 2007.

[46] A. T. Dugbartey, "Neurocognitive aspects of hypothyroidism," *Archives of Internal Medicine*, vol. 158, no. 13, pp. 1413–1418, 1998.

[47] R. Kamil and R. T. Joffe, "Neuroendocrine testing in electroconvulsive therapy," *Psychiatric Clinics of North America*, vol. 14, no. 4, pp. 961–970, 1991.

[48] C. B. Nemeroff and P. T. Loosen, *Handbook of Clinical Psychoneuroendocrinology*, Guilford Press, New York, NY, USA, 1987.

[49] M. P. J. van Boxtel, P. P. C. A. Menheere, O. Bekers, E. Hogervorst, and J. Jolles, "Thyroid function, depressed mood, and cognitive performance in older individuals: the Maastricht Aging Study," *Psychoneuroendocrinology*, vol. 29, no. 7, pp. 891–898, 2004.

[50] P. N. Prinz, J. M. Scanlan, P. P. Vitaliano et al., "Thyroid hormones: positive relationships with cognition in healthy, euthyroid older men," *Journals of Gerontology A*, vol. 54, no. 3, pp. M111–M116, 1999.

[51] S. Volpato, J. M. Guralnik, L. P. Fried, A. T. Remaley, A. R. Cappola, and L. J. Launer, "Serum thyroxine level and cognitive decline in euthyroid older women," *Neurology*, vol. 58, no. 7, pp. 1055–1061, 2002.

[52] Å. Wahlin, T. B. R. Wahlin, B. J. Small, and L. Bäckman, "Influences of thyroid stimulating hormone on cognitive functioning in very old age," *Journals of Gerontology B*, vol. 53, no. 4, pp. P234–P239, 1998.

[53] Å. Wahlin, D. Bunce, and T. B. R. Wahlin, "Longitudinal evidence of the impact of normal thyroid stimulating hormone variations on cognitive functioning in very old age," *Psychoneuroendocrinology*, vol. 30, no. 7, pp. 625–637, 2005.

[54] F. Monzani, P. Del Guerra, N. Caraccio et al., "Subclinical hypothyroidism: neurobehavioral features and beneficial effect of L-thyroxine treatment," *Clinical Investigator*, vol. 71, no. 5, pp. 367–371, 1993.

[55] I. M. Baldini, A. Vita, M. C. Mauri et al., "Psychopathological and cognitive features in subclinical hypothyroidism," *Progress in Neuro-Psychopharmacology and Biological Psychiatry*, vol. 21, no. 6, pp. 925–935, 1997.

[56] T. Del Ser Quijano, C. Delgado, S. Martínez Espinosa, and C. Vázquez, "Cognitive deficiency in mild hypothyroidism," *Neurologia*, vol. 15, no. 5, pp. 193–198, 2000.

[57] S. E. Cook, R. D. Nebes, E. M. Halligan et al., "Memory impairment in elderly individuals with a mildly elevated serum TSH:

the role of processing resources, depression and cerebrovascular disease," *Aging, Neuropsychology, and Cognition*, vol. 9, no. 3, pp. 175–183, 2002.

[58] G. Manciet, J. F. Dartigues, A. Decamps et al., "The PAQUID survey and correlates of subclinical hypothyroidism in elderly community residents in the southwest of France," *Age and Ageing*, vol. 24, no. 3, pp. 235–241, 1995.

[59] D. Osterweil, K. Syndulko, S. N. Cohen et al., "Cognitive function in non-demented older adults with hypothyroidism," *Journal of the American Geriatrics Society*, vol. 40, no. 4, pp. 325–335, 1992.

[60] R. Luboshitzky, A. S. Oberman, N. Kaufman, N. Reichman, and E. Flatau, "Prevalence of cognitive dysfunction and hypothyroidism in an elderly community population," *Israel Journal of Medical Sciences*, vol. 32, no. 1, pp. 60–65, 1996.

[61] Y. J. Park, E. J. Lee, Y. J. Lee et al., "Subclinical hypothyroidism (SCH) is not associated with metabolic derangement, cognitive impairment, depression or poor quality of life (QoL) in elderly subjects," *Archives of Gerontology and Geriatrics*, vol. 50, no. 3, pp. e68–e73, 2010.

[62] R. T. de Jongh, P. Lips, N. M. van Schoor et al., "Endogenous subclinical thyroid disorders, physical and cognitive function, depression, and mortality in older individuals," *European Journal of Endocrinology*, vol. 165, no. 4, pp. 545–554, 2011.

[63] E. Nystrom, K. Caidahl, G. Fager, C. Wikkelso, P. A. Lundberg, and G. Lindstedt, "A double-blind cross-over 12-month study of L-thyroxine treatment of women with 'subclinical' hypothyroidism," *Clinical Endocrinology*, vol. 29, no. 1, pp. 63–75, 1988.

[64] R. Jaeschke, G. Guyatt, H. Gerstein et al., "Does treatment with L-thyroxine influence health status in middle-aged and older adults with subclinical hypothyroidism?" *Journal of General Internal Medicine*, vol. 11, no. 12, pp. 744–749, 1996.

[65] M. H. Samuels, K. G. Schuff, N. E. Carlson, P. Carello, and J. S. Janowsky, "Health status, mood, and cognition in experimentally induced subclinical hypothyroidism," *Journal of Clinical Endocrinology and Metabolism*, vol. 92, no. 7, pp. 2545–2551, 2007.

[66] R. Jorde, K. Waterloo, H. Storhaug, A. Nyrnes, J. Sundsfjord, and T. G. Jenssen, "Neuropsychological function and symptoms in subjects with subclinical hypothyroidism and the effect of thyroxine treatment," *Journal of Clinical Endocrinology and Metabolism*, vol. 91, no. 1, pp. 145–153, 2006.

[67] J. Parle, L. Roberts, S. Wilson et al., "A randomized controlled trial of the effect of thyroxine replacement on cognitive function in community-living elderly subjects with subclinical hypothyroidism: the Birmingham elderly thyroid study," *Journal of Clinical Endocrinology and Metabolism*, vol. 95, no. 8, pp. 3623–3632, 2010.

[68] E. H. Gan and S. H. Pearce, "The thyroid in mind: cognitive function and low thyrotropin in older people," *Journal of Clinical Endocrinology & Metabolism*, vol. 97, no. 10, pp. 3438–3449, 2012.

[69] E. M. Simonsick, A. B. Newman, L. Ferrucci et al., "Subclinical hypothyroidism and functional mobility in older adults," *Archives of Internal Medicine*, vol. 169, no. 21, pp. 2011–2017, 2009.

[70] C. V. Mobbs, G. A. Bray, R. L. Atkinson et al., "Neuroendocrine and pharmacological manipulations to assess how caloric restriction increases life span," *The Journals of Gerontology A*, vol. 56, pp. 34–44, 2001.

[71] V. D. Longo and C. E. Finch, "Evolutionary medicine: from dwarf model systems to healthy centenarians?" *Science*, vol. 299, no. 5611, pp. 1342–1346, 2003.

[72] S. Blanc, D. Schoeller, J. Kemnitz et al., "Energy expenditure of rhesus monkeys subjected to 11 years of dietary restriction," *Journal of Clinical Endocrinology and Metabolism*, vol. 88, no. 1, pp. 16–23, 2003.

[73] G. Atzmon, N. Barzilai, J. G. Hollowell, M. I. Surks, and I. Gabriely, "Extreme Longevity is associated with increased serum thyrotropin," *Journal of Clinical Endocrinology and Metabolism*, vol. 94, no. 4, pp. 1251–1254, 2009.

[74] A. W. van den Beld, T. J. Visser, R. A. Feelders, D. E. Grobbee, and S. W. J. Lamberts, "Thyroid hormone concentrations, disease, physical function, and mortality in elderly men," *Journal of Clinical Endocrinology and Metabolism*, vol. 90, no. 12, pp. 6403–6409, 2005.

[75] A. C. Waring, S. Harrison, M. H. Samuels et al., "Thyroid function and mortality in older men: a prospective study," *Journal of Clinical Endocrinology and Metabolism*, vol. 97, no. 3, pp. 862–870, 2012.

[76] T. B. Robertson, "The influence of thyroid alone and of thyroid administered together with nucleic acids upon the growth and longevity of white mouses," *Australian Journal of Experimental Biology & Medical Science*, vol. 5, pp. 69–74, 1928.

[77] H. Ooka and T. Shinkai, "Effects of chronic hyperthyroidism on the lifespan of the rat," *Mechanisms of Ageing and Development*, vol. 33, no. 3, pp. 275–282, 1986.

[78] H. Ooka, S. Fujita, and E. Yoshimoto, "Pituitary-thyroid activity and longevity in neonatally thyroxine-treated rats," *Mechanisms of Ageing and Development*, vol. 22, no. 2, pp. 113–120, 1983.

[79] H. M. Brown-Borg, "Hormonal regulation of longevity in mammals," *Ageing Research Reviews*, vol. 6, no. 1, pp. 28–45, 2007.

[80] M. P. Rozing, R. G. J. Westendorp, A. J. M. de Craen et al., "Low serum free triiodothyronine levels mark familial longevity: the leiden longevity study," *Journals of Gerontology A*, vol. 65, no. 4, pp. 365–368, 2010.

[81] M. P. Rozing, J. J. Houwing-Duistermaat, P. E. Slagboom et al., "Familial longevity is associated with decreased thyroid function," *Journal of Clinical Endocrinology and Metabolism*, vol. 95, no. 11, pp. 4979–4984, 2010.

[82] G. Atzmon, N. Barzilai, M. I. Surks, and I. Gabriely, "Genetic predisposition to elevated serum thyrotropin is associated with exceptional longevity," *Journal of Clinical Endocrinology and Metabolism*, vol. 94, no. 12, pp. 4768–4775, 2009.

[83] F. D. von Recklinghausen, *Die Fibröse oder deformierende Ostitis, die Osteomalazie und die osteoplastische Carzinose in ihren gegenseitigen Beziehungen*, George Reimer, Berlin, Germany, 1891.

[84] J. M. Britto, A. J. Fenton, W. R. Holloway, and G. C. Nicholson, "Osteoblasts mediate thyroid hormone stimulation of osteoclastic bone resorption," *Endocrinology*, vol. 134, no. 1, pp. 169–176, 1994.

[85] E. Abe, R. C. Marians, W. Yu et al., "TSH is a negative regulator of skeletal remodeling," *Cell*, vol. 115, no. 2, pp. 151–162, 2003.

[86] G. Grimnes, N. Emaus, R. M. Joakimsen, Y. Figenschau, and R. Jorde, "The relationship between serum TSH and bone mineral density in men and postmenopausal women: the Tromsø study," *Thyroid*, vol. 18, no. 11, pp. 1147–1155, 2008.

[87] M. Nagata, A. Suzuki, S. Sekiguchi et al., "Subclinical hypothyroidism is related to lower heel QUS in postmenopausal women," *Endocrine Journal*, vol. 54, no. 4, pp. 625–630, 2007.

Thyroid and Aging or the Aging Thyroid? An Evidence-Based Analysis

73

[88] D. C. Bauer, M. C. Nevitt, B. Ettinger, and K. Stone, "Low thyrotropin levels are not associated with bone loss in older women: a prospective study," *Journal of Clinical Endocrinology and Metabolism*, vol. 82, no. 9, pp. 2931–2936, 1997.

[89] D. C. Bauer, B. Ettinger, M. C. Nevitt, and K. L. Stone, "Risk for fracture in women with low serum levels of thyroid-stimulating hormone," *Annals of Internal Medicine*, vol. 134, no. 7, pp. 561–568, 2001.

[90] J. S. Lee, P. Bůžková, H. A. Fink et al., "Subclinical thyroid dysfunction and incident hip fracture in older adults," *Archives of Internal Medicine*, vol. 170, no. 21, pp. 1876–1883, 2010.

[91] A. C. Waring, S. Harrison, H. A. Fink et al., "A prospective study of thyroid function, bone loss, and fractures in older men: The MrOS study," *Journal of Bone and Mineral Research*, vol. 28, no. 3, pp. 472–479, 2013.

[92] J. Faber and A. M. Galløe, "Changes in bone mass during prolonged subclinical hyperthyroidism due to L-thyroxine treatment: a meta-analysis," *European Journal of Endocrinology*, vol. 130, no. 4, pp. 350–356, 1994.

[93] B. Uzzan, J. Campos, M. Cucherat, P. Nony, J. P. Boissel, and G. Y. Perret, "Effects on bone mass of long term treatment with thyroid hormones: a meta-analysis," *Journal of Clinical Endocrinology and Metabolism*, vol. 81, no. 12, pp. 4278–4289, 1996.

9

Radioiodine Thyroid Remnant Ablation after Recombinant Human Thyrotropin or Thyroid Hormone Withdrawal in Patients with High-Risk Differentiated Thyroid Cancer

Fabián Pitoia,[1] Robert J. Marlowe,[2] Erika Abelleira,[1] Eduardo N. Faure,[3] Fernanda Bueno,[1] Diego Schwarzstein,[4] Rubén Julio Lutfi,[3] and Hugo Niepomniszcze[1]

[1] Division of Endocrinology, Hospital de Clínicas, University of Buenos Aires, Córdoba 2351, 5th Floor, Buenos Aires 1424, Argentina
[2] Division of Medical Editing, Spencer-Fontayne Corporation, 33 Bentley Avenue, Jersey City, NJ 07304-1901, USA
[3] Division of Endocrinology, Hospital Churruca Visca, Uspallata 3400, Buenos Aires 1437, Argentina
[4] Division of Endocrinology, Consultorios Integrados Rosario, Italia 424, Santa Fe, Rosario 2000, Argentina

Correspondence should be addressed to Fabián Pitoia, fpitoia@intramed.net

Academic Editor: Daniele Barbaro

To supplement limited relevant literature, we retrospectively compared ablation and disease outcomes in high-risk differentiated thyroid carcinoma (DTC) patients undergoing radioiodine thyroid remnant ablation aided by recombinant human thyrotropin (rhTSH) versus thyroid hormone withdrawal/withholding (THW). Our cohort was 45 consecutive antithyroglobulin antibody- (TgAb-) negative, T3-T4/N0-N1-Nx/M0 adults ablated with high activities at three referral centers. Ablation success comprised negative (<1 μg/L) stimulated serum thyroglobulin (Tg) and TgAb, with absent or <0.1% scintigraphic thyroid bed uptake. "No evidence of disease" (NED) comprised negative unstimulated/stimulated Tg and no suspicious neck ultrasonography or pathological imaging or biopsy. "Persistent disease" was failure to achieve NED, "recurrence," loss of NED status. rhTSH patients ($n = 18$) were oftener ≥45 years old and higher stage ($P = 0.01$), but otherwise not different than THW patients ($n = 27$) at baseline. rhTSH patients were significantly oftener successfully ablated compared to THW patients (83% versus 67%, $P < 0.02$). After respective 3.3 yr and 4.5 yr mean follow-ups ($P = 0.02$), NED was achieved oftener (72% versus 59%) and persistent disease was less frequent in rhTSH patients (22% versus 33%) (both comparisons $P = 0.03$). rhTSH stimulation is associated with at least as good outcomes as is THW in ablation of high-risk DTC patients.

1. Introduction

Postsurgical thyroid remnant ablation with radioiodine (131-iodine, ^{131}I) in low-risk patients with differentiated thyroid carcinoma (DTC) has engendered considerable controversy [1]. However, current guidelines and consensus strongly favor the procedure in high-risk patients [2, 3].

Thyroid-stimulating hormone (TSH) elevation is believed to be necessary to optimize ablative radioiodine uptake and organification [2]. The traditional method to obtain such elevation is endogenously, through thyroid hormone withdrawal or withholding (THW), with resultant hypothyroidism. An alternative to THW, available since 2001 in our country, Argentina, is exogenous TSH elevation via recombinant human TSH (rhTSH) administration [2, 4–8].

Numerous published comparisons [4, 9–16] have confirmed that rhTSH-aided ablation achieves high remnant eradication rates that are not statistically inferior to those attained with THW-assisted ablation. At the same time, relative to THW, rhTSH use avoids hypothyroid morbidity, improving patient quality-of-life [4, 14, 15, 17–19]. Compared to THW, rhTSH use also lessens extra-thyroidal radiation exposure [20, 21], improving safety [22]. Additionally, a number of published comparisons have documented statistically not different, modest DTC recurrence rates after rhTSH- or THW-aided ablation [9–11, 14, 16, 23]. rhTSH has a relatively high acquisition cost. However, the literature suggests that from the societal and patient/family perspectives, this cost may be balanced by the benefits of shorter hospital length-of-stay (where this variable is determined by whole-body dose rate), shorter absence from work, and improved on-the-job performance. These advantages are related to the preservation of euthyroidism and hence, of cognitive and physical function, when rhTSH is used [24–28]. One study also suggests that from an institutional perspective, the rhTSH acquisition cost may at least partly be offset by increased "patient throughput," that is, more efficient use of radioiodine treatment rooms [28].

However, the preponderance of patients in publications regarding rhTSH-assisted versus THW-assisted ablation had low-intermediate postsurgical DTC recurrence risk; only two groups have published comparisons of the two modalities with respect to remnant eradication and disease persistence or recurrence focusing all or in part on high-risk DTC [9, 29–31].

The larger, more invasive primary tumors often characterizing high-risk disease might render complete cancer excision more difficult. Higher stage DTC also might be associated with increased risk of occult malignancy. Because of these challenges, it is important to compare outcomes in the postsurgical high-risk setting with rhTSH-aided versus with THW-aided ablation. We therefore undertook the present retrospective analysis.

2. Materials and Methods

2.1. Endpoints, Patients, and Ethics. We examined rates of ablation success and of disease outcomes after medium-term follow-up according to the TSH preparation method for ablation in 45 consecutive adults ablated at any of three Argentine referral centers from March 2002 to June 2009. This cohort had initial T3-T4/N0-N1-Nx/M0 staging according to the American Joint Committee on Cancer/Union Internationale Contre le Cancer (AJCC/UICC) system, 6th edition [32], with undetectable antithyroglobulin antibodies (TgAb) by immunometric assay at the time of ablation. All T3 patients had gross invasion and the entire cohort had high recurrence risk according to the Latin American Thyroid Society (LATS) classification [3] and intermediate or high risk according to the American Thyroid Association (ATA) classification [2]. M0 status was confirmed by postablation whole-body scintigraphy (WBS).

All patients were totally thyroidectomized in a specialized center. Thirty-six (80%) also underwent lymph node dissection. In 10 of the 36 (28% of the subgroup), central and lateral neck dissection was performed when intrasurgical anatomopathological frozen section analysis verified lymph node metastasis. In the remaining 26 of the 36 (72% of the subgroup), central neck (level VI) dissection was mostly indicated after T3 status confirmation, when suspicious lymph nodes were noted during surgery, or when both conditions pertained.

Based on postsurgical histological analysis, 7 of these 26 patients eventually were found to have microscopic central lymph node metastasis. Therefore, of the 36 patients undergoing lymph node dissection, 17, or 47%, ultimately had confirmed nodal involvement.

Among the 45 patients in the overall cohort, ablation was aided by rhTSH (Thyrogen, thyrotropin alfa, Genzyme,

Cambridge, MA, USA) in 18 (40%) and by THW in 27 (60%). The choice between rhTSH and THW was individualized according to physician and patient preferences and the patient's circumstances. Among the 18 rhTSH patients, indications for such preparation included poor general physical condition or advanced age ($n = 6$), patient preference ($n = 6$), generally due to desire to avoid hypothyroid morbidity or to decrease time missed from work or study, depression ($n = 5$), or cardiac disease ($n = 1$).

Tables 1(a) and 1(b) summarize key baseline patient characteristics by treatment group. rhTSH patients were on average a decade younger at DTC diagnosis than were their THW counterparts, a statistically significant difference. Nonetheless, the rhTSH group had a significantly greater proportion of patients ≥45 years old (Table 1(a)). Moreover, although there were no significant intergroup differences when T or N classifications were considered as individual categories for patients of all ages (Table 1(a)), patients aged ≥45 years tended to have more advanced T and N classifications, and thus, later AJCC/UICC stages, in the rhTSH group than in the THW group (Table 1(b)). The rhTSH patients were similar to their THW counterparts with respect to all other tested baseline variables.

Institutional review board approvals were obtained for the study.

2.2. Ablation Protocol. Our ablation protocol used fixed radioiodine activities based on the extent of initial disease, without adjustment according to the TSH preparation. Patients typically received 3.70 GBq (100 mCi) [131]I for T3 disease with gross extension beyond the thyroid capsule and N0 status, 5.55 GBq (150 mCi) for T3/N1a-N1b disease, and 7.40 GBq (200 mCi) for T4 tumor. T4 patients ($n = 12$) received a second therapeutic ^{131}I activity (mean ± standard deviation [SD] 3.37 ± 0.74 GBq [91 ± 20 mCi]), rhTSH-aided in all cases, a mean ± SD 9 ± 3 months after ablation. A low-iodine diet was prescribed from one week before radioiodine administration through two days afterwards. Pretherapeutic urinary iodine testing was not routine; however, patients were queried about exposure to possible sources of iodine excess, which was not reported in any case, but would have been grounds to delay ^{131}I administration.

To reduce the risk of actinic thyroiditis from administering large amounts of radioiodine to bulky residues, we assessed preablation thyroid remnant size in some patients ($n = 6$) operated on by surgeons with whose thyroid procedure expertise we were unfamiliar. In those patients, a 3.7 MBq (100 μCi) [131]I tracer activity was given the day preceding, and cervical percentage uptake was ascertained just before ablative activity administration [33]. Uptake above our 3%–5% norm would have warranted consideration of a reduced ablative activity or referral for reoperation, but was not seen.

Posttherapy WBS was performed 5–7 days after ablation and any second radioiodine therapy.

2.3. TSH Preparation. rhTSH was given as two consecutive daily 0.9 mg intramuscular injections, with the tracer activity

TABLE 1: (a) Selected patient characteristics by treatment group. (b) Basis for AJCC/UICC staging in the study cohort.

(a)

Variable	rhTSH group ($n = 18$)	THW group ($n = 27$)	P
Age at DTC diagnosis			
Mean ± SD years	41 ± 16	51 ± 14	0.03
≥45 years old, % (n)	78% (14)	37% (10)	0.01
Female, % (n)	83% (15)	78% (21)	0.30
Histological classification, % (n)			
Papillary, classical variant	78% (14)	82% (22)	
Papillary, follicular variant	6% (1)	11% (3)	0.08
Follicular	16% (3)	7% (2)	
T classification[a], % (n)			
T3	72% (13)	74% (20)	
T4a	22% (4)	19% (5)	0.53
T4b	6% (1)	7% (2)	
N classification[a], % (n)			
N0/Nx	67% (12)	66% (16)	
N1a	27% (5)	22% (6)	0.08
N1b	6% (1)	18% (5)	
Patients with vascular invasion, % (n)	22% (4)	26% (7)	0.33
AJCC/UICC stage[ab], % (n)			
I	22% (4)	63% (17)	
II	0% (0)	0% (0)	
III	50% (9)	33% (9)	0.01
IVa	11% (2)	4% (1)	
IVb	17% (3)	0% (0)	
IVc	0% (0)	0% (0)	
Lymph node dissection, n (%)	78% (14)	81% (22)	0.49

AJCC: American Joint Committee on Cancer; DTC: differentiated thyroid carcinoma; rhTSH: recombinant human thyroid-stimulating hormone; SD: standard deviation; UICC: Union Internationale Contre le Cancer; THW: thyroid hormone withdrawal or withholding.
[a]According to AJCC/UICC classification, 6th edition of 2002 [32]; all patients had M0 staging confirmed by the postablation whole-body scan.
[b]See Table 1(b) for explanation of the basis of staging in this cohort.

(b)

TN status[a], n	AJCC/UICC stage[a]	rhTSH group ($n = 18$)	THW group ($n = 27$)
		Age < 45 years	
T3N0	I	2	3
T3Nx	I	0	2
T3N1a	I	2	2
T3N1b	I	0	4
T4aN0	I	0	4
T4bN1a	I	0	1
T4bN1b	I	0	1
		Age ≥ 45 years	
T3N0	III	7	4
T3Nx	III	0	2
T3N1a	III	2	3
T4aN0	IVa	0	1
T4bN0	IVb	3	0

(b) Continued.

TN status [a], n	AJCC/UICC stage[a]	rhTSH group ($n = 18$)	THW group ($n = 27$)
T4bN1a	IVa	1	0
T4bN1b	IVa	1	0

AJCC: American Joint Committee on Cancer; DTC: differentiated thyroid carcinoma; rhTSH: recombinant human thyroid-stimulating hormone; UICC: Union Internationale Contre le Cancer; THW: thyroid hormone withdrawal or withholding.

[a]According to AJCC/UICC classification, 6th edition of 2002 [32]; all patients had M0 staging confirmed by the postablation whole-body scan.

(when applied) administered at the time of the second injection and the ablative activity or second radioiodine therapy (T4 patients only) administered ~24 hr after the second injection. rhTSH was given while patients were euthyroid with suppressed TSH and receiving levothyroxine, except that this hormone was briefly withdrawn, from 2 days before through 2 days after radioiodine therapy administration, to reduce the risk of iodine interference [34].

THW comprised at least 3 weeks without thyroid hormone, starting from thyroidectomy. Radioiodine was administered following that interval, in all cases with TSH levels above 50 mIU/L.

2.4. Thyroglobulin (Tg)/TgAb Measurement.
Samples for Tg and TgAb measurement were taken on day 5 after the first rhTSH injection in the rhTSH group and on the day of ablative radioiodine administration in the THW group. Tg and TgAb levels were assessed in one of three reference laboratories (depending on the center), using either of two commercial immunometric assays; the same laboratory and assay were used throughout a patient's follow-up. Tg assays comprised the Elecsys Tg Electrochemiluminescence Immunoassay (Roche Diagnostics GmbH, Mannheim, Germany), which has a 0.5 μg/L detection limit, or the Immulite 2000 Tg Chemiluminiscence Assay (Siemens Corp., Los Angeles, CA, USA), with a 0.2 μg/L analytical sensitivity. TgAb assays comprised the Elecsys Anti-Tg Electrochemiluminescence Immunoassay (RSR Ltd., Pentwyn, Cardiff, UK), or the Immulite 2000 Anti-TG Ab chemiluminescent immunometric assay method (Siemens). For both TgAb assays, values >20 IU/mL were considered to be positive, and to render Tg measurements uninterpretable.

2.5. Follow-Up Including Ablation Success Assessment.
Figure 1 represents our protocol for initial treatment and follow-up. After ablation, all patients started (THW group) or restarted (rhTSH group) suppressive thyroid hormone therapy (target TSH: <0.01 mIU/L).

Ablation status was assessed using rhTSH-stimulated Tg testing and rhTSH-stimulated diagnostic WBS (dxWBS; 150 MBq [4 mCi] activity) performed 6–12 (mean ± SD 9 ± 4) months after ablation. Ablation success was defined as negative stimulated Tg (<1 μg/L) in the absence of TgAb, plus absent or <0.1% thyroid bed uptake on dxWBS.

Neck ultrasonography (US) using an 11 MHz linear array transducer was performed every 6 months after ablation. Patients with measurable stimulated or unstimulated Tg, suspicious neck US findings, or both during follow-up underwent morphological or functional imaging or both,

including computed tomography (CT) ($n = 7$ [39%] in the rhTSH group; $n = 13$ [48%] in the THW group) or 18-fluorodeoxyglucose positron emission tomography (FDG-PET) ($n = 6$ [33%] in the rhTSH group; $n = 4$ [15%] in the THW group). All ultrasonographically suspicious nodules ≥1 cm in diameter underwent fine needle aspiration with measurement of Tg in the aspirate.

2.6. Disease Status Definitions.
We defined disease status according to the latest LATS [3] and ATA guidelines [2]. Patients had "no evidence of disease" (NED) when unstimulated and stimulated Tg were negative (<1 μg/L), TgAb were negative (<20 IU/mL), neck US was free of suspicious signs, and there were no pathological findings on any other imaging (WBS, radiography, CT, FDG-PET, or any other modality) or in any biopsy specimen. However, patients with a single stimulated Tg measurement ≥1 to ≤2 μg/L without additional signs of DTC were considered to have indeterminate status until a subsequent stimulated Tg measurement became negative or exceeded 2 μg/L; the latter increase was considered a sign of disease. Patients who never attained NED status were classified as having "persistent disease," while those who lost NED status were defined as having "recurrent disease." Disease sites were classified as local (thyroid bed), lymph node (metastasis confirmed by fine-needle aspiration biopsy with positive cytology), distant (metastasis confirmed by imaging), or unknown ("biochemical only") (stimulated Tg >2 μg/L without structural evidence of disease).

2.7. Statistics.
Data are expressed as mean ± SD unless otherwise noted. Categorical comparisons were made using chi-square testing with the Fisher's exact test when appropriate. Analysis was performed using SPSS software (version 15.0.0: SPSS, Inc., Chicago, IL, USA). P values ≤ 0.05 were considered to be statistically significant.

3. Results

Table 2 provides key data regarding ablation and ablation success for both treatment groups. On average, the treatment groups did not differ regarding the ablative activity, the proportions of patients in different activity categories or receiving a second therapy, the cumulative activity, or the interval between ablation and ablation success assessment. However, successful remnant ablation was observed in a significantly greater proportion of the rhTSH group than of the THW group (83% versus 67%, $P = 0.02$).

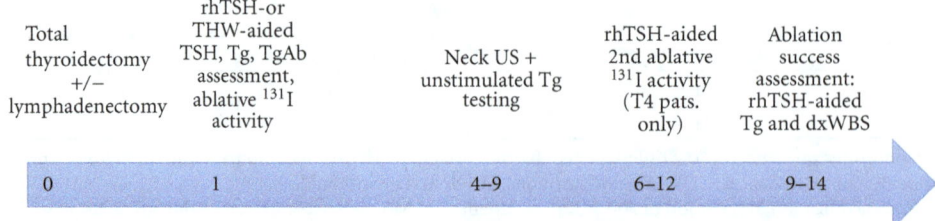

FIGURE 1: Initial treatment and follow-up regimen in patients with thyroid cancer included in the study. Thyroid surgery represents time zero; other numbers refer to months after surgery. Dx, diagnostic; rhTSH, recombinant human thyrotropin; Tg, thyroglobulin; TgAb, antithyroglobulin antibodies; TSH, thyroid-stimulating hormone; US, ultrasonography.

TABLE 2: Ablation characteristics by patient group.

Variable	rhTSH group ($n = 18$)	THW group ($n = 27$)	P
Cumulative radioiodine activity before ablation success evaluation, GBq (mCi), mean ± SD	5.62 ± 1.30 (152 ± 35)	5.85 ± 1.22 (158 ± 33)	0.34
Ablation activity, GBq (mCi), mean ± SD	4.70 ± 1.41 (127 ± 38)	4.85 ± 1.11 (131 ± 29)	0.32
Ablation activity category, n			
3.70 GBq (100 mCi)	9	11	
5.55 GBq (150 mCi)	4	9	0.08
7.40 GBq (200 mCi)	5	7	
Patients receiving 1 additional radioiodine therapy before ablation success evaluation, % (n)	28% (5)	26% (7)	0.43
Timing of ablation success evaluation, months after ablation, mean ± SD	10 ± 3	9 ± 5	0.18
Ablation status, % (n)			
Success	83% (15)	67% (18)	0.02
Failure	17% (3)	33% (9)	

dxWBS: diagnostic whole-body scintigraphy; rhTSH: recombinant human thyroid-stimulating hormone; rxWBS: posttherapy whole-body scintigraphy; SD: standard deviation; Tg: serum thyroglobulin; THW: thyroid hormone withdrawal or withholding; TSH: thyrotropin.

Table 3 highlights the disease status at the end of follow-up according to the treatment group. The mean duration of follow-up was approximately 3 1/3 years in the rhTSH group and a year longer than that in the THW group, a statistically significant difference ($P = 0.02$). The rhTSH patients achieved NED status significantly more often and showed persistent disease significantly less often than did their THW counterparts. The groups did not differ with respect to recurrence rates. No patient developed TgAb or received more than the planned one (T3 patients) or two (T4 patients) ablative radioiodine therapies during follow-up.

Sites of persistence and recurrence appeared to have a roughly similar distribution in the treatment groups; all recurrences affected lymph nodes, and there was no structural evidence of distant recurrence. The times to recurrence detection were 22 months in the rhTSH patient and 19 and 20 months, respectively, in the THW patients who lost NED status. Patients with neck lymph node metastases or recurrence in the neck lymph nodes were reoperated. The patients were reevaluated at 6 ± 4 months after reoperation with rhTSH-stimulated Tg testing and all had biochemical persistence without structural evidence of disease at the latest follow-up.

4. Discussion

This retrospective analysis in DTC patients with an high recurrence risk but no known distant metastases had three main findings regarding rhTSH versus THW stimulation of radioiodine thyroid remnant ablation. rhTSH use was associated with firstly, a significantly higher ablation success rate, and secondly, significantly more frequent favorable medium-term disease outcomes, that is, more frequent NED status and less frequent persistent disease. Thirdly, despite our cohort's high-risk status, both TSH preparation methods appeared to be associated with modest medium-term recurrence rates that did not differ statistically. It is worth noting the context of these observations: more than double the proportion of the rhTSH group than of the THW group was ≥45 years old (78% versus 37%, Table 1(a)), and the rhTSH patients ≥45 years old tended to have more advanced T and N stages than did their THW counterparts (Table 1(b)), even though the groups did not differ significantly when T or N stages were considered as individual categories for patients of all ages (Table 1(a)).

Our findings confirm those of the Santa Casa do Belo Horizonte [9] and Memorial Sloan Kettering Cancer

TABLE 3: Disease status at the end of followup.

Variable	rhTSH group ($n = 18$)	THW group ($n = 27$)	P
Postablation followup, months, mean ± SD	40 ± 16	54 ± 40	0.02
Disease status[a] at the end of followup, % (n)			
NED	72% (13)	59% (16)	0.03
Persistent disease	22% (4)	33% (9)	0.03
Recurrent disease	6% (1)	7% (2)	NS
Sites of persistent disease, n			
Local	0	2	
Lymph nodes	1	3	Not tested
Unknown (biochemical only)[b]	3	4	
Sites of recurrence, n			
Local	0	0	
Lymph nodes	1	2	Not tested
Unknown (biochemical only)[b]	0	0	

NED: no evidence of disease; rhTSH: recombinant human thyroid-stimulating hormone; SD: standard deviation; THW: thyroid hormone withdrawal or withholding.
[a]Please refer to "Materials and Methods" section for a description of potential disease states.
[b]Refers to elevated stimulated Tg ($>2\,\mu$g/L) without structural evidence of disease.

Center (MSKCC) groups [29–31] of numerically similar or statistically not different or superior ablation success and disease outcome rates associated with rhTSH versus THW preparation of ablation in initial high-risk DTC patients. Regarding ablation success, the Belo Horizonte investigators noted respective 80% versus 79% rates (68% and 67% in patients with Tg $> 1\,\mu$g/L at ablation) in the rhTSH ($n = 77$) and THW subgroups ($n = 198$) of a slightly lower risk cohort than ours (T3/N0-N1 but no T4 patients) [9]. The MSKCC investigators reported respective 16% versus 9% rates of "excellent" response to initial therapy and respective 13% versus 7% rates of "acceptable" response in their rhTSH ($n = 69$) and THW subgroups ($n = 92$) of patients with initial ATA high-risk classification; these rates did not significantly differ [30]. Our ablation success rates were 83% for the rhTSH group ($n = 18$) versus 67% for the THW group ($P = 0.02$) (Table 2). It should be noted that the MSKCC "response to initial therapy" variable encompassed a longer postablation follow-up (2 years) than did our or the Brazilian investigators' "ablation success" variables (6–12 and 9–12 months, resp.). Additionally, both the Belo Horizonte and MSKCC groups included ultrasonographic findings in their assessment of response to ablation or "initial treatment," while we did not.

With respect to disease outcome, the Belo Horizonte investigators observed numerically similar, low 9–12-month disease persistence rates in rhTSH patients ($n = 70$) and THW patients ($n = 169$) whose M0 status was confirmed by the postablation WBS: 7.1% versus 7.7%. After a presumably much longer follow-up (median not reported for the initial ATA high-risk patients, but 9 years for their overall cohort [$N = 586$]), the MSKCC group noted statistically not different disease outcomes for rhTSH and THW patients with initial ATA high-risk status: 17.1% NED, 82.6% disease persistence, and 0% recurrence rates for the rhTSH patients

versus 15.2%, 83.7%, and 1.1%, respectively, in their THW counterparts. In our study sample, after a mean follow-up of ~3.3 years in the rhTSH patients and ~4.5 years in the THW patients, the NED rate was significantly higher (72% versus 59%, $P = 0.03$) and the disease persistence rate was significantly lower (22% versus 33%, $P = 0.03$) in the rhTSH group (Table 3). The differences in ablation success and disease outcomes among the Belo Horizonte, MSKCC, and our groups may be attributable to one or more of (1) different follow-up durations; (2) noninclusion of US findings among our ablation success criteria; (3) lack of T4 patients in the Belo Horizonte group; (4) inclusion of only N1 patients with especially extensive neck nodal involvement in the MSKCC cohort; (5) somewhat higher (by ~700 MBq, ~19 mCi) mean cumulative ^{131}I activities in our patients than in their Belo Horizonte counterparts—and perhaps also the MSKCC initial ATA high-risk patients (mean cumulative activity not reported for the latter subgroup, but ~500 MBq [~14 mCi] lower in the overall MSKCC study sample than in our cohort) [9, 30].

Limitations of our study should be noted. Among these were its retrospective nature (shared with the Belo Horizonte and MSKCC studies), relatively small patient cohort, and discrepant mean follow-up durations for the treatment groups. Regarding the first of these limitations, our rhTSH and THW patients nonetheless had quite similar tested baseline and treatment characteristics; key characteristics that differed significantly (proportion of patients ≥45 years old, AJCC/UICC stage) presumably would have favored the THW group. Regarding the follow-up length, which was on average significantly shorter in rhTSH patients (Table 3), one would expect this difference to be relevant mainly to the observed DTC recurrence rate, which did not differ between the treatment groups, rather than to the NED or disease persistence rates, which differed in favor of rhTSH.

5. Conclusion

In a cohort of adult referral center patients with LATS and ATA initial high-risk DTC without known distant metastases, rhTSH-stimulated radioiodine thyroid remnant ablation was associated with significantly greater ablation success rates than was THW-aided ablation. Additionally, after medium-term follow-up, rhTSH stimulation was associated with significantly more frequent NED status, significantly less frequent disease persistence, and statistically not different, low DTC recurrence rates. These results suggest that patients and clinicians do not have to consider initial disease classification in their choice of TSH preparation for postsurgical ablation in DTC without distant metastasis; these observations should be prospectively confirmed.

Acknowledgments

The editorial work on this paper by one of the authors, R. J. Marlowe, was supported, and the Journal of Thyroid Research article processing/open access charges were defrayed in full, by a grant from Genzyme, a Sanofi company, the rhTSH manufacturer. No additional grant support or other funding for the present analysis and paper was received from any commercial source. R. J. Marlowe has received and is receiving support from Genzyme for editorial work on additional manuscripts. F. Pitoia, E. N. Faure, and D. Schwarzstein have received honoraria as advisors to and speakers for Genzyme. The other authors declare no potential conflict of interests.

References

[1] E. L. Mazzaferri, "What is the optimal initial treatment of low-risk papillary thyroid cancer (and why is it controversial)?" *Oncology*, vol. 23, no. 7, pp. 579–588, 2009.

[2] D. S. Cooper, G. M. Doherty, B. R. Haugen et al., "Revised American Thyroid Association management guidelines for patients with thyroid nodules and differentiated thyroid cancer," *Thyroid*, vol. 19, no. 11, pp. 1167–1214, 2009.

[3] F. Pitoia, L. Ward, N. Wohllk et al., "Recommendations of the Latin American Thyroid Society on diagnosis and management of differentiated thyroid cancer," *Arquivos Brasileiros de Endocrinologia e Metabologia*, vol. 53, no. 7, pp. 884–897, 2009.

[4] F. Pacini, P. W. Ladenson, M. Schlumberger et al., "Radioiodine ablation of thyroid remnants after preparation with recombinant human thyrotropin in differentiated thyroid carcinoma: results of an international, randomized, controlled study," *Journal of Clinical Endocrinology and Metabolism*, vol. 91, no. 3, pp. 926–932, 2006.

[5] F. Pitoia and H. Niepomniszcze, "Recombinant human TSH: the Argentinean experience," *Thyroid*, vol. 19, no. 7, p. 799, 2009.

[6] F. Pitoia, E. El Tamer, D. B. Schere, M. Passerieu, O. D. Bruno, and H. Niepomniszcze, "Usefulness of recombinant human TSH aided radioiodine doses administered in patients with differentiated thyroid carcinoma," *Medicina*, vol. 66, no. 2, pp. 125–130, 2006.

[7] S. Iorcansky, V. Herzovich, R. R. Qualey, and R. M. Tuttle, "Serum thyrotropin (TSH) levels after recombinant human TSH injections in children and teenagers with papillary thyroid cancer," *Journal of Clinical Endocrinology and Metabolism*, vol. 90, no. 12, pp. 6553–6555, 2005.

[8] F. Pitoia, V. Ilera, M. B. Zanchetta, A. Foffano, and H. Niepomniszcze, "Optimum recombinant human thyrotropin dose in patients with differentiated thyroid carcinoma and end-stage renal disease," *Endocrine Practice*, vol. 14, no. 8, pp. 961–966, 2008.

[9] P. W. Rosário, A. C. M. Xavier, and M. R. Calsolari, "Recombinant human thyrotropin in thyroid remnant ablation with 131-iodine in high-risk patients," *Thyroid*, vol. 20, no. 11, pp. 1247–1252, 2010.

[10] P. W. Rosário and A. C. M. Xavier, "Recombinant human thyroid stimulating hormone in thyroid remnant ablation with 1.1 GBq 131iodine in low-risk patients," *American Journal of Clinical Oncology*, vol. 35, no. 2, pp. 101–104, 2011.

[11] R. M. Tuttle, M. Brokhin, G. Omry et al., "Recombinant human TSH-assisted radioactive iodine remnant ablation achieves short-term clinical recurrence rates similar to those of traditional thyroid hormone withdrawal," *Journal of Nuclear Medicine*, vol. 49, no. 5, pp. 764–770, 2008.

[12] H. P. Tala Jury, M. G. Castagna, C. Fioravanti, C. Cipri, E. Brianzoni, and F. Pacini, "Lack of association between urinary iodine excretion and successful thyroid ablation in thyroid cancer patients," *Journal of Clinical Endocrinology and Metabolism*, vol. 95, no. 1, pp. 230–237, 2010.

[13] M. Chianelli, V. Todino, F. M. Graziano et al., "Low-activity (2.0 GBq; 54 mCi) radioiodine post-surgical remnant ablation in thyroid cancer: comparison between hormone withdrawal and use of rhTSH in low-risk patients," *European Journal of Endocrinology*, vol. 160, no. 3, pp. 431–436, 2009.

[14] U. Mallick, C. Harmer, B. Yap et al., "Ablation with low-dose radioiodine and thyrotropin alfa in thyroid cancer," *New England Journal of Medicine*, vol. 366, no. 18, pp. 1674–1685, 2012.

[15] M. Schlumberger, B. Catargi, I. Borget et al., "Strategies of radioiodine ablation in patients with low-risk thyroid cancer," *New England Journal of Medicine*, vol. 366, no. 18, pp. 1663–1673, 2012.

[16] J. Clerc, M. Bienvenu-Perrard, C. P. de Malleray et al., "Outpatient thyroid remnant ablation using repeated low 131-iodine activities (740 MBq/20 mCix2) in patients with low-risk differentiated thyroid cancer," *Journal of Clinical Endocrinology and Metabolism*, vol. 97, no. 3, pp. 871–880, 2012.

[17] D. Taïeb, K. Baumstarck-Barrau, F. Sebag et al., "Heath-related quality of life in thyroid cancer patients following radioiodine ablation," *Health and Quality of Life Outcomes*, vol. 9, article 33, 2011.

[18] J. Lee, M. J. Yun, K. H. Nam, W. Y. Chung, E. Y. Soh, and C. S. Park, "Quality of life and effectiveness comparisons of thyroxine withdrawal, triiodothyronine withdrawal, and recombinant thyroid-stimulating hormone administration for low-dose radioiodine remnant ablation of differentiated thyroid carcinoma," *Thyroid*, vol. 20, no. 2, pp. 173–179, 2010.

[19] F. Pitoia and S. Licht, "Evaluation of the effect of thyroid hormone withdrawal on quality of life in patients with differentiated thyroid carcinoma," *Glándulas Tiroides y Paratiroides*, vol. 16, pp. 25–29, 2007 (Spanish).

[20] H. Hänscheid, M. Lassmann, M. Luster et al., "Iodine biokinetics and dosimetry in radioiodine therapy of thyroid cancer: procedures and results of a prospective international controlled study of ablation after rhTSH or hormone withdrawal," *Journal of Nuclear Medicine*, vol. 47, no. 4, pp. 648–654, 2006.

[21] H. Remy, I. Borget, S. Leboulleux et al., "131I effective half-life and dosimetry in thyroid cancer patients," *Journal of Nuclear Medicine*, vol. 49, no. 9, pp. 1445–1450, 2008.

[22] P. W. Rosário, M. A. R. Borges, and S. Purisch, "Preparation with recombinant human thyroid-stimulating hormone for thyroid remnant ablation with 131I is associated with lowered radiotoxicity," *Journal of Nuclear Medicine*, vol. 49, no. 11, pp. 1776–1782, 2008.

[23] R. Elisei, M. Schlumberger, A. Driedger et al., "Follow-up of low-risk differentiated thyroid cancer patients who underwent radioiodine ablation of postsurgical thyroid remnants after either recombinant human thyrotropin or thyroid hormone withdrawal," *Journal of Clinical Endocrinology and Metabolism*, vol. 94, no. 11, pp. 4171–4179, 2009.

[24] I. Borget, C. Corone, M. Nocaudie et al., "Sick leave for follow-up control in thyroid cancer patients: comparison between stimulation with Thyrogen and thyroid hormone withdrawal," *European Journal of Endocrinology*, vol. 156, no. 5, pp. 531–538, 2007.

[25] I. Borget, M. Schlumberger, M. Allyn, G. De Pouvoirville, H. Remy, and M. Ricard, "Radioiodine ablation in thyroid cancer patients: comparison of length and cost of hospital stay between preparation by thyroid hormone withdrawal and Thyrogen," *European Journal of Endocrinology*, vol. 35, no. 8, pp. 1457–1463, 2008.

[26] T. F. Nijhuis, W. van Wepperen, and J. M. H. de Klerk, "Costs associated with the withdrawal of thyroid hormone suppression therapy during the follow-up treatment of well-differentiated thyroid cancer," *Tijdschrift voor Nucleaire Geneeskunde*, vol. 21, pp. 98–100, 1999.

[27] M. Luster, R. Felbinger, M. Dietlein, and C. Reiners, "Thyroid hormone withdrawal in patients with differentiated thyroid carcinoma: a one hundred thirty-patient pilot survey on consequences of hypothyroidism and a pharmacoeconomic comparison to recombinant thyrotropin administration," *Thyroid*, vol. 15, no. 10, pp. 1147–1155, 2005.

[28] J. A. Vallejo Casas, L. M. Mena Bares, M. A. Galvez, R. J. Marlowe, J. M. Latre Romero, and M. Martínez-Paredes, "Treatment room length-of-stay and patient throughput with radioiodine thyroid remnant ablation in differentiated thyroid cancer: comparison of thyroid-stimulating hormone stimulation methods," *Nuclear Medicine Communications*, vol. 32, no. 9, pp. 840–846, 2011.

[29] R. M. Tuttle, N. Lopez, R. Leboeuf et al., "Radioactive iodine administered for thyroid remnant ablation following recombinant human thyroid stimulating hormone preparation also has an important adjuvant therapy function," *Thyroid*, vol. 20, no. 3, pp. 257–263, 2010.

[30] J. Hugo, E. Robenshtok, R. Grewal, S. M. Larson, and R. M. Tuttle, "Recombinant human TSH-assisted radioactive iodine remnant ablation in thyroid cancer patients at intermediate to high risk of recurrence," *Thyroid*, vol. 22, no. 10, pp. 1007–1015, 2012.

[31] H. Tala and R. M. Tuttle, "Contemporary post surgical management of differentiated thyroid carcinoma," *Clinical Oncology*, vol. 22, no. 6, pp. 419–429, 2010.

[32] F. Green, D. L. Page, I. D. Fleming et al., *AJCC Cancer Staging Manual*, Springer, Chicago, Ill, USA, 6th edition, 2002.

[33] F. Pitoia, E. El Tamer, M. E. Salvai, and H. Niepomniszcze, "Protocol for thyroid remnant ablation after recombinant TSH in thyroid carcinoma," *Medicina*, vol. 69, no. 1, pp. 148–152, 2009.

[34] D. Barbaro, G. Boni, G. Meucci et al., "Radioiodine treatment with 30 mCi after recombinant human thyrotropin stimulation in thyroid cancer: effectiveness for postsurgical remnants ablation and possible role of iodine content in L-thyroxine in the outcome of ablation," *Journal of Clinical Endocrinology and Metabolism*, vol. 88, no. 9, pp. 4110–4115, 2003.

10

First- and Second-Trimester Reference Intervals for Thyroid Hormones during Pregnancy in "Rhea" Mother-Child Cohort, Crete, Greece

Polyxeni Karakosta,[1,2] **Leda Chatzi,**[1] **Emmanouil Bagkeris,**[1] **Vasiliki Daraki,**[3] **Dimitris Alegakis,**[1] **Elias Castanas,**[2] **Manolis Kogevinas,**[4,5] **and Marilena Kampa**[2]

[1] Department of Social Medicine, Faculty of Medicine, University of Crete, P.O. Box 2208, 71003 Heraklion, Greece
[2] Department of Experimental Endocrinology, Faculty of Medicine, University of Crete, P.O. Box 2208, 71003 Heraklion, Greece
[3] Department of Endocrinology, Faculty of Medicine, University of Crete, 71003 Heraklion, Greece
[4] Centre for Research in Environmental Epidemiology (CREAL), Doctor Aiguader, 88, 08003 Barcelona, Spain
[5] National School of Public Health, Alexandras Avenue 196, 115 21 Athens, Greece

Correspondence should be addressed to Polyxeni Karakosta, p_karakosta@hotmail.com

Academic Editor: Duncan Topliss

Estimation and interpretation of thyroid function tests in pregnant women is of utmost importance for maternal, fetal and neonatal health. Our objective was to calculate laboratory- and geography-specific reference intervals for thyroid hormones during pregnancy in an iodine-sufficient area of the Mediterranean, Crete, Greece. This project was performed in the context of "Rhea" mother-child cohort. Fulfillment of extensive questionnaires and estimation of free triiodothyronine (fT3), free thyroxine (fT4), thyroid-stimulating hormone (TSH), and antithyroid antibodies were performed. The reference population was defined using inclusion criteria regarding thyroidal, obstetric, and general medical status of women. Reference interval for TSH was 0.05–2.53 μIU/mL for the first and 0.18–2.73 μIU/mL for the second trimester. 6,8% and 5,9% of women in the first and second trimester, respectively, had TSH higher than the upper reference limit. These trimester-specific population-based reference ranges are essential in everyday clinical practice for the correct interpretation of thyroid hormone values and accurate classification of thyroid disorders.

1. Introduction

Pregnancy is a period of significant hormonal changes and metabolic demands which result in complex effects on thyroid function [1–3]. More specifically, alterations in iodine metabolism [1], production of β-chorionic gonadotropin (β-hCG), and increases in both thyroid hormone-binding proteins and thyroid hormones *per se* [4, 5] are some of the physiologic changes that occur during normal pregnancy. At the same time, thyroid hormones play a critical role in neonatal and child neurodevelopment [6], and maternal thyroid disorders can lead to obstetric complications and irreversible effects on the fetus [7]. These findings point out the need for all pregnant women to be screened for thyroid disorders with a valid biomarker with distinct reference ranges.

In the past years, a number of studies from different regions have developed reference ranges for thyroid hormones during pregnancy women [8–31]; however these results should not be extrapolated due to differences in ethnicity, iodine intake, and immunometric assay applied in each study. Moreover, the methodology used for the determination of the reference population (choice of reference population, sample size, assessment of outliers) differs across studies resulting in a variation of absolute reference limits.

The aim of this study was to develop laboratory- and geography-specific reference intervals for thyroid hormones (thyroid-stimulating hormone (TSH), and free triiodothyronine (free T3), free thyroxine (free T4)) during pregnancy in an iodine-sufficient area of the Mediterranean, Crete, Greece.

2. Materials and Methods

2.1. Study Population. This project utilized data from the Rhea mother-child cohort, in the island of Crete, Greece. The mother-child "Rhea" study is a prospective cohort study examining a population sample of pregnant women and their children in a prefecture of southern Greece. Pregnant women, who became pregnant within one year, starting February 2007, participated in the study. The first contact was done at the time of the first major ultrasound, and women were divided in trimesters of pregnancy, according to gestational age which was defined by last menstrual period and ultrasound (first: <13 weeks, second: 13–27 weeks, and third trimester: >28 weeks). Participants were interviewed, and blood samples were collected and stored in −80°C. Extensive questionnaires were completed, and standardized information from ultrasounds was collected together with data from clinical records during pregnancy and birth. The study was approved by the corresponding ethical committees, and all participants provided written informed consent.

From the entire population of the Rhea cohort ($n = 1610$), all available serum samples were analyzed for thyroid hormone measurements ($n = 1300$). According to the recommendations of the National Academy of Clinical Biochemistry (NACB) [32], we subsequently excluded women with a self-reported thyroidal dysfunction (goiter, cancer, hyper-, and hypo-thyroidism), a laboratory diagnosis of overt hypo- or hyperthyroidism (i.e., abnormal values of TSH and FT4 using the reference ranges of the assay used), evidence for autoimmune thyroid disease (elevated anti-TPO and anti-Tg), past or present use of thyroid medications, parental history of any thyroid illness, and women with incomplete information regarding thyroid function. In addition, women with multiple or complicated pregnancies (hyperemesis, gestational diabetes or hypertension, perinatal infections, and stillbirths), clinical diagnosis of a chronic or autoimmune disease (diabetes, hypertension, asthma, inflammatory bowel disease, tumors, and others), and a past history of spontaneous abortions were also removed from the reference population (Figure 1).

2.2. Laboratory Analysis. For each sample, TSH, free thyroxine (free T4), free triiodothyronine (free T3), and antithyroid antibodies (antithyroperoxidase [anti-TPO] and antithyroglobulin [anti-Tg]) were measured by IMMULITE 2000 immunoassay system (Siemens Healthcare Diagnostics, ILL 60015-0778, USA). For TSH, inter- and intra-assay variability were <5.3% and <6.4%, respectively, for levels of 0.32–39 mIU/mL. Accordingly, for free T4 these values were <7.8% and <7.1% for the level of 0.51–4.82 ng/dL (6.56–62.03 pmol/L), for free T3 < 9.1% & <10% for the level of 2.5–13 pg/mL (3.84–19.96 pmol/L), for anti-Tg < 4.9% and <5.8%, and for anti-TPO < 7.4% and 7.2%. The proposed reference limits of the manufacturer for normal euthyroid

adults were: free T3: 1.8–4.2 pg/mL (2.76–6.45 pmol/L), free T4: 0.89–1.76 ng/dL (11.5–22.7 pmol/L), and TSH: 0.4–4 μIU/mL. Anti-TPO and anti-Tg were considered elevated if levels were ≥35 IU/mL and >40 IU/mL, respectively.

2.3. Statistical Analysis. All data were analyzed by SPSS 17 for windows. The nature of the underlying distribution of free T3, free T4, and TSH for the reference population was examined by inspecting normality tests, histograms and P-plots. In case of a significant variation from normal distribution, a logarithm transformation (log and ln) was applied to achieve normality. Outliers were identified using box plots. For the identified outliers Dixon's Q test was applied to the least extreme; if the test rejects the least extreme outlier, then the more extreme outliers are also rejected. Continuously, when the data followed a Gaussian distribution or were transformed to a normal distribution, reference intervals were computed as follows: mean ± 1.96 × standard deviation. If normality was not achieved, even after transformation or after the outlier deletion, a nonparametric method was applied to estimate the reference intervals, by computing the rank numbers of 2.5th and the 97.5th percentiles to estimate the lower and the higher limits of the reference interval, respectively.

Thyroid hormones were expressed as mean, median, standard deviation, 2.5th and 97.5th percentile for the 1st and 2nd trimester. The Mann-Whitney U test was used to compare differences for the 2 trimesters for a level of significance of $P < 0.05$.

3. Results

3.1. Total Study Population. Starting from a total cohort population of 1610 pregnant women, 1300 samples were available for thyroid function and antibody analyses. Of them, 35.2% were in the first (<13 weeks), 61% in the second (13–27 weeks), and 3.7% in the third trimester (>28 weeks) of pregnancy (Table 1). The age of the mothers varied from 15 to 45 years, and the majority of mothers were of Greek origin (85.3%). History of spontaneous miscarriages was present in 223 women (17.2%). Considering thyroid function, 389 (29.9%) of mothers had a positive family history of thyroidal disease, while 165 (12.7%) and 87 (6.7%) women had elevated levels of anti-TPO and anti-TG antibodies, respectively.

3.2. Reference Population. After implementation of the aforementioned exclusion criteria, a total of 875 women were excluded from the study (Figure 1, Table 1), resulting to a final population of 425 women (1st trimester: 143, 2nd trimester: 260, 3rd trimester: 22). Women in the third trimester ($n = 22$) were excluded from the analysis, since the sample size was not adequate for the estimation of reference intervals to a reasonable degree of precision. The final population (403 women) was used to determine the reference limits and the 95% confidence intervals for TSH, free T4, and free T3 for the first and second trimester of pregnancy.

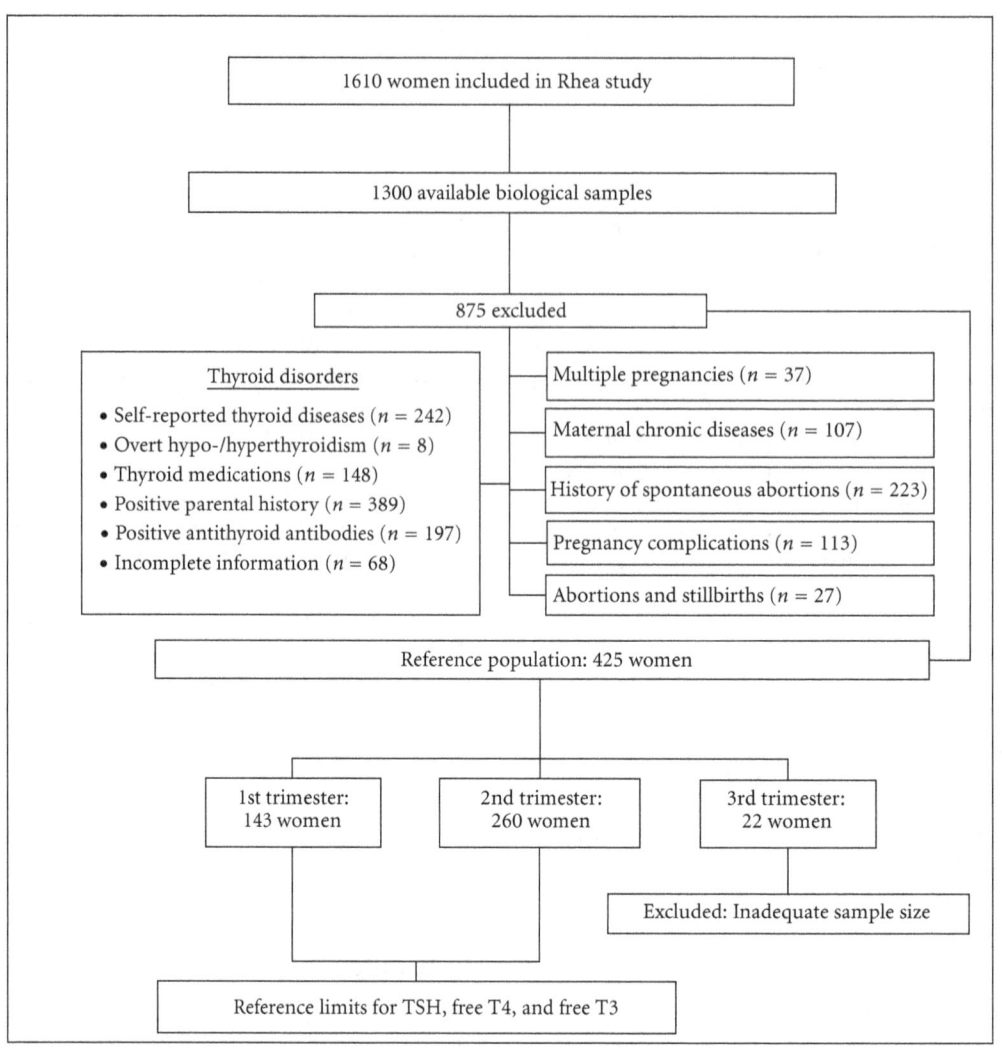

FIGURE 1: Flow diagram of the study process for the determination of the reference population.

TABLE 1: Demographic data for pregnant women in total and reference study population.

| | Total study population[a] | | | Reference population | |
	1st trimester	2nd trimester	3rd trimester	1st trimester	2nd trimester
Sample size (n)	458	794	48	143	260
Age (years)[b]	29.16 (5.12)	28.98 (5.19)	28.37 (4.61)	28.50 (5.09)	27.79 (4.95)
Greek origin n (%)	369 (80.6)	698 (87.9)	42 (87.5)	114 (79.7)	221 (85)

[a] Women with available biological samples.
[b] Values are expressed as mean (SD).

3.3. Reference Values for Thyroid Hormones. Figure 2 shows the box plots for TSH, free T3, and free T4 for first and second trimester after the outlier assessment. Additionally, mean values, standard deviations, medians, and the 2.5th and 97.5th percentiles for all thyroid hormones according to trimester are shown in Table 2.

According to our results (Tables 2 and 3), the reference intervals of serum TSH levels for the first trimester were 0.05–2.53 μIU/mL, of free T3 1.54–5.22 pg/mL (2.37–8.02 pmol/L), and of free T4 0.95–1.53 ng/dL (12.23–19.69 pmol/L). For the second trimester, respective reference intervals were: 0.18–2.73 μIU/mL for TSH, 1.78–5.29 pg/mL (2.73–8.13 pmol/L) for free T3, and 0.87–1.45 ng/dL (11.20–18.66 pmol/L) for free T4. Median TSH and free T3 values showed a slight increase in 2nd trimester, while median free T4 values fell as gestational age advanced.

Mann Whitney U test revealed significant differences between trimesters for free T4 (P value < 0.001), while respective P values for TSH and free T3 were 0.058 and 0.054. These findings justify the separation of groups into different trimesters (Table 2, Figure 2).

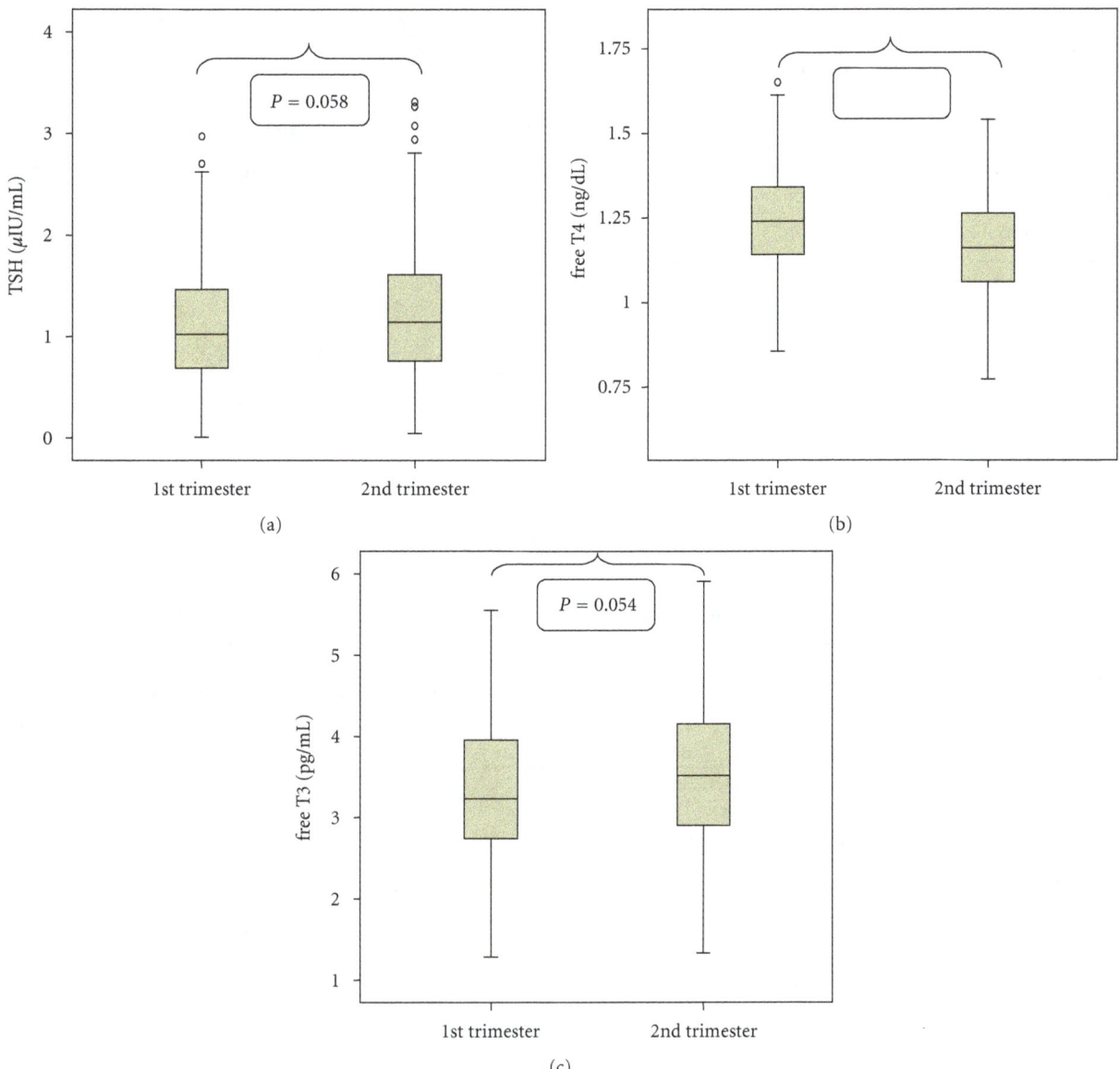

FIGURE 2: Box plot of TSH, free T3, and free T4 concentrations in the reference population during the 1st and 2nd trimester of gestation. TSH: thyroid-stimulating hormone; Free T3: free triiodothyronine; free T4: free thyroxine Differences between first and second trimester are shown with P values ($P = 0.058$ for TSH, $P = 0.054$ for free T3, $P < 0.001$ for free T4).

As shown in Table 4, if the reference limits of the manufacturer were applied to our entire cohort, misclassification of maternal thyroid clinical entities would occur. More specifically, 47 and 43 women with TSH concentrations that are normal for the first and second trimester, respectively would have been misclassified as having subclinical hyperthyroidism. Conversely, 25 and 29 women with a TSH above the first and second trimester-specific upper reference limit would not have been identified as subclinical hypothyroidism.

4. Discussion

During pregnancy several hormonal changes and metabolic demands occur, resulting in complex effects on thyroid function [3]. Alterations in the pituitary-thyroid axis include an

increase in thyroid hormone-binding globulin along with increases in total T4, T3 as well as serum thyroglobulin (TG). Additionally, iodine clearance by the kidneys is enhanced during gestation, while the mild thyrotropic effects of rising β-hCG may exert negative feedback on TSH secretion [33] wrongly suggesting hyperthyroidism in normal pregnant women of the 1st trimester [1].

The incidence of overt and subclinical hypothyroidism in pregnant women has been estimated to be around 0.3–0.5 and 2-3%, respectively [34]. Recent studies have shown that untreated hypothyroidism during pregnancy increases the incidence of maternal anemia, preeclampsia, postpartum hemorrhage, placental abruption, and spontaneous abortion and may cause low birth weight, prematurity, congenital malformations, and impaired fetal brain development with

TABLE 2: Thyroid hormones according to gestational age, Rhea mother-child cohort, Crete, Greece.

	N	Distribution	2.5th percentiles	97.5th percentile	Median	Mean	SD	Reference range
1st trimester								
TSH[a] μIU/mL	141	Not normal	0.05	2.53	1.02	1.08	0.61	0.05–2.53
free T3[b] pg/mL (pmol/L)	141	Normal[d]	1.84 (2.83)	5.39 (8.28)	3.21 (4.93)	3.38 (5.19)	0.94 (1.44)	1.54–5.22 (2.37–8.02)
free T4[c] ng/dL (pmol/L)	139	Normal[e]	0.96 (12.36)	1.60 (20.59)	1.24 (15.96)	1.24 (15.96)	0.15 (1.93)	0.95–1.53 (12.23–19.69)
2nd trimester								
TSH[a] μIU/mL	257	Not normal	0.18	2.73	1.14	1.23	0.65	0.18–2.73
free T3[b] pg/mL (pmol/L)	256	Normal	1.99 (3.06)	5.30 (8.14)	3.52 (5.41)	3.55 (5.45)	0.87 (1.34)	1.78–5.29 (2.73–8.13)
free T4[c] ng/dL (pmol/L)	258	Normal	0.84 (10.81)	1.44 (18.53)	1.16 (14.93)	1.16 (14.93)	0.15 (1.93)	0.87–1.45 (11.20–18.66)

TSH: thyroid-stimulating hormone; free T3: free triiodothyronine; free T4: free thyroxine.
[a]Difference between first and second trimester: $P = 0.058$.
[b]Difference between first and second trimester: $P = 0.054$.
[c]Difference between first and second trimester: $P < 0.001$.
[d]After outlier deletion and log transformation.
[e]After outlier deletion.

TABLE 3: Comparison between reference ranges for thyroid hormones as calculated by our analysis and those proposed by the manufacturer.

Reference ranges	TSH (μIU/mL)		free T4 (ng/dL)		free T3 (pg/mL)	
	1st trimester	2nd trimester	1st trimester	2nd trimester	1st trimester	2nd trimester
Rhea cohort	0.05–2.53	0.18–2.73	0.95–1.53	0.87–1.45	1.54–5.22	1.78–5.29
Manufacturer	0.4–4		0.89–1.76		1.8–4.2	

TSH: thyroid-stimulating hormone; free T3: free triiodothyronine; free T4: free thyroxine.

TABLE 4: Thyroid clinical entities in the general population of Rhea mother-child cohort based on: (i) the manufacturer's and (ii) the derived reference limits.

Trimester	Reference limits	Normal thyroid function n (%)[a]	Subclinical hypothyroidism n (%)[b]	Clinical hypothyroidism n (%)[c]	Subclinical hyperthyroidism n (%)[d]	Clinical hyper-thyroidism n (%)[e]
1st	Manufacturer	386 (84.3)	6 (1.3)	0 (0)	48 (10.5)	7 (1.5)
	Rhea cohort	371 (81.0)	31 (6.8)	0 (0)	1 (0.2)	10 (2.2)
2nd	Manufacturer	680 (86.6)	18 (2.3)	1 (0.1)	61 (7.7)	1 (0.1)
	Rhea Cohort	653 (82.2)	47 (5.9)	0 (0)	18 (2.3)	9 (1,1)

[a]TSH between reference limits and free T4 between reference limits.
[b]TSH over the upper limit of reference limits and free T4 between reference limits.
[c]TSH over the upper limit of reference limits and free T4 under the lower limit of reference limits.
[d]TSH under the lower limit of reference limits and free T4 between reference limits.
[e]TSH under the lower limit of reference limits and free T4 over the upper limit of reference limits.

decreased intelligence quotient (IQ) of children [35]. Conversely, hyperthyroidism has been described in about 0.2% of women during pregnancy [36] and may lead to preeclampsia, stillbirths, preterm delivery, intrauterine growth retardation, and low birth weight [7]. Withstanding the above, the serial changes in serum thyroid hormone levels imply the need to better define "pregnancy-specific" normative reference ranges for thyroid function tests for early diagnosis of hyper- and hypothyroidism during pregnancy.

Our study represents the first study performed in a Mediterranean area, the island of Crete, within an iodine-suf-

ficient country, Greece [37]. It provides reference ranges for thyroid hormones during the first and second trimester of pregnancy. International guidelines recommend determining serum TSH as the first-line screening variable for thyroid dysfunction before conception [38] and during pregnancy [3, 39]. According to our results and in agreement with previous studies [40], the derived reference intervals for TSH were different (narrower and lower) from those proposed by the manufacturer. More specifically, our TSH reference intervals were 0.05–2.53 and 0.18–2.73 μIU/mL for the first trimester and second trimester, respectively, compared

TABLE 5: Worldwide summary of studies reporting 1st and 2nd trimester-specific reference intervals for thyroid hormones during pregnancy.

Study	Country (subgroups)	Sample size	Exclusion criteria	Assay used/test (units)	Reference limits 1st trimester	Reference limits 2nd trimester
Price et al., 2001 [23]	UK (Caucasians/Asians)	120	(i) Serious gestational events (ii) Endocrinological medication	CL (ACS 180, Bayer) TSH (mIU/L) Free T4 (pmol/L)	Caucasians ($n = 50$): TSH: 0.7–1.1 Free T4: 12.0–12.8 Asians ($n = 20$): TSH: 0.6–1.3 Free T4: 11.8–13.4	Caucasians ($n = 50$): TSH: 1.2–1.5 Free T4: 11.2–11.8 Asians ($n = 20$): TSH: 1.0–1.8 Free T4: 10.9–12.1
Panesar et al., 2001 [9]	China	406	(i) Thyroid disease (ii) Serious gestational events (incl. hyperemesis, trophoblastic disease, preeclampsia)	CL (ACS 180, Chiron Diagn.) TSH (mIU/L) Free T4 (pmol/L) Free T3 (pmol/L)	—[a]	—[a]
Haddow et al., 2004 [13]	USA	1126	(i) Thyroid Ab(+)	CL (Immulite, Siemens) TSH (mIU/L)	($n = 1005$) TSH: 0.08–2.73	($n = 1005$) TSH: 0.39–2.70
Kurioka et al., 2005 [14]	Japan	522	(i) Multiple pregnancies	ECL (Elecsys, Roche) TSH mIU/mL Free T4 (ng/dL) Free T3 (pg/mL)	($n = 119$) TSH: 0.04–3.39 Free T4: 1.16–1.95 Free T3: 2.68–4.59	($n = 132$) TSH: 0.17–3.72 Free T4: 0.89–1.39 Free T3: 2.56–4.11
Dhatt et al., 2006 [24]	United Arab Emirates (United Arabs/Other Arabs/Asians)	1140	(i) Multiple pregnancies (ii) Thyroid Ab(+) (iii) Thyroid disease (iv) Thyroid medication (v) Serious gestational events (incl. hyperemesis)	CL (Architect, Abbott) TSH (mIU/L) Free T4 (pmol/L)	United Arabs ($n = 97$): TSH: 0.06–8.3 Free T4: 8.9–24.6 Other Arabs ($n = 122$): TSH: 0.04–9.3 Free T4: 10.5–22.3 Asians ($n = 79$): TSH: 0.12–7.4 Free T4: 11.3–2.19	United Arabs ($n = 252$): TSH: 0.17–5.9 Free T4: 8.4–19.3 Other Arabs ($n = 283$): TSH: 0.23–5.7 Free T4: 9.5–18.7 Asians ($n = 174$): TSH: 0.3–5.5 Free T4: 9.7–18.5
Stricker et al., 2007 [12]	Switzerland	2272	(i) Thyroid Ab(+) (ii) Thyroid medication (iii) Miscarriage (iv) Fetal genetic abnormality	CL (Architect, Abbott) TSH (mIU/L) Free T4 (pmol/L) Free T3 (pmol/L)	($n = 783$) TSH: 0.0888–2.8293 Free T4: 10.53–18.28 Free T3: 3.52–6.22	($n = 528$) TSH: 0.1998–2.7915 Free T4: 9.53–15.68 Free T3: 3.41–5.78
La'ulu and Roberts, 2007 [19]	USA (Asians/Blacks/ Hispanics/Whites)	3064	(i) Thyroid Ab(+)	CL (Architect, Abbott) TSH (mIU/L) Free T4 (pmol/L) Free T3 (pmol/L)	—	($n = 2683$)[b] TSH: 0.15–3.11 Free T4: 9.3–15.2 Free T3: 3.83–5.96

TABLE 5: Continued.

Study	Country (subgroups)	Sample size	Exclusion criteria	Assay used/test (units)	Reference limits 1st trimester	Reference limits 2nd trimester
Cotzias et al., 2008 [15]	UK	335	(i) Multiple pregnancies (ii) Thyroid/endocrine disease (iii) Serious gestational events (incl. preeclampsia, hyperemesis) (iv) Medication (v) Age < 15 & >45	CL (Advia Centaur, Siemens) TSH (mIU/L), Free T4 (pmol/L), Free T3 (pmol/L)	—[a]	—[a]
Lambert-Messerlian et al., 2008 [16]	USA	9562	(i) Multiple pregnancies (ii) Thyroid disease	CL (Immulite, Siemens) TSH (mIU/L)	(n = 9562) TSH: 0.13–4.15	(n = 9562) TSH: 0.36–3.77
Gong and Hoffman, 2008 [17]	Canada	340	(i) Thyroid Ab(+) (ii) TSH < 0.1 mIU/L (iii) TSH > 2.5 mIU/L (1st trimester) (iv) TSH > 3.0 mIU/L (2nd trimester) (v) TSH > 3.5 mIU/L (3rd trimester)	ECL (Modular E170, Roche) Free T4 (pmol/L)	(n = 224) Free T4: 11–19	(n = 240) Free T4: 9.7–17.5
Pearce et al., 2008 [25]	USA	668	(i) Multiple pregnancies (ii) Thyroid Ab(+) (iii) Thyroid disease (iv) Thyroid medication (v) TSH >5.5 mIU/L in Ab(−) women (vi) Miscarriages/fetal death	CL (Advia Centaur, Bayer) TSH (mIU/L)	(n = 585) TSH: 0.04–3.6	—
Marwaha et al., 2008 [11]	India	541	(i) Thyroid Ab(+) (ii) Thyroid disease (iii) Thyroid medication (iv) Family history of thyroid disease (v) Thyroid hypoechogenicity/nodularity (US) (vi) History of abortions and hyperemesis	ECL (Elecsys, Roche) TSH (mIU/mL), Free (T4 pmol/L), Free (T3 pmol/L)	(n = 107) TSH: 0.6–5.0, Free T4: 12–19.45, Free T3: 1.92–5.86	(n = 137) TSH: 0.435–5.78, Free T4: 9.48–19.58, Free T3: 3.2–5.7
Gilbert et al., 2008 [26]	Australia	2159	(i) Thyroid Ab(+) (ii) Thyroid disease	CL (Architect, Abbott) TSH (mIU/L), Free T4 (pmol/L), Free T3 (pmol/L)	(n = 1817) TSH: 0.02–2.15, Free T4: 10.4–17.8, Free T3: 3.3–5.7	—

TABLE 5: Continued.

Study	Country (subgroups)	Sample size	Exclusion criteria	Assay used/test (units)	Reference limits 1st trimester	Reference limits 2nd trimester
Springer et al., 2009 [18]	Czech republic	5520	(i) Thyroid Ab(+) (ii) Thyroid diseases (iii) β-HCG > 56 mg/L	CL (Advia Centaur, Siemens) TSH (mIU/L)	(n = 4337) TSH: 0.06–3.67	—
Bocos-Terraz et al, 2009 [10]	Spain	1198	(i) Thyroid Ab(+) (ii) Thyroid disease	CL (Architect, Abbott) TSH (μIU/mL) Free T4 (ng/dL) Free T3 (pg/mL)	—[a]	—
Ashoor et al., 2010 [27]	UK (Blacks/Whites)	4318	(i) Multiple pregnancies (ii) Thyroid Ab(+) (iii) Thyroid disease (iv) Serious gestational events (incl. preeclampsia, miscarriage/fetal death, delivery <34 weeks) (v) Major fetal abnormalities (vi) Birth weight < 5th percentile	CL (Advia Centaur, Siemens) TSH (mIU/L) Free T4 (pmol/L) Free T3 (pmol/L)	—[a]	—
Garía de Guadiana Romualdo et al, 2010 [29]	Spain	441	(i) Thyroid Ab(+) (ii) Thyroid disease incl. goiter (iii) Thyroid medication	ECL (Cobas, Roche) TSH (mUI/L) Free T4 (ng/dL)	(n = 400) TSH: 0.130–3.710 Free T4: 0.89–1.50	—
Yu et al., 2010 [30]	China	538	(i) Multiple pregnancies (ii) Thyroid disease incl. goiter (iii) Thyroid Ab(+) (iv) History of autoimmune diseases (v) Serious gestational events (incl. hyperemesis, hypertension, gestational diabetes, premature delivery) (vi) Medical history affecting thyroid function (vii) Abnormal urinary iodine	ECL (Cobas, Roche) TSH (mUI/L) Free T4 (pmol/L)	(n = 301) TSH: 0.02–3.65 Free T4: 11.85–21.51	(n = 301) TSH: 0.36– 3.46 Free T4: 9.45–16.26
Männistö et al., 2011 [31]	Finland	5805	(i) Multiple pregnancies (ii) Thyroid Ab(+) (iii) Thyroid disease (iv) Thyroid medication	CL (Architect, Abbott) TSH (mIU/L) Free T4 (pmol/L) Free T3 (pmol/L)	—[a]	—[a]

TABLE 5: Continued.

Study	Country (subgroups)	Sample size	Exclusion criteria	Assay used/test (units)	Reference limits 1st trimester	Reference limits 2nd trimester
Yan et al., 2011 [8]	China	505	(i) Multiple pregnancies (ii) Thyroid Ab(+) (iii) Thyroid disease incl. goitre (iv) Family history of thyroid disease (v) TSH > 5.0 mIU/l (vi) Serious gestational events (vii) Endocrinological medication	CL (Advia Centaur, Bayer) TSH (mIU/L) Free T4 (pmol/L) Free T3 (pmol/L)	(n = 168) TSH: 0.03–4.51 Free T4: 11.8–21 Free T3: 3.57– 5.61	(n = 168) TSH: 0.05–4.50 Free T4: 10.6–17.6 Free T3: 3.55– 5.25
Santiago et al., 2011 [28]	Spain	429	(i) Thyroid Ab(+) (ii) TSH > 5 μIU/mL (iii) Major health problems	CL (Beckman access) TSH (μIU/mL) Free T4 (ng/dL) Free T3 (pg/mL)	(n = 279) TSH: 0.23– 4.18 Free T4: 0.60–1.06 Free T3: 2.33–3.84	(n = 210) TSH: 0.36–3.89 Free T4: 0.43–0.85 Free T3: 2.04–3.51

[a] reference intervals other than trimester-specific (data not shown);

[b] combined reference interval for all ethnicities; reference intervals also provided for ethnicity subgroups (data not shown).

CL: Chemiluminescence assay; ECL: Electrochemiluminescence assay; TSH; thyroid-stimulating hormone; Free T4; serum-free thyroxine; Free T3; serum-free triiodothyronine;

To convert to SI units, for

FT4: pmol/L = ng/dL x12.87

FT3: pmol/L = pg/mL x1.536.

to 0.4–4 µIU/mL. Consequently, women with subclinical hypothyroidism would not have been identified, and normal women would have been misclassified as having subclinical hyperthyroidism if the manufacturer's TSH limits were used. Regarding free T4, and free T3, our intervals were only slightly different.

Many cross-sectional studies have reported trimester-specific reference ranges for free T3, free T4, and TSH among pregnant women [8–31]. However these reported reference ranges vary due to differences in ethnicity, iodine intake, sample size, assessment of reference population, and immunometric assay used among studies. Table 5 summarizes 1st and 2nd trimester-specific reference intervals for thyroid hormones from 21 studies worldwide. Ethnic disparities along with variations in iodine nutrition characteristics result in geographic variability of hormonal values. In addition, different reagents used by laboratories recognize distinct circulating TSH isoforms with resulting fluctuations even for the same sample [41]. Therefore, there is a growing need for laboratory- and geography- specific reference intervals [42]. Moreover, the methodology used by the published studies to date varies in terms of inclusion criteria for the determination of reference population, sample size, and assessment of outliers. More specifically, most studies used nonparametric methods in order to provide reference intervals without reporting the underlying distribution [10, 12, 14, 19], did not mention whether outliers were detected and removed [10–20], and most importantly, in some cases, have not applied strict criteria to obtain a well-defined healthy population [13, 14, 16, 17]. According to the National Academy of Clinical Biochemistry (NACB) [32] and the National Health and Nutrition Examination Survey (NHANES), this well-defined healthy population should be based on specific exclusion criteria and represents the most important prerequisite for the determination of reference intervals [43, 44].

Based on the above, we selected our reference population from a large pool of Rhea mother-child cohort in Crete, after implementation of stringent criteria. Initially, we excluded all mothers with any kind of thyroid abnormality since women positive for thyroid autoantibodies typically have higher TSH values and therefore affect and skew the upper reference limit [45, 46]. In addition, women with twin pregnancies or with hyperemesis gravidum were also removed from the reference population due to their potential for low TSH values (higher serum hCG) and interference with the lower limit of TSH reference range [22, 47, 48]. Based on the association between autoimmunity and thyroid dysfunction [49], we also excluded mothers with positive history of autoimmune diseases. The final strictly defined reference population of 403 women was considered adequate for the estimation of reference intervals fulfilling the sample size requirements of Clinical Laboratory Standards (NCCLS) [43]. Additional methodological strengths of our study include examination of distributions and respective application of parametric or nonparametric methods, assessment of outliers, and use of a statistical test to resolve whether separate reference intervals

should be calculated for the first and second trimester. Results from this test confirmed the need for trimester-specific reference ranges in agreement to the existing literature and as indicated by normal physiology.

Our study is limited by lack of data concerning the third trimester. Pregnant women were partitioned into trimesters upon entering the study, and thus the resulting sample size (n = 22) was not adequate for the estimation of reference intervals to a reasonable degree of precision. However, during the second half of gestation TSH levels return to pre-pregnancy levels and remain stable [50]. In addition, there was only a small number of women (n = 12) in less than 8 weeks of gestation, when hCG has a minimal effect on thyroid. Contrary to The National Health and Nutrition Examination Survey in the USA [36], some studies propose that thyroid ultrasound should be used as an additional exclusion criterion to rule out thyroid pathology [51]. In our study, we did not include thyroid ultrasound for the detection of goiter or presence of hypoechogenicity and nodularity of thyroid, since these data were not collected. Finally, an important limitation is the assumption of iodine sufficiency in all women, as we did not evaluate iodine status by urine iodine estimation. However, median urinary iodine excretion (the best parameter to evaluate the adequacy of iodine nutrition in a population) during the last two decades in Greece has been estimated to be over 200 µg/g Cr [52, 53], which is well within normal limits [54]. These findings indicate that, at present, Greece may be considered as an iodine-sufficient country.

5. Conclusion

Data from this study establish reference values for Greek Cretan pregnant women and point out the need for laboratory- and geography-specific reference ranges in an effort to detect overt and subclinical thyroid disorders and to evaluate the risk for both obstetric complications and impaired fetal development.

Acknowledgment

Dr. Leda Chatzi was supported by the EU Integrated Project NewGeneris, 6th Framework Programme, Priority 5: Food Quality and Safety (Contract no. FOOD-CT-2005-016320). NewGeneris is the acronym of the project "Newborns and Genotoxic exposure risks" http://www.newgeneris.org.

References

[1] D. Glinoer, "The regulation of thyroid function in pregnancy: pathways of endocrine adaptation from physiology to pathology," *Endocrine Reviews*, vol. 18, no. 3, pp. 404–433, 1997.

[2] C. R. Fantz, S. Dagogo-Jack, J. H. Ladenson, and A. M. Gronowski, "Thyroid function during pregnancy," *Clinical Chemistry*, vol. 45, no. 12, pp. 2250–2258, 1999.

[3] M. Abalovich, N. Amino, L. A. Barbour et al., "Management of thyroid dysfunction during pregnancy and postpartum: an

Endocrine Society Clinical Practice Guideline," *The Journal of Clinical Endocrinology and Metabolism*, vol. 92, supplement 8, pp. S1–S47, 2007.

[4] L. Skjoldebrand, J. Brundin, A. Carlstrom, and T. Pettersson, "Thyroid associated components in serum during normal pregnancy," *Acta Endocrinologica*, vol. 100, no. 4, pp. 504–511, 1982.

[5] J. Guillaume, G. C. Schussler, and J. Goldman, "Components of the total serum thyroid hormone concentrations during pregnancy: high free thyroxine and blunted thyrotropin (TSH) response to TSH-releasing hormone in the first trimester," *Journal of Clinical Endocrinology and Metabolism*, vol. 60, no. 4, pp. 678–684, 1985.

[6] R. D. Utiger, "Maternal hypothyroidism and fetal development," *New England Journal of Medicine*, vol. 341, no. 8, pp. 601–602, 1999.

[7] J. H. Metsman, "Hyperthyroidism in pregnancy," *Best Practice and Research*, vol. 18, no. 2, pp. 267–288, 2004.

[8] Y. Q. Yan, Z. L. Dong, L. Dong et al., "Trimester-and method-specific reference intervals for thyroid tests in pregnant Chinese women: methodology, euthyroid definition and iodine status can influence the setting of reference intervals," *Clinical Endocrinology*, vol. 74, no. 2, pp. 262–269, 2011.

[9] N. S. Panesar, C. Y. Li, and M. S. Rogers, "Reference intervals for thyroid hormones in pregnant Chinese women," *Annals of Clinical Biochemistry*, vol. 38, no. 4, pp. 329–332, 2001.

[10] J. P. Bocos-Terraz, S. Izquierdo-Álvarez, J. Bancalero-Flores et al., "Thyroid hormones according to gestational age in pregnant Spanish women," *BMC Research Notes*, vol. 2, article 237, 2009.

[11] R. K. Marwaha, S. Chopra, S. Gopalakrishnan et al., "Establishment of reference range for thyroid hormones in normal pregnant Indian women," *An International Journal of Obstetrics and Gynaecology*, vol. 115, no. 5, pp. 602–606, 2008.

[12] R. Stricker, M. Echenard, R. Eberhart et al., "Evaluation of maternal thyroid function during pregnancy: the importance of using gestational age-specific reference intervals," *European Journal of Endocrinology*, vol. 157, no. 4, pp. 509–514, 2007.

[13] J. E. Haddow, G. J. Knight, G. E. Palomaki, M. R. McClain, and A. J. Pulkkinen, "The reference range and within-person variability of thyroid stimulating hormone during the first and second trimesters of pregnancy," *Journal of Medical Screening*, vol. 11, no. 4, pp. 170–174, 2004.

[14] H. Kurioka, K. Takahashi, and K. Miyazaki, "Maternal thyroid function during pregnancy and puerperal period," *Endocrine Journal*, vol. 52, no. 5, pp. 587–591, 2005.

[15] C. Cotzias, S. J. Wong, E. Taylor, P. Seed, and J. Girling, "A study to establish gestation-specific reference intervals for thyroid function tests in normal singleton pregnancy," *European Journal of Obstetrics Gynecology and Reproductive Biology*, vol. 137, no. 1, pp. 61–66, 2008.

[16] G. Lambert-Messerlian, M. McClain, J. E. Haddow et al., "First- and second-trimester thyroid hormone reference data in pregnant women: a FaSTER (First- and Second-Trimester Evaluation of Risk for aneuploidy) Research Consortium study," *American Journal of Obstetrics and Gynecology*, vol. 199, no. 1, pp. 62.e1–62.e6, 2008.

[17] Y. Gong and B. R. Hoffman, "Free thyroxine reference interval in each trimester of pregnancy determined with the Roche Modular E-170 electrochemiluminescent immunoassay," *Clinical Biochemistry*, vol. 41, no. 10-11, pp. 902–906, 2008.

[18] D. Springer, T. Zima, and Z. Limanova, "Reference intervals in evaluation of maternal thyroid function during the first trimester of pregnancy," *European Journal of Endocrinology*, vol. 160, no. 5, pp. 791–797, 2009.

[19] S. L. La'ulu and W. L. Roberts, "Second-trimester reference intervals for thyroid tests: the role of ethnicity," *Clinical Chemistry*, vol. 53, no. 9, pp. 1658–1664, 2007.

[20] T. Yamamoto, N. Amino, and O. Tanizawa, "Longitudinal study of serum thyroid hormones, chorionic gonadotrophin and thyrotrophin during and after normal pregnancy," *Clinical Endocrinology*, vol. 10, no. 5, pp. 459–468, 1979.

[21] O. P. Soldin, D. Soldin, and M. Sastoque, "Gestation-specific thyroxine and thyroid stimulating hormone levels in the United States and worldwide," *Therapeutic Drug Monitoring*, vol. 29, no. 5, pp. 553–559, 2007.

[22] J. S. Dashe, B. M. Casey, C. E. Wells et al., "Thyroid-stimulating hormone in singleton and twin pregnancy: importance of gestational age-specific reference ranges," *Obstetrics and Gynecology*, vol. 106, no. 4, pp. 753–757, 2005.

[23] A. Price, O. Obel, J. Cresswell et al., "Comparison of thyroid function in pregnant and non-pregnant Asian and western Caucasian women," *Clinica Chimica Acta*, vol. 308, no. 1-2, pp. 91–98, 2001.

[24] G. S. Dhatt, G. Griffin, and M. M. Agarwal, "Thyroid hormone reference intervals in an ambulatory Arab population on the Abbott Architect i2000 immunoassay analyzer," *Clinica Chimica Acta*, vol. 364, no. 1-2, pp. 226–229, 2006.

[25] E. N. Pearce, E. Oken, M. W. Gillman et al., "Association of first-trimester thyroid function test values with thyroperoxidase antibody status, smoking, and multivitamin use," *Endocrine Practice*, vol. 14, no. 1, pp. 33–39, 2008.

[26] R. M. Gilbert, N. C. Hadlow, J. P. Walsh et al., "Assessment of thyroid function during pregnancy: first-trimester (weeks 9–13) reference intervals derived from Western Australian women," *Medical Journal of Australia*, vol. 189, no. 5, pp. 250–253, 2008.

[27] G. Ashoor, N. A. Kametas, R. Akolekar, J. Guisado, and K. H. Nicolaides, "Maternal thyroid function at 11–13 weeks of gestation," *Fetal Diagnosis and Therapy*, vol. 27, no. 3, pp. 156–163, 2010.

[28] P. Santiago, M. Berrio, P. Olmedo et al., "Reference values for thyroid hormones in the population of pregnant women in jaen (Spain)," *Endocrinologia y Nutricion*, vol. 58, no. 2, pp. 62–67, 2011.

[29] L. García de Guadiana Romualdo, M. González Morales, M. D. C. Martín-Ondarza González et al., "Evaluation of thyroid function during pregnancy: first-trimester reference intervals for thyroid-stimulating hormone and free thyroxine," *Endocrinologia y Nutricion*, vol. 57, no. 7, pp. 290–295, 2010.

[30] B. Yu, Q. W. Wang, R. P. Huang et al., "Establishment of self-sequential longitudinal reference intervals of maternal thyroid function during pregnancy," *Experimental Biology and Medicine*, vol. 235, no. 10, pp. 1212–1215, 2010.

[31] T. Männistö, H. M. Surcel, A. Ruokonen et al., "Early pregnancy reference intervals of thyroid hormone concentrations in a thyroid antibody-negative pregnant population," *Thyroid*, vol. 21, no. 3, pp. 291–298, 2011.

[32] Z. Baloch, P. Carayon, B. Conte-Devolx et al., "Laboratory medicine practice guidelines. Laboratory support for the diagnosis and monitoring of thyroid disease," *Thyroid*, vol. 13, no. 1, pp. 3–126, 2003.

[33] M. Yoshimura and J. M. Hershman, "Thyrotropic action of human chorionic gonadotropin," *Thyroid*, vol. 5, no. 5, pp. 425–434, 1995.

[34] R. Z. Klein, J. E. Haddow, J. D. Faix et al., "Prevalence of thyroid deficiency in pregnant women," *Clinical Endocrinology*, vol. 35, no. 1, pp. 41–46, 1991.

[35] L. E. Davis, K. J. Leveno, and F. G. Cunningham, "Hypothyroidism complicating pregnancy," *Obstetrics and Gynecology*, vol. 72, no. 1, pp. 108–112, 1988.

[36] J. G. Hollowell, N. W. Staehling, W. Dana Flanders et al., "Serum TSH, T4, and thyroid antibodies in the United States population (1988 to 1994): National Health and Nutrition Examination Survey (NHANES III)," *Journal of Clinical Endocrinology and Metabolism*, vol. 87, no. 2, pp. 489–499, 2002.

[37] D. A. Koutras, M. Alevizaki, A. Tsatsoulis, and A. G. Vagenakis, "Greece is iodine sufficient," *The Lancet*, vol. 362, no. 9381, pp. 405–406, 2003.

[38] C. A. Spencer, J. S. LoPresti, A. Patel et al., "Applications of a new chemiluminometric thyrotropin assay to subnormal measurement," *Journal of Clinical Endocrinology and Metabolism*, vol. 70, no. 2, pp. 453–460, 1990.

[39] B. Vaidya, S. Anthony, M. Bilous et al., "Brief report: detection of thyroid dysfunction in early pregnancy: universal screening or targeted high-risk case finding?" *Journal of Clinical Endocrinology and Metabolism*, vol. 92, no. 1, pp. 203–207, 2007.

[40] D. Glinoer and C. A. Spencer, "Serum TSH determinations in pregnancy: how, when and why?" *Nature Reviews Endocrinology*, vol. 6, no. 9, pp. 526–529, 2010.

[41] R. Silvio, K. J. Swapp, S. L. La'ulu, K. Hansen-Suchy, and W. L. Roberts, "Method specific second-trimester reference intervals for thyroid-stimulating hormone and free thyroxine," *Clinical Biochemistry*, vol. 42, no. 7-8, pp. 750–753, 2009.

[42] U. Feldt-Rasmussen, A. S. Bliddal Mortensen, A. K. Rasmussen, M. Boas, L. Hilsted, and K. Main, "Challenges in interpretation of thyroid function tests in pregnant women with autoimmune thyroid disease," *Journal of Thyroid Research*, vol. 2011, Article ID 598712, 2011.

[43] P. S. Horn and A. J. Pesce, "Reference intervals: an update," *Clinica Chimica Acta*, vol. 334, no. 1-2, pp. 5–23, 2003.

[44] NCCLS, "How to define and determine reference intervals in the clinical laboratory: approved guideline," NCCLS Document C28-A and C28-A2, Villanova, Pa, USA.

[45] D. Glinoer, M. Riahi, J. P. Grun, and J. Kinthaert, "Risk of subclinical hypothyroidism in pregnant women with asymptomatic autoimmune thyroid disorders," *Journal of Clinical Endocrinology and Metabolism*, vol. 79, no. 1, pp. 197–204, 1994.

[46] C. A. Spencer, J. G. Hollowell, M. Kazarosyan, and L. E. Braverman, "National Health and Nutrition Examination Survey III Thyroid-Stimulating Hormone (TSH)-thyroperoxidase antibody relationships demonstrate that TSH upper reference limits may be skewed by occult thyroid dysfunction," *Journal of Clinical Endocrinology and Metabolism*, vol. 92, no. 11, pp. 4236–4240, 2007.

[47] J. P. Grün, S. Meuris, P. De Nayer, and D. Glinoer, "The thyrotrophic role of human chorionic gonadotrophin (hCG) in the early stages of twin (versus single) pregnancies," *Clinical Endocrinology*, vol. 46, no. 6, pp. 719–725, 1997.

[48] M. R. McClain, G. Lambert-Messerlian, J. E. Haddow et al., "Sequential first- and second-trimester TSH, free thyroxine, and thyroid antibody measurements in women with known hypothyroidism: a FaSTER trial study," *American Journal of Obstetrics and Gynecology*, vol. 199, no. 2, pp. 129.e1–129.e6, 2008.

[49] K. Boelaert, P. R. Newby, M. J. Simmonds et al., "Prevalence and relative risk of other autoimmune diseases in subjects with autoimmune thyroid disease," *American Journal of Medicine*, vol. 123, no. 2, pp. 183.e1–183.e9, 2010.

[50] D. Glinoer and F. Delange, "The potential repercussions of maternal, fetal, and neonatal hypothyroxinemia on the progeny," *Thyroid*, vol. 10, no. 10, pp. 871–887, 2000.

[51] J. Kratzsch, G. M. Fiedler, A. Leichtle et al., "New reference intervals for thyrotropin and thyroid hormones based on national academy of clinical biochemistry criteria and regular ultrasonography of the thyroid," *Clinical Chemistry*, vol. 51, no. 8, pp. 1480–1486, 2005.

[52] A. G. Doufas, G. Mastorakos, S. Chatziioannou et al., "The predominant form of non-toxic goiter in Greece is now autoimmune thyroiditis," *European Journal of Endocrinology*, vol. 140, no. 6, pp. 505–511, 1999.

[53] C. Zois, I. Stavrou, C. Kalogera et al., "High prevalence of autoimmune thyroiditis in schoolchildren after elimination of iodine deficiency in northwestern Greece," *Thyroid*, vol. 13, no. 5, pp. 485–489, 2003.

[54] F. Delange, "Iodine requirements during pregnancy, lactation and the neonatal period and indicators of optimal iodine nutrition," *Public Health Nutrition*, vol. 10, no. 12, pp. 1571–1583, 2007.

11

Myxedema Coma: A New Look into an Old Crisis

**Vivek Mathew, Raiz Ahmad Misgar, Sujoy Ghosh,
Pradip Mukhopadhyay, Pradip Roychowdhury, Kaushik Pandit,
Satinath Mukhopadhyay, and Subhankar Chowdhury**

Institute of Post-Graduate Medical Education & Research, Calcutta 700020, India

Correspondence should be addressed to Sujoy Ghosh, drsujoyghosh@rediffmail.com

Academic Editor: Masanobu Yamada

Myxedema crisis is a severe life threatening form of decompensated hypothyroidism which is associated with a high mortality rate. Infections and discontinuation of thyroid supplements are the major precipitating factors while hypothermia may not play a major role in tropical countries. Low intracellular T3 leads to cardiogenic shock, respiratory depression, hypothermia and coma. Patients are identified on the basis of a low index of suspicion with a careful history and examination focused on features of hypothyroidism and precipitating factors. Arrythmias and coagulation disorders are increasingly being identified in myxedema crisis. Thyroid replacement should be initiated as early as possible with careful attention to hypotension, fluid replacement and steroid replacement in an intensive care facility. Studies have shown that replacement of thyroid hormone through ryles tube with a loading dose and maintenance therapy is as efficacious as intravenous therapy. In many countries T3 is not available and oral therapy with T4 can be used effectively without major significant difference in outcomes. Hypotension, bradycardia at presentation, need for mechanical ventilation, hypothermia unresponsive to treatment, sepsis, intake of sedative drugs, lower GCS and high APACHE II scores and Sequential Organ Failure Assessment (SOFA) scores more than 6 are significant predictors of mortality in myxedema crisis. Early intervention in hypothyroid patients developing sepsis and other precipitating factors and ensuring continued intake of thyroid supplements may prevent mortality and morbidity associated with myxedema crisis.

> *"No decision is easy, Sue.*
> *It only looks that way when you're young.*
> *When you're older, everything is complicated.*
> *There is no black and white, only grey."*
> —Dr. George A. Harris in the movie Coma 1978.

1. Introduction

Myxedema coma is a severe and life-threatening form of decompensated hypothyroidism with an underlying precipitating factor. The mortality rates may be as high as 25–60% even with best possible treatment [1–5]. The term myxedema coma is a misnomer, and myxedema crisis may be an apt term as quite a few patients are obtunded, rather than frankly comatose. As the disease is rare and unrecognized, we only have a few isolated case reports and case series, and there is a dearth of randomized controlled trials in the field of myxedema crisis. At present there are over 300 cases reported in literature [6–8]. In this paper we discuss the standard clinical presentation, treatment, predictors of mortality, and controversies that overshadow the current concepts in the management of myxedema crisis.

The need of the hour is to find answers to some burning questions which may change the way we manage myxedema crisis. Some of these questions include the following:

(a) what are the preventable precipitating factors in myxedema crisis?

(b) are there any geographical variations involved in the presentation?

(c) how can we identify myxedema crisis at an early stage?

(d) are there ways by which we can identify patients at risk of dying?

(e) what is the status of intravenous and oral replacement therapy with T4 and T3?

At present, we need more well-designed studies to address some of these questions.

1.1. Epidemiology. Case series and case reports from western world tell us that the incidence of myxedema crisis is about 0.22 million per year, but there is a scarcity for such epidemiological data from countries that lie around the equator [9]. Epidemiology of myxedema crisis follows the same pattern as in hypothyroidism and is more common in women and elderly.

1.2. Precipitating Events. Literature reveals that most cases present in winter, and hypothermia is a common manifestation. Low ambient temperature may alter thermoregulatory mechanisms and hence will lower the threshold for encephalopathy [1]. However, in our own experience, the presentation may be only slightly more in winter months, and the incidence of severe hypothermia may be lower in tropical countries such as ours as temperatures below 10 degree Celsius are rare, and ambient temperature may influence the degree of hypothermia (unpublished data). In our experience quite a few patients with myxedema crisis have temperatures 2-3° F below normal although we also see patients with severe hypothermia.

Infections and septicemia are the leading precipitating factors [2, 3]. Typical infections include pneumonia, urinary tract infections, and cellulitis. Cerebrovascular accidents, congestive cardiac failure, road traffic accidents, gastrointestinal bleeding, and various sedative drugs may play a role in precipitating myxedema crisis. Diuretics may mask some of the myxedematous features, and they may also aggravate the hyponatremia associated with myxedema crisis.

Recently, Chu and Seltzer reported a case of myxedema crisis precipitated by consumption of raw bok choy [10]. Bok choy or Chinese white cabbage contains glucosinolates. Some of the breakdown products of glucosinolates, such as thiocyanates, nitriles, and oxazolidines, have been implicated for their inhibitory effects on the thyroid as they may inhibit the uptake of iodine. When eaten raw, brassica vegetables release the enzyme myrosinase, which accelerates the hydrolysis of glucosinolates. Cooking deactivates myrosinase.

A commonly ignored background factor in myxedema crisis is the discontinuation of thyroid supplements in critically ill patients. This is possibly due to the fact that attention may be focused on presenting features and precipitating factors, and associated hypothyroidism is generally ignored (Box 1).

2. Pathogenesis of Myxedema Crisis

Low intracellular T3 secondary to hypothyroidism is the basic underlying pathology in myxedema crisis which leads

---

Hypothermia
Infections and septicaemia
Cerebrovascular accidents
Congestive heart failure
Gastrointestinal bleeding
Consumption of raw bok choy
Trauma and fractures
Drugs—anaesthetics, sedatives, tranquilizers, narcotics, amiodarone, and lithium
Withdrawal of thyroid supplements

Box 1: Precipitating factors of myxedema crisis.

---

to hypothermia and suppression of cardiac activity. The body tries to compensate by neurovascular adaptations including chronic peripheral vasoconstriction, mild diastolic hypertension, and diminished blood volume.

Decreased central nervous system sensitivity to hypoxia and hypercapnia leads to respiratory failure [11, 12]. Other factors contributing to respiratory failure include respiratory muscle dysfunction, obesity, pleural effusions, macroglossia, reduced lung volume, myxedema of the nasopharynx and larynx (reduces the effective airway opening), pneumonia, and aspiration [12–14].

Altered vascular permeability leads to effusions and anasarca. Water retention and hyponatremia occurs secondary to reduced glomerular filtration rate, decreased delivery to the distal nephron [15], and excess vasopressin [16, 17] (Figure 1).

Low intracellular T3 leads to depressed cardiac functions with decreased inotropism and chronotropism with vasoconstriction. The hypothyroid heart tries to perform more work at a given amount of oxygen by better coupling of ATP to contractile events. A precipitating factor pushes this precarious balance over the brink [18]. In the decompensated state, low cardiac output and hypotension will result in cardiogenic shock which may not be responsive to vasopressors without thyroid hormone replacement [11].

Decreased gluconeogenesis, precipitating factors like sepsis and concomitant adrenal insufficiency, may contribute to hypoglycemia. In addition to the generalized depression of cerebral function, hyponatremia, hypoglycemia, hypoxemia, and reduced cerebral blood flow can precipitate focal or generalized seizures and worsen the level of consciousness.

3. Clinical Features

A low index of suspicion and a search for precipitating factors should be initial step in dealing with myxedema crisis at an earlier stage. History should focus on the presence of thyroid dysfunction, dose of thyroid hormone, discontinuation of thyroid supplements, thyroid surgery, radioactive iodine ablation, and a detailed record of drug intake for background diseases. Central hypothyroidism may constitute about 5% of all the cases of myxedema crisis [1]. Physical examination should focus on features of severe hypothyroidism like dry skin, sparse hair, a hoarse voice, hypothermia, delayed tendon reflexes, macroglossia, nonpitting edema, goiter, and

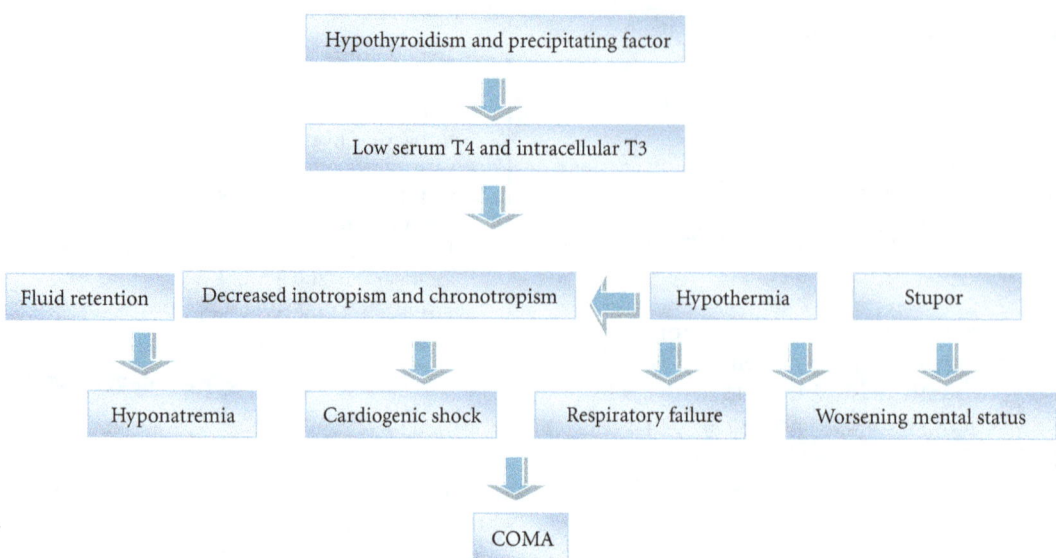

FIGURE 1: Pathogenesis of myxedema crisis.

surgical scar of thyroidectomy in addition to recording vital functions and level of consciousness. Presence of orbitopathy may be a subtle clue to underlying Graves's disease which may have been treated with radioiodine or surgery.

Dutta et al. studied 23 patients with myxedema crisis and found that 39% of them had hypothyroidism detected only at the time of crisis. It should be noted that 17% of these patients had central hypothyroidism which was higher than the previous reported percentage of 5%. Sepsis was the most common precipitating factor, and a significant proportion of patients (61%) had defaulted on thyroid supplements [4]. Reinhardt and Mann reported hypoxemia in 80%, hypercapnia in 54%, and hypothermia with a temperature less than 94°F in 88% of all the patients with myxedema crisis [5].

Sinus bradycardia, low voltage complexes, bundle branch blocks, complete heart blocks, and nonspecific ST-T changes in electrocardiogram have been recorded in myxedema crisis [4, 19]. Schenck et al. reported a patient with severe hypothyroidism who presented with presyncope, prolongation of the QT interval, and polymorphic ventricular tachycardia (torsades de pointes) which reversed with thyroid hormone supplementation [20]. Prolongation of QT interval and increased QT dispersion, a marker of electrical instability [21, 22], have been documented in severe hypothyroidism [23]. These anomalies have been shown to be reversible in subclinical hypothyroidism [24]. Increased myocardial fibrosis in severe hypothyroidism may lead to a resistance in improvement of QT dispersion with thyroid hormone supplementation [24]. The study of heart rate variability parameters also indicate that hypothyroidism leads to a sympathovagal imbalanced state, characterized by both decreased cardiovascular sympathetic and vagal modulation [23]. The occurrence of malignant arrhythmias needs to be recognized in long-standing hypothyroidism and myxedema crisis [19, 23, 25] (Table 1).

An important practical aspect may be the identification of pericardial effusion and myocardial infarction in a setting of myxedema crisis. Low-voltage complexes and nonspecific ST-T changes can be seen in pericardial effusion. Cardiac enzymes should be done with a suspicion of myocardial infarction.

Patients with myxedema crisis may have normocytic normochromic anemia which may be secondary to decreased oxygen requirement and erythropoietin [26]. Macrocytic blood picture may be seen with associated low folate absorption and pernicious anemia [27–29]. Severely hypothyroid patients may have bleeding manifestations, and investigations reveal prolonged bleeding time and clotting time, decreased platelet adhesiveness, elevated APTT, and low or normal factor VIII activity. Acquired von Willebrand's disease is also reported in hypothyroidism with decreased von Willebrand factor antigen and activity [30]. Acquired von Willebrand's disease is very likely to be type 1 in all cases because of a normal ratio of von Willebrand's factor antigen to ristocetin cofactor r [31]. The underlying defect could possibly be a decreased synthesis of von Willebrand factor in the absence of adequate levels of thyroxine [32], and thyroxine replacement corrects these abnormalities [31, 33]. Erfurth and group have demonstrated that desmopressin immediately reduced bleeding time, enhanced platelet adhesiveness, and significantly increased plasma concentrations of factor VIII and von Willebrand's factor and hence may be valuable for the acute treatment of bleeding or as cover for surgery in a setting of myxedema crisis or severe hypothyroidism [33].

Other common biochemical anomalies in myxedema crisis include increased levels of creatine phosphokinase, lactate dehydrogenase, aspartate transaminase, and hypercholesterolemia (elevated LDL) [34].

4. Diagnosis

Patients with altered sensorium, hypothermia, or absence of fever despite infectious disease, clinical and biochemical

TABLE 1: Clinical and laboratory features of myxedema crisis.

Cardiovascular	Neuropsychiatric
Bradycardia and hypotension	Confusion and obtundation
Cardiomegaly	Lethargy
Low cardiac output	Coma
Pericardial effusion	Seizures
Cardiogenic shock	Poor cognitive function
Bundle branch blocks and arrhythmias	Depression and psychosis
Nonspecific ECG findings	
Respiratory	Renal and water metabolism
Hypoxia	Fluid retention
Hypercarbia	Anasarca
Myxedema of larynx	Hyponatremia
Pleural effusion	Bladder atony
Pneumonia (precipitating factor)	Urine sodium normal or increased
	Urine osmolality > serum osmolality
Gastrointestinal	Metabolic
Anorexia and nausea	Hypothermia
Abdominal pain	Hypoglycemia
Constipation	
Paralytic ileus	
Toxic megacolon	
Gastric atony	
Neurogenic oropharyngeal dysphagia	

features of hypothyroidism, those who had a history of hypothyroidism and are currently not on treatment, in the setting of a precipitating factor, should be identified with a high index of suspicion. The treating physician should not hesitate in starting replacement therapy while waiting for serum TSH and serum T4. An active search for precipitating causes should be initiated, and appropriate investigations should be ordered based on patient's clinical presentation. White blood cell counts, urine routine and microscopy, blood and urine culture, serum electrolytes, serum creatinine, chest X-ray, and electrocardiogram should be obtained.

Clinician may face multiple diagnostic dilemmas. First, in central hypothyroidism, TSH may be unusually low. The deciding factor here will be associated pituitary hormone deficiencies as isolated central hypothyroidism is rare. In the second situation, the systemic illness will produce a picture akin to sick euthyroid syndrome, and the elevation in TSH may not be as high as expected, but the T3 levels here may be unusually low as there is decreased conversion of T4 to T3 [34, 35] with elevated reverse T3. Finally, the presenting features of myxedema crisis may also be commonly seen with associated sepsis, stroke, and dyselectrolytemia, and hence the diagnosis is often delayed.

It may be appropriate at this juncture to discuss the rare entity of Hashimoto's encephalopathy which is a rare complication of Hashimoto's thyroiditis [36]. The condition may present as a subacute or acute encephalopathy with seizures, stroke-like episodes, myoclonus, and tremor [37]. Patients will have elevated thyroid-specific autoantibodies

(Anti-TPO), elevated cerebrospinal fluid protein without pleocytosis, and abnormal electroencephalogram [38]. The key points to consider here is that most patients are euthyroid and the condition is steroid responsive [39].

5. Treatment of Myxedema Crisis

Treatment of myxedema crisis should be prompt and multidimensional with attention to the following principles:

(a) intensive care treatment with ventilator support, central venous pressure monitoring, and pulmonary capillary wedge pressure if feasible in patients with cardiac disease,

(b) appropriate fluid management and correction of hypotension and dyselectrolytemia,

(c) aggressive management of precipitating factors and steroid supplementation if required,

(d) thyroid hormone replacement.

6. General Measures in Management

Management of airway and airway protection from aspiration in case of patients with poor consciousness level should be the utmost priority. Endotracheal intubation or tracheostomy with mechanical ventilation may be performed. Arterial blood gas should be monitored frequently to ensure adequate oxygenation and correction of hypercarbia.

Sedatives and other drugs may exacerbate the respiratory depression and may delay the weaning of ventilator support [40].

Fluid management evokes a Damocles sword type situation in myxedema crisis where the choice is between fluid supplementation for hypotension and fluid restriction for hyponatremia. A pragmatic approach in mild hyponatremia will be to advice fluid restriction with replacement to cover the daily losses taking care to supplement glucose, sodium, and potassium [41]. In a situation of severe hyponatremia, it may be prudent to administer 3% sodium chloride along with furosemide, so that serum sodium may be elevated by 3-4 meq/L to tide over the immediate crisis [42]. A rapid correction of chronic hyponatremia might put patients at risk for central pontine myelinolysis [43, 44]. Treatment with furosemide will prevent fluid overloading associated with hypertonic saline. In experimental hypothyroidism, the impaired response to an acute water load was shown to be reversed by a Vasopressin receptor antagonist (V2R antagonist) [17]. Future research with V2R antagonists in treating hyponatremia associated with myxedema crisis may prove to be interesting.

Hypothermia may be managed by external warming, but the accompanying vasodilatation may precipitate hypotension. Hypotension requires careful infusion of dextrose saline solutions and vasopressors if required. A search for other causes of hypotension like sepsis, myocardial infarction, pericardial effusion, and occult bleeding should be initiated. In a setting of concomitant adrenal insufficiency, hydrocortisone supplementation is also required for correction of hypotension.

Hypocortisolemia may be due to primary or secondary adrenal insufficiency. The clinical features of myxedema crisis and cortisol deficiency may overlap. Hyperpigmentation, hyperkalemia, hypercalcemia, and previous history of on and off steroid use must be sought. Thyroid hormone replacement may increase cortisol clearance and may aggravate cortisol deficiency. If the facilities for HPA axis evaluation are not available on an emergency basis, steroid therapy may start and a formal evaluation of axis is done at a later date when patient is stable. Intravenous hydrocortisone is preferred at a rate of 50 mg every 6 hours.

It cannot be overemphasized that the precipitating factors require urgent attention with antibiotics in case of infection, hemodialysis for associated renal failure, and comprehensive care of multiorgan dysfunction.

7. Thyroid Hormone Therapy

Thyroid hormone therapy is the backbone of treatment of patients with myxedema crisis. The main considerations with thyroid hormone replacement are the absorption and distribution of administered hormone preparation, the onset of action and efficacy of the preparation, and finally the safety. At present, oral and intravenous T4 and T3 are used. The major considerations are the dose, route of administration, and frequency of administration.

T4 therapy provides a steady, smooth, and slow onset of action with relatively few adverse events. In many countries, T3 may not be available, but T4 is easily available at hand. T4 therapy avoids major peaks and troughs in body, and values of serum T4 may be easy to interpret [1]. However, T3 is the active hormone in the body, and in a setting of severe illness there may be a decreased conversion of T4 to T3 [34]. Parenteral T4 may be used at a dose of 300–500 μg as bolus to saturate the body pool. The usual protocol then is to continue T4 at a dose of 50–100 μg daily. There are enough studies that have used a large bolus dose of T4 as described earlier, and they demonstrate good results [45, 46]. T4 concentrations rise acutely to levels above normal and slowly gets converted to T3 [46].

Oral administration of T4 through Ryles tube has proved to be equally effective with a drawback that gastric atony may prevent absorption and put the patient at risk for aspiration. Dutta and colleagues compared 500 μg of oral loading dose of T4 with 150 μg of maintenance dose orally and 200 μg of T4 intravenously followed by 100 μg T4 intravenously until they regained their vital functions and were able to take oral medications in patients with myxedema crisis and did not find any difference in outcome among the patients [4].

Advantages of using T3 include a rapid onset of action, an earlier beneficial effect on neuropsychiatric symptoms, and significant clinical improvement within 24 hours. T3 may be given at a dose of 10 to 20 μg, followed by 10 μg every 4 hours for the first 24 hours and then 10 μg every 6 hours for 1 or 2 days till the patient is alert enough to continue therapy through oral route. Measurable increases in body temperature and oxygen consumption occur within 2 to 3 hours after intravenous administration of T3 but may take 8 to 14 hours or longer after intravenous administration of T4 [1, 47]. However, poor availability of T3, fluctuations in serum levels of T3, and adverse cardiac effects may limit the use of T3. Yamamoto et al. reported that doses of LT4 more than 500 μg per day and LT3 more than 75 μg/day were associated with increased mortality [3].

Combined therapy of T4 and T3 may also prove to be useful. T4 may be initiated at a dose of 4 μg/kg of lean body weight, followed by 100 μg 24 hours later and then 50 μg daily intravenously or orally. T3 may also be started simultaneously with T4 at a dose of 10 μg iv, and the same dose is given every 8 to 12 hours until the patient can take maintenance oral doses of T4 [1].

8. Factors Predicting the Mortality in Myxedema Crisis

Dutta and colleagues looked at the predictors of outcome in myxedema crisis and found that hypotension, bradycardia at presentation, need for mechanical ventilation, hypothermia unresponsive to treatment, sepsis, intake of sedative drugs, lower GCS, and high APACHE II scores were significant predictors of mortality. Sequential organ failure assessment (SOFA) score was more effective than other predictive models. Baseline and day 3 SOFA scores of more than 6 were highly predictive of poor outcome. They also demonstrated that treatment defaulters presented early to the hospital and had more severe manifestations than *de novo* patients [4].

Rodríguez and colleagues showed that those patients with coma at the time of presentation, low Glasgow coma scale scores, and higher APACHE II scores had considerably poor outcome [2]. Studies have also shown that higher doses of T3 are associated with increased mortality, and lower doses of T3 and T4 may be associated with favorable prognosis [3, 47, 48]. Other factors associated with mortality include advanced age and cardiovascular disease [1, 3].

9. Summary

Myxedema crisis is a life-threatening extreme form of hypothyroidism with a high mortality rate if left untreated. Myxedema crisis is commonly seen in older patients, especially women, and is associated with signs of hypothyroidism, hypothermia, hyponatremia, hypercarbia, and hypoxemia. There may be a significant delay in diagnosis which may adversely affect the prognosis. Patients should be provided with intensive care facilities with prompt attention to ventilation, hypotension, hypothermia, steroid replacement, and thyroid hormone supplementation. SOFA scoring system may help us to identify patients at risk of mortality at an earlier stage. Early medical attention in hypothyroid patients developing serious illness especially sepsis and ensuring continuation of thyroid supplements may prevent significant morbidity and mortality.

References

[1] L. Wartofsky, "Myxoedema coma," *Endocrinology Metabolism Clinics of North America*, vol. 35, pp. 687–698, 2006.

[2] I. Rodríguez, E. Fluiters, L. F. Pérez-Méndez, R. Luna, C. Páramo, and R. V. García-Mayor, "Factors associated with mortality of patients with myxoedema coma: prospective study in 11 cases treated in a single institution," *Journal of Endocrinology*, vol. 180, no. 2, pp. 347–350, 2004.

[3] T. Yamamoto, J. Fukuyama, and A. Fujiyoshi, "Factors associated with mortality of myxedema coma: report of eight cases and literature survey," *Thyroid*, vol. 9, no. 12, pp. 1167–1174, 1999.

[4] P. Dutta, A. Bhansali, S. Masoodi, S. Bhadada, N. Sharma, and R. Rajput, "Predictors of outcome in myxoedema coma: a study from a tertiary care centre," *Critical Care*, vol. 12, no. 1, p. R1, 2008.

[5] W. Reinhardt and K. Mann, "Incidence, clinical picture, and treatment of hypothyroid coma: results of a survey," *Medizinische Klinik*, vol. 92, pp. 521–524, 1997.

[6] *Report of a Committee of the Clinical Society of London to Investigate the Subject of Myxedema*, vol. 21, Transactions Clinical Society, London, UK, 1888.

[7] C. R. Wall, "Myxedema coma: diagnosis and treatment," *American Family Physician*, vol. 62, no. 11, pp. 2485–2490, 2000.

[8] J. T. Nicoloff and J. S. LoPresti, "Myxedema coma: a form of decompensated hypothyroidism," *Endocrinology and Metabolism Clinics of North America*, vol. 22, no. 2, pp. 279–290, 1993.

[9] J. C. Galofré and R. V. García-Mayor, "Densidad de incidencia del coma mixedematoso," *Endocrinologia*, vol. 44, pp. 103–104, 1997.

[10] M. Chu and T. F. Seltzer, "Myxedema coma induced by ingestion of raw bok choy," *New England Journal of Medicine*, vol. 362, no. 20, pp. 1945–1946, 2010.

[11] D. G. Gardner, "Endocrine emergencies," in *Greenspan's Basic and Clinical Endocrinology*, D. G. Gardner and D. Shoback, Eds., McGraw-Hill, New York, NY, USA, 8th edition, 2007.

[12] P. W. Ladenson, P. D. Goldenheim, and E. C. Ridgway, "Prediction and reversal of blunted ventilatory responsiveness in patients with hypothyroidism," *American Journal of Medicine*, vol. 84, no. 5, pp. 877–883, 1988.

[13] W. R. Wilson and G. N. Bedell, "The pulmonary abnormalities in myxedema," *The Journal of Clinical Investigation*, vol. 39, pp. 42–55, 1960.

[14] R. A. Massumi and J. L. Winnacker, "Severe depression of the respiratory center in myxedema," *The American Journal of Medicine*, vol. 36, no. 6, pp. 876–882, 1964.

[15] F. R. Derubertis Jr., M. F. Michelis, M. E. Bloom, D. H. Mintz, J. B. Field, and B. B. Davis, "Impaired water excretion in myxedema," *The American Journal of Medicine*, vol. 51, no. 1, pp. 41–53, 1971.

[16] W. R. Skowsky and T. A. Kikuchi, "The role of vasopressin in the impaired water excretion of myxedema," *American Journal of Medicine*, vol. 64, no. 4, pp. 613–621, 1978.

[17] Y. C. Chen, M. A. Cadnapaphornchai, J. Yang et al., "Nonosmotic release of vasopressin and renal aquaporins in impaired urinary dilution in hypothyroidism," *American Journal of Physiology—Renal Physiology*, vol. 289, no. 4, pp. F672–F678, 2005.

[18] W. M. Weirsinga, "Hypothyroidism and myxedema coma," in *Endocrinology Adult and Pediatric*, J. L. Jameson and L. J. Legroot, Eds., Saunders, Philadelphia, Pa, USA, 6th edition, 2010.

[19] R. Polikar, A. G. Burger, U. Scherrer, and P. Nicod, "The thyroid and the heart," *Circulation*, vol. 87, no. 5, pp. 1435–1441, 1993.

[20] J. B. Schenck, A. A. Rizvi, and T. Lin, "Severe primary hypothyroidism manifesting with torsades de pointes," *American Journal of the Medical Sciences*, vol. 331, no. 3, pp. 154–156, 2006.

[21] C. G. Roberts and P. W. Ladenson, "Hypothyroidism," *Lancet*, vol. 363, no. 9411, pp. 793–803, 2004.

[22] Y. D. Tang, J. A. Kuzman, S. Said, B. E. Anderson, X. Wang, and A. M. Gerdes, "Low thyroid function leads to cardiac atrophy with chamber dilatation, impaired myocardial blood flow, loss of arterioles, and severe systolic dysfunction," *Circulation*, vol. 112, no. 20, pp. 3122–3130, 2005.

[23] F. Galetta, F. Franzoni, P. Fallahi et al., "Changes in heart rate variability andQT dispersion in patients with overt hypothyroidism," *European Journal of Endocrinology*, vol. 158, pp. 85–90, 2008.

[24] F. Galetta, F. Franzoni, P. Fallahi et al., "Heart rate variability and QT dispersion in patients with subclinical hypothyroidism," *Biomedicine and Pharmacotherapy*, vol. 60, no. 8, pp. 425–430, 2006.

[25] L. A. Osborn, B. Skipper, I. Arellano, S. D. MacKerrow, and M. H. Crawford, "Results of resting and ambulatory electrocardiograms in patients with hypothyroidism and after return to euthyroid status," *Heart Disease*, vol. 1, no. 1, pp. 8–11, 1999.

[26] K. C. Das, M. Mukherjee, T. K. Sarkar et al., "Erythropoiesis and erythropoietin in hypo- and hyperthyroidism," *Journal of Clinical Endocrinology and Metabolism*, vol. 40, no. 2, pp. 211–220, 1975.

[27] J. D. Hines, C. H. Halsted, R. C. Griggs, and J. W. Harris, "Megaloblastic anemia secondary to folate deficiency associated with hypothyroidism," *Annals of Internal Medicine*, vol. 68, no. 4, pp. 792–805, 1968.

[28] R. Carmel and C. A. Spencer, "Clinical and subclinical thyroid disorders associated with pernicious anemia," *Archives of Internal Medicine*, vol. 142, no. 8, pp. 1465–1469, 1982.

[29] G. R. Tudhope and G. M. Wilson, "Deficiency of vitamin b12 in hypothyroidism," *The Lancet*, vol. 279, no. 7232, pp. 703–706, 1962.

[30] H. C. Ford and J. M. Carter, "Haemostasis in hypothyroidism," *Postgraduate Medical Journal*, vol. 66, no. 774, pp. 280–284, 1990.

[31] J. J. Michiels, W. Schroyens, Z. Berneman, and M. van der Planken, "Acquired von Willebrand syndrome type 1 in hypothyroidism: reversal after treatment with thyroxine," *Clinical and Applied Thrombosis/Hemostasis*, vol. 7, no. 2, pp. 113–115, 2001.

[32] I. C. Nitu-Whalley and C. A. Lee, "Acquired von Willebrand syndrome—report of 10 cases and review of the literature," *Haemophilia*, vol. 5, no. 5, pp. 318–326, 1999.

[33] E. M. Erfurth, U. B. Ericsson, K. Egervallah, and S. R. Lethagen, "Effect of acute desmopressin and of long-term thyroxine replacement onhaemostasis in hypothyroidism," *Clinical Endocrinology*, vol. 42, pp. 373–378, 1995.

[34] L. Wartofsky and K. D. Burman, "Alterations in thyroid function in patients with systemic illness: the euthyroid sick syndrome," *Endocrine Reviews*, vol. 3, no. 2, pp. 164–217, 1982.

[35] M. J. Hooper, "Diminished T.S.H. secretion during acute non thyroidal illness in untreated primary hypothyroidism," *Lancet*, vol. 1, no. 7949, pp. 48–49, 1976.

[36] L. Brain, E. H. Jellinek, and K. Ball, "Hashimoto's disease and encephalopathy," *Lancet*, vol. 2, no. 7462, pp. 512–514, 1966.

[37] P. Pozo-Rosich, P. Villoslada, A. Canton, R. Simo, A. Rovira, and X. Montalban, "Reversible white matter alterations in encephalopathy associated with autoimmune thyroid disease," *Journal of Neurology*, vol. 249, no. 8, pp. 1063–1065, 2002.

[38] A. Canton, O. de Fabregas, M. Tintore et al., "Encephalopathy associated to autoimmune thyroid disease: a more appropriate termfor an underestimated condition?" *Journal of the Neurological Sciences*, vol. 176, pp. 65–69, 2000.

[39] R. Peschen-Rosin, M. Schabet, and J. Dichgans, "Manifestation of Hashimoto's encephalopathy years before onset of thyroid disease," *European Neurology*, vol. 41, no. 2, pp. 79–84, 1999.

[40] T. Yamamoto, "Delayed respiratory failure during the treatment of myxedema coma," *Endocrinologia Japonica*, vol. 31, no. 6, pp. 769–775, 1984.

[41] J. G. Verbalis, S. R. Goldsmith, A. Greenberg, R. W. Schrier, and R. H. Sterns, "Hyponatremia treatment guidelines 2007: expert panel recommendations," *American Journal of Medicine*, vol. 120, no. 11, pp. S1–S21, 2007.

[42] V. G. Pereira, E. S. Haron, N. Lima Neto, and G. A. Medeiros Nets, "Management of myxedema coma: report on three successfully treated cases with nasogastric or intravenous administration of triiodothyronine," *Journal of Endocrinological Investigation*, vol. 5, no. 5, pp. 331–334, 1982.

[43] R. H. Sterns, J. D. Cappuccio, S. M. Silver, and E. P. Cohen, "Neurologic sequelae after treatment of severe hyponatremia: a multicenter perspective," *Journal of the American Society of Nephrology*, vol. 4, no. 8, pp. 1522–1530, 1994.

[44] J. E. Brunner, J. M. Redmond, A. M. Haggar, D. F. Kruger, and S. B. Elias, "Central pontine myelinolysis and pontine lesions after rapid correction of hyponatremia: a prospective magnetic resonance imaging study," *Annals of Neurology*, vol. 27, no. 1, pp. 61–66, 1990.

[45] D. N. Holvey, C. J. Goodner, J. T. Nicoloff, and J. T. Dowling, "Treatment of myxedema coma with intravenous thyroxine," *Archives of Internal Medicine*, vol. 113, pp. 89–96, 1964.

[46] E. C. Ridgway, J. A. McCammon, J. Benotti, and F. Maloof, "Acute metabolic responses in myxedema to large doses of intravenous L-thyroxine," *Annals of Internal Medicine*, vol. 77, no. 4, pp. 549–555, 1972.

[47] S. D. MacKerrow, L. A. Osborn, H. Levy, R. P. Eaton, and P. Economou, "Myxedema-associated cardiogenic shock treated with intravenous triiodothyronine," *Annals of Internal Medicine*, vol. 117, no. 12, pp. 1014–1015, 1992.

[48] B. Hylander and U. Rosenqvist, "Treatment of myxoedema coma—factors associated with fatal outcome," *Acta Endocrinologica*, vol. 108, no. 1, pp. 65–71, 1985.

12

Prevalence and Predictors of Thyroid Dysfunction in Patients with HIV Infection and Acquired Immunodeficiency Syndrome

Neera Sharma,[1] Lokesh Kumar Sharma,[1] Deep Dutta,[2] Adesh Kisanji Gadpayle,[3] Atul Anand,[4] Kumar Gaurav,[2] Sabyasachi Mukherjee,[2] and Rahul Bansal[2]

[1]Department of Biochemistry, Post Graduate Institute of Medical Education & Research (PGIMER) and Dr. Ram Manohar Lohia (RML) Hospital, 1 Baba Kharak Singh Marg, New Delhi 110001, India
[2]Department of Endocrinology, Post Graduate Institute of Medical Education & Research (PGIMER) and Dr. Ram Manohar Lohia (RML) Hospital, 1 Baba Kharak Singh Marg, New Delhi 110001, India
[3]Post Graduate Institute of Medical Education & Research (PGIMER) and Dr. Ram Manohar Lohia (RML) Hospital, 1 Baba Kharak Singh Marg, New Delhi 110001, India
[4]Anti-Retroviral Therapy Clinic, Post Graduate Institute of Medical Education & Research (PGIMER) and Dr. Ram Manohar Lohia (RML) Hospital, 1 Baba Kharak Singh Marg, New Delhi 110001, India

Correspondence should be addressed to Deep Dutta; deepdutta2000@yahoo.com

Academic Editor: Noriyuki Koibuchi

Background. Predictors of thyroid dysfunction in HIV are not well determined. This study aimed to determine the prevalence and predictors of thyroid dysfunction in HIV infected Indians. *Methods.* Consecutive HIV patients, 18–70 years of age, without any severe comorbid state, having at least 1-year follow-up at the antiretroviral therapy clinic, underwent clinical assessment and hormone assays. *Results.* From initially screened 527 patients, 359 patients (61.44 ± 39.42 months' disease duration), having good immune function [CD4 count >200 cell/mm^3: 90.25%; highly active antiretroviral therapy (HAART): 88.58%], were analyzed. Subclinical hypothyroidism (ScH) was the commonest thyroid dysfunction (14.76%) followed by sick euthyroid syndrome (SES) (5.29%) and isolated low TSH (3.1%). Anti-TPO antibody (TPOAb) was positive in 3.90%. Baseline CD4 count had inverse correlation with TPOAb after adjusting for age and body mass index. Stepwise linear regression revealed baseline CD4 count, TPOAb, and tuberculosis to be best predictors of ScH after adjusting for age, weight, duration of HIV, and history of opportunistic fungal and viral infections. *Conclusion.* Burden of thyroid dysfunction in chronic HIV infection with stable immune function is lower compared to pre-HAART era. Thyroid dysfunction is primarily of nonautoimmune origin, predominantly ScH. Severe immunodeficiency at disease onset, TPOAb positivity, and tuberculosis were best predictors of ScH.

1. Introduction

Dramatic improvements in survival following institution of highly active antiretroviral therapy (HAART) have given rise to increased occurrence of endocrinopathies in HIV infected patients in the last two decades, which are associated with significant morbidity. Thyroid dysfunction is among the commonest endocrinopathies in HIV. Undiagnosed thyroid dysfunction, even subclinical hypothyroidism, is associated

with significant morbidity and poor quality of life [1–4]. Subtle thyroid dysfunction is common, believed to occur in as many as 35% of all HIV infected individuals [5–7]. In contrast overt thyroid dysfunction is less common, believed to involve 1-2% of all patients [6, 7]. Prevalence of overt primary hypothyroidism in the general population and HIV infected individuals from different studies across the globe has been reported to be 0.3% and 0–2.6%, respectively [6–9]. Similarly the prevalence of subclinical hypothyroidism has also reported to be higher in HIV infected individuals as compared to the general population (4.3% versus 3.5–12.2%) in different studies [6–9]. Most of the hypothyroidism in general population is believed to be of autoimmune etiology, in contrast to HIV, where a majority is believed to be of nonautoimmune origin [8, 9]. Stavudine has been linked with hypothyroidism in some studies [8, 9]. However the data on the prevalence of thyroid dysfunction in HIV infected patients from India is scant. Also factors, which determine the occurrence of thyroid dysfunction, have not been well determined. Patients with HIV infection often have associated comorbidities like infections, malignancies that are associated with significant stress, which may have an impact on hypothalamic-pituitary-thyroid axis making interpretation of thyroid function tests difficult. Hence the aim of this study was to determine the prevalence and predictors of the entire spectrum of thyroid dysfunction (overt hypothyroidism, subclinical hypothyroidism, subclinical hyperthyroidism, overt hyperthyroidism, and sick euthyroid syndrome) in stable ambulatory patients with HIV infection.

2. Methods

Antiretroviral therapy (ART) clinic at our institute has been functional since 2004, established by the National AIDS Control Organization (NACO), India, and the World Health Organization (WHO). The clinic provides for all the necessary investigations, medications (including highly active antiretroviral therapy [HAART]), counseling, and education to all patients with HIV infection. Consecutive ambulatory patients, 18–70 years of age, with serologically documented HIV infection, in stable clinical condition without any acute, severe illness, attending the ART clinic of our hospital were considered. Severely ill patients with multiple comorbid states, which would warrant hospital admission, were excluded. Patients with vitamin-D and/or calcium supplementation in the last 6 months were excluded. Patient records were reviewed and patients having clinical data of at least 1 year of follow-up were further evaluated. Patients whose CD4 cell count records at diagnosis and at least one follow-up (6–12 months after diagnosis) available were included in the study. The study protocol was explained to the considered patients and only those who gave informed written consent were included. The institutional ethics committee approved the study protocol. The period of the study was from August 2014 till September 2015.

Data were collected from the patients and their records regarding the duration of diagnosis of HIV infection and details of HAART. Data was also collected regarding past or current evidence of infections including opportunistic infections (bacterial, viral, and fungal). History of clinical features suggestive of hypothyroidism or hyperthyroidism was taken. All patients underwent detailed clinical assessment, including anthropometry. The patients were called the subsequent day in fasting state for blood sampling. Blood samples of 5 mL each were collected in plain and EDTA Vacutainer (Becton Dickinson). Serum was separated from blood collected in plain Vacutainer and processed immediately for routine biochemical analysis and one aliquot of serum was

stored at −20 degrees' Celsius for specific immunological (hormonal) assays. EDTA sample was processed for hematological analysis.

Chemiluminescent microparticle immunoassay (VITROS ECiQ Immunodiagnostic System, Johnson & Johnson, USA) was used for estimation of free tri-iodothyronine (fT3), free tetraiodothyronine (fT4), thyroid stimulation hormone (TSH), and 25-hydroxy-vitamin-D. FT3 assay had analytical sensitivity of 0.50 pg/mL, analytical range of 0.50–22.8 pg/mL, and intra- and interassay coefficient of variation (CV) of 2.2% and 6.3%, respectively. FT4 assay had analytical sensitivity of 0.07 ng/dL and analytical range of 0.07–6.99 ng/dL with intra- and interassay coefficient of variation (CV) of 2.4% and 5.8%, respectively. TSH assay had analytical sensitivity of 0.015 mIU/L and analytical range of 0.015–100 mIU/L with intra- and interassay coefficient of variation (CV) of 3.3% and 7.2%, respectively. Serum 25-hydroxy-vitamin-D (25OHD) assay had analytical sensitivity of 8.0 ng/mL, analytical range of 8–150 ng/mL, and intra- and interassay coefficient of variation (CV) of 3.4% and 5.5%, respectively. Antithyroid peroxidase antibody (anti-TPO) levels were measured by solid phase immunosorbent assay (AutoSTAT II anti-TPO, HYCOR Biomedical) and had analytical sensitivity of 1.81 U/mL and analytical range of 35–1500 U/mL with intra- and interassay coefficient of variation (CV) of 3.7% and 7.5%, respectively. CD4 cell count was performed using flow cytometry (Becton Dickinson Immunocytochemistry Systems, San Jose, CA). Serum calcium, phosphate, alkaline phosphate, and renal function tests were done using clinical chemistry autoanalyzer based on dry chemistry microslide technology (VITROS 350 chemistry system, Johnson & Johnson, USA).

The reference range of fT3, fT4, and TSH in our laboratory is 2–4.4 pg/mL, 0.6–2.2 ng/dL, and 0.5–5 mIU/L, respectively. Anti-TPO antibody titer <50 IU/mL is considered to be negative or normal. In accordance with previous literature, primary overt hypothyroidism was defined as patients having elevated TSH along with low fT4 [5, 6]. Subclinical hypothyroidism was defined as patients having elevated TSH along with normal thyroid hormone levels. Subclinical hyperthyroidism was defined as patients having suppressed TSH levels with normal thyroid hormone levels [5, 6]. Overt hyperthyroidism was defined as patients having suppressed TSH levels along with elevated fT4 and/or fT3. Sick euthyroid syndrome, a physiological adaptive phenomenon to conserve energy during periods of extreme stress and infection, was defined as patients having isolated low fT3 or low fT4 with low fT3 levels, along with low or normal TSH levels [10]. Euthyroidism was defined as clinically asymptomatic patients having normal fT3, fT4, and TSH levels. It has been reported that 1.3–6.8% HIV infected patients have isolated low TSH with normal thyroid hormone levels [11]. Hence, patients with normal fT3 and fT4 with low TSH were grouped separately. A few studies have also noted isolated low fT4 (up to 6.8% patients), a pattern distinct from sick euthyroid syndrome in patients with HIV infection, which is believed to be due to an alternation in hypothalamic-pituitary-thyroid axis [6]. Hence these patients were also grouped separately in our study. Serum 25-hydroxy-vitamin-D (25OHD) levels ≥30 ng/mL were defined as vitamin-D sufficiency, 20–30 ng/mL as vitamin-D insufficiency, and <20 ng/mL as vitamin-D deficiency [12].

Immune reconstitution inflammatory syndrome (IRIS) in HIV infected patients is characterized by clinical deterioration in a patient secondary reestablishment of immunity following initiation of HAART [13]. It is usually observed in patients with low baseline CD4 count, which increases rapidly following initiation of HAART. HAART has been linked to increased occurrence of autoimmunity and autoimmune disorders [13, 14]. IRIS has been defined as an increased CD4 count above 200 cells/mm^3 in patients who previously had CD4 counts lower than 100–200 cells/mm^3 [15, 16]. Hence patients in our study with baseline CD4 counts less than 200 cells/mm^3, which increased to >200 cells/mm^3 at the first follow-up following initiation of HAART, were defined to have IRIS. Parameters like age, duration of HIV infection, occurrence of opportunistic infections, baseline and posttreatment CD4 counts, IRIS, antiretroviral drugs used, vitamin-D status, and autoimmunity (anti-TPO antibody) were evaluated for their role in predicting the occurrence of thyroid dysfunction.

Subtle thyroid dysfunction is common in HIV infected individuals, believed to involve as many as 35% of all individuals [5–7]. Hence for keeping a power of 80% and type-I error at 5%, it has been calculated that we need to recruit at least 246 patients in our study for accurate assessment of thyroid dysfunction.

3. Statistical Analysis

Normality of the distribution of variables was assessed using the Kolmogorov-Smirnov test. Independent t-test and Wilcoxon rank sum test were done for normally distributed and skewed variables, respectively. Chi-square tests were used for categorical variables. Pearson's or Spearman's correlation coefficient was calculated for normally distributed and skewed variables, respectively. Multiple linear regression analyses were done to determine variables that independently influenced the occurrence of thyroid dysfunction after adjusting for factors in different models. A P value <0.05 was considered statistically significant. SPSS version 20 was used for analyses.

4. Results

Five hundred and twenty-seven consecutive patients with HIV infection were screened at the ART clinic, of which 370 patients who fulfilled all criteria were considered for inclusion into the study. Reasons for exclusion from the study included severe associated illness ($n = 23$), multiple comorbid states like chronic liver disease, chronic kidney disease ($n = 11$), previous steroid use ($n = 25$), and history of calcium or vitamin-D supplementation in last 6 months ($n = 41$). Forty-six patients were excluded because of less than 1-year follow-up and 11 were excluded due to incomplete records. Of the 370 considered patients, 11 refused to consent to the study. Hence 359 patients (225 males and 134 females) who fulfilled all criteria and gave informed written consent

underwent clinical assessment, hormonal evaluation, and analysis. Prevalence of vitamin-D deficiency (<20 ng/mL) and insufficiency (<30 ng/mL) among the study cohort was 55.71% (200/359) and 89.69% (322/359), respectively. Severe vitamin-D deficiency (<10 ng/mL) was observed in 9.19% (33/359) patients. At the time of diagnosis of HIV infection, 60.20% (216/359), 32.60% (117/359), and 7.20% (26/359) patients had CD4 count <200 cell/mm^3, 200–500 cell/mm^3, and >500 cell/mm^3, respectively. The mean duration of HIV infection was 61.44 ± 39.42 months. Three hundred and nineteen (88.86%) patients were on HAART at the time of inclusion into the study. At the time of hormonal analysis, 9.75% (35/359), 58.50% (210/359), and 31.75% (114/359) patients had CD4 count <200 cell/mm^3, 200–500 cell/mm^3, and >500 cell/mm^3, respectively. One hundred and forty-five patients (40.39%) had history of tuberculosis. None of the patients in this study had active tuberculosis at the time of recruitment. Six patients were on isoniazid and rifampicin at the time of recruitment as a part of maintenance phase of antitubercular therapy.

Subclinical hypothyroidism was the most common thyroid dysfunction observed in 53 (14.76%) patients. Sick euthyroid syndrome, isolated low TSH, and isolated low T4 were observed in 16 (4.45%), 11 (3.06%), and 3 (0.84%) patients, respectively. Overt hypothyroidism and hyperthyroidism were observed in 5 (1.39%) and 2 (0.01%) patients, respectively. Anti-TPO antibody titers were positive in 3.90% (14/359) patients (Table 1). Occurrence of thyroid dysfunction, especially sick euthyroid syndrome, was significantly more common in females than males (Table 1). Males were significantly older ($P = 0.001$) and had significantly lower BMI ($P = 0.016$), baseline CD4 count ($P = 0.001$), and current CD4 count ($P = 0.001$) along with significantly higher history of IRIS ($P = 0.008$) (Table 1).

Patients with history of IRIS were older ($P = 0.049$), were more likely to be males ($P = 0.007$), had lower BMI ($P = 0.002$), higher history of tuberculosis ($P = 0.002$), and higher use of protease inhibitors ($P < 0.001$), and had significantly lower baseline ($P < 0.001$) and current CD4 cell counts ($P = 0.005$) (Table 2). Serum fT3 was significantly higher in patients with history of IRIS ($P = 0.036$) (Table 2). The occurrence of different types of thyroid dysfunction was comparable in patients with history of IRIS as compared to those without (Table 2).

An inverse correlation was observed between baseline CD4 count ($P = 0.031$) and anti-TPO antibody titers, which persisted even after adjusting for age and body mass index ($P = 0.032$) (Table 3). Similarly an inverse correlation was observed in CD4 count at present with TSH levels, both at baseline ($P = 0.043$) and after adjusting for age and body mass index ($P = 0.049$) (Table 3). Stepwise linear regression analysis revealed that anti-TPO antibody titers and CD4 cell count at the time of initial diagnosis of HIV infection were the 2 best predictors of occurrence of subclinical hypothyroidism, at baseline (Model-1), after adjusting for age and duration of HIV infection (Model-2), and after adjusting for variables in Model-2 plus weight and history of opportunistic fungal and viral infections (Model-3) (Table 4). Increased anti-TPO antibody titers and lower baseline CD4 count

TABLE 1: Clinical, biochemical, and thyroid function profile of males as compared to females with HIV infection.

Parameter	Males ($n = 225$)	Females ($n = 134$)	P value
Age (years)[a]	39 [49]	35 [39]	0.001
Duration of HIV infection (months)[a]	58 [168]	53 [137]	0.333
Body mass index (kg/m^2)[a]	21.64 (4.88)	22.91 (4.09)	0.016
History of tuberculosis	97 (43.11%)	48 (35.82%)	0.173[#]
History of opportunistic fungal infections	4 (1.78%)	0	—
History of viral infections[*]	7 (3.11%)	1 (0.75%)	0.150[#]
HAART	199	120	0.747[#]
Nature of HAART			
NRTI	198	120	0.654[#]
NNRTI	193	112	0.574[#]
PI	11	8	0.658[#]
IRIS	99	40	0.008[#]
CD4 cell count (at diagnosis)[a]	168 [1242]	195 [1922]	0.001
CD4 cell count (6–12 months after diagnosis)[a]	274 [947]	311 [1598]	0.010
CD4 cell count (at present)[a]	389 [1000]	458 [1355]	0.001
Free T3 (pg/mL)	3.51 (0.58)	3.49 (0.72)	0.741
Free T4 (ng/dl)	0.87 (0.16)	0.87 (0.28)	0.827
TSH (mIU/L)[a]	2.77 [18.57]	3.14 [26.9]	0.353
Anti-TPO antibody (U/mL)[a]	31 [175.75]	33 [164.7]	0.375
Anti-TPO positivity (>50 IU/L)	9 (4%)	5 (3.73%)	0.999[#]
Calcium (mg/dL)	9.17 (0.56)	9.19 (0.59)	0.812
Phosphate (mg/dL)	3.58 (0.59)	3.78 (0.60)	0.017
ALP (U/L)	133.2 (58.61)	118.16 (40.34)	0.045
25OHD (ng/mL)[a]	19.22 [75.70]	18.99 [61.5]	0.097
Euthyroidism	180 (80%)	89 (66.41%)	0.004
Overt primary hypothyroidism	2	3	0.291[#]
Subclinical hypothyroidism	31 (13.78%)	22 (16.41%)	0.495[#]
Subclinical hyperthyroidism	0	0	—
Overt hyperthyroidism	0	2 (1.49%)	—
Sick euthyroid syndrome/central hypothyroidism	6 (2.67%)	10 (7.46%)	0.033[#]
Low TSH with normal free T4	5 (2.22%)	6 (4.48%)	0.230[#]
Isolated low free T4	1 (0.44%)	2 (1.49%)	0.291[#]

All continuous variables expressed as mean (standard deviation); [a]all nonnormally distributed variable expressed as median [range]; all discrete variables have been expressed as absolute numbers (percentage); Wilcoxon rank sum test was done for analysis; normally distributed continuous variables were analyzed using unpaired t-test; normality checked using Kolmogorov-Smirnov test; $P < 0.05$ considered statistically significant; [#]P value calculated using Chi-square test; [*]viral infections include hepatitis-B, hepatitis-C; HAART: highly active antiretroviral therapy; NRTI: nucleoside reverse transcriptase inhibitors; NNRTI: nonnucleoside reverse transcriptase inhibitor; PI: protease inhibitors; zidovudine (AZT), lamivudine (3TC), stavudine (d4T), and/or tenofovir (TDF) were the NRTIs received by the patients; nevirapine (NVP) or efavirinez (EFV) was NNRTIs received by the patients; atazanavir (ATV) or ritonavir (RTV) was the PI received by the patients; 25OHD: 25-hydroxy-vitamin-D; IRIS: immune reconstitution inflammatory syndrome; ALP: alkaline phosphate.

were independent predictors of increased occurrence of subclinical hypothyroidism. Previous history of tuberculosis tended to be a good predictor of subclinical hypothyroidism later in life both at baseline ($P = 0.084$) and after adjusting for variables in Model-2 ($P = 0.087$) and Model-3 ($P = 0.065$) (Table 4).

5. Discussion

The occurrence of sick euthyroid syndrome among HIV infected patients is highly variable ranging from 1.3% to 11.6% in different studies [11, 16–19]. Stable, ambulatory,

asymptomatic patients, with a large majority being on HAART (88.86%) with stable immune function (as evidenced by only 9.75% patients having CD4 count <200 cell/mm^3 at the time of recruitment into this study and hormonal assessment) may explain the low occurrence of sick euthyroid syndrome in our study cohort. Heterogeneity in the disease profile of the patients evaluated in different studies (duration of infection, severity of immunodeficiency, in-patient versus out-patient, associated comorbidities, and functional status) may explain this variation.

A pilot study from central India reported a high prevalence of subclinical (30%) and overt hypothyroidism (10.66%)

TABLE 2: Thyroid function profile of patients with immune reconstitution activation syndrome (IRIS) as compared to those without.

Parameter	History of IRIS (n = 139)	Patients without history of IRIS (n = 220)	P value
Age (years)[a]	39 [41]	36 [49]	0.049
Sex (male : female)	99 : 40	126 : 94	0.007[#]
Duration of HIV infection (months)[a]	56 [168]	55 [137]	0.667
Body mass index (kg/m^2)[a]	21.58 [23.81]	21.94 [30.48]	0.002
History of tuberculosis	70 (50.36%)	75 (34.09%)	0.002[#]
History of opportunistic fungal infections	3 (2.16%)	1 (0.45%)	0.134[#]
History of viral infections*	1 (0.72%)	7 (3.18%)	0.123[#]
HAART	124	195	0.867[#]
Nature of HAART			
NRTI	123	195	1[#]
NNRTI	118	187	1[#]
PI	16	3	<0.001[#]
CD4 cell count (at diagnosis)[a]	135 [192]	258 [1922]	<0.001
CD4 cell count (6–12 months after diagnosis)[a]	311 [657]	266 [1625]	0.144
CD4 cell count (at present)[a]	439 [1068]	389 [1355]	0.005
Free T3 (pg/mL)	3.53 (0.67)	3.41 (0.58)	0.036
Free T4 (ng/dL)	0.87 (0.23)	0.87 (0.17)	0.933
TSH (mIU/L)[a]	2.77 [26.72]	2.99 [19]	0.334
Anti-TPO antibody (U/mL)[a]	33 [175.75]	31 [144.59]	0.431
Anti-TPO positivity (>50 U/mL)	6 (4.32%)	8 (7.27%)	0.745
Calcium (mg/dL)	9.2 (0.56)	9.15 (0.59)	0.530
Phosphate (mg/dL)	3.71 (0.61)	3.53 (0.56)	0.031
ALP (U/L)	131 (60.41)	123.22 (39.26)	0.291
25OHD (ng/mL)[a]	18.23 [74.9]	19.7 [62]	0.335
Euthyroidism	107 (76.98%)	162 (73.64%)	0.477[#]
Overt primary hypothyroidism	1 (0.72%)	4 (1.82%)	0.386[#]
Subclinical hypothyroidism	18 (12.95%)	35 (15.91%)	0.441[#]
Subclinical hyperthyroidism	0	0	—
Overt hyperthyroidism	0	2 (0.91%)	—
Sick euthyroid syndrome/central hypothyroidism	7 (5.04%)	9 (4.09%)	0.666[#]
Low TSH with normal free T4	5 (3.60%)	6 (2.73%)	0.641[#]
Isolated low free T4	1 (0.72%)	2 (0.91%)	0.848[#]

All continuous variables expressed as mean (standard deviation); [a]all nonnormally distributed variable expressed as median [range]; all discreet variables have been expressed as absolute numbers (percentage); Wilcoxon rank sum test was done for analysis; normally distributed continuous variables were analyzed using unpaired t-test; normality checked using Kolmogorov-Smirnov test; P < 0.05 considered statistically significant; [#]P value calculated using Chi-square test; *viral infections include hepatitis-B, hepatitis-C; HAART: highly active antiretroviral therapy; NRTI: nucleoside reverse transcriptase inhibitors; NNRTI: nonnucleoside reverse transcriptase inhibitor; PI: protease inhibitors; zidovudine (AZT), lamivudine (3TC), stavudine (d4T), and/or tenofovir (TDF) were the NRTIs received by the patients; nevirapine (NVP) or efavirinez (EFV) was NNRTIs received by the patients; atazanavir (ATV) or ritonavir (RTV) was the PI received by the patients; 25OHD: 25-hydroxy-vitamin-D; IRIS: immune reconstitution inflammatory syndrome; ALP: alkaline phosphate.

in a cohort of 150 HAART naïve newly diagnosed HIV infected patients [17]. Subclinical hypothyroidism was the commonest type of thyroid dysfunction observed in our study cohort documented in 14.76% patients. The prevalence is comparable to previous reports from other countries [6–9]. However this is in contrast to a previous report from our institute where a very high occurrence of subclinical hypothyroidism (53%) was documented in patients newly diagnosed with HIV infection [20]. It is important to highlight that the patients evaluated in that study were newly diagnosed with HIV infection, had advanced immunodeficiency (mean CD4 count: 147.1 ± 84 cell/mm^3, 70.1% had CD4 count <200 cell/mm^3), and were HAART naïve [20]. This is consistent with data reported from pre-HAART era and from patients newly diagnosed with HIV infection not on HAART, where the occurrence of thyroid dysfunction has been reported to be higher ranging from 10 to 40% [17, 21]. This is in contrast to our patients having mean disease duration of 5 years, with a large majority being on HAART (88.6%), being clinically stable, asymptomatic, and ambulatory with good immune function (90.25% having CD4 count >200 cell/mm^3; 31.75% having CD4 count >500 cell/mm^3).

TABLE 3: Correlation between thyroid function parameters, CD4 cell count parameters, and vitamin-D in patients with HIV infection ($n = 359$).

	Free T3		Free T4		TSH		Anti-TPO antibody	
	Model-1	Model-2	Model-1	Model-2	Model-1	Model-2	Model-1	Model-2
CD4 count (baseline)[a]	0.016 (0.759)	−0.004 (0.947)	0.004 (0.939)	0.063 (0.271)	0.024 (0.646)	0.012 (0.836)	**−0.114 (0.031)**	**−0.123 (<0.032)**
CD4 count (6–12-month follow-up)[a]	−0.008 (0.878)	−0.37 (0.520)	0.041 (0.448)	0.105 (0.067)	−0.063 (0.237)	−0.094 (0.101)	−0.085 (0.113)	−0.086 (0.131)
CD4 count (current)[a]	−0.085 (0.123)	−0.098 (0.086)	0.012 (0.833)	0.045 (0.433)	**−0.111 (0.043)**	**−0.113 (0.049)**	0.001 (0.981)	−0.015 (0.789)
Serum 25OHD[a]	0.024 (0.651)	0.028 (0.625)	0.048 (0.368)	−0.01 (0.856)	−0.007 (0.900)	−0.003 (0.952)	−0.066 (0.216)	−0.098 (0.086)

Model-1: without adjustment for any variable; Model-2: after adjustment for age and body mass index; [a] not normally distributed; Spearman's correlation coefficient calculated. All values expressed as correlation coefficient (P value); $P < 0.05$ considered statistically significant; TSH: thyroid stimulation hormone; TPO: thyroid peroxidase; T3: tri-iodothyronine; T4: tetraiodothyronine.

TABLE 4: Regression analysis showing parameters that are predictors of subclinical hypothyroidism in patients with HIV infection.

Variable	Model-1[a]		Model-2[b]		Model-3[c]	
	Standardized coefficient (β)	P value	Standardized coefficient (β)	P value	Standardized coefficient (β)	P value
Anti-TPO antibody	**0.245**	**<0.001**	**0.247**	**<0.001**	**0.239**	**<0.001**
CD4 count (baseline)	**−0.178**	**0.012**	**−0.175**	**0.018**	**−0.185**	**0.013**
CD4 cell count (6–12 months after diagnosis)[a]	−0.099	0.216	−0.094	0.242	−0.125	0.130
CD4 cell count (at present)[a]	−0.138	0.059	−0.138	0.062	−0.130	0.078
25OHD	−0.027	0.644	−0.025	0.679	−0.018	0.770
Tuberculosis	0.109	0.084	0.108	0.087	0.117	0.065
Lamivudine	−0.032	0.622	−0.030	0.653	−0.022	0.741
Stavudine	0.000	0.996	−0.010	0.903	−0.012	0.880
Tenofovir	−0.006	0.932	−0.001	0.991	0.009	0.904
Efavirinez	−0.126	0.053	−0.125	0.056	−0.125	0.056

Linear regression was initially performed with all parameters which are likely to influence serum testosterone levels [age, weight, duration of HIV infection, antithyroid peroxidase (TPO) antibody titer, baseline CD4 count, CD4 count (6–12 months after diagnosis), CD4 count at the time of recruitment into the study, hemoglobin, erythrocytic sedimentation rate, history of tuberculosis, opportunistic fungal infections, viral infections (hepatitis-B and hepatitis-C), serum 25-hydroxy-vitamin-D (25OHD), and individual antiretroviral agents received by the patient] to evaluate their role in the occurrence of subclinical hypothyroidism. [a,b,c]Parameters with $P < 0.2$ were included into the stepwise forward line regression analysis without adjustment for any variables (Model-1), after adjustment for age and duration of HIV infection (Model-2) and after adjustment for variables in Model-2 plus weight and history of opportunistic fungal infections and viral infections (Model-3). Standardized coefficient (β): change in odds ratio with 1 unit change in predictor variable; for the tuberculosis variable, patients without tuberculosis were taken as reference group.

Anti-TPO antibody titers, baseline CD4 counts, and history of tuberculosis were the best predictors of subclinical hypothyroidism in HIV infected patients in our study. Anti-TPO antibody positivity has previously been documented to be predictors of subclinical and overt hypothyroidism in normal and postpartum individuals [22, 23]. However it needs to be emphasized that, in spite of being a good predictor of subclinical hypothyroidism in our study, the prevalence of elevated anti-TPO antibody titers in our cohort was only 3.9%, which is lower than that observed in the general population (3–15%) [24]. A previous study of 642 normal individuals from northern India revealed the prevalence of anti-TPO positivity to be 21% [25].

The inverse relation observed between current CD4 count and TSH even after adjusting for variables highlights the possible link between increased immunodeficiency and elevated TSH. Further, in the setting of low prevalence of elevated anti-TPO antibody titers, low baseline CD4 count being a strong independent predictor of subclinical hypothyroidism highlights the importance of early immunodeficiency and HIV infection per se having an important role in the genesis of subclinical hypothyroidism later in life. It is likely that patients with lower CD4 counts had higher viral load. However, HIV viral load was not evaluated in our study and is a limitation of this report. Previous history of tuberculosis being an important independent predictor of hypothyroidism in our study also highlights the importance of immunodeficiency in the pathogenesis of thyroid dysfunction (as tuberculosis is more common in the immunodeficient state). A high rate of hypothyroidism (54%) was reported from 69 HIV infected patients with multidrug resistant (MDR) tuberculosis from Mumbai, India [26]. Use of rifampicin, para-aminosalicylate (PAS), and ethionamide for treating

tuberculosis has been linked to the increased occurrence of hypothyroidism in these patients [26].

The inverse relationship observed between baseline CD4 count and anti-TPO antibody titers raises the possibility of increased immunodeficiency early in the course of disease being linked to increased occurrence of autoimmunity later. Increased autoantibody expression has previously been documented in patients of HIV infection with lower CD4+ cell counts, believed to be the result of a direct effect of the virus on endothelium, hematopoietic cells, and different tissues leading to enhancement of the cytotoxic activity of immune cells and autoantigen expression [27, 28]. Induction of immune restoration by HAART has been linked to thyroid dysfunction in some studies [29, 30]. This was primarily observed with regard to occurrence of hyperthyroidism and Graves' disease [17, 29, 30]. Graves' disease has most commonly been reported 12–36 months after HAART initiation [17]. Subclinical hyperthyroidism was not observed in our study. Also the occurrence of overt hyperthyroidism was too low in our study (0.01%) to be able to evaluate the factors responsible for their occurrence. In our study, IRIS was not a predictor of thyroid dysfunction.

In our study, none of the antiretroviral agents were predictors of occurrence of subclinical hypothyroidism. Studies evaluating the link between HAART and thyroid dysfunction have given conflicting results, with some but not all studies observing a link [6, 7]. A large cross-sectional study in 350 patients did not observe any link between HAART and occurrence of subclinical hypothyroidism [6]. Afhami et al. documented similar observations in a cross-sectional study of 85 HIV infected patients [31]. A higher than expected incidence of hypothyroidism (10.7 per 1000 treated patient years) but not hyperthyroidism (3.7 per 1000 treated patient years) was observed in a large study of 2437 HIV infected patients evaluated over 11-year period from 1995 to 2006 in United Kingdom [32]. Isolated low TSH was observed in 3.1% of patients in our cohort, which is in accordance with previous reports, which have documented a 1.3–6.8% prevalence of this condition [11]. The cause for this isolated low TSH is not well known. It may represent a spectrum of sick euthyroid syndrome. Increased endogenous cortisol tone, secondary to stress of HIV and associated comorbidities, may explain the isolated suppressed TSH levels [16]. In contrast to few previous reports, isolated low fT4 was uncommon in our study observed in only 0.84% of study patients. The cause for this isolated low fT4 is not well known. It is believed that these patients have intact response to TRH stimulation test in contrast to sick euthyroid syndrome [6, 33].

HIV infection has been linked to increased circulating levels of globulins including thyroid binding globulin, cortisol binding globulin, and sex-hormone binding globulin [34]. The cause for this phenomenon is not known. Hence total hormone (T3 and T4) may be falsely elevated in HIV patients. This was the rationale for measuring free T3 and free T4 in our study.

6. Conclusion

To summarize, it may be said that the burden of thyroid dysfunction in patients with chronic HIV infection with stable immune function (secondary to use of HAART) is lower compared to the pre-HAART era and newly diagnosed HAART naïve HIV infected patients. Subclinical hypothyroidism is the commonest type of thyroid dysfunction followed by sick euthyroid syndrome. Patients with more severe immunodeficiency (lower CD4 count) at disease onset and history of tuberculosis were more likely to have subclinical hypothyroidism later in life. Our study reiterated that thyroid dysfunction in HIV is primarily of nonautoimmune origin. However presence of elevated anti-TPO antibody titers in HIV was also independently associated with subclinical hypothyroidism similar to the normal population.

Acknowledgments

The authors are indebted to the participants in the study that made this study possible. Assistance of the staff of the Antiretroviral Therapy (ART) Clinic and laboratory technicians of the Nursing Home Laboratory of the Department of Biochemistry is deeply appreciated.

References

[1] D. Biswas, D. Dutta, I. Maisnam, S. Mukhopadhyay, and S. Chowdhury, "Occurrence of osteoporosis & factors determining bone mineral loss in young adults with Graves' disease," *Indian Journal of Medical Research*, vol. 141, no. 3, pp. 322–329, 2015.

[2] S. Razvi, L. Ingoe, G. Keeka, C. Oates, C. McMillan, and J. U. Weaver, "The beneficial effect of L-thyroxine on cardiovascular risk factors, endothelial function, and quality of life in subclinical hypothyroidism: randomized, crossover trial," *The Journal of Clinical Endocrinology & Metabolism*, vol. 92, no. 5, pp. 1715–1723, 2007.

[3] J. Leclère, C. Cousty, J.-L. Schlienger, and J.-L. Wémeau, "Subclinical hypothyroidism and quality of life of women aged 50 or more with hypercholesterolemia: results of the HYOGA study," *Presse Medicale*, vol. 37, no. 11, pp. 1538–1546, 2008.

[4] V. S. Reuters, C. D. P. Almeida, P. D. F. D. S. Teixeira et al., "Effects of subclinical hypothyroidism treatment on psychiatric symptoms, muscular complaints, and quality of life," *Arquivos Brasileiros de Endocrinologia e Metabologia*, vol. 56, no. 2, pp. 128–136, 2012.

[5] L. Calza, R. Manfredi, and F. Chiodo, "Subclinical hypothyroidism in HIV-infected patients receiving highly active antiretroviral therapy," *Journal of Acquired Immune Deficiency Syndromes*, vol. 31, no. 3, pp. 361–363, 2002.

[6] S. Beltran, F.-X. Lescure, R. Desailloud et al., "Increased prevalence of hypothyroidism among human immunodeficiency virus-infected patients: a need for screening," *Clinical Infectious Diseases*, vol. 37, no. 4, pp. 579–583, 2003.

[7] G. Madeddu, A. Spanu, F. Chessa et al., "Thyroid function in human immunodeficiency virus patients treated with highly active antiretroviral therapy (HAART): a longitudinal study," *Clinical Endocrinology*, vol. 64, no. 4, pp. 375–383, 2006.

[8] M. Grappin, L. Piroth, B. Verges et al., "Increased prevalence of subclinical hypothyroidism in HIV patients treated with highly active antiretroviral therapy," *AIDS*, vol. 14, no. 8, pp. 1070–1072, 2000.

[9] J. Collazos, S. Ibarra, and J. Mayo, "Thyroid hormones in HIV-infected patients in the highly active antiretroviral therapy era: evidence of an interrelation between the thyroid axis and the immune system," *AIDS*, vol. 17, no. 5, pp. 763–765, 2003.

[10] J. S. LoPresti, J. C. Fried, C. A. Spencer, and J. T. Nicoloff, "Unique alterations of thyroid hormone indices in the acquired immunodeficiency syndrome (AIDS)," *Annals of Internal Medicine*, vol. 110, no. 12, pp. 970–975, 1989.

[11] S. Beltran, F.-X. Lescure, I. El Esper, J.-L. Schmit, and R. Desailloud, "Subclinical hypothyroidism in HIV-infected patients is not an autoimmune disease," *Hormone Research*, vol. 66, no. 1, pp. 21–26, 2006.

[12] D. Dutta, S. A. Mondal, S. Choudhuri et al., "Vitamin-D supplementation in prediabetes reduced progression to type 2 diabetes and was associated with decreased insulin resistance and systemic inflammation: an open label randomized prospective study from Eastern India," *Diabetes Research and Clinical Practice*, vol. 103, no. 3, pp. e18–e23, 2014.

[13] J. D. Reveille, "The changing spectrum of rheumatic disease in human immunodeficiency virus infection," *Seminars in Arthritis and Rheumatism*, vol. 30, no. 3, pp. 147–166, 2000.

[14] M. L. Cuellar, "HIV infection-associated inflammatory musculoskeletal disorders," *Rheumatic Disease Clinics of North America*, vol. 24, no. 2, pp. 403–421, 1998.

[15] A. Wren, "How best to approach endocrine evaluation in patients with HIV in the era of combined antiretroviral therapy?" *Clinical Endocrinology*, vol. 79, no. 3, pp. 310–313, 2013.

[16] G. A. R. da Silva, M. C. T. Andrade, D. de Alvarenga Salém Sugui et al., "Association between antiretrovirals and thyroid diseases: a cross-sectional study," *Archives of Endocrinology and Metabolism*, vol. 59, no. 2, pp. 116–122, 2015.

[17] L. P. Meena, M. Rai, S. K. Singh et al., "Endocrine changes in male HIV patients," *Journal of Association of Physicians of India*, vol. 59, no. 6, pp. 365–366, 2011.

[18] C. J. Hoffmann and T. T. Brown, "Thyroid function abnormalities in HIV-infected patients," *Clinical Infectious Diseases*, vol. 45, no. 4, pp. 488–494, 2007.

[19] D. E. Sellmeyer and C. Grunfeld, "Endocrine and metabolic disturbances in human immunodeficiency virus infection and the acquired immune deficiency syndrome," *Endocrine Reviews*, vol. 17, no. 5, pp. 518–532, 1996.

[20] N. Dev, R. Sahoo, B. Kulshreshtha, A. K. Gadpayle, and S. C. Sharma, "Prevalence of thyroid dysfunction and its correlation with CD4 count in newly-diagnosed HIV-positive adults—a cross-sectional study," *International Journal of STD & AIDS*, vol. 26, no. 13, pp. 965–970, 2015.

[21] M. Bongiovanni, F. Adorni, M. Casana et al., "Subclinical hypothyroidism in HIV-infected subjects," *Journal of Antimicrobial Chemotherapy*, vol. 58, no. 5, pp. 1086–1089, 2006.

[22] B. G. A. Stuckey, G. N. Kent, L. C. Ward, S. J. Brown, and J. P. Walsh, "Postpartum thyroid dysfunction and the long-term risk of hypothyroidism: results from a 12-year follow-up study of women with and without postpartum thyroid dysfunction," *Clinical Endocrinology*, vol. 73, no. 3, pp. 389–395, 2010.

[23] P. W. Rosario, M. Carvalho, and M. R. Calsolari, "Natural history of subclinical hypothyroidism with TSH ≤10 mIU/l: a prospective study," *Clinical Endocrinology*, 2015.

[24] V. Deshmukh, A. Behl, V. Iyer, H. Joshi, J. P. Dholye, and P. K. Varthakavi, "Prevalence, clinical and biochemical profile of subclinical hypothyroidism in normal population in Mumbai," *Indian Journal of Endocrinology and Metabolism*, vol. 17, no. 3, pp. 454–459, 2013.

[25] R. Goswami, R. K. Marwaha, N. Gupta et al., "Prevalence of vitamin D deficiency and its relationship with thyroid autoimmunity in Asian Indians: a community-based survey," *British Journal of Nutrition*, vol. 102, no. 3, pp. 382–386, 2009.

[26] A. Andries, P. Isaakidis, M. Das et al., "High rate of hypothyroidism in multidrug-resistant tuberculosis patients co-infected with HIV in Mumbai, India," *PLoS ONE*, vol. 8, no. 10, Article ID e78313, 2013.

[27] G. Zandman-Goddard and Y. Shoenfeld, "HIV and autoimmunity," *Autoimmunity Reviews*, vol. 1, no. 6, pp. 329–337, 2002.

[28] P. S. Massabki, C. Accetturi, I. A. Nishie, N. P. da Silva, E. I. Sato, and L. E. C. Andrade, "Clinical implications of autoantibodies in HIV infection," *AIDS*, vol. 11, no. 15, pp. 1845–1850, 1997.

[29] N. F. Crum, A. Ganesan, S. T. Johns, and M. R. Wallace, "Graves disease: an increasingly recognized immune reconstitution syndrome," *AIDS*, vol. 20, no. 3, pp. 466–469, 2006.

[30] B. Knysz, M. Bolanowski, M. Klimczak, A. Gladysz, and K. Zwolinska, "Graves' disease as an immune reconstitution syndrome in an HIV-1-positive patient commencing effective antiretroviral therapy: case report and literature review," *Viral Immunology*, vol. 19, no. 1, pp. 102–107, 2006.

[31] S. Afhami, V. Haghpanah, R. Heshmat et al., "Assessment of the factors involving in the development of hypothyroidism in HIV-infected patients: a case-control study," *Infection*, vol. 35, no. 5, pp. 334–338, 2007.

[32] M. Nelson, T. Powles, A. Zeitlin et al., "Thyroid dysfunction and relationship to antiretroviral therapy in hiv-positive individuals in the HAART era," *Journal of Acquired Immune Deficiency Syndromes*, vol. 50, no. 1, pp. 113–114, 2009.

[33] M. J. T. Hommes, J. A. Romijn, E. Endert et al., "Hypothyroid-like regulation of the pituitary-thyroid axis in stable human immunodeficiency virus infection," *Metabolism*, vol. 42, no. 5, pp. 556–561, 1993.

[34] A. P. Weetman, "Thyroid abnormalities," *Endocrinology and Metabolism Clinics of North America*, vol. 43, no. 3, pp. 781–790, 2014.

13

Influence of a Medium-Impact Exercise Program on Health-Related Quality of Life and Cardiorespiratory Fitness in Females with Subclinical Hypothyroidism

Andrea Garces-Arteaga,[1] Nataly Nieto-Garcia,[1] Freddy Suarez-Sanchez,[1] Héctor Reynaldo Triana-Reina,[1] and Robinson Ramírez-Vélez[2]

[1] Departamento de Educación Física y Deporte, Universidad del Valle, Meléndez Cali, Colombia
[2] Grupo GICAEDS, Facultad de Cultura Física, Deporte y Recreación, Universidad Santo Tomás, Carrera 9 N° 51-23, Bogotá, DC, Colombia

Correspondence should be addressed to Robinson Ramírez-Vélez; robin640@hotmail.com

Academic Editor: Noriyuki Koibuchi

Objective. To examine the influence of a medium-impact exercise program (MIEP) on health-related quality of life (HRQoL) and cardiorespiratory fitness ($VO_{2\,max}$) in females with subclinical hypothyroidism (sHT). *Materials and Methods.* We selected 17 sedentary women with sHT (mean age: 43.1 (standard deviation: 9.7) years). Participants carried out an MIEP consisting of 3 weekly sessions of 60 minutes during 12 weeks. Before and after the exercise program HRQoL was assessed by the SF-12v2 questionnaire, and $VO_{2\,max}$ was evaluated by Rockport walk test. *Results.* After the 12-week intervention, the participants that performed an MIEP showed improvements in HRQoL in most domains, particularly the vitality domain by 7 points, the social functioning domain by 10 points, the mental health domain by 7 points, and the mental component summary by 7 points. One of the four domains within the physical component summary (general health domain) showed significant effect of the exercise intervention: 6 points. Moreover, the participants that performed exercise showed a higher $VO_{2\,max}$ (28%; $P < 0.01$). *Conclusion.* After 12 weeks of medium-impact exercise program, there were remarkable improvements in HRQoL in most domains. Moreover, this exercise program proved to have a positive influence on cardiorespiratory fitness.

1. Introduction

Prevalence of subclinical hypothyroidism (sHT), defined as elevated thyroid stimulating hormone (TSH) with free thyroxine (fT4) in the normal range, increases with age affecting about 6% of individuals aged 70 to 79 years and 10% of those aged 80 or older [1, 2]. Patients with sHT are associated with increased prevalence of atherosclerotic lesions and cardiovascular events [3, 4]. Besides, thyroid hormone deficiency may also interfere substantially with various aspects of physical, mental, and social well being [5] and many studies showed changes in functional status (i.e., mobility limitation, disability, and poor fitness level) in patients with sHT [6, 7].

On the other hand, the evidence for improvement of psychiatric symptoms with hormonal treatment (levothyroxine) of OH and the use of triiodothyronine (T3) to potentiate the response to treatment of depressive disorders suggests a direct relationship between thyroid hormones and psychiatric symptoms [8, 9]. Neurobiological evidence seems to corroborate the hypothesis of an organic basis of the effects of thyroid hormone on the brain and on psychiatric symptoms [9].

Interventions for sHT have included pharmacologic agents (i.e., hormonal treatment), psychotherapy, alternative therapies, and physical activity which can improve cardiovascular health, psychiatric symptoms, and health-related quality of life (HRQoL) [10, 11]. To date, few studies on HRQoL in subjects with sHT in response to exercise program have been reported [12, 13].

It has been proved that regular exercise positively affects the mechanisms of action associated with the physiologic deterioration and transition from subclinical thyroid disease [14]. Several authors recommended exercise to be performed within an intensity range of 40–85% of maximum oxygen consumption by $VO_{2\,max}$. Nevertheless, more recent studies emphasize the necessity of exploring the effects of intensity [15, 16]. Clinical thyroid disease is associated with changes in the cardiovascular system, including changes in heart rate during exercise. Considering this, we hypothesized that medium-impact exercise program would provide a more adequate exercise stimulus for improving a number of metabolic factors in females at risk for thyroid disease. Therefore, we hypothesized that a medium-impact exercise program can also improve HRQoL and cardiorespiratory fitness in females with sHT.

2. Materials and Methods

2.1. Subjects. From January 2012 to September 2012, 17 sedentary Colombian women with sHT (physical exercise less than once a week) were referred to our hospital for health examination (Servicio Medico Universidad del Valle). Subjects studied were between 40 and 65 years of age, mean age 43.1 ± 9.7 years. All patients with sHT were newly diagnosed and were positive for both antithyroid peroxidase (TPO-Ab) and antithyroglobulin (Tg-Ab) antibodies. The diagnosis of sHT was established on the basis of the elevated TSH levels and normal fT3 and fT4 values. In patients with sHT, laboratory tests were performed 1–3 days before and 12 weeks after the initiation of the training program. Obese subjects (body mass index (BMI) > $30 kg.m^{-2}$), smokers, and individuals with hypertension, clinical detectable coronary artery disease, and other diseases were excluded from the study. None of the patients were taking any medicine, such as estrogen supplements, T4, diuretics, antihypertensive, or hypolipidemic drugs. The University of Valle Research Ethics Committee approved this study. Informed consent was gained from all participants before the data collection began.

2.2. Medium-Impact Exercise Program. Preparatory training phase (weeks 1–6): the present study began with a 6-week preparatory phase of training to bring all participants up their 12 kcal/kg/wk goal. To accomplish this, all participants began their exercise program at a selected intensity set at a heart corresponding to 40–55% of $VO_{2\,max}$ and a frequency of 3 times per week.

Implementation of medium-impact exercise program (weeks 7–12): exercise prescription was standardized to body weight, and it was estimated that 180 minutes per week of moderate intensity exercise was equivalent to 10 to 12 kcal/kg of body weight per week. Exercise intensity was defined between 55% and 80% of $VO_{2\,max}$. An aerobic dose of

12 kcal/kg per week was selected for the aerobic group. Participants were weighed weekly to calculate their kcal/kg per week target. American College of Sports Medicine equations (ACSM) were used to estimate caloric expenditure rate and time required per session [17]. The exercise prescription used was established from the participants baseline exercise test and corresponded to a speed and grade associated with an upper intensity working level of 50% to 80% $VO_{2\,max}$ followed by recovery level of 30% $VO_{2\,max}$. Each session included a 30 min aerobic circuit training guided by an audio recording (tropical and latin music). The entire workout lasted about 30 minutes that, depending on the number of exercise (10 stations), were usually repeated three times. During 15 and 30 minutes throughout the routine, participants were instructed to check their pulse to ensure that they were working within their target heart rate range. Each session was preceded and followed by a gradual warm-up and cool down period, both of 10 minutes duration and consisting of walking and light, static stretching (avoiding muscle pain) of most muscle groups (upper and lower limbs, neck, and trunk muscles). The cool-down period also included relaxation and stretching exercises. Resistance exercises were performed through the full range of motion normally associated with correct technique for each exercise and engaged the major muscle groups (abdominal, dorsal, shoulder, and upper and lower limb muscles). They included 5 exercise group circuit training (50 repetitions of each) using barbells (1–3 kg/exercise) or low-to-medium resistance bands (therabands and balls). Each type of exercise on the back was performed for 2 min.

Adherence to the exercise program was encouraged by the exercise trainer and the physician who supervised each of the group sessions. Trainers were physical educators with experience in developing and monitoring exercise programs among clinical populations. In order to maximise adherence to the training program, exercise classes consisted of relevant activities for the group, 3–5 participants were accompanied by music dancing and performed in a spacious, air-conditioned room (08:00 am). Each participant met with the study dietician for nutrition assessment and counselling, and an individualized nutrition intervention plan was developed from the baseline food intake assessment, participant preferences, and the meal plan [18].

2.3. Health-Related Quality of Life Assessment. The Colombian standard version of the Medical Outcome Study Short-Form Health Survey (SF-12 version 2) is a questionnaire comprising 12 questions grouped into eight different domains of health: physical functioning, role limitation due to physical problems, bodily pain, general health perception, vitality, social function, role limitation due to emotional problems, and mental health. These eight scales are further clustered into the physical component summary (comprising physical function, role-physical, bodily pain and general health) and mental component summary (comprising vitality, social function, role-emotional, and mental health) [19]. The quantification of the mentioned dimensions is values varying from 0 to 100, where 0 corresponds to "worse health" and 100 to "better health."

TABLE 1: Baseline characteristics in females with subclinical hypo-thyroidism.

Variable	Mean (SD)
Age (years)	43.1 (9.7)
Weight (kg)	73.57 (13.54)
BMI (kg/m^2)	29.99 (4.48)
Waist circumference (cm)	93.47 (10.39)
Hip circumference (cm)	109.65 (10.51)
Systolic BP (mm Hg)	109.36 (8.74)
Diastolic BP (mm Hg)	66.68 (6.98)
Submaximal oxygen consumption by VO$_{2\,max}$	17.85 (8.40)
Maximum heart rate (beats/min)	151.56 (16.48)
Total cholesterol (mg/dL)	218.88 (25.55)
Triglycerides (mg/dL)	137.4 (64.4)
HDL-C (mg/dL)	57.18 (13.97)
LDL-C (mg/dL)	134.24 (23.26)
Glucose (mg/dL)	84.65 (11.68)
TSH (mIU/L)	2.90 (1.56)

2.4. Cardiorespiratory Fitness Evaluation. Submaximal oxygen consumption (VO$_{2\,max}$) was assessed with the Rockport walking test. During the test, heart rate was monitored electronically using a Polar A-5 pulse meter (Polar Electro Oy, Kempele, Finland). The cardiorespiratory fitness was calculated by VO$_{2\,max}$ via the ACSM equation [17]:

$$VO_{2\,max} \left(mL \cdot Kg \cdot min^{-1} \right)$$
$$= 132.853 - 0.0769 \times weight - 0.3877$$
$$\times height + 6.315 \times 0 - 3.2649 \tag{1}$$
$$\times time - 1565 \times heart\ rate.$$

Statistical Methods. It was sought to detect a between-group difference in the change of the SF-12v2 score of 4 points (mental component summary) as it was considered clinically important. Assuming that the standard deviation in this score would be 6, similar to what was observed in a similar sample of patients [20], a total sample size of 15 would provide 80% power to detect a difference of 4 points as statistically significant. The normality of the distribution of scores was confirmed with the *Kolmogorov-Smirnov* test. The paired *t*-test was later used to estimate the difference in each outcome. The significance level was set at $P < 0.05$. All analyses were carried out by using the statistical package SPSS 16 (Chicago, IL, USA).

3. Results

The mean and standard deviation of patients' age was 43.10 ± 9.70. All subjects were nonsmokers and had a sedentary lifestyle. 90% of patients were females and in the reproductive age group. The anthropometric, cardiorespiratory fitness, and metabolic profile data are listed in Table 1.

After the 12-week intervention, the participants that performed of a medium-impact exercise program showed

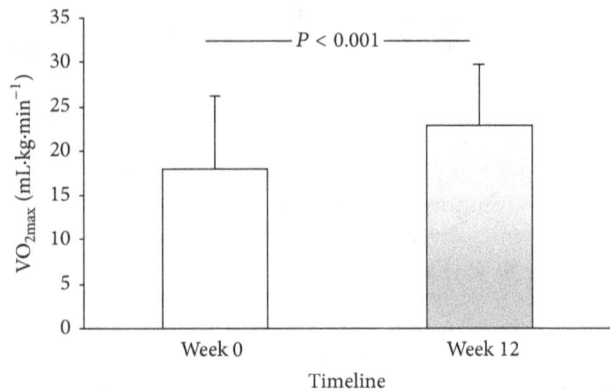

FIGURE 1: Influence of a medium-impact exercise program on cardiorespiratory fitness by submaximal VO$_{2\,max}$.

improvements in HRQoL in most domains, particularly the vitality domain by 7 points (95% CI 2 to 11), the social functioning domain by 10 points (95% CI 4 to 15), the mental health domain by 7 points (95% CI 1 to 12), and mental component summary by 7 points (95% CI 2 to 11). One of the four domains within the physical component summary (general health domain) showed significant effect of the exercise intervention: 6 points (95% CI 1 to 11), Table 2.

The paired *t*-test analysis revealed that the participants had a greater cardiorespiratory fitness at the end of the intervention, measured by Rockport walk test ($P = 0.01$) and by the submaximal VO$_{2\,max}$ (28%; $P < 0.001$), Figure 1.

Finally, the subjects participated 28.9 out of 36 (SD 3.2) sessions over the 12 weeks. No adverse events occurred during or after the exercise in any participant.

4. Discussion

The purpose of this study was to examine the influence of a medium-impact exercise program on HRQoL and cardiorespiratory fitness in females with sHT. To the authors' knowledge, this is the first systematic study evaluating the potential effectiveness of exercise program in sHT on HRQoL and VO$_{2\,max}$. In our clinical experience, we consider that an improvement of 4 points on the SF-12v2 resulting from this intervention is clinically important. However, no threshold has been established empirically for the amount of improvement in the SF-12v2 score that women typically feel makes aerobic training worthwhile. Our estimation of the average effect of the training had some uncertainty, with a 95% CI ranging from 1 to 10 points. Therefore, even if 4 points is a valid estimate for the smallest worthwhile effect, it must be acknowledged that it is uncertain whether the statistically significant effect of exercise is clinically worthwhile.

The median mental component summary and general health scores observed in the present study of women were similar to other studies of patient populations with conditions such as overweight [21] or sedentary [22]. There are very few studies that evaluated HRQoL in sHT [9, 10], and none included cardiorespiratory fitness and health

TABLE 2: Influence of a medium-impact exercise program on health-related quality of life (SF-12v2).

	Timeline mean (SD)		Difference mean (SD)	95% CI
	Week 0	Week 12		
Physical component summary (0 to 100)	43 (7)	46 (6)	3 (10)	−8 to 2
Physical function	47 (9)	48 (9)	1 (11)	−6 to 4
Role-physical	27 (4)	28 (3)	2 (4)	−4 to 1
Bodily pain	45 (12)	52 (10)	7 (17)	−15 to 1
General health	42 (8)	48 (5)	6 (11)	1 to 11
Mental component summary (0 to 100)	40 (8)	47 (7)	7 (9)	2 to 11
Vitality	57 (9)	63 (7)	7 (12)	2 to 11
Social functioning	43 (9)	54 (6)	10 (10)	4 to 15
Role-emotional	19 (5)	21 (4)	2 (6)	−5 to 1
Mental health	48 (9)	55 (9)	7 (11)	1 to 12

SF-12v2: Colombian standard version of the Medical Outcome Study Short-Form Health Survey.

status in the same study. It is believed that some psychological aspects of thyroid hypofunction, when present in sHT, may be influenced by physical findings, as suggested by the association between physical aspects of quality of life, in the SF-12 evaluation and cardiorespiratory fitness, specially $VO_{2\,max}$, in the present study. One of the primary consequences of thyroid dysfunction is lower tolerance to physical exertion, because of its implications involving the muscle and cardiovascular systems. This interferes directly with the patient's ability to perform daily activities, thereby reducing his quality of life. The study performed by Kahaly et al. [23] showed that subjects with thyroid dysfunction have reduced workload tolerance at the anaerobic threshold, compared to euthyroid subjects. According to these authors, in hyperthyroidism this exercise intolerance is caused by mitochondria oxidative dysfunction and in hypothyroidism, by inadequate cardiovascular support.

Following the 12-week exercise program, trends to improvement were seen in most domains of the HRQoL questionnaire, with statistically significant changes in the mental component summary and several of its domains. The confidence intervals were not narrow enough to confirm that the benefits would be worth the effort of exercising for these women. Nevertheless, given the other benefits of exercise in females with sHT, physicians can prescribe exercise expecting that it will improve quality of life. The recommended levels of physical activity were positively associated with one or more domains of health-related quality of life [19, 24]. In particular, physical functioning, general health, vitality, social functioning, and mental health are critically affected by the recommended level of physical activity [19]. In the current study, the physical aspects of HRQoL, such as mental component summary and general health, seemed to be more closely associated with the amount of physical activity than the physical aspects are. This finding is consistent with several previous studies [19, 20].

The intervention showed better cardiorespiratory fitness results similar to those previously reported in healthy women with high levels of physical activity [3, 6, 7]. Interestingly, it was observed that the $VO_{2\,max}$ diminishes progressively during thyroid hormone deficiency. So one might speculate

that the increase of $VO_{2\,max}$ observed in the training group could have a beneficial effect in patients with thyroid disease occuring as a result of metabolic status.

The main limitation of this study is its uncontrolled design. This study, however, was conceived as preliminary research aiming to evaluate the potential usefulness of exercise in patients with sHT. Nevertheless, the finding that sHT mental symptoms were those showing greater improvement is a fact that argues against a possible placebo effect despite the lack of a control group. Investigation of other intervention components, such as behavior therapy, is also needed. In addition, future randomized controlled trials should study the effects of exercise in patients with disorders secondary to thyroid function variations and their implication, as well as therapeutic options for this highly prevalent disease.

In summary, a supervised 12-week program of primarily medium-impact exercise in females with sHT improves health-related quality of life. Moreover, this exercise program proved to have a positive influence on the functional capacity of the subjects, being effective in improving cardiorespiratory fitness.

References

[1] M. I. Surks and J. G. Hollowell, "Age-specific distribution of serum thyrotropin and antithyroid antibodies in the U.S. population: implications for the prevalence of subclinical hypothyroidism," *Journal of Clinical Endocrinology and Metabolism*, vol. 92, no. 12, pp. 4575–4582, 2007.

[2] P. M. Yen, "Physiological and molecular basis of thyroid hormone action," *Physiological Reviews*, vol. 81, no. 3, pp. 1097–1142, 2001.

[3] G.-D. Xiang, J. Pu, H. Sun, L. Zhao, L. Yue, and J. Hou, "Regular aerobic exercise training improves endothelium-dependent arterial dilation in patients with subclinical hypothyroidism," *European Journal of Endocrinology*, vol. 161, no. 5, pp. 755–761, 2009.

[4] J. Kvetny, P. E. Heldgaard, E. M. Bladbjerg, and J. Gram, "Subclinical hypothyroidism is associated with a low-grade inflammation, increased triglyceride levels and predicts cardio-

vascular disease in males below 50 years," *Clinical Endocrinology*, vol. 61, no. 2, pp. 232–238, 2004.

[5] C. F. A. Eustatia-Rutten, E. P. M. Corssmit, A. M. Pereira et al., "Quality of life in longterm exogenous subclinical hyperthyroidism and the effects of restoration of euthyroidism, a randomized controlled trial," *Clinical Endocrinology*, vol. 64, no. 3, pp. 284–291, 2006.

[6] A. B. Newman, E. M. Simonsick, B. L. Naydeck et al., "Association of long-distance corridor walk performance with mortality, cardiovascular disease, mobility limitation, and disability," *Journal of the American Medical Association*, vol. 295, no. 17, pp. 2018–2026, 2006.

[7] J. M. Guralnik, L. Ferrucci, E. M. Simonsick, M. E. Salive, and R. B. Wallace, "Lower-extremity function in persons over the age of 70 years as a predictor of subsequent disability," *The New England Journal of Medicine*, vol. 332, no. 9, pp. 556–561, 1995.

[8] J. W. Smith, A. T. Evans, B. Costall, and J. W. Smythe, "Thyroid hormones, brain function and cognition: a brief review," *Neuroscience and Biobehavioral Reviews*, vol. 26, no. 1, pp. 45–60, 2002.

[9] V. S. Reuters, P. Almeida Cde, F. Teixeira Pde et al., "Effects of subclinical hypothyroidism treatment on psychiatric symptoms, muscular complaints, and quality of life," *Arquivos Brasileiros de Endocrinologia e Metabologia*, vol. 56, no. 2, pp. 128–136, 2012.

[10] R. S. Fortunato, D. L. Ignácio, Á. S. Padron et al., "The effect of acute exercise session on thyroid hormone economy in rats," *Journal of Endocrinology*, vol. 198, no. 2, pp. 347–353, 2008.

[11] A. R. Cappola, L. P. Fried, A. M. Arnold et al., "Thyroid status, cardiovascular risk, and mortality in older adults," *Journal of the American Medical Association*, vol. 295, no. 9, pp. 1033–1041, 2006.

[12] R. M. McAllister, M. D. Delp, and M. H. Laughlin, "Thyroid status and exercise tolerance. Cardiovascular and metabolic considerations," *Sports Medicine*, vol. 20, no. 3, pp. 189–198, 1995.

[13] A. Gonçalves, E. S. Resende, M. L. M. P. Fernandes, and A. M. da Costa, "Effect of thyroid hormones on cardiovascular and muscle systems and on exercise tolerance: a brief review," *Arquivos Brasileiros de Cardiologia*, vol. 87, no. 3, pp. e45–e47, 2006.

[14] A. C. Hackney, A. Kallman, K. P. Hosick, D. A. Rubin, and C. L. Battaglini, "Thyroid hormonal responses to intensive interval versus steady-state endurance exercise sessions," *Hormones*, vol. 11, no. 1, pp. 54–60, 2012.

[15] E. Maor, S. Kivity, E. Kopel et al., "Differences in heart rate profile during exercise among subjects with subclinicalthyroid disease," *Thyroid*, vol. 23, pp. 1226–1232, 2013.

[16] Sunita, A. S. Mahajan, A. Jain, N. Singh, and T. Mishra, "Heart rate and blood pressure response to exercise and recovery in subclinical hypothyroid patients," *International Journal of Applied and Basic Medical Research*, vol. 3, pp. 106–110, 2013.

[17] American College of Sports Medicine (ACSM), *Guidelines for Exercise Testing and Prescription*, Lippincott Williams & Wilkins, Philadelphia, Pa, USA, 6th edition, 2000.

[18] M. F. Mottola, I. Giroux, R. Gratton et al., "Nutrition and exercise prevent excess weight gain in overweight pregnant women," *Medicine and Science in Sports and Exercise*, vol. 42, no. 2, pp. 265–272, 2010.

[19] R. Ramírez-Vélez, R. A. Agredo-Zuñiga, and A. M. Jerez-Valderrama, "The reliability of preliminary normative values from the short form health survey (SF-12) questionnaire regarding colombian adults," *Revista de Salud Publica*, vol. 12, no. 5, pp. 807–819, 2010.

[20] H. Sato, N. Nakamura, S. Harada, N. Kakee, and N. Sasaki, "Quality of life of young adults with congenital hypothyroidism," *Pediatrics International*, vol. 51, no. 1, pp. 126–131, 2009.

[21] S. Grant, K. Todd, T. C. Aitchison, P. Kelly, and D. Stoddart, "The effects of a 12-week group exercise programme on physiological and psychological variables and function in overweight women," *Public Health*, vol. 118, no. 1, pp. 31–42, 2004.

[22] J. M. S. Garcia, Sanchez EDLC, A. D. S. Garcia, Y. E. Gonzalez, and S. T. Piles, "Influence of a circuit-training programme on health-related fitness and quality of life in sedentary women of over 70 years," *Fitness & Performance Journal*, vol. 6, pp. 14–19, 2007.

[23] G. J. Kahaly, C. Kampmann, and S. Mohr-Kahaly, "Cardiovascular hemodynamics and exercise tolerance in thyroid disease," *Thyroid*, vol. 12, no. 6, pp. 473–481, 2002.

[24] A. V. Montoya Arizabaleta, L. Orozco Buitrago, A. C. Aguilar de Plata, M. Mosquera Escudero, and R. Ramírez-Vélez, "Aerobic exercise during pregnancy improves health-related quality of life: a randomised trial," *Journal of Physiotherapy*, vol. 56, no. 4, pp. 253–258, 2010.

14

Clinical and Economic Outcomes of Thyroid Surgery in Elderly Patients

Michael C. Sullivan, Sanziana A. Roman, and Julie A. Sosa

Department of Surgery, Yale School of Medicine, New Haven, CT 06520, USA

Correspondence should be addressed to Julie A. Sosa, julie.sosa@yale.edu

Academic Editor: Juan José Diez

The U.S. population is undergoing a dramatic shift in demographics, with a rise in the proportion of elderly Americans. Given an increased prevalence of thyroid disease and malignancy with age, understanding the safety of thyroid surgery in this age group is increasingly pertinent. There remains disagreement regarding the clinical outcomes of elderly patients after thyroidectomy and the applicability of single-institution cohorts to the population at large. This paper reviews the epidemiology of thyroid disease in the elderly, current surgical indications and practice patterns, and the clinical and economic outcomes of elderly patients with thyroid disease after surgical intervention.

1. Introduction

The U.S. population is rapidly changing. According to Census Bureau projections, the number of elderly Americans will double to 80 million by 2050; the most expeditious growth is expected to occur between 2010 and 2030, when the number of Americans aged >65 years will increase by 2.8% annually [1]. The "oldest old," or individuals >85 years, are the most rapidly expanding subgroup of elderly citizens. Numbering 3 million in 1994, they represented 10% of the elderly and 1% of the overall population; by 2050, an estimated 19 million individuals >85 years are projected to comprise 24% of elderly Americans, and 5% of the total population [1].

Approximately 50% of all surgical procedures are performed on patients >65 years [2]; according to the National Hospital Discharge Survey, elderly patients represented 39% of discharges from short-stay hospitals and 45% of days of inpatient care in 2009 [3]. Given increasing life expectancy and a generalized expansion of surgical indications, the elderly will likely account for a significant proportion of the anticipated 14–47% increase in demand for surgical services by 2020 [2, 4]. For surgical oncologists, this increase is estimated to be 42.7% and 25.4% for selected inpatient and outpatient procedures, respectively [5].

The prevalence of thyroid disease and thyroid malignancy increases with age [6–8]. Common surgical indications in the elderly include hyperthyroidism resistant to medical management, symptoms of compression due to retrosternal goiter extension, suspicion of a malignant nodule requiring histologic diagnosis, or thyroid carcinoma [9, 10]. While age itself is not a contraindication for major surgery [8, 10], controversy remains regarding the safety of surgical interventions for thyroid disease in aging Americans.

2. Epidemiology

Thyroid gland dysfunction is common among older patients, and can lead to significant morbidity when left untreated. For hyperthyroidism, the prevalence of overt disease in the elderly is estimated to be 0.5–4%, with subclinical hyperthyroidism having a prevalence of 3–8% [6]. Inciting causes of thyrotoxicosis most frequently include toxic multinodular goiter (MNG) and Graves disease [11–13], with the prevalence of both toxic adenomas and MNG increasing with age [6]. While many patients demonstrate classic signs of sympathetic overactivity, a proportion of elderly patients will present with "masked" or "apathetic" thyrotoxicosis [14, 15]. Nonspecific symptoms that can be attributed to the aging process or previously diagnosed health issues, such as weight loss, muscle weakness, loss of appetite, and apathy, can delay diagnosis and may compromise outcomes [16]. In a cross-sectional study involving 3,049 patients, those >60 years most frequently reported 0–2 symptoms of hyperthyroidism at diagnosis (54.4%, $P < .001$ across all age groups) and were least likely to report ≥5 symptoms (14.8%, $P < .001$ across all age groups) [17].

The prevalence of thyroid nodules increases with age; almost 50% of patients ≥65 years demonstrate nodules on ultrasound examination [18], with a similar prevalence among autopsies performed for the general population [19, 20]. Further, there is an established association between age and the malignant potential of thyroid nodules [21, 22]. Thyroid carcinoma represents approximately 1% of all U.S. cancers, with an estimated 0.1% of adults aged 50–70 years having clinically apparent disease [6]. The Centers for Disease Control (CDC) estimates there will be 56,460 incident cases and 1,780 deaths from thyroid cancer in 2012 [23]. Well-differentiated thyroid cancer (DTC), comprised of papillary, follicular, and Hürthle cell histologic subtypes, accounts for >90% of all diagnoses; poorly differentiated, medullary, and anaplastic thyroid cancers comprise a much smaller percentage of cases [24, 25].

While women are afflicted by thyroid cancer two to three times more frequently than men, this gender disparity appears to decline among elderly patients [26, 27]. At the same time, older age is associated with changes in the incidence and behavior of thyroid cancer subtypes. Papillary thyroid cancer behaves more aggressively among elderly patients, with more frequent extrathyroidal spread and distant metastases [28, 29]. Previous research examining 30,504 patients with papillary thyroid cancer from the Surveillance, Epidemiology, and End Results (SEER) registry found that cervical lymph node metastases did not affect survival among patients aged <45 years ($P = .535$), but they conferred a 46% increased risk of death to those individuals ≥45 years ($P < .001$) [30]. Among all differentiated cancers, age >60 years has been associated with an increase in cause-specific mortality and failure of surgical extirpation [31, 32].

For medullary cancer, older age is more closely associated with sporadic than hereditary tumors; it also has been cited as a poor prognostic factor [33]. Anaplastic thyroid cancer represents 2–5% of all thyroid tumors and has a peak incidence in the 6th-7th decades of life [34]. Generally arising in the setting of a goiter or DTC, this disease is almost uniformly fatal.

3. Surgical Indications and Practice Patterns

Because of an elevated risk for perioperative morbidity among elderly patients undergoing surgical procedures, indications for thyroidectomy in this population are often restricted to overt compressive symptoms or a strong suspicion for malignancy [8]. Lang and Lo studied patients undergoing total thyroidectomy for MNG and found that 38.2% of elderly patients (age ≥ 70 years) had compressive symptoms as their principal indication for surgery [35]. They were more likely than younger patients to have as an indication thyrotoxicosis (30.9% versus 11.6%, $P < .001$) or

recent gland enlargement (27.3% versus 7.9%, $P < .001$). Passler et al. reported that patients ≥75 years were more likely to undergo thyroid surgery for suspected or verified malignancy (52.7% versus 30.3%, $P < .001$) or compressive symptoms (38.2% versus 3.1%, $P < .001$), but significantly less likely to have surgery for a noncompressive benign goiter (9.1% versus 66.6%, $P < .001$) [36]. In neither study did the type/extent of procedure significantly differ between age groups. These findings are partially supported by Rios et al. who reviewed 591 patients (81 patients >65 years) receiving treatment for MNG [8]. Elderly patients were more likely than their younger counterparts to have compressive symptoms (43% versus 21%, $P = .001$) and less likely to have concern for malignancy (19% versus 29%, $P = .031$), recent goiter growth (1% versus 6%, $P = .021$), or patient request (4% versus 12%, $P = .001$).

For patients >45 years with DTC that is ≥1 cm in size, current American Thyroid Association (ATA) guidelines recommend near-total or total thyroidectomy with adjuvant radioiodine ablation (RAI) for patients with metastases or a functional thyroid remnant [37]. Park et al. used SEER to describe the treatment patterns of elderly Americans with DTC for which the ATA guidelines would suggest surgery and RAI. Among 8,899 patients (45–64 years: 6,184; 65–79 years: 2,271; ≥80 years: 444), 78% received near-total or total thyroidectomy, 21% lobectomy, and 1% no surgery; 52% of all patients received adjuvant RAI [25]. Patients ≥65 years demonstrated more aggressive disease with multiple, larger tumors and more advanced-stage disease, nonpapillary histology, and extrathyroidal extension (all $P < .001$). Nevertheless, elderly patients were less likely to undergo near-total or total thyroidectomy, lymphadenectomy, or radiation treatment (all $P < .001$). Elderly patients were observed to undergo less aggressive treatment than that recommended by the ATA for all stages of disease; on multivariate analysis, older age was associated with less aggressive surgery (65–79 years: OR—1.27, ≥80 years: OR—2.32) and failure to receive RAI (65–79 years: OR—1.16, ≥80 years: OR—2.45).

Similar findings have been reported for MTC. Panigrahi et al. retrospectively examined the treatment experiences of 2,033 patients with MTC using SEER [38]. Among all patients ($n = 1,344$) without local invasion or distant metastases, only 59% underwent total thyroidectomy and central compartment neck dissection, as recommended by the ATA [39]; when stratified by age, older patients were less likely to receive appropriate treatment (age <40 years: 65%, 40–65 years: 62%, >65 years: 45%, $P < .001$). On multivariate regression analysis, age >65 years was independently associated with a patient receiving care that was out of step with ATA guidelines (OR: 3.1); on Kaplan-Meier survival analysis, this was associated with compromised disease-specific survival ($P < .05$) [38].

4. Clinical Outcomes

There is evidence from single institution analyses to support the safety of thyroid surgery in the elderly. Passler et al. reviewed the experiences of 738 patients (55 aged ≥75 years) undergoing thyroid surgery over a 5-year study period [36]. The elderly cohort was more likely to undergo remedial thyroid surgery (18.2% versus 6.7%, $P = .006$). The rate of early postoperative complications (elderly: 25.5% versus younger: 21.8%), including hypocalcemia and recurrent laryngeal nerve (RLN) injury, did not differ between age groups. There was no 30-day mortality. Notably, 12.7% of elderly patients were admitted to the ICU for postoperative care; among all elderly patients, the mean preoperative and total hospital length of stays (LOS) were exceptionally long compared to conventional standards at 4.3 and 14.2 days, respectively. The authors acknowledge that each patient underwent operative intervention because of an "absolute necessity," thus representing a carefully selected cohort. Seybt et al. compared the post-thyroidectomy experiences of 86 young patients (aged 21–35 years) and 44 elderly patients (aged ≥65 years) [40]. While patient comorbidities and operative details (including the procedure performed) were not provided, the rates of transient postoperative hypocalcemia, true vocal cord paralysis, and complications were similar between age groups. Due to small sample size, the study might not have been adequately powered to detect meaningful differences in outcomes based on age; for example, the elderly cohort demonstrated an almost fourfold higher rate of readmission, but this was not significant (4.5% versus 1.2%, $P = .26$).

Bliss et al. presented a single institution series of 1,631 patients who underwent 1,673 thyroid procedures; patients were divided into three age groups: 50–60 years (725 patients), 61–74 years (685 patients), and ≥75 years (221 patients) [10]. The most common indication for surgery in all groups was retrosternal goiter causing compression, although this was least frequent in patients ≥75 years ($P < .001$). Of note, elderly patients were most likely to undergo remedial thyroid surgery ($P = .003$). While hematoma formation was more common in patients aged 61–74 years than those ≥75 years ($P = .02$), the rates of other complications and postoperative death did not differ between groups. Reeve et al. reviewed 575 patients aged >60 years at a single institution [41]. The most frequent operations included thyroid lobectomy (185 cases, 32%) and subtotal thyroidectomy (148 cases, 26%); pathology demonstrated a malignancy rate of 14%. The authors report an "acceptably low" frequency of complications, as the rate of RLN injury and hypoparathyroidism were 1.0% and 0.2%, respectively. However, a total of 68 postoperative events were reported, including hemorrhage requiring reoperation, hematoma, tracheostomy, respiratory problems, myocardial infarction, arrhythmias, and seizures. The authors assert that such general complications "were those expected in an elderly population with multiple pathology"; however, such events highlight the inherent risk assumed by elderly patients undergoing surgery.

In another single institution series, Rafaelli et al. described the experiences of 320 patients ≥70 years who underwent thyroid surgery [9]. Indications for surgery included bilateral nodular goiter (53.5%), suspicious nodule/confirmed malignancy (28.1%), and toxic goiter (18.4%); 64% of patients presented with ≥1 comorbidity (72.5% of patients of ASA class II). Postoperatively, 23 (7%) patients

required ICU admission for management of a concomitant disorder, and average LOS was 3.3 days. Early complications occurred in 39% of patients, including 104 cases of hypocalcemia; hypoparathyroidism and permanent RLN injury were seen in 1.6% and 0.3% of patients, respectively.

In 279 patients who underwent a total thyroidectomy for MNG at a single institution, Lang and Lo found that patients aged ≥70 years ($n = 55$) were more likely to have retrosternal goiters (76.4% versus 24.4%, $P < .001$), larger goiters (164.1 g versus 100.5 g, $P < .001$), longer operating times (148.9 min versus 136.5, $P = .023$), greater blood loss (102.1 mL versus 66.2 mL, $P = .030$), and fewer parathyroid glands visualized (2.9 versus 3.3, $P < .001$) [35]. While the rate of surgical complications was similar between age groups, the rate of nonsurgical complications was higher in patients ≥70 years (5.5% versus 0.4%, $P = .021$). LOS also was longer among elderly patients (6.4 days versus 3.7 days, $P < .001$). Of note, 31 of 55 elderly patients were ASA class I, 13 were ASA class II, and 11 were ASA class III. Among these individuals, the number of comorbidities was directly correlated to total LOS: 0 comorbidities (4.7 days) versus ≥3 comorbidities (11.0 days).

An additional review of geriatric thyroidectomy for MNG was performed by Rios et al. The experiences of 591 patients (81 patients aged >65 years) were compared over 30 years [8]. Elderly patients sustained more complications (40% versus 28%, $P = .011$), including transient hypoparathyroidism ($P = .003$) and hematomas ($P = .034$). There were no complications among 8 patients ≥80 years. The authors conclude that surgery for MNG in elderly patients is indicated restrictively.

Other investigations have focused on the superelderly, or patients ≥80 years. Miccoli et al. reported on 12 patients (mean age 81.4 years) undergoing thyroid procedures for a diagnosis of malignancy or "dramatic" evidence of airway compression [42]. There were no instances of postoperative hemorrhage, RLN injury, or hypoparathyroidism. Mekel et al. described 90 consecutive patients ≥80 years (mean age 83.2 years; range 80–94) who underwent thyroid surgery, and compared them to a randomly selected cohort of 242 individuals aged 18–79 years (mean age 50.1 years; range, 18–79) [43]. No between-group differences were noted with regard to gender, body mass index, previous thyroid operations, principal diagnosis, or final pathology. Of note, octogenarians had higher mean Charlson comorbidity index scores (1.08 versus 0.38, $P < .001$) and ASA scores ($P < .001$). Octogenarians had a higher rate of complications (24% versus 9%, $P < .001$), although there was no difference in the frequency of thyroid-specific complications; there was no mortality in the series. On multivariate analysis, age was not associated with developing a complication. The authors recommend avoiding unnecessary surgery in the elderly, with more strict criteria applied to the biopsy of thyroid nodules.

5. Population Studies: Combined Clinical and Economic Outcomes

While some single institution reports have produced encouraging results regarding the safety of thyroid surgery in the elderly, recent population-level analyses regarding short-term clinical and economic outcomes in geriatric patients have diverged.

Sosa et al. used the Healthcare Cost and Utilization Project Nationwide Inpatient Sample (HCUP-NIS) to study 22,848 patients undergoing thyroid procedures in the U.S. in 2003-2004; there were 4,092 patients aged 65–79 years and 744 ≥80 years [44]. Older age was associated with a lower likelihood of total thyroidectomy (18–44 y: 44.2%, 45–64 y: 41.1%, 65–79 y: 36.9%, and ≥80 y: 37.1%, $P < .001$ across all ages and procedures), an increased frequency of a substernal component (2.7% versus 3.7% versus 6.3% versus 8.7%, $P < .001$), an increase in the severity of illness ($P < .001$), and an increase in the likelihood of a nonelective hospital admission ($P < .001$). Clear differences in clinical outcomes were noted. In comparison to younger age groups, elderly patients had higher rates of endocrine-specific and overall complications and in-hospital mortality; after adjustment, they also had longer mean LOS and higher costs (all $P < .001$, resp.). These findings were especially pronounced among the superelderly; compared to similar patients aged 65–79 years, patients aged ≥80 years had a 34% increase in complications, a 60% longer inpatient LOS, and a 28% increase in costs. These findings are supported by those of Sosa et al., in their analysis of Maryland Health Services Cost Review Commission data for 5,860 patients undergoing thyroid procedures [45]. After adjustment for patient, surgeon, and hospital characteristics, patients aged ≥70 years had significantly longer LOS, more complications, and greater total hospital charges.

The SEER-Medicare linked database provides a unique opportunity to follow the incident cancer diagnoses and the subsequent cancer-directed surgeries of Medicare beneficiaries in a SEER registry in a longitudinal fashion, through both administrative records and comprehensive clinical data [46]. Information regarding patient demographics and comorbidities, physician and hospital characteristics, tumor histology, index hospitalization, adjuvant therapy, and complications of treatment are accessible [47]. Tuggle et al. examined the frequency of unplanned hospital readmission within 30 days of discharge among 2,127 elderly patients who underwent thyroidectomy for thyroid cancer in this database [46]. In all, 171 patients (8%) required 185 readmissions, at a mean time of 15.8 days after discharge. Those experiencing a complication during their index hospitalization (22%) were more likely to require an unplanned readmission; the most common reason for rehospitalization was endocrine-specific complications (47%), followed by "other" (25%) and pulmonary complications (17%). The mean LOS for all unplanned readmissions was 3.5 days, with a mean cost of $5,921. Patients who were rehospitalized had a significantly increased risk of death at one year (18% versus 6%, $P < .001$), particularly among those who suffered a pulmonary-related complication (38%). After adjustment, metastatic disease, an increased number of comorbidities, longer index LOS, and having ≥1 postoperative complication at the time of index hospitalization were independently associated with having an unplanned readmission.

Tuggle et al. also examined the effect of outpatient follow-up on the rate of unplanned readmission. Among the 1,131 patients (53%) seen by a healthcare provider (general practitioner or specialist) after discharge from index hospitalization (mean time to visit: 13.6 days), there was a significantly lower likelihood of readmission than those without prompt physician follow-up (5.1% versus 11.4%, $P < .001$) [46]. As such, the authors emphasize the importance of continuity during the transition from an inpatient to outpatient care setting, especially among elderly patients at high risk for rehospitalization.

6. Discussion

Surgical management of elderly patients presents a unique set of challenges, including overcoming compromised access to appropriate care and high-volume surgeons, and increased patient complexity and severity of illness [44]. To date, the majority of studies regarding outcomes for elderly patients undergoing thyroid surgery have been largely limited to the single institution experiences of high-volume, tertiary care centers. It is not surprising that many of these small series have demonstrated superlative outcomes; previous population-level analyses have delineated a positive association between increased surgeon and hospital case volume and patient outcomes, including those performed on children [48], pregnant women [49, 50], and the elderly [51]. For thyroid surgery in an elderly population, the use of a representative national database supports this notion [44, 45]. Therefore, small published case series may underestimate the true risks of surgery for the average elderly patient with thyroid pathology, potentially limiting external validity.

Using the HCUP-NIS database, Sosa et al. found that, among all age groups (18–44 y, 45–64 y, 65–79 y, and ≥80 y) surgeons performing >100 thyroidectomies/year had shorter LOS and lower complication rates than their lower-volume colleagues [44]. When patients were stratified by age and comorbidities, elderly and superelderly patients who underwent thyroidectomy by high-volume surgeons (≥30 cases/year) had shorter LOS and lower-complication rates than patients who had surgery by low-volume surgeons; high-volume surgeons also had lower total costs in all groups except healthy superelderly patients. These results were particularly pronounced among superelderly patients with multiple comorbidities, where high-volume surgeons had lower rates of complications than their low-volume colleagues (11% versus 25%), shorter LOS (2.2 versus 7.7 days), and lower total costs ($5,140 versus $12,541).

Despite these findings, low-volume surgeons continue to perform the overwhelming majority of thyroid surgery, particularly among elderly patients. Using data from the 1988–2000 HCUP-NIS, Saunders et al. found that 82% of all thyroidectomies were performed by surgeons with a practice composed of <25% endocrine procedures; surgeons with a practice consisting of >75% endocrine procedures performed just 3% of all thyroidectomies [52]. Sosa et al. found that not only did lowest volume surgeons (1–9 cases/year) account for the largest proportion of thyroidectomies among all patient age groups examined, but that this trend increased with patient age (18–44 y: 47%, 45–64 y: 46%, 65–79 y: 52%, and ≥80 y: 58%, $P < .001$); for surgeons performing >30 thyroidectomies/year, the reverse trend was noted (18–44 y: 29%, 45–64 y: 29%, 65–79 y: 23%, and ≥80 y: 16%, $P < .001$) [44]. This is a finding of concern, and may partially explain why the outcomes of elderly patients undergoing thyroid surgery on a national scale appear to be inferior to those from select high-volume institutional cohorts.

A majority of published single-institution case series have found no effect of age on the risks of thyroid surgery. However, given their small sample sizes and thus the risk of associated type II error, it is possible that these studies have been underpowered to adequately test the hypothesis of interest. Underpowered studies, which frequently fail to calculate or report power analyses, are prevalent in the surgical literature [53–55]. In a review of randomized control trials in the surgical literature, Maggard et al. found that only 38% reported sample size calculations; among all studies, 81% did not have a large enough sample size to detect a 20% outcome difference, with 55% of the these studies requiring a 10-fold increase in sample size [55].

Observational studies assessing comparative effectiveness or safety of different treatment strategies can suffer from confounding by indication [56]. Analytic tools such as propensity scores are being employed more and more in surgical health services research to account for residual selection bias, especially when the outcomes of interest are rare, as morbidity and mortality can be in endocrine surgery [57]. As evidence-based practice continues to drive clinical and operative decision-making, it is critical to understand the strength of conclusions to be drawn from studies regarding surgical outcomes.

Thyroid surgery presents distinct risks for elderly patients; on a national scale, the clinical and economic outcomes for many of these individuals appear to be compromised compared to younger patients. Thyroid surgery in this population should be applied selectively, and undertaken after meticulous preoperative medical optimization. Given the correlation between surgeon caseload and postoperative morbidity, strong consideration should be given for referral of elderly patients to high-volume surgeons, especially among individuals with complex or malignant thyroid pathology. Attention also should be paid to ensure the surgical care of elderly patients follows current practice guidelines, and aggressive postoperative follow-up should be standardized to minimize the risk of costly, unplanned hospital readmissions. Future areas of analysis could include a further clarification of indications for thyroid surgery in this population, as well as outcome measures such as long-term survival and quality of life.

References

[1] "Sixty-five plus in the United States," U.S. Census Bureau, 2011, http://www.census.gov/population/socdemo/statbriefs/agebrief.html.

[2] C. Christmas, M. A. Makary, and J. R. Burton, "Medical considerations in older surgical patients," *Journal of the American College of Surgeons*, vol. 203, no. 5, pp. 746–751, 2006.

[3] "National Hospital Discharge Survey," Centers for Disease Control and Prevention, 2012, http://www.cdc.gov/nchs/nhds/nhds_tables.htm#number.

[4] D. A. Etzioni, J. H. Liu, M. A. Maggard, and C. Y. Ko, "The aging population and its impact on the surgery workforce," *Annals of Surgery*, vol. 238, no. 2, pp. 170–177, 2003.

[5] D. A. Etzioni, J. H. Liu, M. A. Maggard, J. B. O'Connell, and C. Y. Ko, "Workload projections for surgical oncology: will we need more surgeons?" *Annals of Surgical Oncology*, vol. 10, no. 9, pp. 1112–1117, 2003.

[6] M. Papaleontiou and M. R. Haymart, "Approach to and treatment of thyroid disorders in the elderly," *Medical Clinics of North America*, vol. 96, no. 2, pp. 297–310, 2012.

[7] S. U. Rehman, D. W. Cope, A. D. Senseney, and W. Brzezinski, "Thyroid disorders in elderly patients," *Southern Medical Journal*, vol. 98, no. 5, pp. 543–549, 2005.

[8] A. Rios, J. M. Rodriguez, P. J. Galindo, M. Canteras, and P. Parrilla, "Surgical treatment for multinodular goitres in geriatric patients," *Langenbeck's Archives of Surgery*, vol. 390, no. 3, pp. 236–242, 2005.

[9] M. Raffaelli, R. Bellantone, P. Princi et al., "Surgical treatment of thyroid diseases in elderly patients," *American Journal of Surgery*, vol. 200, no. 4, pp. 467–472, 2010.

[10] R. Bliss, N. Patel, A. Guinea, T. S. Reeve, and L. Delbridge, "Age is no contraindication to thyroid surgery," *Age and Ageing*, vol. 28, no. 4, pp. 363–366, 1999.

[11] P. A. Singer, D. S. Cooper, E. G. Levy et al., "Treatment guidelines for patients with hyperthyroidism and hypothyroidism. Standards of Care Committee, American Thyroid Association," *The Journal of the American Medical Association*, vol. 273, no. 10, pp. 808–812, 1995.

[12] S. Morganti, G. P. Ceda, M. Saccani et al., "Thyroid disease in the elderly: sex-related differences in clinical expression," *Journal of Endocrinological Investigation*, vol. 28, no. 11, pp. 101–104, 2005.

[13] A. Faggiano, M. Del Prete, F. Marciello, V. Marotta, V. Ramundo, and A. Colao, "Thyroid diseases in elderly," *Minerva Endocrinologica*, vol. 36, pp. 211–231, 2011.

[14] P. Mitrou, S. A. Raptis, and G. Dimitriadis, "Thyroid disease in older people," *Maturitas*, vol. 70, no. 1, pp. 5–9, 2011.

[15] J. J. Diez, "Hyperthyroidism in patients older than 55 years: an analysis of the etiology and management," *Gerontology*, vol. 49, no. 5, pp. 316–323, 2003.

[16] C. Trivalle, J. Doucet, P. Chassagne et al., "Differences in the signs and symptoms of hyperthyroidism in older and younger patients," *Journal of the American Geriatrics Society*, vol. 44, no. 1, pp. 50–53, 1996.

[17] K. Boelaert, B. Torlinska, R. L. Holder, and J. A. Franklyn, "Older subjects with hyperthyroidism present with a paucity of symptoms and signs: a large cross-sectional study," *Journal of Clinical Endocrinology and Metabolism*, vol. 95, no. 6, pp. 2715–2726, 2010.

[18] E. L. Mazzaferri, "Management of a solitary thyroid nodule," *The New England Journal of Medicine*, vol. 328, no. 8, pp. 553–559, 1993.

[19] M. Shirodkar and S. A. Jabbour, "Endocrine incidentalomas," *International Journal of Clinical Practice*, vol. 62, no. 9, pp. 1423–1431, 2008.

[20] J. D. Mortensen, L. B. Woolner, and W. A. Bennett, "Gross and microscopic findings in clinically normal thyroid glands," *The Journal of Clinical Endocrinology and Metabolism*, vol. 15, no. 10, pp. 1270–1280, 1955.

[21] A. Belfiore, G. L. La Rosa, G. A. La Porta et al., "Cancer risk in patients with cold thyroid nodules: relevance of iodine intake,

sex, age, and multinodularity," *American Journal of Medicine*, vol. 93, no. 4, pp. 363–369, 1992.

[22] J. D. Lin, T. C. Chao, B. Y. Huang, S. T. Chen, H. Y. Chang, and C. Hsueh, "Thyroid cancer in the thyroid nodules evaluated by ultrasonography and fine-needle aspiration cytology," *Thyroid*, vol. 15, no. 7, pp. 708–717, 2005.

[23] "Thyroid Cancer," National Cancer Institute, 2012, http://www.cancer.gov/cancertopics/types/thyroid.

[24] L. Davies and H. G. Welch, "Increasing incidence of thyroid cancer in the United States, 1973–2002," *Journal of the American Medical Association*, vol. 295, no. 18, pp. 2164–2167, 2006.

[25] H. S. Park, S. A. Roman, and J. A. Sosa, "Treatment patterns of aging americans with differentiated thyroid cancer," *Cancer*, vol. 116, no. 1, pp. 20–30, 2010.

[26] B. A. Kilfoy, S. S. Devesa, M. H. Ward et al., "Gender is an age-specific effect modifier for papillary cancers of the thyroid gland," *Cancer Epidemiology Biomarkers and Prevention*, vol. 18, no. 4, pp. 1092–1100, 2009.

[27] B. Aschebrook-Kilfoy, M. H. Ward, M. M. Sabra, and S. S. Devesa, "Thyroid cancer incidence patterns in the United States by histologic type, 1992–2006," *Thyroid*, vol. 21, no. 2, pp. 125–134, 2011.

[28] A. Toniato, C. Bernardi, A. Piotto, D. Rubello, and M. R. Pelizzo, "Features of papillary thyroid carcinoma in patients older than 75 years," *Updates in Surgery*, vol. 63, no. 2, pp. 115–118, 2011.

[29] L. Vini, S. L. Hyer, J. Marshall, R. A'Hern, and C. Harmer, "Long-term results in elderly patients with differentiated thyroid carcinoma," *Cancer*, vol. 97, no. 11, pp. 2736–2742, 2003.

[30] V. Zaydfudim, I. D. Feurer, M. R. Griffin, and J. E. Phay, "The impact of lymph node involvement on survival in patients with papillary and follicular thyroid carcinoma," *Surgery*, vol. 144, no. 6, pp. 1070–1078, 2008.

[31] E. L. Mazzaferri, "Long-term outcome of patients with differentiated thyroid carcinoma: effect of therapy," *Endocrine Practice*, vol. 6, no. 6, pp. 469–476, 2000.

[32] R. W. Tsang, J. D. Brierley, W. J. Simpson, T. Panzarella, M. K. Gospodarowicz, and S. B. Sutcliffe, "The effects of surgery, radioiodine, and external radiation therapy on the clinical outcome of patients with differentiated thyroid carcinoma," *Cancer*, vol. 82, no. 2, pp. 375–388, 1998.

[33] E. Kebebew, P. H. Ituarte, A. E. Siperstein, Q. Y. Duh, and O. H. Clark, "Medullary thyroid carcinoma: clinical characteristics, treatment, prognostic factors, and a comparison of staging systems," *Cancer*, vol. 88, no. 5, pp. 1139–1148, 2000.

[34] S. Chiacchio, A. Lorenzoni, G. Boni, D. Rubello, R. Elisei, and G. Mariani, "Anaplastic thyroid cancer: prevalence, diagnosis and treatment," *Minerva Endocrinologica*, vol. 33, no. 4, pp. 341–357, 2008.

[35] B. H. H. Lang and C. Y. Lo, "Total thyroidectomy for multinodular goiter in the elderly," *American Journal of Surgery*, vol. 190, no. 3, pp. 418–423, 2005.

[36] C. Passler, R. Avanessian, K. Kaczirek, G. Prager, C. Scheuba, and B. Niederle, "Thyroid surgery in the geriatric patient," *Archives of Surgery*, vol. 137, no. 11, pp. 1243–1248, 2002.

[37] D. S. Cooper, G. M. Doherty, B. R. Haugen et al., "Management guidelines for patients with thyroid nodules and differentiated thyroid cancer," *Thyroid*, vol. 16, no. 2, pp. 109–142, 2006.

[38] B. Panigrahi, S. A. Roman, and J. A. Sosa, "Medullary thyroid cancer: are practice patterns in the united states discordant

from american thyroid association guidelines?" *Annals of Surgical Oncology*, vol. 17, no. 6, pp. 1490–1498, 2010.

[39] R. T. Kloos, C. Eng, D. B. Evans et al., "Medullary thyroid cancer: management guidelines of the American Thyroid Association," *Thyroid*, vol. 19, no. 6, pp. 565–612, 2009.

[40] M. W. Seybt, S. Khichi, and D. J. Terris, "Geriatric thyroidectomy: safety of thyroid surgery in an aging population," *Archives of Otolaryngology*, vol. 135, no. 10, pp. 1041–1044, 2009.

[41] T. S. Reeve, L. Delbridge, and P. Crummer, "Thyroid surgery in the elderly," *Annals of the Academy of Medicine Singapore*, vol. 16, no. 1, pp. 54–57, 1987.

[42] P. Miccoli, P. Iacconi, G. M. Cecchini et al., "Thyroid surgery in patients aged over 80 years," *Acta Chirurgica Belgica*, vol. 94, no. 4, pp. 222–223, 1994.

[43] M. Mekel, A. E. Stephen, R. D. Gaz, Z. H. Perry, R. A. Hodin, and S. Parangi, "Thyroid surgery in octogenarians is associated with higher complication rates," *Surgery*, vol. 146, no. 5, pp. 913–921, 2009.

[44] J. A. Sosa, P. J. Mehta, T. S. Wang, L. Boudourakis, and S. A. Roman, "A population-based study of outcomes from thyroidectomy in aging Americans: at what cost?" *Journal of the American College of Surgeons*, vol. 206, no. 6, pp. 1097–1105, 2008.

[45] J. A. Sosa, H. M. Bowman, J. M. Tielsch, N. R. Powe, T. A. Gordon, and R. Udelsman, "The importance of surgeon experience for clinical and economic outcomes from thyroidectomy," *Annals of Surgery*, vol. 228, no. 3, pp. 320–330, 1998.

[46] C. T. Tuggle, L. S. Park, S. Roman, R. Udelsman, and J. A. Sosa, "Rehospitalization among elderly patients with thyroid cancer after thyroidectomy are prevalent and costly," *Annals of Surgical Oncology*, vol. 17, no. 11, pp. 2816–2823, 2010.

[47] "SEER-Medicare: Measurements and Methods," National Cancer Institute, 2010, http://healthservices.cancer.gov/seer-medicare/considerations/methods.html.

[48] J. A. Sosa, C. T. Tuggle, T. S. Wang et al., "Clinical and economic outcomes of thyroid and parathyroid surgery in children," *Journal of Clinical Endocrinology and Metabolism*, vol. 93, no. 8, pp. 3058–3065, 2008.

[49] S. Kuy, S. A. Roman, R. Desai, and J. A. Sosa, "Outcomes following thyroid and parathyroid surgery in pregnant women," *Archives of Surgery*, vol. 144, no. 5, pp. 399–406, 2009.

[50] S. Kuy, S. A. Roman, R. Desai, and J. A. Sosa, "Outcomes following cholecystectomy in pregnant and nonpregnant women," *Surgery*, vol. 146, no. 2, pp. 358–366, 2009.

[51] J. D. Birkmeyer, T. A. Stukel, A. E. Siewers, P. P. Goodney, D. E. Wennberg, and F. L. Lucas, "Surgeon volume and operative mortality in the United States," *The New England Journal of Medicine*, vol. 349, no. 22, pp. 2117–2127, 2003.

[52] B. D. Saunders, R. M. Wainess, J. B. Dimick, G. M. Doherty, G. R. Upchurch, and P. G. Gauger, "Who performs endocrine operations in the United States?" *Surgery*, vol. 134, no. 6, pp. 924–931, 2003.

[53] R. M. Christley, "Power and error: increased risk of false positive results in underpowered studies," *The Open Epidemiology Journal*, vol. 3, pp. 16–19, 2010.

[54] A. W. Chan and D. G. Altman, "Epidemiology and reporting of randomised trials published in PubMed journals," *The Lancet*, vol. 365, no. 9465, pp. 1159–1162, 2005.

[55] M. A. Maggard, J. B. O'Connell, J. H. Liu, D. A. Etzioni, and C. Y. Ko, "Sample size calculations in surgery: are they done correctly?" *Surgery*, vol. 134, no. 2, pp. 275–279, 2003.

[56] B. M. Psaty and D. S. Siscovick, "Minimizing bias due to confounding by indication in comparative effectiveness research: the importance of restriction," *The Journal of the American Medical Association*, vol. 304, no. 8, pp. 897–898, 2010.

[57] M. Adamina, U. Guller, W. P. Weber, and D. Oertli, "Propensity scores and the surgeon," *British Journal of Surgery*, vol. 93, no. 4, pp. 389–394, 2006.

15

Antitumor Activity of Lenvatinib (E7080): An Angiogenesis Inhibitor that Targets Multiple Receptor Tyrosine Kinases in Preclinical Human Thyroid Cancer Models

Osamu Tohyama,[1] Junji Matsui,[2] Kotaro Kodama,[2] Naoko Hata-Sugi,[2] Takayuki Kimura,[1] Kiyoshi Okamoto,[2] Yukinori Minoshima,[2] Masao Iwata,[2] and Yasuhiro Funahashi[3]

[1] *Biomarkers and Personalized Medicine Core Function Unit, Eisai Co., Ltd, Tsukuba, Ibaraki 300-2635, Japan*
[2] *Discovery Biology, Oncology Product Creation Unit, Eisai Co., Ltd, Tsukuba, Ibaraki 300-2635, Japan*
[3] *Biomarkers and Personalized Medicine Core Function Unit, Eisai Inc., 4 Corporate Drive, Andover, MA 01810, USA*

Correspondence should be addressed to Yasuhiro Funahashi; yasuhiro_funahashi@eisai.com

Academic Editor: Giovanni Tallini

Inhibition of tumor angiogenesis by blockading the vascular endothelial growth factor (VEGF) signaling pathway is a promising therapeutic strategy for thyroid cancer. Lenvatinib mesilate (lenvatinib) is a potent inhibitor of VEGF receptors (VEGFR1–3) and other prooncogenic and prooncogenic receptor tyrosine kinases, including fibroblast growth factor receptors (FGFR1–4), platelet derived growth factor receptor α (PDGFRα), KIT, and RET. We examined the antitumor activity of lenvatinib against human thyroid cancer xenograft models in nude mice. Orally administered lenvatinib showed significant antitumor activity in 5 differentiated thyroid cancer (DTC), 5 anaplastic thyroid cancer (ATC), and 1 medullary thyroid cancer (MTC) xenograft models. Lenvatinib also showed antiangiogenesis activity against 5 DTC and 5 ATC xenografts, while lenvatinib showed in vitro antiproliferative activity against only 2 of 11 thyroid cancer cell lines: that is, RO82-W-1 and TT cells. Western blot analysis showed that cultured RO82-W-1 cells overexpressed FGFR1 and that lenvatinib inhibited the phosphorylation of FGFR1 and its downstream effector FRS2. Lenvatinib also inhibited the phosphorylation of RET with the activated mutation C634W in TT cells. These data demonstrate that lenvatinib provides antitumor activity mainly via angiogenesis inhibition but also inhibits FGFR and RET signaling pathway in preclinical human thyroid cancer models.

1. Introduction

Thyroid cancer is a common malignant endocrine tumor, the incidence of which has recently been increasing. More than 90% of thyroid cancers are the follicular or papillary types known as differentiated thyroid cancer (DTC) [1], which comprises 1% of all cancers globally. Ninety percent of patients with DTC survive at least 10 years [2]; however, DTC patients with radioactive iodine- (RAI-) refractory disease have a median survival of 2.5 to 3.5 years from detection of distant metastases [3, 4]. The cytotoxic agents used to treat RAI refractory disease have been universally classified as having only marginal efficacy and substantial toxicity [5, 6]. Approximately 10% of all thyroid cancers are

medullary thyroid cancer (MTC) [7], which is a distinct C-cell tumor of the thyroid. MTC occurs in both sporadic (75% of patients) and hereditary settings, and the latter includes three distinct inherited cancer syndromes: familial MTC, multiple endocrine neoplasia type 2A (MEN2A), and MEN2B [8]. MTC is associated with a favorable prognosis (i.e., 10-year survival rate, ~70%) in the case that the disease is treated at an early stage, but the prognosis is poor (i.e., 10-year survival rate, <50%) in patients with distant metastatic disease [9]. Anaplastic thyroid cancer (ATC) remains one of the most deadly human diseases but accounts for fewer than 2% of all thyroid cancers [10, 11]. Average survival after diagnosis is only 4 to 6 months [10, 12], and the tumor is usually well advanced by the time of diagnosis. ATC tumors are generally resistant to chemotherapy, and currently there is no effective therapeutic regimen for the treatment of ATC.

Various genetic alterations participate in the tumorigenesis of thyroid cancer [13]. BRAF V600E is one of the most frequent mutations, occurring in approximately 45% of papillary thyroid cancers (PTCs) [14] and 26% of ATCs [14, 15]. Other genetic alterations in PTC are point mutations in RAS [13, 16] and rearrangement of RET [17]. In follicular thyroid carcinoma (FTC), mutations in RAS [18, 19] and rearrangement of the PPARγ and PAX8 genes [18] are also common. Germline mutations in the RET proto-oncogene cause hereditary MTC [20–22], and approximately 50% of patients with sporadic MTC have somatic RET mutations [23, 24]. Accordingly, new molecularly targeted therapies are needed for the treatment of thyroid cancer.

Tumor angiogenesis—the formation of blood vessels within tumors—plays a key role in cancer cell survival, local tumor growth, and the development of distant metastases [25–28]. Numerous angiogenic factors have been identified, including VEGF, basic fibroblast growth factor (bFGF), hepatocyte growth factor, interleukin-8, and PDGF. VEGF is a crucial regulator of both physiologic and pathologic angiogenesis via its binding to the cognate receptor VEGFR2. Since increased VEGF expression is significantly associated with advanced-stage thyroid cancer [29], the use of inhibitors against VEGFR2 signaling pathway may represent a viable approach to controlling malignant thyroid cancer [30]. Inhibitors of the VEGFR2 signaling pathway show antitumor activity against various types of tumors, and consequently many of them are now in clinical use [31]. In phase 2 clinical trials of thyroid cancers motesanib, axitinib, and pazopanib, which are multiple receptor-tyrosine kinase inhibitors, have shown promising antitumor activity [32]. The US FDA recently approved sorafenib for the treatment of patients with locally recurrent or metastatic, progressive DTC that is refractory to RAI treatment [33]. Vandetanib [34] and cabozantinib have been approved for use in the treatment of advanced or metastatic MTC. Therefore, molecularly targeted agents for the VEGFR2 signaling pathway are expected as new thyroid cancer therapy. Beside VEGFR2 signaling pathway, other receptor tyrosine kinases (RTKs) have significant roles in thyroid cancer. Overexpression of fibroblast growth factor receptor [35] and mutations of RET [23, 24] are reported to participate in the development and aggressive phenotypes of thyroid cancers. Given that the most of VEGFR2 inhibitors which target multiple receptors, inhibition of those RTKs could improve thyroid cancer therapy in addition to targeting the VEGFR2 signaling pathway.

Lenvatinib mesilate (lenvatinib) inhibits the multiple RTKs that target VEGF receptors (VEGFR1–3), FGF receptors (FGFR1–4), PDGF receptor α (PDGFRα), KIT, and RET [36]. Besides its antiangiogenesis activity based on VEGFR2 inhibition [36], lenvatinib has also shown antitumor activity based on inhibition of RET phosphorylation in PTC carrying RET/PCT fusion genes [37]. Lenvatinib has shown antitumor activity against multiple tumor types, such as DTC, MTC, melanoma, endometrial and hepatocellular [38, 39]. The purpose of this study was to assess the antitumor activity of lenvatinib and explore its mode of action in preclinical human thyroid cancer models, using DTC, MTC, and ATC cell lines. Here, we describe how lenvatinib inhibited in vivo tumor growth and tumor-induced angiogenesis in various human thyroid cancer xenograft models. We also show that lenvatinib directly inhibits the in vitro proliferation of thyroid cancer cell lines carrying mutations that activate RET or in which FGFR1 is overexpressed.

2. Materials and Methods

2.1. Compounds. Lenvatinib mesilate (lenvatinib), PD166866, PD173074, imatinib, and Ki6783 were synthesized at Eisai Co., Ltd. (Ibaraki, Japan). Sorafenib was purchased from Bayer (Tokyo, Japan).

2.2. Cell Free Kinase Inhibition Assay. The kinase inhibitory activities of lenvatinib and sorafenib against 66 purified recombinant protein kinases (including tyrosine kinases and serine threonine kinases) were examined by using an ELISA and an Off-Chip Mobility Shift Assay (MSA) from Carna Biosciences, Inc. (Kobe, Japan). Briefly, each test compound was mixed with enzyme, substrate, ATP, and Mg under appropriate buffer conditions for the ELISA or MSA. The readout value of the reaction control (complete reaction mixture) was set as 0% inhibition, and the readout value of the background (Enzyme (−)) was set as 100% inhibition; the percent inhibition of each test solution was then calculated. IC_{50} values (the half maximal inhibitory concentration) were calculated from concentrations versus % inhibition curves.

2.3. Cells. The human DTC cell lines K1, FTC-133, FTC-236, FTC-238, and RO82-W-1 and the human thyroid follicular epithelial cell line Nthy-ori 3-1 were obtained from DS Pharma Biomedical Co., Ltd. (Osaka, Japan). The human MTC cell line TT was obtained from the American Type Culture Collection (Manassas, VA). The human ATC cell lines 8305C, 8505C, HTC/C3, KHM-5M, and TCO-1 were obtained from the Japanese Collection of Research Bioresources Cell Bank (Osaka, Japan). K1 and RO82-W-1 cells were cultured in a mixture of Dulbecco's Modified Eagle Medium (DMEM), Ham's F12 medium, and MCDB 105 medium (2:1:1, v/v/v) with 10% FBS; FTC-133, FTC-236, and FTC-238 cells were cultured in a mixture of DMEM and Ham's F12 medium (1:1, v/v) with 10% FBS, Nthy-ori 3-1 cells were cultured in RPMI-1640 medium with 10% FBS, TT cells were cultured in RPMI-1640 medium with 15% FBS, TCO-1 cells were cultured in DMEM with 10% FCS, and 8305C and 8505C cells were cultured in Eagle's minimal essential medium (EMEM) supplemented with 10% FBS. KHM-5M cells were cultured in RPMI-1640 medium with 15% FBS. HTC/C3 cells were cultured in DMEM supplemented with 4,500 mg/L glucose and 10% FBS. All cells were grown at 5% CO_2 and 37°C. DMEM, EMEM, Ham's F12 medium, and RPMI-1640 medium were purchased from Wako (Osaka, Japan). MCDB 105 medium was purchased from Sigma-Aldrich (St. Louis, MO).

2.4. Animals. Nude mice (CAnN.Cg-Foxn1nu/CrlCrlj, female, 5-6 weeks old) were obtained from Charles River Laboratories Japan (Kanagawa, Japan). Mice were maintained under specific pathogen-free conditions and housed in barrier facilities on a 12 h light/dark cycle, with food and water ad libitum. All procedures using laboratory animals were done in accordance with all applicable institutional and government regulatory guidelines and policies and were performed in an animal facility accredited by the Center for Accreditation of Laboratory Animal Care of the Japan Health Sciences Foundation.

2.5. Human Thyroid Cancer Xenograft Models. Tumor cells were cultured in appropriate culture mediums. Cells were harvested with 0.05% or 0.25% (w/v) trypsin/EDTA and suspended with 50% (v/v) BD Matrigel (BD Biosciences, San Jose, CA) in the mixture of culture mediums at a density of $5-10 \times 10^7$ cells/mL. Then, 0.1-0.2 mL of the cell suspension was inoculated subcutaneously into the right flank region of each mouse. When the tumor volume reached between 100 and 300 mm^3, mice were selected based on their tumor volumes, tumor shapes, physical condition, and body weights to be randomly split into each treatment group: vehicle, lenvatinib, PD173074, or sorafenib ($n = 5$ per group). Lenvatinib, PD173074, and sorafenib were dissolved in sterile distilled water, sterile distilled water containing equimolar hydrochloric acid, and distilled water containing 12.5% (v/v) ethanol and 12.5% (v/v) Cremophor EL, respectively, and administered orally once daily. The tumor size was measured in two dimensions by using a caliper, and the volume was calculated by using the formula: tumor volume (mm^3) = 1/2 length (mm) $\times$ [width (mm)]^2. The change in tumor volume in the treated group relative to that in the control group was calculated according to the following formula: $\Delta T/C = (\Delta T/\Delta C) \times 100\%$, where ΔT and ΔC are the change in tumor volume (i.e., growth) for the treated and vehicle control group, respectively. The percentage of tumor growth inhibition (%TGI) was calculated from the formula: $[(1 - \Delta T/\Delta C) \times 100]$.

2.6. Quantitative RT-PCR. Cells (5×10^6) were seeded and cultured in 6-well culture plates. After overnight culture, total RNA was isolated from the cultured cells by using an RNeasy Mini Kit (Qiagen, Hilden, Germany) according to the manufacturer's protocol. Reverse transcription was carried out with purified RNA by using a High Capacity cDNA Reverse Transcription Kit (Life Technologies, Carlsbad, CA). Synthesized cDNA was used as a template for quantitative polymerase chain reaction (PCR) assays using TaqMan Universal PCR Master Mix (Life Technologies), AmpErase UNG (Life Technologies), and TaqMan probes [*FGFR1* (Hs 00241111), *FGFR2* (Hs 01552926), *FGFR3* (Hs 00179829), *FGFR4* (Hs 00242558), *VEGFR1* (Hs 01904119), *VEGFR2* (Hs 00176676), *VEGFR3* (Hs 01047687), *KIT* (Hs 00174029), *EGFR* (Hs 00193306), *PDGFRA* (Hs 00183486), *PDGFRB* (Hs 00182163), *MET* (Hs 01565580), *RET* (Hs 01120032), *18S rRNA* (Hs 99999901)] (Life Technologies, Carlsbad, CA) in an ABI 7900 PCR system (Life Technologies). A standard curve was

used to determine PCR efficiency. Cycle threshold (Ct) values were determined by using SDS software (Life Technologies). Relative gene expression was normalized to a housekeeping gene (18S rRNA).

2.7. Plasmid Construction. The human full-length KIF5B-RET gene [37] was chemically synthesized by GenScript Corp. (Piscataway, NJ) and then amplified by polymerase chain reaction (PCR) using a primer set containing attB recombination sequences. ENTRY vectors for the Gateway cloning system (Life Technologies) were generated via the BP Clonase reaction using the PCR products and the plasmid pDONR221. The expression vector pCLxIP KIF5B-RET was generated via the LR Clonase reaction between each ENTRY vector and the destination vector pCLxIP-DEST [37]. Expression vectors for KIF5B-RET M918T were generated by introducing a point mutation into the pCLxIP KIF5B-RET expression vector.

2.8. Western Blot Analysis. Cells (1×10^5 to 3×10^6) were seeded and cultured to subconfluency in 6-well, 100mm, or 150mm cell culture plates in appropriate culture mediums overnight. RO82-W-1 cells were lysed in RIPA buffer (50 mM HEPES [pH 7.4], 150 mM NaCl, 1.5 mM MgCl$_2$, 10% [v/v] glycerol, 1% [v/v] Triton X-100, EDTA-free Protease Inhibitor Cocktail (Roche, Mannheim, Germany), Phosphatase Inhibitor Cocktail 2 (Sigma-Aldrich), and Phosphatase Inhibitor Cocktail 3 (Sigma-Aldrich)). TT cells were lysed in lysis buffer (50 mM HEPES [pH 7.4], 150 mM NaCl, 1 mM MgCl$_2$, 10% [v/v] glycerol, 1% [v/v] Triton X-100, 1 mM EDTA [pH 8.0], 100 mM NaF, 1 mM phenylmethylsulfonyl fluoride, 1 mM sodium orthovanadate, 10 μg/mL aprotinin, 50 μg/mL leupeptin, and 1 μg/mL pepstatin A). RO82-W-1 cells were starved overnight in culture medium containing 0.5% (w/v) bovine serum albumin (BSA), treated with PD173074, lenvatinib, or sorafenib for 1 h at the indicated concentrations and then stimulated for 10 min with bFGF (20 ng/mL; R&D Systems, Minneapolis, MN) and heparin (Sigma-Aldrich) before being lysed. Cultured TT cells were treated with lenvatinib for 1 h at the indicated concentrations before being lysed. Nthy-ori 3-1 cells were transfected with either KIF5B-RET- or KIF5B-RET M918T-expressing plasmids by using X-tremeGENE9 (Roche Diagnostics K. K., Tokyo, Japan). The next day, the transfected cells were treated with lenvatinib for 1 h before being lysed. Lysates from RO82-W-1 cells were immunoprecipitated with an anti-FGFR1 monoclonal antibody (WH0002260M3[5E9], Sigma-Aldrich). Nude mice bearing RO82-W-1 or TT xenografts were treated once orally with either vehicle or lenvatinib at 3, 10, 30, and 100 mg/kg. Nude mice bearing RO82-W-1 were also treated with sorafenib at 100 mg/kg. Tumors were collected 2 h after administration for RO82-W-1 xenografts and 2, 8, 12, and 24 h after administration for TT xenografts and were then lysed with RIPA buffer or lysis buffer, respectively. Lysed RO82-W-1 xenografts treated with lenvatinib at 30 and 100 mg/kg and sorafenib were immunoprecipitated with an anti-FRS2-α polyclonal antibody (FRS2, AF4069; R&D Systems). Immunoprecipitated samples and lysed samples

(20–30 μg of protein in 10 μL) were electrophoresed in 5%–20% or 4%–20% (for RET detection) polyacrylamide gels. Separated proteins were transferred onto PVDF membranes (Millipore, Bedford, MA) or Hybond-P (GE Healthcare Life Sciences, Uppsala, Sweden) and the membranes were incubated with the following primary antibodies: FGFR1 (ab76464; abcam, Cambridge, MA), FGFR1 (#3472; Cell Signaling, Beverly, MA) for immunoprecipitated samples, FGFR2 (MAB6842; R&D systems), FGFR3 (#4574; Cell Signaling), FGFR4 (SC-136988; Santa Cruz, Dallas, TX), phospho-FGFR1 (SC-30262R; Santa Cruz), FRS2-α (FRS2, SC-8318; Santa Cruz) for cell lysates, FRS2-α (FRS2, AF4069; R&D Systems) for tumor tissue lysates, phospho-FRS2-α [Thr196] (phospho-FRS2, #3864; Cell Signaling), RET (sc-1290; Sigma-Aldrich), phospho-RET (#3221, Cell Signaling), MEK1/2 (#9122, Cell Signaling), phospho-MEK [Ser217/221] (#9121, Cell Signaling), ERK1/2 (#9102, Cell Signaling), and phospho-ERK1/2 (#9101, Cell Signaling). Blots were detected with an ECL Prime Western Blotting Detection System (GE Healthcare Life Sciences) or with a SuperSignal Enhanced Chemiluminescence Kit (Pierce, Rockford, IL). Immunoreactive bands were visualized by using an LAS-4000 luminescent image analyzer (Fuji Film, Tokyo, Japan), Image Master (GE Healthcare Life Sciences), or Chemi Doc XRS (BioRad, Hercules, CA).

2.9. Antiproliferation Assay. Cells (1,000–3,000/well) were seeded and cultured in 96-well culture plates. After overnight culture, the cells were incubated with various concentrations of compounds for 3 days (10 days for TT cells). Cell numbers were determined by using WST-8 (Dojindo, Kumamoto, Japan); 10 μL of WST-8 was added to each well, and absorbance was measured at a wavelength of 450 nm and compared with a reference measurement at 660 or 665 nm by using an MTP-500 microplate reader (Corona Electric, Ibaraki, Japan) or an EnVision Multilabel Reader (Perkin Elmer, Turku, Finland). IC_{50} were graphically obtained from the dose-response curves.

2.10. Immunohistochemical Analysis. Tumor tissues were resected from nude mice, embedded in Optimal Cutting Temperature (OCT) compound (Sakura Finetek Japan, Tokyo, Japan), frozen in dry ice-acetone, and then sectioned (8 μm), or they were embedded in paraffin, fixed overnight in immunohistochemical (IHC) Zinc Fixative (BD Biosciences), and then sectioned (6 μm). Tumor microvessels were stained by the indirect immunoperoxidase method with a rat anti-mouse CD31 monoclonal antibody (clone MEC13.3, BD Biosciences) and then visualized by using Vectastain ABC (Dako, Tokyo, Japan). Pericyte was stained by the indirect alkaline phosphatase method with an anti-α smooth muscle actin (SMA) antibody conjugated alkaline phosphatase (A 5691, Sigma-Aldrich) and visualized by using Simple Stain AP(R) (Nichirei Biosciences Inc, Tokyo, Japan). Adjacent sections were stained with Hematoxylin-Eosin. Microvessel density (MVD) was determined as described previously [40]. Each section was scanned by using a microscope (VANOX AHBS3, Olympus, Tokyo, Japan) at low magnification to identify 5 areas with the highest densities of CD31-stained microvessels.

The microvessels in the selected areas were then counted at 400x magnification. MVD was recorded as the number of microvessels per mm^2. In the DTC xenografts, the percentage of pericyte-covered microvessels was analyzed. Pericyte-covered vessels were identified by examining the colocalization of CD31- (endothelial cells-) positive vessels and αSMA- (pericytes-) positive cells. The number of pericyte-covered vessels was counted in the selected area and then compared with the total number of CD31-stained microvessels in the same area. The percentage of pericyte-covered microvessels was calculated as the number of pericyte-covered microvessels/total number of microvessels $\times$ 100 in the selected area. The MVD in the ATC xenograft models was determined by using the digital pathology system ScanScope XT (Aperio, Vista, CA). Briefly, CD31-stained whole tissue slices were scanned on the ScanScope system (Aperio) to generate high-resolution digital slides. By using a digital slide viewer, Aperio ImageScope (v10.0.36.1805, Aperio), 5 regions of interest (ROIs: each 500 μm square) were manually selected as areas with the highest densities of CD31-stained microvessels in each tumor slice. The number of microvessels in each ROI was measured by using Microvessel Analysis Algorithm v1.0 (Aperio), which automatically detects and quantifies microvessels on slides stained with endothelial markers. MVD was expressed as the number of microvessels per mm^2. The mean MVD of 5 ROIs was defined as the MVD of the tumor. The percentage of microvessel inhibition (%MVI) was calculated from the microvessel density (MVD) according to the following formula: [(1 − MVD of tumor in each compound-treated animal/Mean MVD of tumors in the vehicle control-treated group) $\times$ 100].

2.11. Gene Mutation Analysis. Cells (2×10^6) were seeded and cultured in 6-well culture plates. After overnight culture, genomic DNA was isolated from the cultured cells (K1, RO82-W-1, FTC-133, FTC-236, and FTC-238) by using the DNeasy Blood & Tissue kit (Qiagen). Mutation analysis for 443 mutations among 32 genes [ABL1, AKT1, AKT2, APC, BRAF, CDK4, CDKN2A, CSF1R, CTNNB1, EGFR, FGFR1, FGFR3, FLT3, HRAS, JAK2, JAK3, KIT, KRAS, MET, MLH1, NRAS, P53, PDGFRA, PIK3CA, PTEN, RB1, RET, SRC, STK11, VH1] was performed by using the MassARRAY System (Sequenom, San Diego, CA) with OncoCarta Panel versions 1.0 and 3.0.

2.12. Statistical Analysis. All statistical analyses were performed by using GraphPad Prism 6.0 Software (GraphPad Software, Inc., La Jolla, CA). The significance of the differences between the vehicle and treated groups in terms of both antitumor and antiangiogenesis activity in the human tumor xenograft models was determined by using Dunnett's multiple comparison test. Results were considered significant at $P < 0.05$. To analyze the relationship between antitumor activity (%TGI) and antivascular activity (%MVI), average %TGI and %MVI values were plotted on X- and Y-axes, respectively. Analysis of covariance (ANCOVA) for %TGI was examined by using %MVI as the covariate.

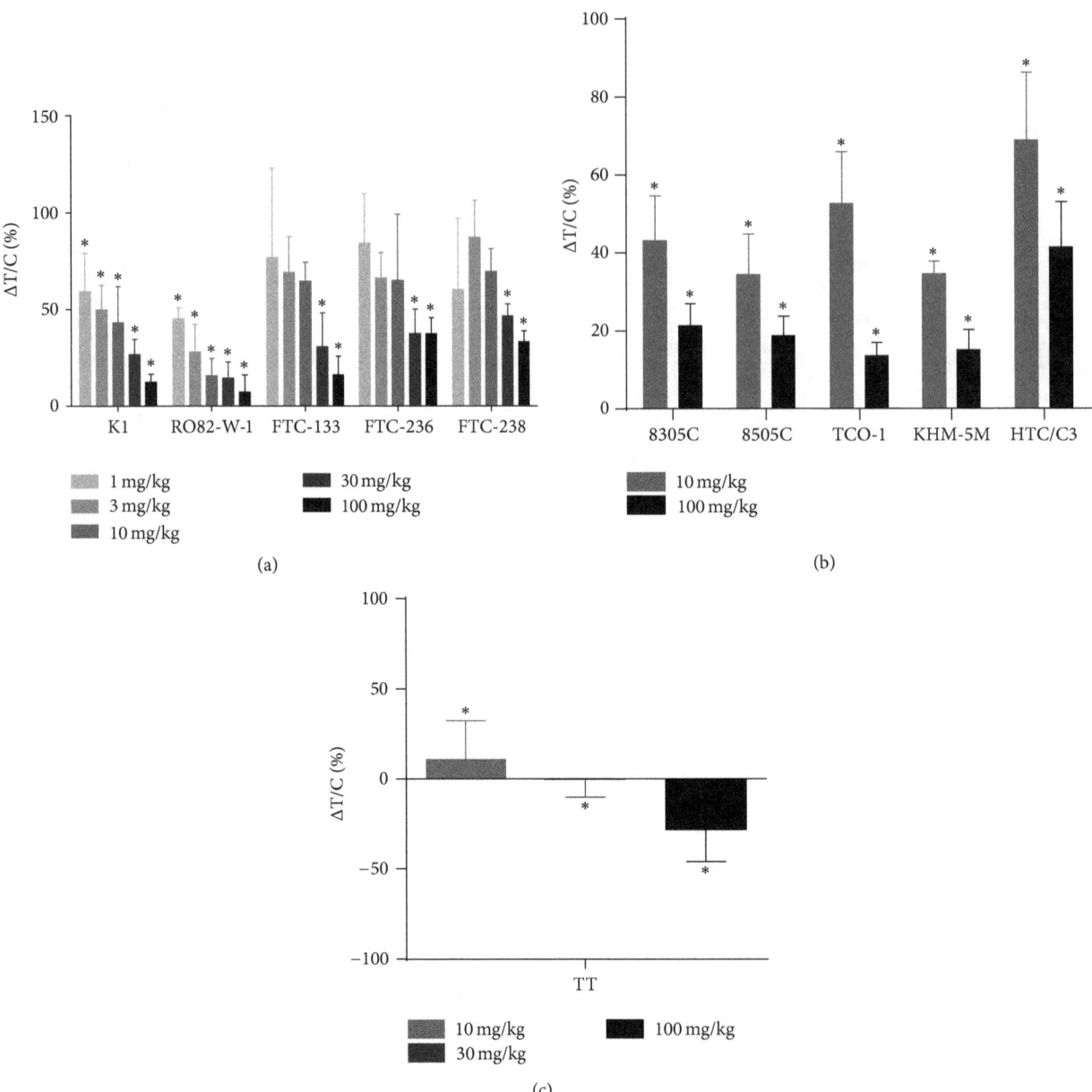

FIGURE 1: Antitumor activity of lenvatinib in human thyroid cancer xenograft models in nude mice. Nude mice bearing tumor xenografts were treated orally once daily with either vehicle or lenvatinib at the indicated doses when tumor volumes reached between 100 and 300 mm^3 (day 1). Each group consisted of 5 mice. The change in tumor volume in the treated group relative to that in the control group $\Delta T/C$ (%) was calculated as $(\Delta T/\Delta C) \times 100\%$, where ΔT and ΔC are the change in tumor volume for the treated and vehicle control group, respectively. (a) DTC xenograft models. $\Delta T/C$ on day 15. (b) ATC xenograft models. $\Delta T/C$ on day 15. (c) TT xenograft model. $\Delta T/C$ on day 29. Data are shown as means ± SD. $^*P < 0.05$ compared with vehicle-treated mice.

3. Results

3.1. Antitumor Activity of Lenvatinib in Human Thyroid Cancer Xenograft Models in Nude Mice. We examined the antitumor activity of lenvatinib in 11 human thyroid cancer xenograft models with 3 types of histology, such as DTC, MTC, and ATC. Five DTC cell lines [1 papillary thyroid cancer line (K1) and 4 follicular thyroid cancer cell lines (RO82-W-1, FTC-133, FTC-236, and FTC-238)], 1 MTC cell line (TT), and 5 ATC cell lines (8305C, 8505C, TCO-1, KHM-5M, and HTC/C3) were examined. Tumor cells were subcutaneously

inoculated into the hind flank region of nude mice. Tumors were allowed to grow to sizes of between 100 and 300 mm^3 before initiation of daily oral treatment with lenvatinib for 14 days (TT cells were treated for 29 days). During treatment with lenvatinib, no macroscopic changes or loss of body weight were observed (data not shown). Lenvatinib showed significant antitumor activity at 30 and 100 mg/kg in all 5 DTC xenograft models and at lower doses (1, 3, and 10 mg/kg) in the K1 and RO82-W-1 xenograft models (Figure 1(a), Supplementary Figure S1(a) in the Supplementary Material

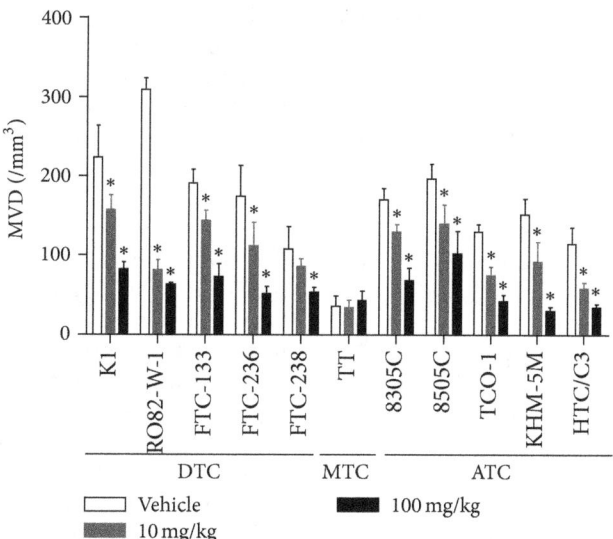

FIGURE 2: Antiangiogenesis activity of lenvatinib in human thyroid cancer xenograft models in nude mice. Nude mice bearing tumor xenografts were treated orally once daily with either vehicle or lenvatinib at the indicated doses when tumor volumes reached between 100 and 300 mm^3 (day 1). Microvessel density (MVD) was analyzed by immunohistochemical staining of endothelial cells with an anti-mouse CD31 antibody within the resected tumor xenografts as described in Section 2. MVD is expressed as the average number of microvessels per mm^2 in 5 regions of interest (ROIs). Each group consisted of 5 mice. Data are shown as means ± SD. $^*P < 0.05$ compared with vehicle-treated mice. DTC: differentiated thyroid cancer, MTC: medullary thyroid cancer, and ATC: anaplastic thyroid cancer.

available online at http://dx.doi.org/10.1155/2014/638747). Lenvatinib also showed significant antitumor activity in all 5 ATC xenograft models at doses of 10 and 100 mg/kg (Figure 1(b), Supplementary Figure S1(b)). In addition, lenvatinib inhibited in vivo tumor growth of TT xenografts in a dose-dependent manner at 10, 30, and 100 mg/kg, causing tumor shrinkage at 100 mg/kg (Figure 1(c), Supplementary Figure S1(c)). These results demonstrate that lenvatinib shows the significant antitumor activity in a panel of 11 human thyroid cancer xenograft models with different histology of thyroid cancers.

3.2. Antiangiogenesis Activity of Lenvatinib in Human Thyroid Cancer Xenograft Models in Nude Mice.

The antiangiogenesis activity of lenvatinib was evaluated by using the same 11 human thyroid cancer xenograft models that were examined for antitumor activity. For immunohistochemical analysis tumor tissues were resected next days after the last administration from nude mice bearing tumor xenografts that had been treated with lenvatinib at a dose of either 10 or 100 mg/kg. Tumor microvessels were stained immunohistochemically with an antibody against endothelial cell marker CD31, and MVD within tumor tissues was analyzed (Figure 2). MVD was significantly decreased in 4 of the 5 DTC xenografts treated with lenvatinib at 10 mg/kg and in all of the 5 DTC xenografts that received lenvatinib at 100 mg/kg. The MVDs in the human MTC TT xenografts were the lowest with vehicle treatments among the 11 human thyroid cancer xenograft models tested, and lenvatinib did not decrease the MVDs within the TT xenografts. The MVDs in all 5 ATC xenograft models decreased significantly with lenvatinib treatments at both 10 and 100 mg/kg. These results

demonstrate that lenvatinib shows antiangiogenesis activity in almost all DTC and ATC models but not in MTC one. This antiangiogenesis activity may explain the mechanism of action of lenvatinib's antitumor activity observed in Figure 1. However, another mechanism may also contribute to the antitumor activity of lenvatinib against the human MTC TT model, because lenvatinib did not decrease the MVD in this model.

We performed immunohistochemical analyses in 5 DTC xenograft models by staining pericytes and endothelial cells with an anti-αSMA antibody and anti-CD31 antibody, respectively (Supplementary Figure S2), because treatment with a VEGF signal inhibitor was reported to increase the association of pericytes with endothelial cells (pericyte coverage), an event related to the acquisition of resistance [41]. The percentage of pericyte coverage in K1 and RO82-W1 cells was lower than that in the other 3 DTC cell types (Supplementary Figure S3). Interestingly, K1 and RO82-W-1 also have higher MVDs (>200/mm^3) than the other 3 DTC cell lines (<200/mm^3) among 5 DTC xenograft models (Figure 2). Lenvatinib showed significant antitumor activity in the K1 and RO82-W-1 models at the lower doses of between 1 and 10 mg/kg. These vascular parameters (low pericyte coverage and high MVD) together with the antitumor activity of lenvatinib suggest that the antiangiogenesis activity of lenvatinib is the mechanism of action behind the antitumor effects of lenvatinib in these models.

3.3. Antiproliferative Activity of Lenvatinib against Human Thyroid Cancer Cell Lines In Vitro.

We examined the antiproliferative activity of lenvatinib against 11 human thyroid cancer cell lines to determine whether the RTK signaling pathway

TABLE 1: In vitro antiproliferative activity of lenvatinib against human thyroid cancer cells.

Tissue type	Cell line	Lenvatinib	
		IC_{50}[1] (μM)	T/N[2]
Normal	Nthy-ori 3-1	15	—
DTC[3]	K1	22	1.47
	RO82-W-1	3.8	0.25
	FTC-133	24	1.6
	FTC-236	17	1.13
	FTC-238	18	1.2
MTC[4]	TT	0.078	0.01
ATC[5]	8305C	26	1.73
	8505C	26	1.73
	TCO-1	28	1.87
	KHM-5M	28	1.87
	HTC/C3	28	2.53

[1] The half maximal inhibitory concentration.
[2] T/N: ratio of IC_{50} values of thyroid cancer cell lines to that of Nthy-ori 3-1 cells.
[3] DTC: differentiated thyroid cancer.
[4] MTC: medullary thyroid cancer.
[5] ATC: anaplastic thyroid cancer.

has a role in the in vitro proliferation of human thyroid cancer cell lines. Antiproliferative activity of lenvatinib was evaluated by using IC_{50} values and the ratios of the IC_{50} values of the thyroid cancer cell lines relative to that of Nthy-ori 3-1 cells (Table 1). Lenvatinib did not show the potent in vitro antiproliferative activity for 9 out of the 11 cell lines with IC_{50} values being greater than 10 μM (Supplementary Figure S4). Lenvatinib did, however, show antiproliferative activity against the human DTC RO82-W-1 and MTC TT cell lines, with IC_{50} values of 3.8 and 0.078 μM, respectively; moreover, it was selective against these two DTC cell lines compared with normal thyroid cells (T/N = 0.25 and 0.01, resp.). These data suggest that RTK signaling pathways may have roles in oncogenic proliferation of these two human thyroid cancer cells lines.

3.4. Antiproliferative Activity of Selective Receptor Tyrosine Kinase Inhibitors against Human DTC Cell Lines In Vitro. To investigate which RTK signaling pathways participate in the proliferation of RO82-W-1 cells, we tested the activity of selective RTK inhibitors [42–46] targeting VEGFR (sorafenib), FGFR (PD166866 and PD173074), KIT (imatinib), and PDGFR (Ki6783) against 5 DTC cell lines including RO82-W-1 (Table 2), because lenvatinib inhibited these RTKs at IC_{50} values of less than 100 nM (Supplementary Table S1) and RO82-W-1 cells express the mRNA of some of these RTKs (Supplementary Figure S5). The inhibitory activity of each RTK inhibitor varied against normal thyroid cells (Nthy-ori 3-1). We first determined the IC_{50} values against thyroid cancer cell lines and Nthy-ori 3-1, and then, we compared the ratio of the IC_{50} values between the tumor cells and the normal cells (i.e., T/N). Among the 5 DTC cell lines, the RO82-W-1 cell line showed selective sensitivity (T/N $\leq$ 0.5)

to FGFR inhibitors (T/N = 0.14 for both PD166866 and PD173074). No cell lines showed selective sensitivity to any of the RTK inhibitors we examined except for PD166866, PD173074, and lenvatinib (T/N = 0.26) against RO82-W-1 cells; thus, lenvatinib might target the FGFR signaling pathway to inhibit the proliferation of RO82-W-1 cells.

3.5. Effect of the Selective FGFR Kinase Inhibitor PD173074 on the FGFR Signaling Pathway in Human DTC RO82-W-1 Cells. Our data suggested a role of the FGFR signaling pathway in the in vitro proliferation of RO82-W-1 cells. Therefore, we performed western blot analysis to examine whether the expression levels of FGFR1–4 were upregulated in RO82-W-1 cells compared with normal thyroid cells (Figure 3(a)), because quantitative RT-PCR suggested overexpression of some of FGFRs (Supplementary Figure S5). Among the 4 FGFRs, the expression of FGFR1 was upregulated in RO82-W-1 cells compared with that in normal thyroid cells, whereas FGFR2 and FGFR3 protein expression was downregulated. FGFR4 protein was expressed at similar levels in RO82-W-1 and normal thyroid cells. Next, we examined whether PD173074, a selective FGFR kinase inhibitor, affected FGFR1-mediated signaling pathways in RO82-W-1 cells in vitro by performing western blot analysis to evaluate the phosphorylation status of FGFR1 and its downstream effectors (i.e., FRS2, MEK, and ERK) (Figure 3(b)). PD173074 inhibited the bFGF-induced phosphorylation of FGFR1, FRS2, MEK, and ERK in a concentration-dependent manner, suggesting that the FGFR1 signaling pathway is active in RO82-W-1 cell lines. To evaluate the role of FGFR signaling in the tumorigenesis of the RO82-W-1 cell line, we examined the antitumor effect of PD173074 against the in vivo tumor growth of RO82-W-1 xenografts in nude mice (Figure 3(c)). Daily oral administration of PD173074 for 14 days led to significant antitumor activity in the RO82-W-1 xenograft models. These results indicate that the FGFR1 signaling pathway participates in the tumorigenesis of the human DTC RO82-W-1 cell line.

3.6. Effect of Lenvatinib on FGFR1 Signaling Pathway in the Human DTC RO82-W-1 Model. We examined whether lenvatinib inhibited FGFR1 signaling pathways in RO82-W-1 cells in vitro by performing western blot analysis to evaluate the phosphorylation status of FGFR1 and its downstream effectors (Figure 4). Lenvatinib inhibited the phosphorylation of FGFR1 and of FRS2, MEK, and ERK, in a concentration-dependent manner at a similar concentration to that at which it showed antiproliferative activity (3 μM). Lenvatinib-induced inhibition of phosphorylation of FRS2 was also detected as a band-shift of FRS2 in vitro. We also examined whether sorafenib affected the FGFR1 signaling pathway in WO82-W-1 cells as a reference. Sorafenib, another multitargeted kinase inhibitor, targets KIT, FLT-3, RAF1, RET, VEGFR1–3, and PDGFRβ but is not reported to inhibit the FGFR signaling pathway. Sorafenib weakly inhibited phosphorylation of MEK at 10 μM but did not clearly inhibit the phosphorylation of FGFR1 or its other downstream effectors, even though the concentration used

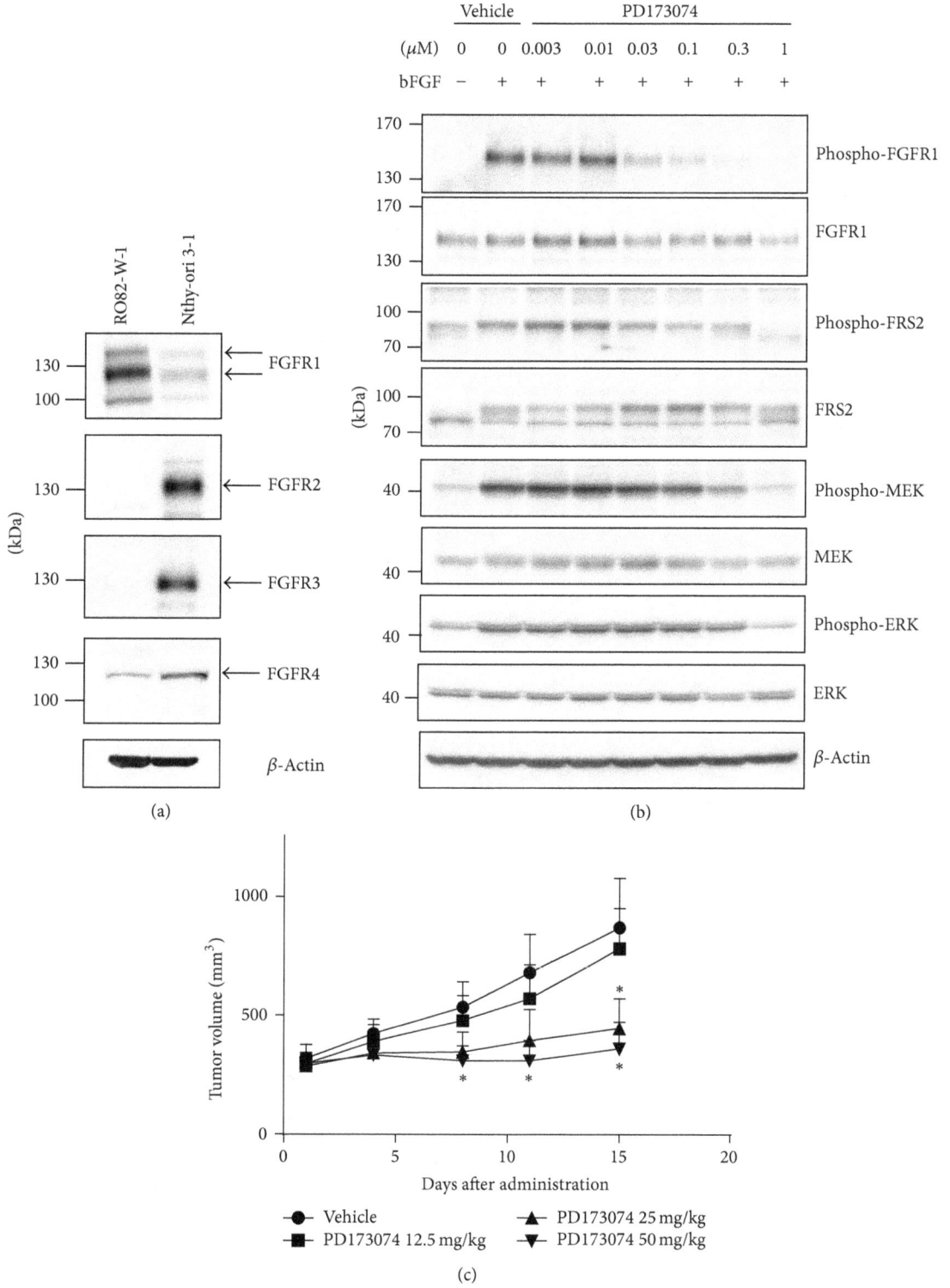

(a)

(b)

(c)

FIGURE 3: Effect of the selective FGFR kinase inhibitor PD173074 on the FGFR signaling pathway in human DTC RO82-W-1 cells. (a) Western blot analysis of the expression of FGF receptors in vitro. Expression levels of FGF receptors in RO82-W-1 cells were compared to those in Nthy-ori 3-1 cells (normal thyroid cells). (b) Western blot analysis of the effects of PD173074 on the phosphorylation of FGFR1 and its downstream effectors. After starvation overnight, RO82-W-1 cells were treated with PD173074 at the indicated concentrations for 1 h and were then stimulated for 10 min with bFGF (20 ng/mL) and heparin before being lysed. (c) Antitumor activity of PD173074 against RO82-W-1 xenografts in nude mice. Nude mice bearing RO82-W-1 xenografts were treated orally once daily for 14 days with either vehicle or PD173074 at the indicated doses when tumor volumes reached about 300 mm^3 (day 1). The tumor volume was measured on the indicated days after administrations. Each group consisted of 5 mice. Data are shown as means ± SD. $^*P < 0.05$ compared with vehicle-treated mice.

TABLE 2: In vitro antiproliferative activity of selective receptor tyrosine kinase inhibitors against human DTC cells.

Tissue type	Cell line	VEGFR2i[1] Sorafenib		FGFRi PD166866		FGFRi PD173074		KITi Glivec		PDGFi Ki6783	
		IC_{50}[3] (μM)	T/N[4]	IC_{50}[3] (μM)	T/N[4]	IC_{50}[3] (μM)	T/N[4]	IC_{50}[3] (μM)	T/N[4]	IC_{50}[3] (μM)	T/N[4]
Normal	Nthy-ori 3-1	5.7	—	14	—	4.6	—	20	—	1.7	—
DTC[2]	K1	5.2	0.91	29	2.07	11	2.39	21	1.1	9.2	5.4
	RO82-W-1	4.2	0.73	1.9	0.14	0.63	0.14	21	1.1	2.5	1.5
	FTC-133	5.5	0.96	23	1.64	9.7	2.11	23	1.2	8	4.7
	FTC-236	7.7	1.35	30<	2.14<	4.3	0.93	30<	2.14<	30<	2.14<
	FTC-238	7.3	1.28	21	1.5	9.4	2.04	24	1.3	2	1.2

[1] Inhibitor.
[2] Differentiated thyroid cancer.
[3] IC_{50}: the half maximal inhibitory concentration.
[4] T/N ratio of IC_{50} values of thyroid cancer cell lines to that of Nthy-ori 3-1 cells.

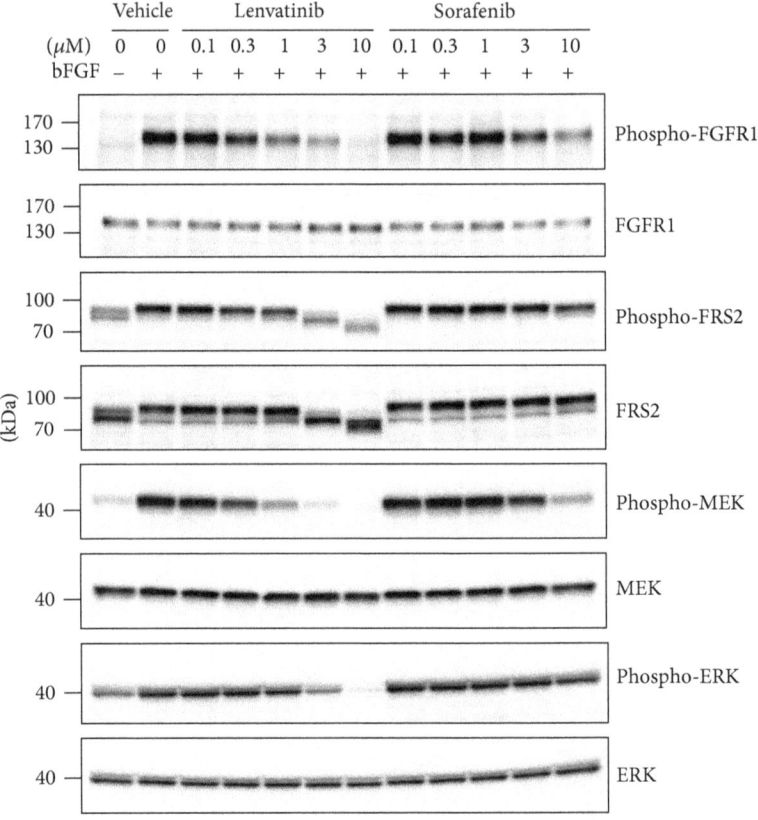

FIGURE 4: Effect of lenvatinib on FGFR1 signaling pathway in human DTC RO82-W-1 cells in vitro. After starvation overnight, RO82-W-1 cells were treated with vehicle (control), lenvatinib or sorafenib at the indicated concentrations for 1 h and were then stimulated for 10 min with bFGF (20 ng/mL) and heparin before being lysed. Western blot analyses of the phosphorylation of FGFR1 and its downstream effectors in RO82-W-1 cells were then performed and representative images were shown.

was sufficient to produce antiproliferative effects in RO82-W-1 cells, with an IC_{50} value 4.2 μM (Table 2). We also tested whether lenvatinib inhibited the phosphorylation of FRS2 in RO82-W-1 xenografts in nude mice (Supplementary Figure S6). Two hours after administration of lenvatinib at 3, 10, 30, or 100 mg/kg, the phosphorylation of FRS2 was decreased in RO82-W-1 xenografts. However, we could not detect a clear decrease in the phosphorylation of FRS2 along with band shift with sorafenib treatment at 100 mg/kg. These

data demonstrate that lenvatinib inhibits the FGFR signaling pathway both in vitro and in vivo and suggest that the antitumor effect of lenvatinib against RO82-W-1 xenografts is attenuated through the inhibition of FGFR signaling in cancer cells, besides antiangiogenic activity through the inhibition of VEGFR2 signaling in endothelial cells. We also examined the activity of sorafenib in the RO82-W-1 DTC model both in vitro and in vivo. Sorafenib did not inhibit the phosphorylation of FGFR1 in RO82-W-1 cells in

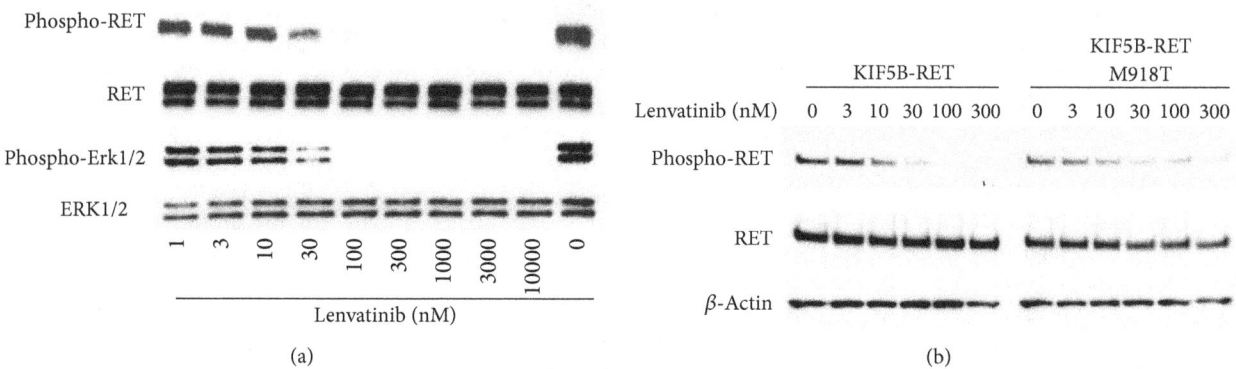

FIGURE 5: Effect of lenvatinib on the phosphorylation of RET with an activating mutation or a rearrangement in vitro. (a) Western blot analyses of the phosphorylation of RET in human medullary thyroid TT cells. TT cells were seeded and cultured overnight. They were then treated with lenvatinib at the indicated concentrations for 1 h before being lysed. (b) Western blot analyses of the phosphorylation of KIF5B-RET fusion proteins in normal thyroid cells; Nthy-ori 3-1 transfectants overexpressing KIF5B-RET (wild-type) or KIF5B-RET (M918T). Nthy-ori 3-1 transfectants were cultured overnight and then treated with lenvatinib at the indicated concentrations for 1 h before being lysed. Western blot analyses of the phosphorylation of RET and its downstream effectors in Nthy-ori 3-1 transfectants were then performed and representative images were shown.

vitro even at concentrations that produced antiproliferative activity (Table 2 and Figure 4). Orally administered sorafenib inhibited tumor growth of RO82-W-1 xenografts in nude mice at doses between 30 and 300 mg/kg (Supplementary Figure S7). At the highest dose of lenvatinib (100 mg/kg) compared with that of sorafenib (300 mg/kg), lenvatinib showed significant potent antitumor activity against tumor growth of RO82-W-1 xenografts in nude mice (Supplementary Figure S7). When we compared antiangiogenesis activity with antitumor activity for each treatment, we found that lenvatinib showed stronger antitumor activity (percentage of tumor growth inhibition, %TGI) than did sorafenib when the two treatments were normalized for angiogenesis inhibition as determined by decreases in MVD (percentage of microvessel inhibition, %MVI) (Supplementary Figure S7). These results suggest that some additional activity of lenvatinib, besides its effect on antiangiogenesis, may contribute to its more potent antitumor activity in RO82-W-1 xenograft models.

3.7. Effects of Lenvatinib on the Activated RET Signaling Pathway in Human MTC TT Cells. Lenvatinib showed potent antiproliferative activity against human MTC TT cells with an IC$_{50}$ value of 0.078 μM in vitro (Table 1). Because TT cells carry the C634W activating mutation of RET [47], lenvatinib might exert an antiproliferative effect on TT cells by inhibiting the RET RTK. To examine whether lenvatinib affects the RET signaling pathway that is activated by C634W mutation we performed western blot analysis to detect phosphorylation of RET and its downstream effector phosphor-ERK1/2 in vitro. Treatments with lenvatinib for 1 h inhibited the phosphorylation of RET and of ERK1/2 in cultured TT cells (Figure 5(a)). In addition, inhibition of RET phosphorylation in TT xenografts was also observed 2 h after oral administrations of lenvatinib (Supplementary Figure S8) at doses that produced antitumor activity as shown in Figure 1(c). We also examined the effect of lenvatinib on the phosphorylation of RET with the M918T mutant. We

generated transfectants overexpressing the fusion genes of KIF-RET (wild-type) and KIF-RET (M918T) in Nthy-ori 3-1 cells to compare the effect of lenvatinib on phosphorylation of wild-type RET and M918T mutant. Lenvatinib inhibited the phosphorylation of both wild-type RET and M918T mutant (Figure 5(b)) at a similar concentration to that which inhibited the phosphorylation of RET (C634W mutant). These data demonstrate that lenvatinib inhibits the RET signaling pathway that is activated by mutations in RET in vitro and lenvatinib thus may show significant antitumor effects in the human MTC TT xenograft model.

3.8. Molecular Mutation Profile of Human DTC Cell Lines. We determined the gene mutation profiles of 5 DTC cell lines by using the MassARRAY System to evaluate 443 mutations in 32 genes. A summary of our mutation analysis is shown in Supplementary Table S2. K1 cells were found to carry the BRAF mutation (V600E) and the PIK3CA mutation (E542K). FTC-133, FTC-236, and FTC-238 cells have a PTEN deletion mutation (R130*) and the TP53 mutation (R273H). We did not detect any RAS mutations among the 5 DTC cell lines.

4. Discussion

In this report, we determined the antitumor and antiangiogenesis activities of lenvatinib, an angiogenesis inhibitor that targets multiple RTKs, in 11 human thyroid cancer xenograft models with 3 types of histology (DTC, MTC, and ATC). Orally administered lenvatinib significantly inhibited tumor growth of 1 PTC (a major type of DTC), 4 FTC (another major type of DTC), 1 MTC, and 5 ATC xenografts in nude mice. Lenvatinib inhibited tumor angiogenesis in 5 DTC and 5 ATC xenograft models as evidenced by a decrease in MVD. Our finding that lenvatinib did not show potent antiproliferative activity against 9 out of 11 human thyroid cancer cell lines in vitro suggests the antitumor activity of lenvatinib against a broad panel of human thyroid cancer models primarily from its antiangiogenic effects.

Lenvatinib inhibited the in vitro proliferation of some of the thyroid cancer cell lines: that is, the RO82-W-1 and TT cell lines. We performed qRT-PCR analysis to examine the mRNA expression levels of 13 RTKs including lenvatinib-targeted RTKs, in 5 DTC cell lines compared with those in normal thyroid cells (Supplementary Figure S5). FGFR1 mRNA levels were upregulated in WO82-W-1 cells compared to Nthy-ori 3-1 and expressed the highest level of FGFR1 mRNA. Both KIT and PDGFα mRNA were highly expressed in RO82-W-1 cells. However, selective RTK inhibitors of KIT (imatinib) and PDGFRα (Ki6783) showed no antiproliferative activity against RO82-W-1, but FGFR inhibitors (PD166866 and PD174073) did. Consistent with these data, western blot analysis showed that RO82-W-1 cells overexpress FGFR1 protein. Together these results suggest a selective role of FGFR signaling pathway in the RO82-W-1 cell line.

Our results showed that lenvatinib inhibited the FGFR signaling pathway in vitro and in vivo (Figure 4 and Supplementary Figure S6). Although lenvatinib showed the inhibitory activity against the VEGFR1–R3, FGFR1–R4, KIT, RET, and PDGFRα tyrosine kinases (Supplementary Table S1), our data suggest that lenvatinib showed direct antitumor activity against RO82-W-1 cell lines by inhibiting the FGFR signaling pathway. FGFR1 and FGFR3 are expressed in well-differentiated thyroid cancers, and ATC cells overexpress FGFR4 [35]. It will be interesting to investigate whether lenvatinib shows antitumor activity against human thyroid cancers with active FGFR signaling pathways.

We found that lenvatinib showed potent antiproliferative activity in vitro (IC_{50} value of $0.078\,\mu M$) against TT MTC cells, in which the RET signaling pathway was activated by a mutation in RET (C634W). As a reference, sorafenib showed antiproliferative activity against TT cells with an IC_{50} value of $0.26\,\mu M$. Lenvatinib inhibited the phosphorylation of RET both in vitro (Figure 5) and in vivo (Supplementary Figure S8). We did not detect a significant decrease in MVD in the TT xenograft models, although lenvatinib showed clear antitumor activity, causing tumor shrinkage at 100 mg/kg (Figure 1). Therefore, the antiproliferative activity of lenvatinib may contribute to its anticancer activity in TT MTC xenograft models. We also examined the effect of lenvatinib on the phosphorylation of RET carrying another activated mutation (M918T) in Nthy-ori 3-1 cells that ectopically expressed either KIF5B-RET (wild-type) or KIF5B-RET (M918T) (Figure 5(b)). Lenvatinib inhibited both the wild-type and M918T mutant RET proteins at similar concentrations in vitro. We previously reported that lenvatinib inhibits the phosphorylation of CCDC-RET and both the in vitro proliferation and in vivo tumor growth of human DTC TPC1 cell lines [37]. These results demonstrate that lenvatinib inhibits RET signaling in the presence of genetic alterations in RET such as an activated mutation or gene rearrangement. In a phase 3 trial in MTC patients, vandetanib, a VEGFR2/RET inhibitor, showed clinical benefits that were independent of RET gene mutation status [34], suggesting that multiple receptor tyrosine kinase inhibitors may be able to show antitumor activity based on antiangiogenesis

activity targeting VEGFR2. In the TT xenograft model, we did not detect a clear decrease in MVD. Lenvatinib showed significant antitumor activity against this model with inhibition of the phosphorylation of RET, suggesting that the antitumor activity of lenvatinib against TT cells was derived from RET inhibition. However, further investigation is needed to determine whether the antiangiogenesis activity of lenvatinib participates in its antitumor activity against MTCs with activated mutations in RET.

Molecular profiling of the 5 DTC cell lines showed that K1 cells carry the BRAF V600E mutation (Supplementary Table S2). Activation of the MAPK pathway due to gene mutations in RAS and BRAF has been associated with malignant phenotypes in thyroid cancer [48]. Because lenvatinib showed antitumor and antiangiogenesis activity in the K1 DTC xenograft model at low doses (between 1 and 10 mg/kg), the activated BRAF mutation might not be involved in resistance to antiangiogenesis therapy in this preclinical model. Taken together, these results suggest that lenvatinib has antitumor activity despite the presence of genetic alterations related to thyroid cancer in the 11 preclinical thyroid cancer models we examined.

In conclusion, lenvatinib showed promising antitumor activity in 11 human thyroid cancer xenograft models derived from DTC, MTC, and ATC cell lines. Lenvatinib showed antitumor activity in most of the human thyroid cancer models tested due to its antiangiogenesis activity. In addition, the activity of lenvatinib through the inhibition of multiple RTKs may contribute to its antitumor activity against thyroid cancer cell lines with gene alterations (e.g., mutations or rearrangements) and overexpression of targeted RTKs, such as RET and FGFR1. Lenvatinib is thus an effective therapeutic agent in most thyroid cancer xenograft models.

Acknowledgments

The authors thank Saori Watanabe-Miyano, Hideki Watanabe, Mai Uesugi, and Hiroyuki Muto for preparing the materials used in this study. They also thank Midori Kawamata, Shizuka Taniguchi, Tomoya Shiina, Yusuke Niwa, and Syugo Hasuike for technical support and Mitsuhiro Ino for help preparing the paper.

References

[1] A. Safavi, A. Vijayasekaran, and M. A. Guerrero, "New insight into the treatment of advanced differentiated thyroid cancer," *Journal of Thyroid Research*, vol. 2012, Article ID 437569, 8 pages, 2012.

[2] K.-P. Wong and B. H.-H. Lang, "New molecular targeted therapy and redifferentiation therapy for radioiodine-refractory advanced papillary thyroid carcinoma: literature review," *Journal of Thyroid Research*, vol. 2012, Article ID 818204, 9 pages, 2012.

[3] N. L. Busaidy and M. E. Cabanillas, "Differentiated thyroid cancer: management of patients with radioiodine nonresponsive disease," *Journal of Thyroid Research*, vol. 2012, Article ID 618985, 12 pages, 2012.

[4] R. J. Robbins, Q. Wan, R. K. Grewal et al., "Real-time prognosis for metastatic thyroid carcinoma based on 2-[^{18}F]fluoro-2-deoxy-D-glucose-positron emission tomography scanning," *The Journal of Clinical Endocrinology & Metabolism*, vol. 91, no. 2, pp. 498–505, 2006.

[5] S. I. Sherman, "Cytotoxic chemotherapy for differentiated thyroid carcinoma," *Clinical Oncology*, vol. 22, no. 6, pp. 464–468, 2010.

[6] F. Pacini, M. G. Castagna, L. Brilli, and G. Pentheroudakis, "Thyroid cancer: ESMO clinical practice guidelines for diagnosis, treatment and follow-up," *Annals of Oncology*, vol. 23, supplement 7, pp. vii110–vii119, 2012.

[7] M. Schlumberger, F. Carlomagno, E. Baudin, J. M. Bidart, and M. Santoro, "New therapeutic approaches to treat medullary thyroid carcinoma," *Nature Clinical Practice Endocrinology & Metabolism*, vol. 4, no. 1, pp. 22–32, 2008.

[8] S. J. Marx, "Molecular genetics of multiple endocrine neoplasia types 1 and 2," *Nature Reviews Cancer*, vol. 5, no. 8, p. 663, 2005.

[9] S. Roman, R. Lin, and J. A. Sosa, "Prognosis of medullary thyroid carcinoma: demographic, clinical, and pathologic predictors of survival in 1252 cases," *Cancer*, vol. 107, no. 9, pp. 2134–2142, 2006.

[10] J. L. Pasieka, "Anaplastic thyroid cancer," *Current Opinion in Oncology*, vol. 15, no. 1, pp. 78–83, 2003.

[11] S. I. Sherman, "Thyroid carcinoma," *The Lancet*, vol. 361, no. 9356, pp. 501–511, 2003.

[12] S. M. Lim, S.-J. Shin, W. Y. Chung et al., "Treatment outcome of patients with anaplastic thyroid cancer: a single center experience," *Yonsei Medical Journal*, vol. 53, no. 2, pp. 352–357, 2012.

[13] M. Xing, "Molecular pathogenesis and mechanisms of thyroid cancer," *Nature Reviews Cancer*, vol. 13, no. 3, pp. 184–199, 2013.

[14] M. Xing, "BRAF mutation in thyroid cancer," *Endocrine-Related Cancer*, vol. 12, no. 2, pp. 245–262, 2005.

[15] R. C. Smallridge, L. A. Marlow, and J. A. Copland, "Anaplastic thyroid cancer: molecular pathogenesis and emerging therapies," *Endocrine-Related Cancer*, vol. 16, no. 1, pp. 17–44, 2009.

[16] H. Namba, S. A. Rubin, and J. A. Fagin, "Point mutations of ras oncogenes are an early event in thyroid tumorigenesis," *Molecular Endocrinology*, vol. 4, no. 10, pp. 1474–1479, 1990.

[17] A. Bounacer, R. Wicker, B. Caillou et al., "High prevalence of activating ret proto-oncogene rearrangements, in thyroid tumors from patients who had received external radiation," *Oncogene*, vol. 15, no. 11, pp. 1263–1273, 1997.

[18] N. L. Eberhardt, S. K. G. Grebe, B. McIver, and H. V. Reddi, "The role of the PAX8/PPARγ fusion oncogene in the pathogenesis of follicular thyroid cancer," *Molecular and Cellular Endocrinology*, vol. 321, no. 1, pp. 50–56, 2010.

[19] V. Vasko, M. Ferrand, J. di Cristofaro, P. Carayon, J. F. Henry, and C. de Micco, "Specific pattern of RAS oncogene mutations in follicular thyroid tumors," *Journal of Clinical Endocrinology and Metabolism*, vol. 88, no. 6, pp. 2745–2752, 2003.

[20] K. M. Carlson, S. Dou, D. Chi et al., "Single missense mutation in the tyrosine kinase catalytic domain of the RET protooncogene is associated with multiple endocrine neoplasia type 2B," *Proceedings of the National Academy of Sciences of the United States of America*, vol. 91, no. 4, pp. 1579–1583, 1994.

[21] H. Donis-Keller, S. Dou, D. Chi et al., "Mutations in the RET proto-oncogene are associated with MEN 2A and FMTC," *Human Molecular Genetics*, vol. 2, no. 7, pp. 851–856, 1993.

[22] L. M. Mulligan, J. B. J. Kwok, C. S. Healey et al., "Germ-line mutations of the RET proto-oncogene in multiple endocrine neoplasia type 2A," *Nature*, vol. 363, no. 6428, pp. 458–460, 1993.

[23] R. Elisei, B. Cosci, C. Romei et al., "Prognostic significance of somatic RET oncogene mutations in sporadic medullary thyroid cancer: a10-year follow-up study," *The Journal of Clinical Endocrinology & Metabolism*, vol. 93, no. 3, pp. 682–687, 2008.

[24] D. J. Marsh, D. L. Learoyd, S. D. Andrew et al., "Somatic mutations in the RET proto-oncogene in sporadic medullary thyroid carcinoma," *Clinical Endocrinology*, vol. 44, no. 3, pp. 249–257, 1996.

[25] P. Carmeliet and R. K. Jain, "Angiogenesis in cancer and other diseases," *Nature*, vol. 407, no. 6801, pp. 249–257, 2000.

[26] J. Folkman and M. Klagsbrun, "Angiogenic factors," *Science*, vol. 235, no. 4787, pp. 442–447, 1987.

[27] J. Folkman, K. Watson, D. Ingber, and D. Hanahan, "Induction of angiogenesis during the transition from hyperplasia to neoplasia," *Nature*, vol. 339, no. 6219, pp. 58–61, 1989.

[28] D. Hanahan and J. Folkman, "Patterns and emerging mechanisms of the angiogenic switch during tumorigenesis," *Cell*, vol. 86, no. 3, pp. 353–364, 1996.

[29] H. Erdem, C. Gündogdu, and S. Üipal, "Correlation of E-cadherin, VEGF, COX-2 expression to prognostic parameters in papillary thyroid carcinoma," *Experimental and Molecular Pathology*, vol. 90, no. 3, pp. 312–317, 2011.

[30] R. T. Anderson, J. E. Linnehan, V. Tongbram, K. Keating, and L. J. Wirth, "Clinical, safety, and economic evidence in radioactive iodine-refractory differentiated thyroid cancer: a systematic literature review," *Thyroid*, vol. 23, no. 4, pp. 392–407, 2013.

[31] B. Sennino and D. M. McDonald, "Controlling escape from angiogenesis inhibitors," *Nature Reviews Cancer*, vol. 12, no. 10, pp. 699–709, 2012.

[32] M. L. Gild, M. Bullock, B. G. Robinson, and R. Clifton-Bligh, "Multikinase inhibitors: a new option for the treatment of thyroid cancer," *Nature Reviews Endocrinology*, vol. 7, no. 10, pp. 617–624, 2011.

[33] M. S. Brose, C. M. Nutting, B. Jarzab et al., "Sorafenib in radioactive iodine-refractory, locally advanced or metastatic differentiated thyroid cancer: a randomised, double-blind, phase 3 trial," *The Lancet*, vol. 384, no. 9940, pp. 319–328, 2014.

[34] S. A. Wells Jr., B. G. Robinson, R. F. Gagel et al., "Vandetanib in patients with locally advanced or metastatic medullary thyroid cancer: a randomized, double-blind phase III trial," *Journal of Clinical Oncology*, vol. 30, no. 2, pp. 134–141, 2012.

[35] R. St. Bernard, L. Zheng, W. Liu, D. Winer, S. L. Asa, and S. Ezzat, "Fibroblast growth factor receptors as molecular targets in thyroid carcinoma," *Endocrinology*, vol. 146, no. 3, pp. 1145–1153, 2005.

[36] Y. Yamamoto, J. Matsui, T. Matsushima et al., "Lenvatinib, an angiogenesis inhibitor targeting VEGFR/FGFR, shows broad antitumor activity in human tumor xenograft models associated with microvessel density and pericyte coverage," *Vascular Cell*, vol. 6, no. 18, 2014.

[37] K. Okamoto, K. Kodama, K. Takase et al., "Antitumor activities of the targeted multi-tyrosine kinase inhibitor lenvatinib (E7080) against RET gene fusion-driven tumor models," *Cancer Letters*, vol. 340, no. 1, pp. 97–103, 2013.

[38] D. S. Boss, H. Glen, J. H. Beijnen et al., "A phase i study of E7080, a multitargeted tyrosine kinase inhibitor, in patients with advanced solid tumours," *British Journal of Cancer*, vol. 106, no. 10, pp. 1598–1604, 2012.

[39] K. Yamada, N. Yamamoto, Y. Yamada et al., "Phase I dose-escalation study and biomarker analysis of E7080 in patients with advanced solid tumors," *Clinical Cancer Research*, vol. 17, no. 8, pp. 2528–2537, 2011.

[40] S. Dalal, A. M. Berry, C. J. Cullinane et al., "Vascular endothelial growth factor: a therapeutic target for tumors of the Ewing's sarcoma Family," *Clinical Cancer Research*, vol. 11, no. 6, pp. 2364–2378, 2005.

[41] N. R. Smith, D. Baker, M. Farren et al., "Tumor stromal architecture can define the intrinsic tumor response to VEGF-targeted therapy," *Clinical Cancer Research*, vol. 19, no. 24, pp. 6943–6956, 2013.

[42] B. J. Druker, S. Tamura, E. Buchdunger et al., "Effects of a selective inhibitor of the Abl tyrosine kinase on the growth of Bcr-Abl positive cells," *Nature Medicine*, vol. 2, no. 5, pp. 561–566, 1996.

[43] M. Mohammadi, S. Froum, J. M. Hamby et al., "Crystal structure of an angiogenesis inhibitor bound to the FGF receptor tyrosine kinase domain," *EMBO Journal*, vol. 17, no. 20, pp. 5896–5904, 1998.

[44] R. L. Panek, G. H. Lu, T. K. Dahring et al., "In vitro biological characterization and antiangiogenic effects of PD 166866, a selective inhibitor of the FGF-1 receptor tyrosine kinase," *Journal of Pharmacology and Experimental Therapeutics*, vol. 286, no. 1, pp. 569–577, 1998.

[45] A. E. Wakeling, S. P. Guy, J. R. Woodburn et al., "ZD1839 (Iressa): an orally active inhibitor of epidermal growth factor signaling with potential for cancer therapy," *Cancer Research*, vol. 62, no. 20, pp. 5749–5754, 2002.

[46] M. Yagi, S. Kato, Y. Kobayashi et al., "Selective inhibition of platelet-derived growth factor (PDGF) receptor autophosphorylation and PDGF-mediated cellular events by a quinoline derivative," *Experimental Cell Research*, vol. 234, no. 2, pp. 285–292, 1997.

[47] M. Drosten, G. Hilken, M. Böckmann et al., "Role of MEN2A-derived RET in maintenace and proliferation of medullary thyroid carcinoma," *Journal of the National Cancer Institute*, vol. 96, no. 16, pp. 1231–1239, 2004.

[48] P. Soares, J. Lima, A. Preto et al., "Genetic alterations in poorly differentiated and undifferentiated thyroid carcinomas," *Current Genomics*, vol. 12, no. 8, pp. 609–617, 2011.

16

Resistant Thyrotoxicosis in a Patient with Graves Disease

Taimur Saleem,[1] Aisha Sheikh,[2] and Qamar Masood[2]

[1] Medical College, Aga Khan University, Stadium Road, Karachi 74800, Pakistan
[2] Section of Diabetes, Endocrinology, and Metabolism, Department of Medicine, Aga Khan University, Stadium Road, Karachi 74800, Pakistan

Correspondence should be addressed to Taimur Saleem, taimur@gmail.com

Academic Editor: Fausto Bogazzi

Background. Conventional management of thyrotoxicosis includes antithyroid drugs, radioactive iodine, and surgery while adjunctive treatment includes beta-blockers, corticosteroids, inorganic iodide and iopanoic acid. Very rarely, patients may be resistant to these modalities and require additional management. *Case Presentation.* A 50-year-old lady presented with weight loss and palpitations diagnosed as atrial fibrillation. Her past history was significant for right thyroid lobectomy for thyrotoxicosis. Thyroid functions tests at this presentation showed free T4 of 6.63 ng/dl (normal range: 0.93–1.7) and TSH of <0.005 μIU/mL (normal range: 0.4–4.0). She was given aspirin, propranolol, heparin and carbimazole; however free T4 failed to normalize. Switching to propylthiouracil (PTU) did not prove successful. She was then given high doses of prednisolone (1 mg/kg/day) and lithium (400 mg twice daily) which prepared the patient for radioactive iodine treatment by reducing free T4 levels (2.82 ng/dl). Two doses of radioactive iodine were then administered 6 months apart. Subsequently she became hypothyroid and was started on thyroid replacement therapy. *Conclusion.* This case highlights management options in patients with resistant thyrotoxicosis. Radioactive iodine and surgery are definitive modes of treatment in such complex cases while steroids and lithium play an important role in preparing patients for more definitive treatment.

1. Background

Thyrotoxicosis affects approximately 2% of women and 0.2% of men [1]. Graves disease is the most common cause of thyrotoxicosis. It is an autoimmune disorder characterized by a constellation of clinical features including hyperthyroidism, diffuse goitre, ophthalmopathy, and dermopathy [2].

Conventional principal management of thyrotoxicosis includes antithyroid drugs, radioactive iodine, and surgery. Adjunctive treatment in the form of beta-blockers, corticosteroids, inorganic iodide, and iopanoic acid may also be used for more prompt control of symptoms [3–6]. However, a few cases may require additional treatment despite these conventional modalities to achieve euthyroid state.

We have described a case of thyrotoxicosis in a patient with Graves disease that was resistant to antithyroid drugs. High-dose steroids and lithium were additionally administered to improve her thyrotoxicosis so that radioactive iodine could be administered later.

2. Case Presentation

A 50-year-old lady from Afghanistan presented to our institution with complaints of undocumented weight loss, palpitations, and anxiety for the past 4 weeks. Her past history was significant for right thyroid lobectomy for thyrotoxicosis more than four years ago. She did not have any history of a recent iodine load. Clinically, she had an irregularly irregular pulse of 110–120 beats per minute. Physical examination showed signs of thyrotoxicosis, a diffusely enlarged left thyroid lobe and thyroid bruit. Her electrocardiograph (ECG) showed atrial fibrillation with rapid ventricular rate (RVR). Thyroid functions tests were ordered which showed severe thyrotoxicosis with free T4 of 6.63 ng/dl (normal range: 0.93–1.7) and TSH of <0.005 μIU/mL (normal range: 0.4–4.0). A diagnosis of Graves disease was made on the basis of high titres of thyroid antibodies (antithyroid peroxidase antibody >1000 IU/mL (normal range: 0–12)). In addition, the presence of a thyroid bruit is also considered pathognomonic for

Graves disease. The patient did not have any signs of Graves ophthalmopathy or dermopathy.

Echocardiography showed moderately dilated right atrium with a severely dilated left atrium and moderate to severe mitral regurgitation and no evidence of a thrombus. Her left ventricular systolic function was moderately reduced with estimated ejection fraction of 35–40%. Ultrasound of the neck showed heterogeneously enlarged left lobe of thyroid gland which measured 4 × 3.5 cm; no discrete nodules were identified.

It was planned that the patient be made euthyroid with free T4 values as near normal as possible, so that radioactive iodine (RAI) could be safely administered without the risk of precipitating thyrotoxic crises. The patient was started on aspirin, propranolol, heparin, and carbimazole. Her initial dose of carbimazole was 30 mg/day but was increased up to 90 mg/day due to no improvement in symptoms. Her free T4 failed to normalize despite maximum doses of carbimazole. Switching to propylthiouracil (PTU) and administering maximum doses had minimal benefit with free T4 values still bordering on 4 ng/dl. The patient was an illiterate lady who was accompanied by her son at every visit. The issue of compliance was thoroughly ascertained through direct questioning and visual inspection of pill bottles at the initial visit and then at every subsequent visit thereafter. The patient appeared to be compliant in taking her medications.

She was then given high doses of prednisolone (1 mg/kg/day) along with lithium (400 mg twice daily) to make her euthyroid so that RAI could be safely given in the future. The patient showed a good response to these treatment modalities, and her free T4 further reduced to 2.82 ng/dl. However, despite intensive medical management, her thyrotoxic symptoms showed little improvement overall.

PTU was stopped 5 days before giving the RAI to enhance its uptake by the thyroid. After a period of 12 weeks from the initial presentation to our institution, the patient was administered 15 mCi of RAI. Unfortunately, measurement of radioactive iodine uptake prior to the administration of RAI is not performed at our institution.

She was then given potassium iodide for the next two weeks. Ross et al. [7] have shown that adjunctive potassium iodide given after RAI has the potential to treat thyrotoxicosis more rapidly than RAI alone without any adverse effect on outcomes at 1 year. Although not standard practice yet, this particular method of treatment [7] has been utilized by at least 19 authors in the management of patients with thyrotoxicosis. As our patient was resistant to antithyroid drugs, we explored all available options including administration of potassium iodide for a short duration of time.

The patient remained stable without the occurrence of thyrotoxic crises. After 3 days, PTU was restarted at a dose of 1200 mg/day. Her free T4 measured at three months after the RAI was 2.93 ng/dl. After 6 months of initial administration of RAI, the patient was still thyrotoxic. A second dose of 20 mCi of RAI was then administered.

Three weeks after receiving the second RAI dose, her free T4 decreased to 1.81 ng/dl. Another repeat measurement in three weeks showed a free T4 value of 0.87 ng/dl. The patient was started on thyroid replacement therapy (at 50 mcg/day)

soon thereafter as she had become hypothyroid. Her clinical condition has remained stable at 6 months followup.

3. Discussion

3.1. Causes of Thyrotoxicosis.
Graves disease is the most common cause of thyrotoxicosis. Thyrotoxicosis can also be associated with other entities such as toxic nodular goiter, human chorionic gonadotropin, pituitary resistance to thyroid hormone regulation, TSH-secreting pituitary adenoma, subacute thyroiditis, ectopic hormone production, or exogenous ingestion of thyroid hormone. In addition, it can also be iodine induced [5] or may occur with postpartum thyroiditis.

3.2. Medical Management of Thyrotoxicosis

3.2.1. Thionamides.
Methimazole/carbimazole are the mainstay of treatment in the majority of patients with Graves-associated thyrotoxicosis. PTU, on the other hand, is considered a second-line agent (except in the first trimester of pregnancy) due to reports of associated severe hepatotoxicity. These drugs decrease thyroid hormone synthesis, and control of hyperthyroidism is usually achieved within several weeks. Large doses of PTU have been reported to decrease the peripheral conversion of T4 to T3 [3]. Thionamides also have an important role in the long-term management of patients with Graves disease. A treatment regime of 12–18 months has been reported to induce remission in 40–60% of patients [8]. Although initially championed with a vogue of enthusiasm, it has now been reported that block-replace regimen (combined thionamide and thyroxine therapy) does not increase the chances of long-term remission in patients [6]. Common side effects of thionamides include fever, urticaria, arthralgias, and mild elevations in transaminase levels while more severe side effects such as agranulocytosis, acute inflammatory hepatitis, and vasculitis are rare [3].

3.2.2. Adjunctive Drugs.
In certain instances, adjunctive drugs may also be required to alleviate severe symptoms or achieve euthyroidism more promptly. Such aggressive management is usually needed in elderly patients as well as patients with thyrotoxic heart disease. Beta-blockers, high-dose glucocorticoids, and iopanoic acid (an oral cholecystographic agent) all inhibit the peripheral conversion of T4 to T3 while inorganic iodide and iopanoic acid decrease synthesis and release of thyroid hormone [3]. Sodium ipodate has been used for the long-term control of Graves thyrotoxicosis and is believed to cause a more rapid fall in thyroid hormone level and provide an easier control of symptoms. However, it may itself rarely cause severe resistant hyperthyroidism when used in the treatment of Graves disease [9].

3.3. Radioactive Iodine Ablation.
[131]I is an effective definitive treatment option for Graves thyrotoxicosis; a single dose is successful in achievement of euthyroid status in the majority of patients within 8 weeks [10]. However, ^{131}I causes permanent hypothyroidism in almost all patients in the long run [3, 6]. Other adverse aspects associated with the use of

[131]I also merit consideration; these include initial worsening of thyrotoxicosis and development or worsening of Graves ophthalmopathy [3]. In our patient, the first dose of RAI was not successful in controlling the hyperthyroid symptoms even after 6 months. Therefore, a second dose of RAI was administered. An expected side effect of this therapy occurred in our patient in the form of hypothyroidism. The patient was then put on thyroid replacement therapy.

3.4. Surgical Management of Thyrotoxicosis. Thyroidectomy is the definitive surgical management for Graves thyrotoxicosis and usually requires a short course of pretreatment with thionamides or inorganic iodine to achieve euthyroid state; this reduces operative complications and thyroid vascularity. Although subtotal thyroidectomy was once practiced, most surgeons now recommend complete thyroidectomy to minimize chances of relapse [3, 6]. The present case also demonstrates why subtotal thyroidectomy in this setting has fallen out of favor. While the procedure is not associated with worsening of Graves ophthalmopathy, it can be complicated by bleeding, infection, recurrent laryngeal nerve injury, hypocalcemia, and permanent hypothyroidism [3].

The modus operandi selected for each patient should be individualized on a case-per-case basis. A consideration should be given to the merits and demerits of the chosen modality. Local and regional trends may also influence this decision. For example, radioiodine is the preferred primary modality in the USA while antithyroid drug therapy is preferred in Europe and Australia [6].

3.5. Resistant Thyrotoxicosis. Majority of the patients respond to the conventional treatments outlined above. However, literature review showed sporadic reports of patients with resistant thyrotoxicosis.

3.5.1. Etiologies of Resistant Thyrotoxicosis. Etiologies of resistant thyrotoxicosis in literature include type I amiodarone-induced thyrotoxicosis (AIT) [11] and Graves disease [12–16]. Refractory cases have mostly shown resistance to high-dose thionamides and beta-blockers; rarely resistance to iodine has also been reported [11–13, 15–18]. In our patient, resistance to two different thionamides was seen. Also, beta-blockers did not improve the thyrotoxic symptoms.

3.5.2. Mechanisms of Resistance. Possible mechanisms mediating resistance in cases refractory to conventional treatment may range from drug malabsorption, rapid drug metabolism, antidrug antibodies, impairment of intrathyroidal drug accumulation or action, and predominant elevation of T3 rather than T4 levels [15].

3.5.3. Workup of Patients with Resistant Thyrotoxicosis. Evaluation of resistant cases should always start with the evaluation of patient compliance [17]. We were attentive to this aspect in the management of our patient and found her to be compliant in taking her medications. This compliance was ascertained through direct questioning at the initial visit and then at every subsequent visit thereafter. Malabsorption should also be ruled out in these patients through careful history taking and physical examination. In our patient, there was nothing remarkable in the history or physical examination to suggest malabsorption as a potential cause for drug resistance. The measurement of drug levels or anti-drug antibodies may then be undertaken. However, these tests are usually not available for routine clinical use; we also did not perform them at our institution due to nonavailability. Alternatively, resistance to drugs can be tested by performing a perchlorate discharge test four hours after drug intake under medical supervision. However, it should be noted that pharmaceutical-grade perchlorate may not be universally available. For example, it is no longer manufactured in the USA. Although not performed in our patient, iodine measurement of urinary iodine excretion may be additionally undertaken to evaluate iodine contamination [19].

3.5.4. Management of Resistant Thyrotoxicosis. Different approaches have been used for the management of resistant thyrotoxicosis. Such patients can either be offered surgery or radioactive iodine ablation as the definitive treatment. However, achievement of a euthyroid state before opting for any of these interventions is recommended in order to minimize potential complications such as precipitation of thyroid crisis [13, 14, 17]. Some authors have advocated the use of iopanoic acid prior to definitive thyroidectomy in patients with drug-resistant Type I AIT. [11] as well as in patients with Graves disease [12]. However, iopanoic acid, like perchlorate, is no longer universally available and is no longer manufactured, for example, in the USA. Although corticosteroids have traditionally been used in the management of thyroid crisis [20], some authors have also reported their use in the management of resistant thyrotoxicosis. Dexamethasone, in conjunction with iopanoic acid, has been used for the rapid preoperative preparation of uncontrolled, resistant thyrotoxicosis [12]. Similarly, prednisolone (20 mg/day), added to antithyroid drugs, has been successfully used to achieve euthyroid state in patients with resistant thyrotoxicosis before administration of radioiodine [17]. Cholestyramine, a bile acid sequestrant, has been shown to cause a dramatic decline in serum thyroid hormone levels in Graves associated thyrotoxicosis resistant to conventional treatment [13].

Lithium, an agent used to treat bipolar affective disorder, has shown favorable response in resistant cases of thyrotoxicosis. Lithium probably increases retention of radioactive iodine in the thyroid in treatment-resistant Graves thyrotoxicosis and has accordingly been used as an adjunct to radioactive iodine in such cases [16, 21–24]. Such use is especially beneficial in patients with underlying cardiovascular disorders in whom even minor elevations of thyroid hormone levels can prove seriously deleterious [24]. We successfully used a combination of lithium and steroids to prepare the patient for the RAI procedure.

4. Conclusion

This case highlights an important yet uncommon clinical entity of resistant thyrotoxicosis. Our patient was resistant to the conventional management including beta-blockers and thyrostatics. We have also discussed the possible management options in such patients. Radioactive iodine or surgery are the definitive modes of treatment in such complex cases while steroids and lithium may play an important part in preparing the patients for more definitive forms of treatment.

Author's Contribution

T. Saleem and Q. Massod collected the data, helped in its interpretation, and drafted the paper. A. Sheikh conceived the study, helped in data collection and interpretation, drafted the paper, and provided overall supervision in the project. All authors read and approved the final paper.

References

[1] J. A. Franklyn, "The management of hyperthyroidism," *The New England Journal of Medicine*, vol. 330, pp. 1731–1738, 2002.

[2] J. Ginsberg, "Diagnosis and management of Graves' disease," *Canadian Medical Association Journal*, vol. 168, no. 5, pp. 575–585, 2003.

[3] E. N. Pearce, "Diagnosis and management of thyrotoxicosis," *British Medical Journal*, vol. 332, no. 7554, pp. 1369–1373, 2006.

[4] J. R. Reid and S. F. Wheeler, "Hyperthyroidism: diagnosis and treatment," *American Family Physician*, vol. 72, no. 4, pp. 623–636, 2005.

[5] J. V. Hennessey, "Diagnosis and management of thyrotoxicosis," *American Family Physician*, vol. 54, no. 4, pp. 1315–1324, 1996.

[6] D. J. Topliss and C. J. Eastman, "Diagnosis and management of hyperthyroidism and hypothyroidism," *Medical Journal of Australia*, vol. 180, no. 4, pp. 186–193, 2004.

[7] D. S. Ross, G. H. Daniels, and P. De Stefano, "Use of adjunctive potassium iodide after radioactive Iodine (131I) treatment of Graves' hyperthyroidism," *Journal of Clinical Endocrinology and Metabolism*, vol. 57, no. 2, pp. 250–253, 1983.

[8] P. Abraham, A. Avenell, W. A. Watson, C. M. Park, and J. S. Bevan, "Antithyroid drug regimen for treating Graves' hyperthyroidism," *Cochrane Database of Systematic Reviews*, no. 2, Article ID CD003420, 2004.

[9] G. Caldwell, M. Errington, and A. D. Toft, "Resistant hyperthyroidism induced by sodium ipodate used as treatment for Graves' disease," *Acta Endocrinologica*, vol. 120, no. 2, pp. 215–216, 1989.

[10] L. E. Holm, G. Lundell, I. Dahlqvist, and A. Israelsson, "Cure rate after 131I therapy for hyperthyroidism," *Acta Radiologica. Oncology Radiation Therapy Physics and Biology*, vol. 20, no. 3, pp. 161–166, 1981.

[11] F. Bogazzi, F. Aghini-Lombardi, C. Cosci et al., "Iopanoic acid rapidly controls Type I amiodarone-induced thyrotoxicosis prior to thyroidectomy," *Journal of Endocrinological Investigation*, vol. 25, no. 2, pp. 176–180, 2002.

[12] C. K. Pandey, M. Raza, S. Dhiraaj, A. Agarwal, and P. K. Singh, "Rapid preparation of severe uncontrolled thyrotoxicosis due to Grave's disease with Iopanoic acid—a case report," *Canadian Journal of Anesthesia*, vol. 51, no. 1, pp. 38–40, 2004.

[13] A. Sebastián-Ochoa, M. Quesada-Charneco, D. Fernández-García, R. Reyes-García, P. Rozas-Moreno, and F. Escobar-Jiménez, "Dramatic response to cholestyramine in a patient with Graves' disease resistant to conventional therapy," *Thyroid*, vol. 18, no. 10, pp. 1115–1117, 2008.

[14] B. Winsa, J. Rastad, E. Larsson et al., "Total thyroidectomy in therapy-resistant Graves' disease," *Surgery*, vol. 116, no. 6, pp. 1068–1075, 1994.

[15] H. Li, J. Okuda, T. Akamizu, and T. Mori, "A hyperthyroid patient with Graves' disease who was strongly resistant to methimazole: investigation on possible mechanisms of the resistance," *Endocrine Journal*, vol. 42, no. 5, pp. 697–704, 1995.

[16] K. Hoogenberg, J. A. M. Beentjes, and D. A. Piers, "Lithium as an adjunct to radioactive iodine in treatment-resistant Graves thyrotoxicosis," *Annals of Internal Medicine*, vol. 129, no. 8, p. 670, 1998.

[17] E. B. Jude, J. Dale, S. Kumar, and P. M. Dodson, "Treatment of thyrotoxicosis resistant to carbimazole with corticosteroids," *Postgraduate Medical Journal*, vol. 72, no. 850, pp. 489–491, 1996.

[18] R. Hall and J. H. Lazarus, "Changing iodine intake and the effect on thyroid disease," *British Medical Journal*, vol. 294, no. 6574, pp. 721–722, 1987.

[19] B. Corvilain and P. Schinohoritis, "Carbimazole—Resistant thyrotoxicosis," *Postgraduate Medical Journal*, vol. 73, no. 864, p. 686, 1997.

[20] J. D. Wilson and D. W. Foster, *Textbook of Endocrinology*, W. B. Saunders, 8th edition, 1992.

[21] J. G. Turner, B. E. W. Brownlie, and T. G. H. Rogers, "Lithium as an adjunct to radioiodine therapy for thyrotoxicosis," *Lancet*, vol. 1, no. 7960, pp. 614–615, 1976.

[22] F. Akin, G. F. Yaylali, and M. Bastemir, "The use of lithium carbonate in the preparation for definitive therapy in hyperthyroid patients," *Medical Principles and Practice*, vol. 17, no. 2, pp. 167–170, 2008.

[23] Y. W. Ng, S. C. Tiu, K. L. Choi et al., "Use of lithium in the treatment of thyrotoxicosis," *Hong Kong Medical Journal*, vol. 12, no. 4, pp. 254–259, 2006.

[24] F. Bogazzi, L. Bartalena, A. Campomori et al., "Treatment with lithium prevents serum thyroid hormone increase after thionamide withdrawal and radioiodine therapy in patients with graves' disease," *Journal of Clinical Endocrinology and Metabolism*, vol. 87, no. 10, pp. 4490–4495, 2002.

17

Shear Wave Elastography may Add a New Dimension to Ultrasound Evaluation of Thyroid Nodules

Rafal Z. Slapa,[1] Antoni Piwowonski,[2] Wieslaw S. Jakubowski,[1] Jacek Bierca,[3] Kazimierz T. Szopinski,[4] Jadwiga Slowinska-Srzednicka,[5] Bartosz Migda,[1] and R. Krzysztof Mlosek[1]

[1] Department of Diagnostic Imaging, Second Faculty of Medicine, Medical University of Warsaw, ul. Kondratowicza 8, 03-242 Warsaw, Poland
[2] NZOZ Almed, 37-500 Jarosław, Poland
[3] Surgery Department, Solec Hospital, 00-382 Warsaw, Poland
[4] Department of Dental and Maxillofacial Radiology, Institute of Stomatology, First Faculty of Medicine, Medical University of Warsaw, 02-006 Warsaw, Poland
[5] Department of Endocrinology, Centre for Postgraduate Medical Education, 01-809 Warsaw, Poland

Correspondence should be addressed to Rafal Z. Slapa, r.slapa@acn.waw.pl

Academic Editor: P. Beck-Peccoz

Although elastography can enhance the differential diagnosis of thyroid nodules, its diagnostic performance is not ideal at present. Further improvements in the technique and creation of robust diagnostic criteria are necessary. The purpose of this study was to compare the usefulness of strain elastography and a new generation of elasticity imaging called supersonic shear wave elastography (SSWE) in differential evaluation of thyroid nodules. Six thyroid nodules in 4 patients were studied. SSWE yielded 1 true-positive and 5 true-negative results. Strain elastography yielded 5 false-positive results and 1 false-negative result. A novel finding appreciated with SSWE, were punctate foci of increased stiffness corresponding to microcalcifications in 4 nodules, some not visible on B-mode ultrasound, as opposed to soft, colloid-inspissated areas visible on B-mode ultrasound in 2 nodules. This preliminary paper indicates that SSWE may outperform strain elastography in differentiation of thyroid nodules with regard to their stiffness. SSWE showed the possibility of differentiation of high echogenic foci into microcalcifications and inspissated colloid, adding a new dimension to thyroid elastography. Further multicenter large-scale studies of thyroid nodules evaluating different elastographic methods are warranted.

1. Introduction

The main reasons for the widespread use of thyroid sonography are availability, low cost, limited discomfort to the patient, and absence of ionizing radiation. Sonography has many favourable features, such as detection of nonpalpable nodules, estimation of nodule size/goiter volume, and guidance for fine needle biopsy (FNB). High-resolution ultrasound is very sensitive in detection of thyroid nodules, enabling differentiation of solid and liquid lesions. Consequently, the interobserver agreement is high [1].

However, with introduction of sonography it became evident that thyroid nodules are very common, with prevalence ranging from 17% to as much as 67% in some cohorts. Nodular goiter does not include thyroid cancer, but one of the main aims of the clinical evaluation is to exclude the risk of overlooking thyroid cancer which is much less prevalent than benign nodules. A hard thyroid nodule on neck palpation is suggestive of thyroid carcinoma [1].

Sonographic characteristics such as hypoechogenicity, microcalcifications, and increased nodular flow visualized by Doppler are all to some extent predictive of malignancy [1].

Microcalcifications visible on ultrasound examination are considered to be a specific feature of thyroid cancer (85,8–95%); however, the sensitivity of this sign is relatively low (29–59%) [2]. Presence of calcifications doubles the risk of malignancy, whereas microcalcifications increase the risk of thyroid cancer three-fold [3]. However, in pathologic examinations of benign thyroid nodules-inspissated colloid, fibrosis, and microcalcifications often coexist [4].

The estimation of tissue hardness is a very ancient diagnostic tool in medicine. Palpation—the earliest and most common form of tissue hardness estimation—was practiced by Egyptian physicians as early as 2600 BC [5].

A more recent and sophisticated method of imaging of tissue hardness is the technique known as elastography. The term "elastography" was coined by Ophir et al. [6] to refer to an ultrasound-based imaging technique, where local axial strains were estimated by computing the gradient of axial shifts in echo arrival times along the ultrasound beam direction following quasistatic tissue deformation. Elastography, however, has now been used as a more general term to identify methods that image tissue stiffness, using different imaging modalities for example, ultrasound, magnetic resonance imaging, optical coherence tomography, different perturbation techniques to deform tissue, based on the elasticity parameter being measured or imaged [7]. Roughly 20 years have elapsed since the first images depicting the local elastic properties of tissues were obtained. The first decade of development produced a remarkable proliferation of techniques and optimization strategies. In the second decade this trend continued, but with an important extension to dedicated platforms for conducting clinical trials in the hands of radiologists and skilled clinicians [8].

There are 3 main types of ultrasound elasticity imaging: elastography that tracks tissue movement during compression to obtain an estimate of strain (quasi-static elastography), sonoelastography that uses color Doppler to generate an image of tissue movement in response to external vibrations (harmonic elastography), and a technique tracking shear wave propagation through tissue to obtain the elastic modulus (transient elastography) [5].

The first commercially available, clinical ultrasound scanners with option of tissue elasticity evaluation were equipped with strain elastography. Application of strain elastography to thyroid nodules examination resulted in different results of evaluation of usefulness of this technique in regard to differential diagnosis of benign and malignant thyroid nodules [9–14]. Diagnostic value of strain elastography is limited in evaluation of small nodules, large nodules (with diameter approaching or exceeding the length of the probe), nodules with calcifications, and nodules with liquid content. Different results are obtained in different anatomical planes (e.g., axial versus sagittal), and the reproducibility is poor. Finally, multinodular goiters with scarce or no normal thyroid tissue for reference are difficult to evaluate [9, 11–16].

The new generation of elasticity imaging called supersonic shear wave elastography (SSWE) has been introduced since 2006 to imaging of superficial organs as breast and thyroid with high-frequency linear probes [17–21]. This type of transient elastography does not require the compression of the tissues during their elasticity examination. The obtained information is based on calculated elastic modulus (described in kPa) of the examined tissues. Based on multinational large-scale studies in the field of breast cancer detection and characterization, SSWE proved to be highly reproducible, and it increased specificity without loss of sensitivity [20, 21]. In the field of thyroid SSWE, it was proved that autoimmune thyroiditis does not hinder the evaluation of elasticity of thyroid nodules [20].

The aim of this study was to compare the usefulness of the new supersonic shear wave imaging elastography with strain elastography in evaluation of thyroid nodules.

2. Methods

During a few weeks trial time in 2010, four consecutive patients with single thyroid nodule ($n = 1$) and nodular goiter ($n = 3$) were evaluated. Approval for this study was obtained from the Ethics Committee of the Medical University of Warsaw, and all patients provided informed consent. The B mode and power Doppler ultrasound of whole thyroid and neck lymph nodes was performed. Six dominant thyroid nodules (in regard to B-mode and power Doppler ultrasound features) were evaluated with shear wave and strain elastography qualitatively and quantitatively as well as some with contrast-enhanced ultrasound (Sonovue (Bracco)). The examinations were performed with following scanner: Aixplorer (Supersonic Imagine Inc. France)—SSWE, Aplio XG (Toshiba, Japan)—strain elastography, Technos (Esaote, Italy)—contrast-enhanced ultrasound, with linear high-resolution transducers: 15–4 MHz, 18–7 MHz, and, 8–3 MHz respectively. For strain elastography, we adopted qualitative scale of Rubaltelli et al. with threshold score of 2/3 [22] and quantitative scale of Cantisani et al. with threshold thyroid tissue/nodule strain ratio of 2 [23] measured with Elasto-Q (Toshiba). For shear wave elastography, we adopted quantitative scale of Sebag et al. with the threshold stiffness (mean elastic modulus) of thyroid nodule of 65 kPa [19]. The final diagnosis was based on clinical evaluation, multiple FNB, 1 year followup, or surgery.

3. Results

Final diagnosis (pathology examination after surgery in 5 nodules, double FNB, and 1 year followup in 1 nodule) was established: 1 papillary carcinoma (Figure 1), 4 colloid nodules, and 1 benign nodule (Figure 2).

Shear weave elastography revealed 1 true positive and 5 true negative diagnoses in regard of thyroid cancer.

Strain elastography revealed 5 false positive and 1 false negative diagnoses.

False positive diagnoses with strain elastography were found in nodules with liquid (not evident on B-mode ultrasound) or degenerative content of the nodules visible on contrast-enhanced ultrasound and/or pathology examination. A novel finding were the punctate increased stiffness foci in microcalcifications seen in 4 nodules, some not visible on B-mode ultrasound as opposed to soft inspissated colloid foci visible on B-mode ultrasound in 2 nodules (Figure 3).

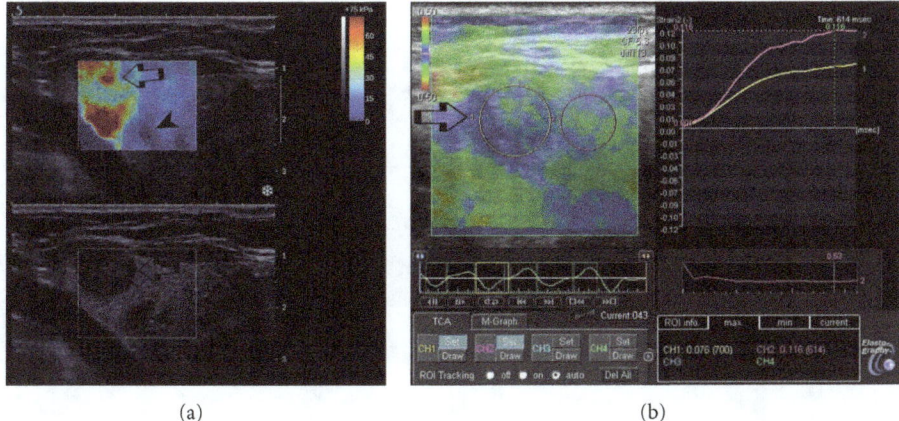

(a) (b)

FIGURE 1: Diffuse sclerosing papillary carcinoma of the left lobe of the thyroid gland (arrow) in patient with multinodular goiter and multiple colloid nodules (arrow head). (a) on B-mode ultrasound (lower image), the cancer is less suspicious than some of the colloid nodules; however, on supersonic shear wave elastography (upper image) the nodule presents areas of high stiffness (over 75 kPa) indicating malignant lesion. The colloid nodule presents as a lesion with low stiffness. (b) on strain elastography, the carcinoma qualitatively and quantitatively presents features of soft lesion falsely indicating benign nature of the lesion.

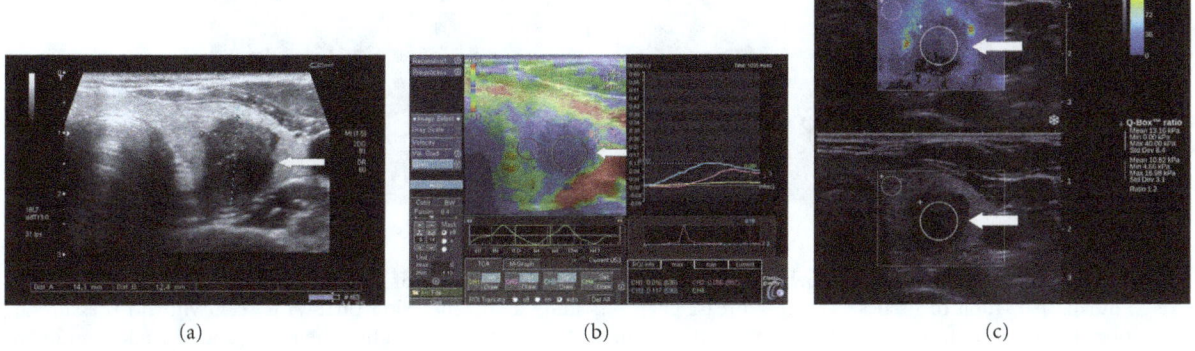

(a) (b) (c)

FIGURE 2: A benign nodule (arrow) of the left lobe of the thyroid gland (with massive degeneration demonstrated on contrast-enhanced ultrasound and in pathologic examination) in patient with multinodular goiter. (a) on B-mode axial section, the nodule is markedly hypoechoic, taller than wide, with somewhat ill-defined margins and high echogenic foci suggesting microcalcifications, a suspicious nodule. (b) on strain elastography, the nodule both qualitatively and quantitatively presents as very hard suspicious of cancer. (c) on supersonic shear wave elastography (upper image), the lesion is very soft, truly indicating its benign nature, with some stiff calcifications in the capsule.

4. Discussion

Supersonic shear weave elastography consists of the generation of remote radiation force by focused ultrasonic beams, the so-called "pushing beams," a patented technology called "Sonic Touch" [19]. Using Sonic Touch, ultrasound beams are successively focused at different depth in tissues. The source is moved at a speed that is higher than the speed of the shear waves that are generated. In this supersonic regime, shear waves are coherently summed in a "Mach cone" shape, which increases their amplitude and improves their propagation distance. For a fixed acoustic power at a given location, Sonic Touch increases shear wave generation efficiency by a factor of 4 to 8 compared to a nonsupersonic source [24]. After generation of this shear wave, an ultrafast echographic imaging sequence is performed to acquire successive raw radiofrequency dots at a very high-frame rate

(up to 20000 frames per second). Based on Young's modulus formula, the assessment of tissue elasticity can be derived from shear wave propagation speed. A color-coded image is displayed, which shows softer tissue in blue and stiffer tissue in red. Quantitative information is delivered; elasticity is expressed in kilo-Pascal (kPa) [19].

This preliminary paper based on small number of cases indicates that SSWE indicated correctly thyroid nodules suspicious for cancer in contrast to strain elastography. False positives on strain elastography could be due to liquid or degenerative content of nodules.

However, imaging with SSWE, as a sensitive method of evaluation of stiffness of human tissue, the operator should be aware of physiological processes influencing the elasticity and easily apply a few rules to avoid artifacts (Figures 4, 5 and 6) (Supplementary material 1-cine loop video). Among well-known artifacts on SSWE that should be mentioned is

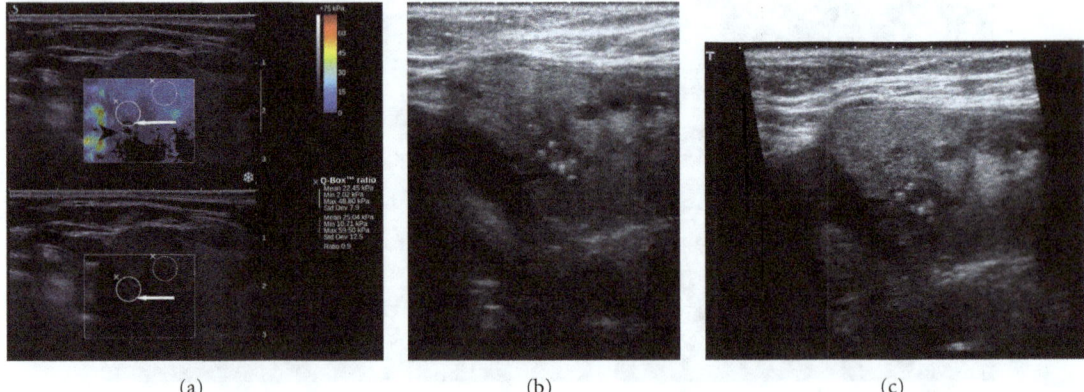

(a)	(b)	(c)

FIGURE 3: A colloid nodule in a patient with nodular goiter and papillary carcinoma. (a) on supersonic shear wave elastography (upper image) the colloid nodule (full circle) is very soft with punctuate increased stiffness (arrow head) representing microcalcifications (some not visible on B-mode lower image), in contrast to bigger high echogenicity foci (arrow), which are soft and represent inspissated colloid as evident on subsequent images. (b) presents comet tail artifacts (arrow heads) that change the direction with steering of ultrasound beam (c) indicating the nature of this artifact that is attributable to inspissated colloid in thyroid nodule.

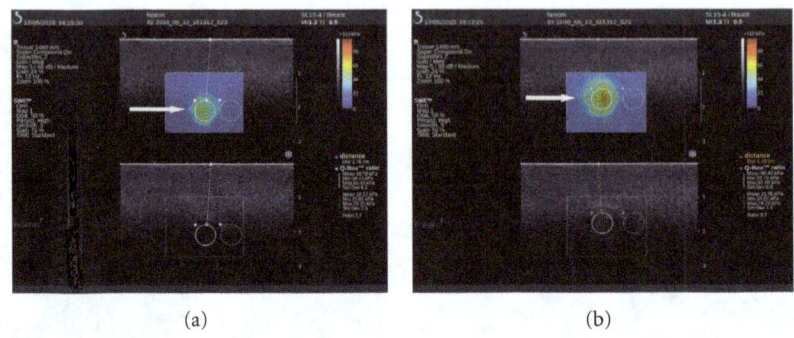

(a)	(b)

FIGURE 4: Phantom studies illustrating well-known physiologic phenomenon of increase of perceived tissue stiffness with applied increased pressure (e.g., during palpation of tissues). (a) on a breast phantom study a stiff inclusion (arrow) is seen with no pressure applied at ultrasound probe. The distance from the surface, the stiffness of the inclusion and surrounding medium (dotted circle) can be measured. (b) with application of pressure on the phantom with ultrasound probe, which is evident as a reduced distance of the inclusion to the surface of the phantom, the stiffness of the inclusion and surrounding medium is increased. Thus, the measurements of stiffness of tissues with supersonic shear wave elastography should be performed in a resting state without pressure on the ultrasound probe to avoid the unpredictable influence of the compression on the stiffness of the tissues.

the one that can be encountered in any region when the SSWE can be applied: the increased stiffness of the structures under externally applied pressure (Figures 4 and 5) (Supplementary material 1-cine loop video) that can be due to nonlinear elastic effects, well explained by theory [25]. Another artifact that can be encountered in thyroid SSWE is one of increased stiffness in the isthmus of the thyroid due to trachea (Figure 6). It can be avoided with imaging in paracoronal plane of the nodule that does not incorporate the trachea. However, it is important to state that these artifacts when properly interpreted do not hinder the accurate diagnosis.

Supersonic shear wave elastography may add a new dimension to ultrasound evaluation of thyroid nodules in several ways, for example:

(a) improve general performance in elasticity differentiation of thyroid nodules over strain elastography due

to its high reproducibility, independence of examiners skill and numeral scale of elasticity measurement in kPa;

(b) overcome the limitations of strain elastography:

 (i) nodules with liquid components or with degenerative changes;

 (ii) small nodules (very good spatial resolution of the technique);

 (iii) large nodules (possibility of subsequent determination of stiff regions even of large nodules, without the need of visualizing the whole nodule on one image);

 (iv) multinodular goiter with no or scarce normal thyroid tissue as a reference;

(c) differentiation between soft-inspissated colloid and stiff microcalcifications;

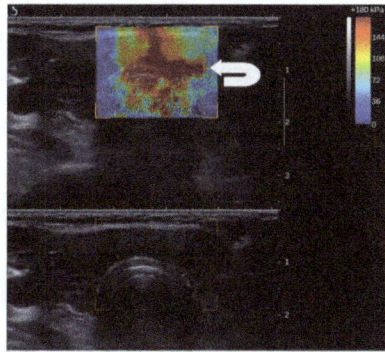

FIGURE 5: An artifact (arrow) from tissue compression on elastogram (upper image) in patient with Hashimoto thyroiditis, with no real focal lesions evident on B-mode ultrasound (lower image). A hard stiff pseudolesion is generated (see also Supplementary material 1 available online on doi: 10.1155/2012/657147). To avoid such artifacts no pressure on the probe during elasticity evaluation should be applied.

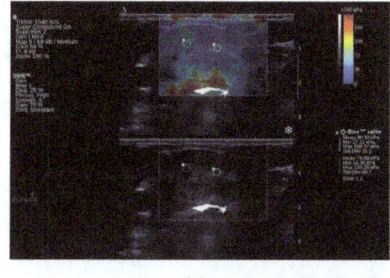

(a)

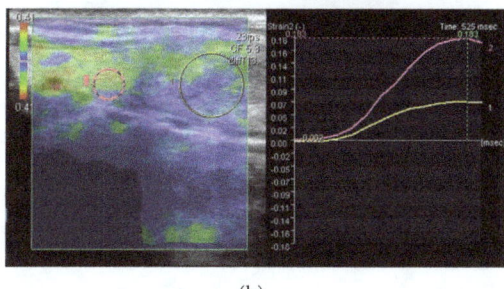

(b)

FIGURE 6: A benign thyroid nodule in a patient with solitary nodule in the thyroid isthmus that was suspicious on power Doppler ultrasound (not shown). The SSWE was true negative and the strain elastography was false positive for thyroid cancer. (a): The thyroid nodule in coronal plane on supersonic shear wave elastography (SSWE) (upper image) and B-mode ultrasound (lower image). The nodule is very soft on SSWE in contradiction to strain elastography (b). In the centre of the circular ROIs punctuate increased stiffness of small calcifications that are also visible on B-mode (lower image) is seen. Also artifacts of increased stiffness in the isthmus of the thyroid are visible. These artifacts are due to trachea (star arrow) and can be avoided with imaging in paracoronal plane of the nodule that does not incorporate the trachea. (b): The thyroid nodule (ROI 1-yellow) on strain elastography in sagittal plane, where the comparison with upper part of normal tissue of isthmus (ROI 2-pink) is possible. The strain color map (left) presents mostly stiff nodule-thyroid nodule score 3. The time-strain graph (right) presents that the lesion is more than 2 times stiffer than thyroid tissue.

(d) visualization of microcalcifications, even not visualized on B-mode imaging (may increase sensitivity and decrease specificity of thyroid cancer diagnosis);

(e) introduction of three-dimensional elastographic images to routine clinical practice and to national thyroid cancer databases [26], as this technique is already available and enables rapid acquisition of 3D ultrasound and elastographic data. This would devoid diagnostic process and data archiving of image selection bias attributable to 2D ultrasound examination.

Further multicenter large scale studies of thyroid nodules evaluating different elastographic methods are warranted, including (a) investigation of developmental models of diseases that link biomechanical properties (elastography findings) with genetic, cellular, biochemical, and gross pathological changes; (b) comparison of accuracy of different elastographic methods; (c) establishment of optimal diagnostic elastographic criteria; (d) establishment of limitations of different elastographic methods in relation to evaluation of thyroid pathology.

Abbreviations

FNB: Fine-needle biopsy
SSWE: Supersonic shear wave elastography
kPa: Kilo-Pascal.

Acknowledgments

This paper and publication was supported by the Grants N N402 476437 (2009–2012) and N N402 481239 (2010–2013) from the Ministry of Science and Higher Education of Poland. The authors thank Miro, Inc., Poland, a representative of Supersonic Imagine, Inc., France for lending the Aixplorer for trial. Material displayed as oral presentation at 10th International Tissue Elasticity Conference, October, 12–15 2011, Arlington, TX, USA.

References

[1] M. Tonacchera, A. Pinchera, and P. Vitti, "Assessment of nodular goiter," *Best Practice & Research*, vol. 24, no. 1, pp. 51–61, 2010.

[2] N. Khati, T. Adamson, K. S. Johnson, and M. C. Hill, "Ultrasound of the thyroid and parathyroid glands," *Ultrasound Quarterly*, vol. 19, no. 4, pp. 162–176, 2003.

[3] M. C. Frates, C. B. Benson, P. M. Doubilet et al., "Prevalence and distribution of carcinoma in patients with solitary and multiple thyroid nodules on sonography," *Journal of Clinical Endocrinology and Metabolism*, vol. 91, no. 9, pp. 3411–3417, 2006.

[4] R. Slapa, W. Jakubowski, J. Slowinska-Srzednicka, J. Bierca, and K. Szopinski, "How can new ultrasound techniques that enhance visualization of calcification/microcalcification-like

echogenic foci influence the ultrasound evaluation of thyroid nodules?" in *Proceedings of the Annual American Institute of Ultrasound in Medicine Convention*, pp. S47–S48, New York, NY, USA, April 2011.

[5] B. S. Garra, "Imaging and estimation of tissue elasticity by ultrasound," *Ultrasound Quarterly*, vol. 23, no. 4, pp. 255–268, 2007.

[6] J. Ophir, I. Cespedes, H. Ponnekanti, Y. Yazdi, and X. Li, "Elastography: a quantitative method for imaging the elasticity of biological tissues," *Ultrasonic Imaging*, vol. 13, no. 2, pp. 111–134, 1991.

[7] T. Varghese, "Quasi-static ultrasound elastography," *Ultrasound Clinics*, vol. 4, no. 3, pp. 323–338, 2009.

[8] K. J. Parker, M. M. Doyley, and D. J. Rubens, "Imaging the elastic properties of tissue: the 20 year perspective," *Physics in Medicine and Biology*, vol. 56, no. 1, pp. R1–R29, 2011.

[9] C. Vorländer, J. Wolff, S. Saalabian, R. H. Lienenlüke, and R. A. Wahl, "Real-time ultrasound elastography-a noninvasive diagnostic procedure for evaluating dominant thyroid nodules," *Langenbeck's Archives of Surgery*, vol. 395, no. 7, pp. 865–871, 2010.

[10] T. Rago, M. Scutari, F. Santini et al., "Real-time elastography: useful tool for refining the presurgical diagnosis in thyroid nodules with inderterminate or nondiagnostic cytology," *The Journal of Clinical Endocrinology & Metabolism*, vol. 95, no. 12, pp. 5274–5280, 2010.

[11] P. V. Lippolis, S. Tognini, G. Materazzi et al., "Is elastography actually useful in presurgical selection of thyroid nodules with indeterminate cytology?" *The Journal of Clinical Endocrinology & Metabolism*, vol. 96, no. 11, pp. E1–E5, 2011.

[12] R. Kagoya, H. Monobe, and H. Tojima, "Utility of elastography for differential diagnosis of benign and malignant thyroid nodules," *Otolaryngology*, vol. 143, no. 2, pp. 230–234, 2010.

[13] K. S. S. Bhatia, D. P. Rasalkar, Y. P. Lee et al., "Cystic change in thyroid nodules: a confounding factor for real-time qualitative thyroid ultrasound elastography," *Clinical Radiology*, vol. 66, no. 9, pp. 799–807, 2011.

[14] R. Z. Slapa, W. S. Jakubowski, J. Bierca, B. Migda, and J. Slowinska-Srzednicka, "Diagnostic performance of strain elastography in multinodular thyroid goiter is unsatisfactory," in *Proceedings of the 10th International Tissue Elasticity Conference*, p. 90, Arlington, Tex, USA, October 2011.

[15] S. H. Park, S. J. Kim, E.-K. Kim, J. K. Min, J. S. Eun, and J. Y. Kwak, "Interobserver agreement in assessing the sonographic and elastographic features of malignant thyroid nodules," *American Journal of Roentgenology*, vol. 193, no. 5, pp. W416–W423, 2009.

[16] B. Cakir, C. Aydin, B. Korukluoglu et al., "Which axis should be performed for elastography scoring in thyroid nodules?" in *Proceedings of the 14th International Thyroid Congress*, Paris, France, September 2010.

[17] M. Tanter, J. Bercoff, A. Athanasiou et al., "Quantitative assessment of breast lesion viscoelasticity: initial clinical results using supersonic shear imaging," *Ultrasound in Medicine and Biology*, vol. 34, no. 9, pp. 1373–1386, 2008.

[18] A. Evans, P. Whelehan, K. Thomson et al., "Quantitative shear wave ultrasound elastography: initial experience in solid breast masses," *Breast Cancer Research*, vol. 12, no. 6, article R104, 2010.

[19] F. Sebag, J. Vaillant-Lombard, J. Berbis et al., "Shear wave elastography: a new ultrasound imaging mode for the differential diagnosis of benign and malignant thyroid nodules," *The Journal of Clinical Endocrinology & Metabolism*, vol. 95, no. 12, pp. 5281–5288, 2010.

[20] D. O. Cosgrove, W. A. Berg, and C. J. Dore, "Shear wave elastography for breast masses is highly reproducible," *European Radiology*, vol. 22, no. 5, pp. 1023–1032, 2012.

[21] W. A. Berg, D. O. Cosgrove, C. J. Dore et al., "Shear-wave elastography improves the specificity of brest US: the BE1 multinational study of 939 masses," *Radiology*, vol. 262, no. 2, pp. 435–449, 2012.

[22] L. Rubaltelli, S. Corradin, A. Dorigo et al., "Differential diagnosis of benign and malignant thyroid nodules at elastosonography," *Ultraschall in der Medizin*, vol. 30, no. 2, pp. 175–179, 2009.

[23] V. Cantisani, P. Ricci, M. Medvedeieva et al., "Prospective evaluation of multiparametric ultrasound and quantitative elastosonography in the differential diagnosis of benign and malignant thyroid nodules," *Insights into Imaging*, vol. 2, supplement 1, p. 180, 2011.

[24] J. Bercoff, "Shear wave elastography," SuperSonic Imagine, 2008, http://www.supersonicimagine.fr/.

[25] J.-L. Gennisson, M. Rénier, S. Catheline et al., "Acoustoelasticity in soft solids: assessment of the nonlinear shear modulus with the acoustic radiation force," *Journal of the Acoustical Society of America*, vol. 122, no. 6, pp. 3211–3219, 2007.

[26] R. Z. Slapa, W. S. Jakubowski, J. Slowinska-Srzednicka, and K. T. Szopinski, "Advantages and disadvantages of 3D ultrasound of thyroid nodules including thin slice volume rendering," *Thyroid Research*, vol. 4, no. 1, 2011.

18

Prognosis of Thyroid Cancer Related to Pregnancy

Gustavo Vasconcelos Alves,[1] Ana Paula Santin,[2] and Tania Weber Furlanetto[2,3]

[1] Oncology Division, Nossa Senhora da Conceição Hospital, Porto Alegre, RS, Brazil
[2] Postgraduation Program in Medicine and Medical Sciences, Universidade Federal do Rio Grande do Sul,
  Rua Ramiro Barcellos 2400, 90035-003 Porto Alegre, RS, Brazil
[3] Internal Medicine Division, Hospital de Clínicas de Porto Alegre, Universidade Federal do Rio Grande do Sul,
  Rua Ramiro Barcellos 2350/700, 90035-003 Porto Alegre, RS, Brazil

Correspondence should be addressed to Tania Weber Furlanetto, taniafurlanetto@gmail.com

Academic Editor: Roberto Negro

Differentiated thyroid cancer (DTC) is the second most common cancer in pregnancy. Its management is a challenge for both doctors and patients, and the best timing for surgery is unclear. A systematic review evaluating the prognosis of DTC in pregnant patients was conducted. After reviewing 401 unique citations and 54 full texts, 4 studies that compared the prognosis of patients with DTC related to pregnancy (DTC diagnosed during pregnancy or within 12 months after childbirth) or not were included. In two studies the primary outcome was overall survival, in one study the primary outcomes were recurrent disease and death related to thyroid cancer, and in one study the primary outcome was recurrent or persistent disease. In the first two studies, there was no difference in overall survival in patients with pregnancy-related DTC, when compared with matched controls; in one study, there was no difference in death caused by DTC nor recurrence in DTC related to pregnancy. Nevertheless, in a recent retrospective study, a higher rate of recurrent or persistent DTC was observed in patients with DTC related to pregnancy. There are not many studies on which to base treatment decisions in pregnant patients with DTC.

1. Introduction

Thyroid cancer currently ranks tenth in incidence among solid organ malignancies. The majority of thyroid cancers are classified as papillary (88%) or follicular (9%); together these two histological types are grouped as differentiated thyroid cancers (DTC) [5]. While the annual rate of cancer incidence is decreasing, there has been a 2.4-fold increase in thyroid cancer from 1973 to 2002 [6].

DTC occurs more commonly in women of child-bearing age with an incidence of 14 per 100,000 live births and represents the second most frequent tumor diagnosed during pregnancy only behind breast cancer [7, 8]. As DTC is commonly found during pregnancy or in the early postpartum period [9], it is possible that physiological changes associated with it, as high levels of estrogen, human chorionic gonadotropin (hCG) and/or others, could create a favorable environment to tumor development and growth. Maternal thyroid gland secretes more thyroid hormone during early pregnancy in response to the thyrotropic activity of hCG that overrides the operation of the hypothalamic-pituitary-thyroid feedback system. This could partially explain an increase in the size of preexisting thyroid nodules as well as new thyroid nodule formation in pregnancy [10–15].

The best treatment option for thyroid cancer in pregnant women or in the early postpartum period should be based on evidence, so the aim of this paper was to evaluate whether the prognosis of DTC associated with pregnancy is similar or not to DTC in nonpregnant women.

2. Methods

2.1. Search Strategy. This literature search was conducted in the PubMed, Cochrane, and Scopus databases, combining the MESH terms: thyroid neoplasms and pregnancy. All studies in English until February 2011 were included.

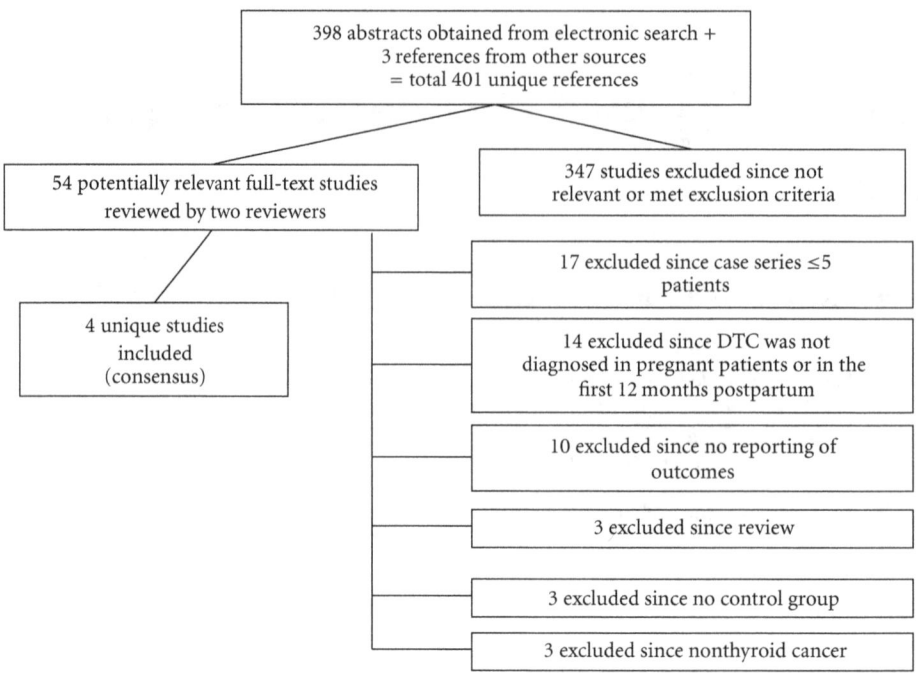

FIGURE 1: Process of study selection for the systematic review.

2.2. Inclusion and Exclusion Criteria for Studies. To be included in this review the original article should describe the comparison between the outcomes in patients diagnosed with DTC during pregnancy or in the first 12 months postpartum (DTC related to pregnancy), with a control group comprising women of child-bearing age, diagnosed with DTC when nonpregnant or at least 12 months after delivery.

Patients should have no prior exposure to radiation or previous malignancies.

2.3. Selection of Studies for Inclusion. All citations and abstracts identified by the electronic search were reviewed by two independent reviewers. Any abstract identified as relevant was analyzed as a full text. Other sources of obtaining papers were used, as cross-referencing texts reviewed.

3. Results and Discussion

After reviewing 398 abstracts from the electronic search and 3 summaries obtained by manual search, 54 articles were reviewed in full-text form. However, after analysis of these studies, several were excluded, for the following reasons: DTC did not occur during pregnancy, there was no control group, there was no reporting of outcomes, or they described small case series, so only four studies were included in this paper, as shown in Figure 1 [1–4]. The characteristics of the studies and the outcomes are described, respectively, in Tables 1 and 2.

There are only a few studies about outcomes of DTC related to pregnancy. As DTC has a good prognosis, the number of patients studied should be large, and the followup

should be very long to detect any difference in survival or even recurrence. Most recurrences of DTC occur within the first five years after initial treatment, but recurrences may occur many years or even decades later, particularly in patients with papillary cancer [16, 17]. In addition to this, decisions about cancer treatment during pregnancy are associated with ethical conflicts between the best option for the mother and for the fetus [18, 19]. The management of pregnant women with cancer should consider the maternal-fetal risk related to treatment, as well as the possibility of tumor progression for postponing treatment or for the tumor being related to pregnancy. During this study we could observe that there is little published data comparing outcomes in patients with DTC related to pregnancy or not. No randomized controlled trial was available.

In the study of Moosa and Mazzaferri there was no impact from pregnancy in DTC-related death [3]; in the studies of Yasmeen et al. and Herzon et al. overall survival was not affected by DTC [2, 4]; when evaluating if the timing of surgical treatment, during pregnancy or after birth, affected the prognosis of patients with DTC detected during pregnancy, Moosa and Mazzaferri and Yasmeen et al. [2, 3] have not shown differences in recurrence rates and, respectively, in DTC-related death and overall survival. Such findings, however, are not in agreement with the study published by Vannucchi et al. They found a strong association of DTC in pregnant women with recurrence or persistence of cancer (60% in pregnant women (group 2) versus 4.2% in women with DTC diagnosed 1 year after delivery (group 1) versus 13.1% in nulliparous patients when diagnosed with DTC (group 3)). After a stepwise logistic regression analysis entering the following variables: extrathyroidal extension,

TABLE 1: Characteristics of the included studies.

Study	Study design	Study population	Control group description	Followup (median)
Vannucchi et al., 2010 [1]	Retrospective cohort in a single institution—1995–2006	14 women (one affected twice), age 32.2 ± 6.4 yr, DTC diagnosed during pregnancy (G2)	47 women, age 36.1 ± 3.6 yr, DTC diagnosed at least one year after delivery (G1), and 61 nulliparous women when diagnosed with DTC, age 34.1 ± 6.2 yr, (G3)	G1: 68.2 months G2: 60.1 months G3: 64.7 months
Yasmeen et al., 2005 [2]	Population-based case control study—California 1991–1999	595 pregnant women with DTC, 129 diagnosed during pregnancy and 466 diagnosed within 12 months postpartum	2270 age-matched nonpregnant women with DTC	Not reported
Moosa and Mazzaferri, 1997 [3]	Case control study—United States Air Force registry	61 pregnant women with DTC, age 26.0 ± 5.9 yr	528 age-matched nonpregnant women with DTC, age 26.3 ± 5.9 yr	22.4 yr in study population and 19.5 yr in control group
Herzon et al., 1994 [4]	Case control study—New Mexico Registry 1970–1991	22 pregnant women with DTC, age 18–46 yr	465 women with DTC in the same database, age 18–46 yr	6 months to 20 years reported for study population

Age (years) is expressed as mean + SD; DTC: differentiated thyroid cancer; G: group.

lymph-node metastases, radioiodine treatment, pregnant or not pregnant status at diagnosis, histotype, and tumor size ≤2 or >2 cm, pregnancy was found to be the most significant predictor for disease recurrence or persistence [1]. As the outcomes and the methodology employed in each study were different, it was not possible to compare their results and to combine the data in a meta-analysis. In the studies of Yasmeen et al. and Herzon et al., the overall survival was the main outcome [2, 4], while the study of Moosa and Mazzaferri had death related to DTC and recurrence, evaluated by biopsy or by ^{131}I uptake in distant sites, as primary outcomes [3], and the more recent study of Vannucchi et al. evaluated persistent/recurrent DTC through more sensible tests such as Tg basal levels and Tg response to rhTSH [1]. Such methods were not used in the study of Moosa and Mazzaferri [3], which could explain some of the discrepancies among them.

In the study of Vannucchi et al. more patients from the pregnant women with DTC had follicular histotype. However, this factor does not seem to explain the worse outcome which has been found on the group of patients with DTC associated to pregnancy, since two of three patients with follicular histology remained in remission [1].

Two studies reported differences among clinical presentation between pregnant and nonpregnant women [1, 3]. In the study of Moosa and Mazzaferri, fewer pregnant patients showed symptoms associated to thyroid nodules (74% versus 43%, $P < 0.01$) [3]. On the other hand, in the study of Vannucchi et al. DTC was less commonly an incidental finding in pregnant patients, probably indicating that these patients had more aggressive disease [1].

A very interesting molecular datum was described by Vannucchi et al. The expression of the estrogen receptor alfa through immunohistochemical analysis was higher in group 2 patients, as compared to groups 1 and 3 [1]. As estrogen probably increases proliferative activity of thyroid follicular cells [20], this hormone could be implicated in a more aggressive pattern of DTC diagnosed in pregnancy.

Other important factor found in this paper refers to the time of followup of the studies. The mean median followup ranged from four to twenty-three years. Considering that DTC is a disease with low lethality and the followup was not very long, it is possible that the full impact of DTC on the patients survival was not evident.

The treatment of choice for both pregnant and nonpregnant patients was thyroidectomy. The central lymphadenectomy (VI-VII levels) was performed on all patients in the cohort described by Vannucchi et al. [1], and, according to clinical judgment, in the other studies [2–4]. There seemed to be no difference on the outcome of DTC during pregnancy whether the surgery took place at the second trimester of pregnancy or after childbirth [2–4]. In contrast to these findings, Kuy et al. compared the risk of thyroid and parathyroid surgery complications in pregnant and nonpregnant women, paired by age, in a retrospective cross-sectional study. A total of 201 pregnant women and 31155 nonpregnant women were included; among the 201 pregnant women, 45.8% have undergone surgery due to thyroid cancer, the others had benign thyroid and parathyroid diseases. Thyroidectomy during pregnancy was associated with an increased surgical complication rate in both malignant (21% to 8%) and benign diseases (27% to 14%), as well as higher endocrine complication rates (15.9% to 8.2%) and treatment costs ($6873 versus $5963) [21].

In summary, there are few studies which give base to the policies about pregnant patients with DTC. Up to present time, data obtained through systematic review show conflicting results when it comes to observed outcomes in this population. There seem to be a higher disease recurrence and persistence rates in this population when current treatment

TABLE 2: Main outcomes in patients with differentiated thyroid cancer (DTC) diagnosed during pregnancy or within 12 months of childbirth.

Study	Timing of surgery (study group)	Outcomes	Main study results	Comments and others outcomes
Vannucchi et al., 2010 [1]	(i) 11 patients operated during pregnancy and (ii) 4 patients operated after delivery[d]	(i) Persistent or recurrent disease detected by highly sensitive Tg and rhTSH (ii) ERα tumor expression by IHC	(i) ↑Persistent/recurrent disease in G2 versus G1 and G3 (60% versus 4.2% and 13.1%)[a] (ii) ↑ERα tumor expression in G2 versus G1 and G3 (87.5% versus 31% and 0%)[b]	(i) PTC more frequent in G1 and G3 versus G2 (97.8% and 98.3% versus 80%)[c] (ii) DTC was an incidental finding more frequently in G1 and G3 (iii) More sensitive methods for detecting recurrence were used in this study when compared with others (iv) Conclusion: pregnancy has a negative impact on the outcome of DTC
Yasmeen et al., 2005 [2]	(i) 96 patients operated during pregnancy and (ii) 27 patients operated after delivery[e]	Overall survival	No difference in survival between pregnancy-associated thyroid cancer and aged-matched nonpregnant women with DTC	Persistent/recurrent disease was not evaluated
Moosa and Mazzaferri, 1997 [3]	(i) 14 patients operated during pregnancy and (ii) 47 patients operated after delivery	(i) Death (ii) Recurrence diagnosed by biopsy, or by 131I uptake in distant site	No difference in cancer recurrence and death in study and control groups	(i) Outcomes similar in patients operated after delivery and during pregnancy (ii) Fewer pregnant patients showed symptoms associated with thyroid nodules when compared with nonpregnant (74% versus 43%)[b]
Herzon et al., 1994 [4]	(i) 6 patients operated during pregnancy and (ii) 16 patients operated after delivery	Overall survival	No difference in survival between pregnancy-associated thyroid cancer and aged-matched nonpregnant women with DTC	

PTC: papillary histotype; Tg: serum thyroglobulin; rhTSH: recombinant human TSH; ERα: estrogen receptor alfa; G: group; G1: DTC diagnosed at least one year after pregnancy, G2: DTC diagnosed during pregnancy, G3: DTC diagnosed in nulliparous women or before pregnancy; [a]$P < 0.0001$; [b]$P = 0.01$; [c]$P < 0.0001$; [d]1 patient was considered twice: she had two tumors in two different pregnancies; [e]In patients with DTC diagnosed during pregnancy.

response evaluation methods are employed. However, the impact on overall survival in the long time appears to be unaltered. There is no evidence to support termination of pregnancy when the diagnosis of DTC is performed. The guidelines of the endocrine society for pregnancy-related DTC recommend thyroidectomy after delivery for patients with no evidence of advanced disease or without rapid progression, and thyroidectomy in the second trimester of pregnancy for the others (USPSTF recommendation level B). Radioactive iodine should only be given after delivery and the ending of breastfeeding [22].

Prospective studies should be done to compare the prognosis of DTC diagnosed during pregnancy or not, as well as the effects of postponing surgery after childbirth in DTC diagnosed during pregnancy.

References

[1] G. Vannucchi, M. Perrino, S. Rossi et al., "Clinical and molecular features of differentiated thyroid cancer diagnosed during pregnancy," *European Journal of Endocrinology*, vol. 162, no. 1, pp. 145–151, 2010.

[2] S. Yasmeen, R. Cress, P. S. Romano et al., "Thyroid cancer in pregnancy," *International Journal of Gynecology and Obstetrics*, vol. 91, no. 1, pp. 15–20, 2005.

[3] M. Moosa and E. L. Mazzaferri, "Outcome of differentiated thyroid cancer diagnosed in pregnant women," *Journal of Clinical Endocrinology and Metabolism*, vol. 82, no. 9, pp. 2862–2866, 1997.

[4] F. S. Herzon, D. M. Morris, M. N. Segal, G. Rauch, and T. Parnell, "Coexistent thyroid cancer and pregnancy," *Archives*

of Otolaryngology—Head and Neck Surgery, vol. 120, no. 11, pp. 1191–1193, 1994.

[5] W. R. Burns and M. A. Zeiger, "Differentiated thyroid cancer," *Seminars in Oncology*, vol. 37, no. 6, pp. 557–566, 2010.

[6] L. Davies and H. G. Welch, "Increasing incidence of thyroid cancer in the United States, 1973–2002," *Journal of the American Medical Association*, vol. 295, no. 18, pp. 2164–2167, 2006.

[7] L. H. Smith, J. L. Dalrymple, G. S. Leiserowitz, B. Danielsen, and W. M. Gilbert, "Obstetrical deliveries associated with maternal malignancy in California, 1992 through 1997," *American Journal of Obstetrics and Gynecology*, vol. 184, no. 7, pp. 1504–1513, 2001.

[8] L. H. Smith, B. Danielsen, M. E. Allen, and R. Cress, "Cancer associated with obstetric delivery: results of linkage with the California cancer registry," *American Journal of Obstetrics and Gynecology*, vol. 189, no. 4, pp. 1128–1135, 2003.

[9] M. Lambe and A. Ekbom, "Cancers coinciding with child-bearing: delayed diagnosis during pregnancy?" *British Medical Journal*, vol. 311, no. 7020, pp. 1607–1608, 1995.

[10] L. A. Akslen, S. Nilssen, and G. Kvale, "Reproductive factors and risk of thyroid cancer. A prospective study of 63,090 women from Norway," *British Journal of Cancer*, vol. 65, no. 5, pp. 772–774, 1992.

[11] M. R. Galanti, M. Lambe, A. Ekbom, P. Sparen, and B. Pettersson, "Parity and risk of thyroid cancer: a nested case-control study of a nationwide Swedish cohort," *Cancer Causes and Control*, vol. 6, no. 1, pp. 37–44, 1995.

[12] M. Yoshimura and J. M. Hershman, "Thyrotropic action of human chorionic gonadotropin," *Thyroid*, vol. 5, no. 5, pp. 425–434, 1995.

[13] I. B. Rosen and P. G. Walfish, "Pregnancy as a predisposing factor in thyroid neoplasia," *Archives of Surgery*, vol. 121, no. 11, pp. 1287–1290, 1986.

[14] M. Hod, R. Sharony, S. Friedman, and J. Ovadia, "Pregnancy and thyroid carcinoma: a review of incidence, course and prognosis," *Obstetrical and Gynecological Survey*, vol. 44, no. 11, pp. 774–779, 1989.

[15] R. E. Neale, S. Darlington, M. F. G. Murphy, P. B. S. Silcocks, D. M. Purdie, and M. Talbäck, "The effects of twins, parity and age at first birth on cancer risk in Swedish women," *Twin Research and Human Genetics*, vol. 8, no. 2, pp. 156–162, 2005.

[16] A. R. Shaha, T. R. Loree, J. P. Shah et al., "Prognostic factors and risk group analysis in follicular carcinoma of the thyroid," *Surgery*, vol. 118, no. 6, pp. 1131–1138, 1995.

[17] E. L. Mazzaferri and S. M. Jhiang, "Long-term impact of initial surgical and medical therapy on papillary and follicular thyroid cancer," *American Journal of Medicine*, vol. 97, no. 5, pp. 418–428, 1994.

[18] F. S. Oduncu, R. Kimmig, H. Hepp, and B. Emmerich, "Cancer in pregnancy: maternal-fetal conflict," *Journal of Cancer Research and Clinical Oncology*, vol. 129, no. 3, pp. 133–146, 2003.

[19] E. L. Mazzaferri, "Approach to the pregnant patient with thyroid cancer," *Journal of Clinical Endocrinology and Metabolism*, vol. 96, no. 2, pp. 265–272, 2011.

[20] A. P. Santin and T. W. Furlanetto, "Role of estrogen on thyroid function and growth regulation," *Journal of Thyroid Research*, vol. 2011, Article ID 875125, 7 pages, 2011.

[21] S. Kuy, S. A. Roman, R. Desai, and J. A. Sosa, "Outcomes following thyroid and parathyroid surgery in pregnant women," *Archives of Surgery*, vol. 144, no. 5, pp. 399–406, 2009.

[22] M. Abalovich, N. Amino, L. A. Barbour et al., "Management of thyroid dysfunction during pregnancy and postpartum: an Endocrine Society Clinical Practice Guideline," *The Journal of Clinical Endocrinology and Metabolism*, vol. 92, no. 8 , supplement, pp. S1–S47, 2007.

19

The Hypothalamic-Pituitary-Thyroid Axis in Infants and Children: Protection from Radioiodines

Jeffrey Fisher,[1] **Xiaoxia Yang,**[1] **Curtis Harris,**[2] **Igor Koturbash,**[3] **and Annie Lumen**[1]

[1] *National Center for Toxicological Research, US FDA, 3900 NCTR Road, Jefferson, AR 72079, USA*
[2] *College of Public Health, University of Georgia, 115 DW Brooks Dr, Barrow Hall, Room 001B, Athens, GA 30602, USA*
[3] *Department of Environmental and Occupational Health, Fay W. Boozman College of Public Health,*
    University of Arkansas for Medical Sciences, 4301 West Markham Street, Slot 820-11, Little Rock, AR 72205, USA

Correspondence should be addressed to Jeffrey Fisher; jeffrey.fisher@fda.hhs.gov

Academic Editor: Massimo Tonacchera

Potassium iodide (KI) is recommended as an emergency treatment for exposure to radioiodines, most commonly associated with nuclear detonation or mishaps at nuclear power plants. Protecting the thyroid gland of infants and children remains a priority because of increased incidence of thyroid cancer in the young exposed to radioiodines (such as ^{131}I and ^{133}I). There is a lack of clinical studies for KI and radioiodines in children or infants to draw definitive conclusions about the effectiveness and safety of KI administration in the young. In this paper, we compare functional aspects of the hypothalamic-pituitary-thyroid (HPT) axis in the young and adults and review the limited studies of KI in children. The HPT axis in the infant and child is hyperactive and therefore will respond less effectively to KI treatment compared to adults. Research on the safety and efficacy of KI in infants and children is needed.

1. Introduction

Several governmental and scientific bodies are dedicated to ensuring protection of the public from radiation. The International Commission on Radiological Protection was created in 1928 by the International Congress of Radiology to advance the science of radiation protection for the public by publishing peer reviewed radiation articles. The United States Atomic Regulatory Commission was established in 1946 with a mission to encourage nuclear power and also protect the public. Eventually strong concerns about the dual roles of the Commission resulted in Congress dissolving this Commission and forming another, the United States Nuclear Regulatory Commission (USNRC). The USNRC began operation in 1975 and is responsible for protection and measurement, with regulatory involvement in nuclear facilities and protection of public health and safety. In 1955, the General Assembly of the United Nations established the United Nations Scientific Committee on the Effects of Atomic Radiation (UNSCEAR), which releases reports on important current topics of concern such as the Fukushima-Daiichi nuclear power plant accident.

In 1964, the US congress chartered the National Council on Radiation Protection and Measurements with a mission to develop and disseminate guidance and recommendations on radiation protection and measurement. This group is well known for producing technical documents concerning a vast array of radiation topics.

Radioisotopes of iodines (stable elemental iodine (^{127}I) and radioactive forms of iodine (such as ^{131}I) are converted in the body to stable iodide (^{127}I$^-$) and radioiodide (^{131}I$^-$), primarily in the gut. Iodine in the diet refers to several inorganic forms (e.g., iodates) that are converted in the body to iodide) are produced in large quantities by fission reactions of uranium atoms in nuclear reactors and either plutonium or uranium atoms in nuclear detonations. The radioisotopes of iodines are subsequently released into the environment. At Three Mile Island, 6×10^{11} Bq was released into the atmosphere over several hours, while at Chernobyl 10×10^{17} Bq was released over a 10-day period, and most recently at Fukushima, several releases occurred totaling 10×10^{16} Bq [33]. Once in the environment, the radioactive iodines can be inhaled or ingested by consumption of contaminated food and milk. The threat of nuclear detonations or nuclear industrial accidents resulted in laboratory experiments to characterize the health hazards of radionuclides throughout the late 1940s into the 1960s [34–37]. Fresh cow's milk was considered to be a primary source of radionuclides after cows forage on contaminated vegetation. The first radioiodine and stable iodine (^{125}I) experiments with cows to simulate a nuclear detonation or nuclear industrial accident were conducted by Bustad et al. [34]. The authors demonstrated that increasing the intake of stable or dietary iodine resulted in less radioiodide dose in the thyroid gland and milk. The use of stable iodine as a blocking agent for thyroidal uptake of radioiodide was an area of active research in the 1950s and 1960s [16, 30, 38]. Unknown at this time, iodide in systemic circulation, radioactive or stable, is sequestered into the thyroid gland and mammary tissue by the sodium iodide symporter protein (NIS), a basolateral transport protein. The stable form of systemic iodide competes with radioiodide for transport into the thyroid gland via the NIS. Additionally excess stable systemic iodide can cause a transient shut-down in the thyroid gland referred to as the Wolff-Chaikoff effect [39]. The mechanism of iodide action may involve posttranslational modification of the NIS [40]. Once in the thyroid gland excess stable iodide can also bind to thyroglobulin, the protein backbone for synthesis of thyroid hormones, and reduce the extent of binding of radioiodides to thyroglobulin.

Thyroid cancer in children and adolescents is one of the most severe health outcomes resulting from releases of radioiodines after a nuclear mishap or detonation [33]. Irradiation of the thyroid gland may also result in nodules or hypothyroidism [41]. Children's increased sensitivity to thyroidal radiation is one of the most important scientific findings from the Chernobyl nuclear accident. The rates of thyroid cancer were greater than expected in children exposed to radioactive isotopes of iodide [42, 43]. A workshop report [44] found evidence for mild goiter in the regions' children suggesting mild to moderate iodide deficiency. Some of the conclusions in the workshop report were that iodide deficient children with goiter may result in less radiation dose per mg weight of the thyroid gland or an altered distribution of radioiodides within the thyroid gland may occur. The report also noted that thyroidal uptake of systemic radioiodide may be greater in iodide deficient children compared to euthyroid children. In addition to radioiodide dosimetry concerns in iodide deficient children the thyroid glands of these children may be more susceptible to exposure of radioiodines. Potassium iodide (KI), a thyroidal radioiodide blocking agent, is recommended by the United States Food and Drug Administration (US FDA) as a drug to reduce the thyroid radioiodide dose in children and adults [45].

In this paper, we integrate interdisciplinary information from health physics, basic and clinical thyroid endocrinology, physiology, public health, and mathematical modeling. This review focuses on the biology of the hypothalamic-pituitary-thyroid (HPT) axis in children, selected clinical and field studies with KI and radioiodine tracer, and current knowledge about KI use in children. Data gaps are identified and research is recommended.

2. Aspects of the HPT Axis in Adults and Children

Protecting children from the potential harmful effects of radioiodines, drugs, or chemicals is not as simple as treating children as "small adults." How children differ from adults in their overall kinetic and dynamic responses to drugs and chemicals remains a concern for conducting appropriate safety or risk assessments [46]. Growth from birth to adolescence alters, to varying degrees, the pharmacokinetics of therapeutic drugs and chemicals [46]. Several physiological processes undergo maturation including breathing rate, cardiac output, blood flows to tissues and organs, and organ or tissue volumes. Table 1 provides examples of some important physiological changes that occur during maturation of infants and children. On a per Kg basis, cardiac output, ventilation rates, blood flow rates to organs, and organ volume are greater in early life (Table 1). Other aspects of physiology gradually increase with age such as glomerular filtration (Table 1) and kidney transporter proteins [47], which both affect the pharmacokinetics of drugs and chemicals. Enzyme maturation can be complex. For example, Cytochrome P450 (CYP) CYP3A is an important drug metabolizing enzyme. One isoform (CYP3A7) is active *in utero* and decreases the first week of life, while another isoform, CYP3A4, increases rapidly the first year of life [48]. Much is known about age-dependent changes in gross physiology; however, no data were found on the blood flow rate to the thyroid gland in infants and children. Measurements of blood flow rate for the thyroid gland in infants and children would help clarify if the rate of delivery of systemic radioiodide to the thyroid gland (normalized to the weight of the thyroid gland) is different than in adults.

Iodine is an essential element for life and its retention in the body is controlled by urinary excretion and sequestration into the thyroid gland by the NIS protein. Iodide can be sequestered into other NIS containing tissues (e.g., mammary tissue and gut lumen), but organification does not take place. Transfer of iodide (and to some degree thyroid hormones) to the nursing infant represents an important physiological process for dietary iodide intake for the nursing infant [49]. In the body, systemic levels of iodide originate from dietary ingestion of iodide and the release of iodide atoms from deiodination of thyroid hormones. The majority of iodide is excreted in urine with a minor loss to feces [50].

The function of the HPT axis has been studied by independently evaluating several aspects of the HPT axis. This includes measuring the uptake of trace amounts of radioiodide into the thyroid gland, intake of stable iodide, the excretion of stable iodide into urine, serum levels of stable iodide, thyroid pools of stable iodide, and rates of thyroid hormone secretion. The state of knowledge about the age-dependent changes in the HPT axis is discussed below.

2.1. Radioactive Iodide Uptake (RAIU) (Table 2). Tracking trace amounts of radioactive iodide uptake (RAIU) into the thyroid gland in a clinical setting is expressed as percent of administered radioiodine dose. This measurement reflects

TABLE 1: Selected physiology values in infants, children, and young adults.

	Age (days)	Value	Age (months)	Value	Age (years)	Value	Age (years)	Value	References
Blood flows (L/hr/kg bw)[a]									
Cardiac output	6	11.1[b]	10.6	8.6[c]	6	11.1	18	8	[1, 2]
Alveolar ventilation	1	13.4	3	8.7	6	6.9	18	6.7[d]	[3]
Glomerular filtration	2	0.09[b]	12	0.18	3	0.17	12	0.13	[4]
Blood flow to brain	1	3.2	12	4.3	5	2.9	15	0.83	[5]
Blood flow to kidney	1	1.9	12	1.4	5	1.8	15	1.1	[5]
Blood flow to thyroid	—	—	—	—	—	—	18	0.13[e]	[6]
Organ volumes (L/kg bw)[a]									
Body weight (Kg)	1	3.4	12	9.8	6	21.1	18	54.4	[7]
Blood	1	0.088	24	0.046	6	0.081	18	0.077	[7]
Brain	1	0.10	12	0.091	6	0.057	18	0.024	[7]
Kidney	1	0.007	12	0.0066	6	0.0052	18	0.0044	[7]
Thyroid	1–30	$0.3\text{–}0.4E-3$	12–24	$0.2\text{–}0.3E-3$	5–9	$0.2\text{–}0.3E-3$	15–19	$0.3E-3$	[8]

[a]Body weight for females at specified ages calculated using equation from [7].
[b]Calculated using body weight at birth.
[c]Calculated using body weight of 1 year old.
[d]Derived values using respiratory frequency, tidal volume, and physiological dead space [3].
[e]Calculated based on reported percentage of blood flow to thyroid in adult humans (1.6% of cardiac output) [6] and cardiac output (8 L/hr/kg bw) in females of 18 years old.

the ability of the thyroid gland to sequester radioiodide and is a fundamental functional aspect of the thyroid gland. The measured fraction of administered radioiodine dose in the thyroid gland is a consequence of NIS mediated transport of radioiodide and its organification.

In a study conducted in the United States, Fields et al. reported a mean 24 hr RAIU value of 31.1% for 60 children [9], which did not differ from the mean 24 hr RAIU value for 64 euthyroid adults (32.2%). The same authors reported a mean 24 hr RAIU value of 76.1% for hyperthyroid adult ($n = 62$), which compares favorably to their findings for hyperthyroid children (87%, $n = 5$). Fields et al. stated that for euthyroid children under the age of 4 increased "hyperactivity" of the thyroid gland was evident and this "hyperactivity" may persist until age 9 [9]. These authors also stated that thyroid activity in older children aged 10 to 18 was similar to adults. Fields et al. also summarized 8 child RAIU studies reported from the late 1940s to early 1950s [9]. In general these earlier studies reported RAIU values less than the values Fields et al. reported [9], except for premature infants and newborns. Van Middleworth reported a mean RAIU value of 69.7% in 7 newborns from the United States [10] and Martmer reported a mean RAIU value of 38.6% for 16 premature infants from the United States [11].

A few RAIU studies have been reported on children since the 1950s. Twenty-four-hour RAIU values for 5 children from the United States, 2 years of age, were reported to range from 15 to 23% [12]. Twenty-six children, aged 9 to 15 years, had a mean 24 hr RAIU value of 52.9% [13]. Ingenbleek and Beckers reported a mean 24 hr RAIU value of 39.6% for children aged 1.5 to 2 years ($n = 6$) from the Republic of Senegal [14].

Cuddihy reported a mean RAIU value of 23.5% in 4 children aged 7 to 9 years from the United States [15].

Sternthal et al. determined a mean 24 hr RAIU value of 20.0% in adults from the United States [16]. Malvaux et al. reported a mean 24 hr RAIU value of 41.7% for Belgium adults [13]. Greer et al. reported a range of RAIU values in 37 adults from the United States of 18.1 to 21.6% [18]. In a recent German study, a mean RAIU value of 24.8% is reported for 27 adults [17].

A wide range of RAIU values are reported for children and adults. RAIU values reflect the ability of the thyroid gland to form precursor thyroid hormones (organify radioiodide) and the functionality of the NIS symporter proteins. Some studies show that the RAIU in the young is greater than in adults (Table 2) suggesting that infants and children may be at a greater risk of radiation exposure. An important confounding factor for interpreting these studies is the dietary iodine status. RAIU is well known to increase with decreasing dietary iodine.

2.2. Thyroidal Clearance of Radioactive Iodide (Table 2). Another measure of thyroidal uptake of radioiodide is the thyroidal clearance of radioiodide, defined as a volume of serum or plasma cleared of radioiodide per unit time and is calculated by monitoring radioiodide uptake into the thyroid gland and clearance of radioiodide from the serum. Malvaux et al. reported thyroidal radioactive iodide clearance values of 30.3 and 25.3 mL/min for adolescents and adults [13] and when expressed as mL/min/kg, the values were 0.80 and 0.35. The authors also calculated 24 hr accumulation rates of dietary (stable) iodine in the

TABLE 2: Radioactive iodide uptake into the thyroid gland (RAIU, expressed as percent of the administered radioactive dose) and thyroidal and renal clearance rates of iodide in infants, children, and adults.

RAIU study	24 hr RAIU % of dose mean	24 hr RAIU % of dose range	Number of volunteers	Location	Reference
Infant and child age					
2 months to 18 years	31.1	17 to 50	60	United States	[9]
9 to 18 years, hyperthyroidism	87	72 to 99	5	United States	[9]
Newborn, 2-3 days, 14[a] hr RAIU	69.7[a]	46 to 97[a]	7	United States	[10]
Premature (2 lb, 4 oz to 5 lb 15 oz)	38.6	28 to 52	16	United States	[11]
2 years	—	15–23	5	United States	[12]
9 to 15 years	52.9	28–52	26	Belgium	[13]
1.5 to 2 years (euthyroid)	39.6	SD ± 3.08	6	Republic of Senegal	[14]
1.5 to 2 years (malnutrition)	23.9	SD ± 6.24	12	Republic of Senegal	[14]
7 to 9 years	23.5	21 to 25	4	United States	[15]
Adults					
Euthyroid	32.2	16 to 50	64	United States	[9]
Hyperthyroid	76.1	34 to 100	62	United States	[9]
23 to 50 years	20.0	17.2 to 21.8	22	United States	[16]
Unknown	41.7	SE ± 1.5	unknown	Belgium	[13]
25 to 46 years	24.8	10–47.8	27	Germany	[17]
18 to 57 years	20.0	SE 1.5 to 3.8	37	United States	[18]
	Mean (mL/min)	Mean (mL/min/kg)	Number of Volunteers	Location	Reference
Thyroidal clearance of iodide					
Children					
Birth to 3 weeks	—	2.52	3	Belgium	[19]
3 weeks to 6 months	—	1.09	4	Belgium	[19]
6 to 12 months	—	0.9	7	Belgium	[19]
1 to 2 years	—	1.7	7	Belgium	[19]
9 to 15 years, normal	30.3	0.80	26	Belgium	[13]
Normal	21.5	—	6	Republic of Senegal	[14]
Malnourished	7.3	—	12	Republic of Senegal	[14]
Adults	25.3	0.35	unknown	Belgium	[13]
Renal clearance of iodide					
Children					
Birth to 3 weeks	—	0.74	3	Belgium	[19]
3 weeks to 6 months	—	1.1	4	Belgium	[19]
6 to 12 months	—	0.73	7	Belgium	[19]
1 to 2 years	—	1.5	7	Belgium	[19]
9 to 15 years	25.5	0.65	26	Belgium	[13]
Adults	29.7	0.41	—	Belgium	[13]

[a]Refers to a 14 hr RAIU value, which is different than all others, which are in the column with a header stating 24 hr RAIU.

thyroid gland of 1.0 and 0.65 µg/kg/day for adolescents and adults. Ponchon et al. investigated the iodide kinetics in 21 newborns and infants [19], and pharmacokinetic parameters were compared to values reported earlier for adolescents and adults [13]. The thyroidal clearance of iodide, expressed in units of mL/min/kg, was found to decrease with increasing age. Ingenbleek and Beckers reported thyroidal radioiodide clearance values of 21.5 mL/min for normal children and 7.3 mL/min for malnourished children [14].

Thyroidal clearance of radioactive iodide (uptake of radioiodide into the thyroid gland and its clearance from blood) appears to be a better measure of the thyroidal uptake of radioiodide than RAIU because the rate at which this happens is captured and can be used in quantitative and dynamic evaluations of radioiodide dosimetry. These studies indicate that the uptake of thyroidal iodide occurs at a faster rate in the young than adults when normalized to body weight.

2.3. Urinary Excretion of Iodide (Table 2). The neonatal kidneys are anatomically and functionally immature, exhibiting a disproportionately low glomerular filtration rate (about 30% of the adult level) and relatively low blood flow compared to the adult [51, 52]. The level of glomerular filtration increases very rapidly, especially within the first three months of life [52].

Age related differences in renal clearance of iodide from the plasma or serum have been documented. Oddie et al. evaluated dietary iodide in many subjects from Australia and the United States, using a linear statistical model [53]. Despite the immature glomerular filtration, the authors concluded that the renal clearance of iodide decreased with increasing age by about 0.7% per year. Also, hypothyroid individuals had a lower renal clearance rate of iodide compared to euthyroid individuals. Malvaux et al. reported renal clearance values of 25.5 and 29.7 mL/min for adolescents and adults and on a mL/min/kg basis, the values were 0.65 and 0.41 for adolescents and adults [13].

Similar to the thyroidal clearance of iodide, the renal clearance of iodide was also found to be higher in the young, particularly between the age of 3 weeks to 6 months [19]. When normalized for body weight, the young excrete iodide in urine at a greater rate than adults, which is inconsistent with maturation of glomerular filtration. These observations suggest that other biological determinants, perhaps age-dependent, are important for kidney function such as protein transporters.

2.4. Iodine Intake. Adequate intake levels for iodine estimated for the first year of life (110 to 130 μg/day, [54]) are not much different than the recommended dietary allowances for adults (150 μg/day, [54]) suggesting that on a body weight basis the HPT axis for the young is "accelerated." In the United States, the pediatric intake of iodine, on a μg/kg/day basis, is greater than adults [55]. In children of 6 years of age or under, the lower and upper bound for iodine intake ranged from 144 to 280 μg/person/day and in adults 40 to 65 years of age, 138 to 284 μg/person/day.

There is a dearth of data on direct measurements of iodide in serum or whole blood. A recent study in the United States [56] using modern analytical methods reported that median serum iodide concentrations were 8 μg/L for fetal cord blood and 2.58 μg/L for maternal blood serum. In China the reverse was reported, using modern analytical methods and whole blood samples. The mean infant iodide blood concentration was 15.7 μg/L (range of 12.5 to 21.7 μg/L) compared to adult mean serum iodide concentration of 110 μg/L (range of 14.1 to 812 μg/L) [57]. During the first year of life for infants in Belgium, the serum iodide levels were 2.2 to 6 μg/L and for adults, near 1 μg/L [19].

The intake of dietary iodine appears to be fairly well established in the young based on urinary excretion of iodide

and iodide in breast milk and formula. The resulting serum levels of iodide in the young are less known because only in the last decade have advanced analytical methods been used to measure the inorganic iodide directly. Understanding the circulating levels of inorganic stable iodide is important for understanding the influence of dietary iodide on the radiation health risks (thyroid radioiodide dose) of infants and children exposed to radioiodine. The dose of radioiodide to the thyroid gland can be predicted mathematically based on competitive inhibition of radioiodide by stable iodide at the NIS protein of the thyroid gland.

2.5. Thyroidal Iodide and HPT Function. There are limited data on the total iodide content of thyroid glands in adults, children, and newborns (Table 3). Iodide content of thyroid glands provides an indicator of the status of the HPT axis. For euthyroid adults the thyroidal iodide stores (organified iodide) are estimated to be between 10 and 20 mg [25]. In Venezuelan population, Zabala et al. reported a median of 15 mg of thyroidal iodide content for adults, with a range of 4 to 37 mg of thyroidal iodide (Table 3) [20]. Fisher and Oddie reported a mean value of 15 mg iodide in thyroids of 8 young adults from the United States with a range of 9.0 to 23.6 [22]. In Russia, where mild iodide deficient conditions exist, lower thyroidal iodide values of 3.9 to 8.3 mg were found for adults and in teenagers, 1.5 mg [21] (Table 3). Thyroidal iodide stores have been measured in premature or term infants who only survived for a short period after birth (Table 3). A mean thyroidal iodide value of 0.29 mg for newborns is reported from Canada, where dietary iodide is sufficient [26]. Other studies in Europe reported thyroidal iodide concentrations of 0.09 and 0.04 mg for term babies [23, 24] (Table 3), where iodide insufficient conditions exist.

Thyroidal iodide stores are useful indicators of the status of the HPT axis, but data is difficult to obtain in humans. More age-specific information is needed on the thyroid gland, including thyroidal iodide content, weight, and the content of thyroid hormones and their precursors.

The HPT axis is very dynamic in the first hours and days after birth (Table 4). At birth serum thyroid stimulating hormone (TSH) and thyroxine (T4) concentrations are very high. This suggests that the negative feedback system is ineffective and that cold stimulation of the newborn may be the dominant factor controlling the HPT axis [58]. The calculated T4 secretion rate from the thyroid gland of the newborn is very high (Table 4). However, this condition is transient and a steady decline in serum TSH and T4 concentrations and T4 secretion occurs over several days after birth and the negative feedback becomes functional. Elevated secretion rates of T4 persist for months after birth.

Establishing population based reference intervals for serums TSH, T4, fT4, and T3 in newborns, infants, and children from the United States is needed along with clinical studies which can be used to quantitatively estimate thyroid secretion rates of thyroid hormones and deiodination rates (thyroid hormone metabolic rates) for euthyroid populations. This information would provide baseline data for better understanding the consequences of KI administration.

TABLE 3: Thyroid gland weights and thyroidal iodide stores in infants, children, and adults.

Subject	Thyroid weight (g)	Thyroidal iodide (mg/g)	Thyroidal iodide (mg)	Location	Reference
Adult males ($n = 50$)	10 ± 2 SD (5.6 to 17.7)	1.4 ± 0.7 median, SD (0.42 to 3.43)	15 ± 8 (4 to 37)	Venezuela	[20]
Age 16 to 85 years, range of mean values ($n = 83$)	13 to 15.3	0.32 to 0.67	3.9 to 8.3	Russia	[21]
Age less than 16 years, 8 years average age ($n = 5$)	6.1 ± 1.0 SE	0.24 ± 0.08 SE	1.5 ± 0.52 SE	Russia	[21]
Young adults ($n = 8$)	14.5 ± 1.2 SE (11.1 to 20.3)	0.97	15.0 ± 1.5 SE (9.0 to 23.6)	United States	[22]
Newborns					
Less than 13-day-old term newborns ($n = 4$)	0.74 ± 0.74 SD	0.060 ± 42.3 SD	0.04	Italy	[23]
Gestation age 22 to 34 weeks preterm ($n = 28$)	0.61 ± 0.35 SD	0.042 ± 0.04 SD	0.03	Italy	[23]
Less than 30-day-old near-term newborns ($n = 15$)	0.93 ± 0.4 SD	0.096 ± 0.034 SD	0.09	Yugoslavia	[24]
Preterm newborns, under 10 days of age ($n = 9$)	—	0.092 ± 0.01 SE 0.049 to 0.166	—	Belgium	[25]
Preterm newborns, under 10 days of age ($n = 8$)	—	0.270 ± 0.05 SE 0.094 to 0.493	—	Canada	[25]
Newborns ($n = 13$)	1.0	—	0.292 ± 0.05 SE	Canada	[26]
Preterm newborns ($n = 17$), under 20 hrs of age*, 1–3 days of age**, and 10 days to 7 weeks of age	0.42 to 1.2	0.06 ± 0.05* 0.09 ± 0.05** 0.26 ± 0.05	—	France	[27]

The use of ** and * is associated with ages of newborns shown to the left, in column 1.

TABLE 4: Estimated secretion rates of thyroxine (T4) and total and free serum concentrations of T4 in infants, children, and adults.

Subject	T4 secretion μg/kg/day	Serum TSH mIU/L	Serum total T4 (nmol/L)/ Serum free T4 (pmol/L)	Reference
Adults	1.5	0.4 to 4.2	55–161/12–32	[28]
	0.75	—	—	[29]
Infant age				
1 to 4 days	10	1 to 39	142–277/28–68	[28]
7 to 28 days	7	1.7 to 9.1	106–221/12–30	[28]
1 to 12 months	6	0.8 to 8.2	76–210/10–23	[28]
Child age				
1 to 15 years	3 to 5	0.7 to 5.7	54–193/10–26	[28]
3 to 9 years	1.29	—	—	[29]

In conclusion, the infant and child homeostatic control of the HPT axis is very different than in the adult. Therefore, when considering the protection of infants and children from the harmful effects of thyroidal radiation, the age-dependent changes in physiology and the dynamic nature of the HPT axis need to be accounted for in estimating thyroidal radioiodine dosimetry.

2.6. KI Treatment (Table 5). Safety concerns have been expressed regarding KI administration to infants and children while also ensuring adequate protection from radioiodine exposure [59]. The effectiveness of KI to reduce systemic radioiodide uptake into the thyroid gland in a clinical environment is inferred by evaluating the reduction in fractional RAIU. The use of KI in the young requires special consideration. The pharmacokinetic profiles for iodide are age-dependent, in part, because of physiological differences, but more importantly, the HPT axis differences between the infant and child and the adult are pronounced as discussed above.

Chronic treatment with iodine for goiter has caused hyperthyroidism [59]. Hypothyroidism has also occurred from chronic treatment with iodine and is associated with autoimmunity [59]. Spallek et al. reviewed the results of adverse effects from repeated doses with KI, iodide deficient population sensitivities to iodine, case studies of adverse

TABLE 5: Inhibition of radioactive iodide uptake (RAIU) into the thyroid gland by potassium or sodium iodide in children and adults.

Subject, KI dose (mg)	RAIU (% thyroidal radiotracer dose)	RAIU inhibition (% of radiotracer dose)	Reference location
Adult	*30 hr RAIU*	*RAIU % inhibition*	
247 ($n = 1$)	38	100 at 30 hr, 16 at 5 days	
124 ($n = 1$)	45	96 at 30 hr, 22 at 5 days	[30]
37 ($n = 1$)	44	86 at 30 hr, 16 at 3 days	England
25 ($n = 1$)	39	97 at 30 hr	
5 ($n = 1$)	52	54 at 30 hr	
Adult	*24 hr RAIU*	*24 hr RAIU % inhibition*	
10 ($n = 5$)	19.4	36	
30 ($n = 15$)	19.4 to 22.6	93 to 96	[16]
50 ($n = 5$)	19.7	92	United States
100 ($n = 5$)	17.2	96	
Adult, NaI	*24 hr RAIU*	*24 hr RAIU inhibition*	
5 ($n = 1$)	33	78	
25 ($n = 1$)	41	96	
50 ($n = 1$)	28	97	[31]
100 ($n = 13$)	28.6	97.8	United States
200 ($n = 10$)	25.9	98.5	
1000 ($n = 1$)	19	99.0	
Adult (hyperthyroidism)	*24 hr RAIU*	*24 hr RAIU inhibition*	
50 ($n = 8$ for both doses)		73.3	[32]
100	65.3 for 8 patients	79.5	Japan
Children	*1-2 day RAIU*	*24 hr RAIU inhibition*	[15]
1.8 ($n = 2, 8,$ and 9 years of age)	21 and 25	33 and 48	United States
Children ($n = 5$, 2 years of age)	*24 hr RAIU*	*24 hr RAIU % inhibition*	
0.3	≈15 to 25	≈20 to 55	[12]
0.6	≈15 to 25	≈47 to 67	United States

effects, and the use of KI in Poland after the Chernobyl nuclear power plant accident [59]. They concluded that newborns and young children are most vulnerable to radioiodines and are also the group who experience a low frequency of adverse effects from KI. The adverse health risks from KI depend on nutritional iodine status. Iodine deficiency is a risk factor. However, the authors state that KI is an underrepresented research topic. Thus, the safe use of KI warrants more attention, particularly in infants.

The blocking effects of stable iodide salts (KI or sodium iodide (NaI)) on RAIU have been evaluated in adult human clinical studies, but clinical studies in children or infants are limited [60]. Ramsden et al. evaluated a few adult individuals with doses of 5 to 247 mg KI (Table 4) and reported greater than 86% RAIU inhibition at 30 hr for all doses except for the 5 mg KI (54% RAIU inhibition) [30]. At 3 or 5 days after dosing, the percent of RAIU inhibition was 16 to 22%. In another study [31] (Table 5) using several adult volunteers, 100 or 200 mg NaI was administered together with tracer radioiodine resulting in average 24 hr RAIU inhibition values ranging from 98 to 99% for both NaI doses. The RAIU inhibition drops to 50% if NaI was administered 3 hr after exposure to radioiodine. The effectiveness of NaI drops substantially after radioiodine is administered because

the thyroidal radioiodide is organified (iodination of thyroglobulin) and stored in the thyroid gland. The iodinated thyroglobulin is transformed into thyroid hormones and slowly secreted from the thyroid gland in adults. The duration of effectiveness of a single dose is less than a day because of the renal clearance of iodide; thus, the authors recommend daily repeated doses of 100 to 200 mg NaI for radiation exposure situations exceeding one day. On a mg/kg body weight basis, this equates to 1.43 to 2.86 mg/kg KI administration for a 70 kg individual. These authors dosed a small number of individuals with other doses of KI (5, 25, 50, and 1000 mg) at the same time as administration of radioiodine. Although the study was not designed for dose-response assessment of KI, all doses were effective except for possibly the 5 mg of KI (RAIU inhibition value of 78%) (Table 5).

Sternthal et al. reported 24 hr RAIU inhibition values of over 92% for KI doses of 30, 50, and 100 mg and 36% RAIU inhibition for 10 mg KI (Table 4) [16]. In a more recent study, Hänscheid et al. reported 24 hr RAIU inhibition values of 64% for 7 individuals administered 100 mg KI 2 hr after administration of radioiodine [17]. The effectiveness of KI plummeted as the time interval was increased between administration of radioiodine and KI. Administration of KI before radioiodine administration was very effective, even 24 hr before administration of radioiodine. Takamura et al.

reported 24 hr RAIU inhibition values of 73 and 80% in 8 hyperthyroid individuals dosed with 50 and 100 mg of KI, respectively [32].

Data on the ability of KI to block thyroidal uptake of radioiodide is considerable in adults, including varying conditions for time intervals between exposure to radioiodines and administration of KI and repeated dosing with KI. KI is very effective at reducing the thyroid gland burden of radioiodines if the treatment is administered within hours as of the exposure to radioiodines. If radioiodine exposure is prolonged repeated treatment with KI may be advantageous. Dose adjustment of KI to account for body weight is probably not needed in healthy nonpregnant, nonlactating adults if kidney function and nutrition are normal (e.g., 130 mg KI [45]).

For pediatric populations, the minimum effective KI dosages required for newborns, infants, and children are less certain because of a lack of adequate clinical studies. A clinical children's study was conducted in the 1960s, during the cold war at a state hospital in the United States, to determine the minimal effective dose of NaI to protect their thyroid glands from radioactive iodide irradiation [12]. Unfortunately the details of the study and study results are sparsely reported. The dose-responses for NaI and RAIU values were reported as μg stable iodide per M^2 skin surface area per day. For five 2-year-old children, baseline 24 hr RAIU values were collected and then over 8 weeks of daily administration of 0.3 mg stable iodide four 24 hr RAIU values were collected before the stable iodide dose was increased to 0.6 mg for a 4-week period in the same children and two 24 hr RAIU values were collected. NaI administration was curtailed and a final RAIU value was determined 2 weeks after NaI administration. RAIU inhibition values ranged from approximately 20 to 55% during 8 weeks of daily doses of 0.3 mg stable iodide and near 47 to 67% during 4 weeks of daily administration of 0.6 mg stable iodide. To convert dosing units from mg/M^2 to body weight (mg/kg) Center for Disease Control and Prevention (CDC) body weight growth charts for children from the United States [61] were used to represent the possible range of body weights. A 5th percentile for a 2-year-old female child (lowest body weight) and a 95th percentile for a 2-year-old male child (largest body weight) were selected to represent the range of body weights of 2-year-old children reported in [12]. Surface area for different age groups per sex was taken from [62]. Three-tenths of one mg stable iodide/child (0.3 mg) equates to a stable iodide dose range of 0.03 to 0.02 mg/kg/day for a 2 yr infant and for 0.6 mg, 0.04 to 0.06 mg/kg/day.

Cuddihy reported that a KI dose of 1.8 mg repeated daily doses for 14 days in two children, 8 and 9 years old, resulted in 24 hr RAIU inhibitions of 33 and 48% [15], which would be for an estimated dose range of 0.05 to 0.06 mg/kg/day (using CDC growth charts). Noteboom et al. performed KI studies in infant chimpanzees as a surrogate for children. Six infant chimpanzees, aged two weeks to 2 years, had baseline RAIU values of 3.1 to 32.8%, with a mean value of 11.5% [63]. Mean RAIU inhibition at 24 hr for doses of 0.5 (n = 4), 1.5 (n = 3), and 5.0 mg/kg (n = 6) of KI was 74, 95, and 93%,

respectively. Body weights were not given for the infant chimpanzees; however assuming a weight range of 2 to 4 kg [64], this equates to doses of 1-2, 3–6, and 10–20 mg of KI, respectively, which resulted in 93 to 95% RAIU inhibition for the 1.5 and 5.0 mg/kg dose groups and 74% for the 0.5 mg/kg dose group.

Single KI doses were administered to 10.5 million children in Poland in response to the Chernobyl nuclear disaster. Newborns received 15 mg iodine, children under 5 years of age were given 50 mg iodine, and all other children were administered 70 mg iodine [65]. KI administration occurred days after the onset of exposure to radioactive iodines. In children of 5 years and younger, RAIU inhibition of inhaled and ingested radioactive iodide-131 (^{131}I) was estimated to range from 40 to 14%. The dose of KI for a newborn was approximately 6.7 to 3.5 mg/kg using a 5th percentile body weight for girls and 95th percentile body weights for boys in the United States. Less than 1% of newborns exhibited hypothyroidism (12 of 3214 babies) or increased serum TSH levels and decreased serum total thyroxine levels [65]. The predominant side effects for children were gastrointestinal (vomiting, stomach ache, and diarrhea), skin rashes, headache, and shortness of breath. Children under one year of age had the highest committed doses of thyroidal ^{131}I$^-$. An increased sensitivity of young children to thyroid cancer was observed [42, 43, 66], although the influence of iodine deficiency may be a contributing factor for thyroid cancer rates [67]. The proceedings from a workshop on iodine nutrition and radioactive iodide after Chernobyl incident state that, for a variety of reasons, it is difficult to determine the influence of iodide nutrition on the risks of thyroid cancer from exposure to radioactive iodine [44].

To better understand the effectiveness and safety of KI administration to infants and children more research is required, perhaps clinical studies. Alternatively, mathematical models have been developed to better understand radioiodine dosimetry in children. Compartmental mathematical models for predicting the dosimetry of radioiodide have existed for decades, primarily for adults [68]. More recently Zanzonico created a compartmental radioiodide model for children [69]. This nonphysiological model uses first order terms to account for age-dependent thyroidal uptake of radioiodide and secretion of organified radioiodide (thyroid hormone) from the thyroid gland. The model predicted that the mean ^{131}I$^-$ absorbed thyroidal dose in newborns is 26 times greater than adults. In another modeling study Jang et al. created a compartmental model for KI and radioiodide in children over 3 months of age [70]. These authors used first order terms to describe thyroidal uptake of stable iodide and radioiodide without considering age-dependent kinetic behavior. A first order term, describing secretion of organified radioiodide (thyroid hormone), was assumed to be age-dependent. The model predicted that KI would be equally effective at blocking thyroidal uptake of radioactive iodide for ages of 3 months to adulthood. Future modeling efforts, using physiological models [71] for the infant and child, and known information about the age-dependent physiology and the HPT axis (Tables 1 to 5) should provide useful insights into the effectiveness of KI as a drug to treat exposure to radioiodines.

2.7. What Do We Know about KI Dosing in Infants and Children? To protect people from radioiodines the US Food and Drug Administration [45] recommends a single oral dose of 16 mg KI for neonates from birth to 1 month of age (7.1 to 3.7 mg/kg KI for 5th percentile female body weight and 95% percentile male body weight), 32 mg KI (7.0 to 3.6 mg/kg KI) for infants 1 month of age to children 3 years of age, and 65 mg KI for children from 3 years of age to up to 18 years old (5.7 to 0.6 mg/kg KI). In the case of adults, 130 mg KI per day is recommended, averaging about 2 mg/kg. The recommended KI dosages for the infant and child, on a mg/kg basis, would typically be greater than for an adult.

The two repeated dosing KI studies in children with small doses of KI [12, 15] are not adequate to draw general conclusions about the safety and efficacy of single high dose KI administration in children. The studies do suggest that small doses of KI result in RAIU inhibition. Since infants and children have a hyperactive HPT axis (Tables 2, 3, and 4), the evaluation of the efficacy of KI in hyperthyroid adults is useful for speculating on the efficacy of KI in children. The baseline RAIU in hyperthyroid, iodide sufficient adults from Japan was 65% of the administered radioiodide dose, while in the United States euthyroid (iodide sufficient) adult baseline RAIU values ranged from 17 to 50% [9, 16, 31]. For hyperthyroid iodide sufficient children from the United States Fields et al. reported RAIU baseline values of 72 to 99%, while several authors report a wide range of baseline RAIU values (40 to 70%) for iodide sufficient euthyroid children (Table 2) [9]. Twenty-four hr RAIU inhibition values of 73 and 80% for KI doses of 50 and 100 mg were reported for iodide sufficient adult hyperthyroid Japanese subjects [32] and 94 to 99% for KI doses of 50 and 100 mg [16, 31] in iodide sufficient euthyroid adult volunteers from the United States.

These results demonstrate that KI is less effective at blocking thyroidal uptake of radioiodide if the HPT axis is hyperactive in adults. By analogy KI is expected to be less effective in infants and children with a "hyperactive HPT axis." The Poland experience, where very large numbers of children were administered doses of 15 to 50 mg KI, resulted in apparently low RAIU inhibition for children less than 5 years of age [65]. Interpreting this study is difficult because of confounding factors. These children may have been iodide deficient, which would further exacerbate the hyperactive HPT axis and further reduce the effectiveness of KI. Also the time lag from the onset of radioiodine exposure to KI treatment was probably detrimental, further reducing the effectiveness of KI. Interestingly the authors of the infant monkey KI study [63] suggest that a dose of at least 1.5 mg/kg (5.1 mg KI for a newborn human) is needed to protect the infant thyroid gland.

3. Recommendations

The US FDA recommended single KI doses for infants may effectively block radioiodides [45]. Clearly, more research is needed to better characterize the safety and effectiveness of KI in infants and children. Several issues need to be considered when addressing administration of KI in the young. A low incidence of thyroid and nonthyroid related side effects may occur. The protective effect of KI will be for a shorter duration than in adults because of the hyperactive nature of the HPT axis. Stable iodide will be excreted into urine more quickly reducing the protective effect of KI. The amount of thyroidal iodide stores is much less in infants than adults. The half-life of organified iodide in the thyroid gland of children (~2.5 or 3 days) is less than the radionuclide decay half-life of ^{131}I (8 days), which is not the case in adults. Thus, radioactive thyroid hormones would be secreted from the thyroid gland and distributed into the body. Radioiodide derived from deiodination of radioactive thyroid hormones would be secreted in urine or recycled back into the thyroid gland, increasing the duration of systemic radioiodide. As the lag time from radioiodine exposure to administration of KI increases, the effectiveness of KI would be expected to decrease at a faster rate than in adults because of the hyperactive nature of the HPT axis, raising an important question about "single versus multiple doses of KI." The iodide nutritional status of the sensitive population is expected to alter the effectiveness of KI.

To conduct KI clinical trials in children seems unattainable; however, the Presidential Commission of Bioethical Issues did recently provide research guidelines to the Secretary of Health and Human Services for considering medical countermeasure pediatric trails for an anthrax vaccine [72]. Preevent pediatric testing of medical countermeasures may be carried out by clinical trials using age deescalation, coupled with previous informative research endeavors such as mathematical modeling, toxicity testing of laboratory animals, and adult human studies.

With over 100 operational nuclear reactors in the USA, continued planning and reevaluation for the possible use for KI is prudent. Advanced research methods for toxicity testing and computational modeling of the thyroid system [71, 73–76] and extrapolation tools [77] can provide useful quantitative predictions of pediatric KI doses which will maximize the blocking effect of KI while protecting against adverse outcomes from KI. These research findings can then be compared to existing recommended pediatric KI doses to ensure the safety of children.

Disclosure

This paper does not necessarily reflect the views of the United States Food and Drug Administration. The authors thank Igor Pogribny, William Tolleson, and Fred Beland for reviewing this paper.

References

[1] G. G. Cayler, A. M. Rudolph, and A. S. Nadas, "Systemic blood flow in infants and children with and without heart disease," *Pediatrics*, vol. 32, no. 2, pp. 186–201, 1963.

[2] G. F. Sholler, "Echo Doppler assessment of cardiac output and its relation to growth in normal infants [correction]," *The American Journal of Cardiology*, vol. 61, no. 10, p. 872, 1988.

[3] K. Price, S. Haddad, and K. Krishnan, "Physiological modeling of age-specific changes in the pharmacokinetics of organic chemicals in children," *Journal of Toxicology and Environmental Health A*, vol. 66, no. 5, pp. 417–433, 2003.

[4] M. I. Rubin, E. Bruck, M. Rapoport, M. Snively, H. McKay, and A. Baumler, "Maturation of renal function in childhood: clearance studies," *The Journal of Clinical Investigation*, vol. 28, no. 5, part 2, pp. 1144–1162, 1949.

[5] A. N. Edginton, W. Schmitt, and S. Willmann, "Development and evaluation of a generic physiologically based pharmacokinetic model for children," *Clinical Pharmacokinetics*, vol. 45, no. 10, pp. 1013–1034, 2006.

[6] R. P. Brown, M. D. Delp, S. L. Lindstedt, L. R. Rhomberg, and R. P. Beliles, "Physiological parameter values for physiologically based pharmacokinetic models," *Toxicology and Industrial Health*, vol. 13, no. 4, pp. 407–484, 1997.

[7] S. Haddad, C. Restieri, and K. Krishnan, "Characterization of age-related changes in body weight and organ weights from birth to adolescence in humans," *Journal of Toxicology and Environmental Health A*, vol. 64, no. 6, pp. 453–464, 2001.

[8] C. Kay, S. Abrahams, and P. McClain, "The weight of normal thyroid glands in children," *Archives of Pathology*, vol. 82, no. 4, pp. 349–352, 1966.

[9] T. Fields, R. M. Kohlenbrener, R. H. Kunstadter, and L. Oliner, "Thyroid function studies in children: normal values for thyroidal I^{131} uptake and PBI^{131} levels up to the age of 18," *The Journal of Clinical Endocrinology & Metabolism*, vol. 17, no. 1, pp. 61–75, 1957.

[10] L. van Middlesworth, "Radioactive iodide uptake of normal newborn infants," *The American Journal of Diseases of Children*, vol. 88, no. 4, pp. 439–442, 1954.

[11] E. E. Martmer, "Radioactive iodine uptake studies in premature infants, preliminary report," *Harper Hospital Bulletin*, vol. 13, no. 3, pp. 108–111, 1955.

[12] K. M. Saxena, E. M. Chapman, and C. V. Pryles, "Minimal dosage of iodide required to suppress uptake of iodine-131 by normal thyroid," *Science*, vol. 138, no. 3538, pp. 430–431, 1962.

[13] P. Malvaux, C. Beckers, and M. Devissher, "Dynamic studies on the inorganic iodine compartment and its exchanges during adolescence," *The Journal of Clinical Endocrinology & Metabolism*, vol. 25, no. 6, pp. 817–822, 1965.

[14] Y. Ingenbleek and C. Beckers, "Thyroidal iodide clearance and radioiodide uptake in protein-calorie malnutrition," *The American Journal of Clinical Nutrition*, vol. 31, no. 3, pp. 408–415, 1978.

[15] R. G. Cuddihy, "Thyroidal iodine-131 uptake, turnover and blocking in adults and adolescents," *Health Physics*, vol. 12, no. 8, pp. 1021–1025, 1966.

[16] E. Sternthal, L. Lipworth, and B. Stanley, "Suppression of thyroid radioiodine uptake by various doses of stable iodide," *The New England Journal of Medicine*, vol. 303, no. 19, pp. 1083–1088, 1980.

[17] H. Hänscheid, C. Reiners, G. Goulko et al., "Facing the nuclear threat: thyroid blocking revisited," *The Journal of Clinical Endocrinology & Metabolism*, vol. 96, no. 11, pp. 3511–3516, 2011.

[18] M. A. Greer, G. Goodman, R. C. Pleus, and S. E. Greer, "Health effects assessment for environmental perchlorate contamination: the dose response for inhibition of thyroidal radioiodine uptake in humans," *Environmental Health Perspectives*, vol. 110, no. 9, pp. 927–937, 2002.

[19] G. Ponchon, C. Beckers, and M. de Visscher, "Iodide kinetic studies in newborns and infants," *The Journal of Clinical Endocrinology & Metabolism*, vol. 26, no. 12, pp. 1392–1394, 1966.

[20] J. Zabala, N. Carrión, M. Murillo et al., "Determination of normal human intrathyroidal iodine in Caracas population," *Journal of Trace Elements in Medicine and Biology*, vol. 23, no. 1, pp. 9–14, 2009.

[21] V. Zaichick and S. Zaichick, "Normal human intrathyroidal iodine," *Science of The Total Environment*, vol. 206, no. 1, pp. 39–56, 1997.

[22] D. A. Fisher and T. H. Oddie, "Thyroid iodine content and turnover in euthyroid subjects: validity of estimation of thyroid iodine accumulation from short-term clearance studies," *The Journal of Clinical Endocrinology & Metabolism*, vol. 29, no. 5, pp. 721–727, 1969.

[23] A. Costa, V. de Filippis, and M. Panizzo, "Development of thyroid function between VI-IX month of fetal life in humans," *Journal of Endocrinological Investigation*, vol. 9, no. 4, pp. 273–280, 1986.

[24] S. Savin, D. Cvejić, O. Nedić, and R. Radosavljević, "Thyroid hormone synthesis and storage in the thyroid gland of human neonates," *The Journal of Pediatric Endocrinology & Metabolism*, vol. 16, no. 4, pp. 521–528, 2003.

[25] F. Delange, "The disorders induced by iodine deficiency," *Thyroid*, vol. 4, no. 1, pp. 107–128, 1994.

[26] F. Delange, "Screening for congenital hypothyroidism used as an indicator of the degree of iodine deficiency and of its control," *Thyroid*, vol. 8, no. 12, pp. 1185–1192, 1998.

[27] N. Etling, "Concentration of thyroglobulin, iodine contents of thyroglobulin and of iodoaminoacids in human neonates thyroid glands," *Acta Paediatrica Scandinavica*, vol. 66, no. 1, pp. 97–102, 1977.

[28] D. A. Fisher, "Physiological variations in thyroid hormones: physiological and pathophysiological considerations," *Clinical Chemistry*, vol. 42, no. 1, pp. 135–139, 1996.

[29] H. M. Haddad, "Rates of I^{131}-labeled thyroxine metabolism in euthyroid children," *The Journal of Clinical Investigation*, vol. 39, no. 10, pp. 1590–1594, 1960.

[30] D. Ramsden, F. H. Passant, C. O. Peabody, and R. G. Speight, "Radioiodine uptakes in the thyroid. Studies of the blocking and subsequent recovery of the gland following the administration of stable iodine," *Health Physics*, vol. 13, no. 6, pp. 633–646, 1967.

[31] M. Blum and M. Eisenbud, "Reduction of thyroid irradiation from 131-I by potassium iodide," *The Journal of the American Medical Association*, vol. 200, no. 12, pp. 1036–1040, 1967.

[32] N. Takamura, Y. Nakamura, K. Ishigaki et al., "Thyroid blockade during a radiation emergency in iodine-rich areas: effect of a stable-iodine dosage," *Journal of Radiation Research*, vol. 45, no. 2, pp. 201–204, 2004.

[33] C. Reiners and R. Schneider, "Potassium iodide (KI) to block the thyroid from exposure to I-131: current questions and answers to be discussed," *Radiation and Environmental Biophysics*, vol. 52, no. 2, pp. 189–193, 2013.

[34] L. K. Bustad, D. H. Wood, E. E. Elefson, H. A. Ragan, and R. O. McClellan, "I^{131} in milk and thyroid of dairy cattle following a single contamination event and prolonged daily administration," *Health Physics*, vol. 9, no. 12, pp. 1231–1234, 1963.

[35] R. O. McClellan, W. J. Clarke, H. A. Ragan, D. H. Wood, and L. K. Bustad, "Comparative effects of I^{131} and X-irradiation on sheep thyroids," *Health Physics*, vol. 9, no. 12, pp. 1363–1368, 1963.

[36] L. K. Bustad, R. O. McClellan, and R. J. Garner, "The significance of radionuclide contamination in ruminants," in *Proceedings of the 2nd International Symposium on the Physiology of Digestion in the Ruminant*, R. W. Dougherty, Ed., Butterworth's, Washington, DC, USA, 1965.

[37] D. H. Wood, E. E. Elefson, V. G. Horstman, and L. K. Bustad, "Thyroid uptake of radioiodine following various routes of administration," *Health Physics*, vol. 9, no. 12, pp. 1217–1220, 1963.

[38] C. A. Adams and J. A. Bonnell, "Administration of stable odide as a means of reducing thyroid irradiation resulting from inhalation of radioactive iodine," *Health Physics*, vol. 7, no. 3-4, pp. 127–149, 1962.

[39] J. Wolff and I. L. Chaikoff, "Plasma inorganic iodide, a chemical regulator of normal thyroid function," *Endocrinology*, vol. 42, no. 6, pp. 468–471, 1948.

[40] C. Serrano-Nascimento, J. Calil-Silveira, and M. T. Nunes, "Posttranscriptional regulation of sodium-iodide symporter mRNA expression in the rat thyroid gland by acute iodide administration," *American Journal of Physiology: Cell Physiology*, vol. 298, no. 4, pp. C893–C899, 2010.

[41] P. B. Zanzonico and D. V. Becker, "Effects of time of administration and dietary iodine levels on potassium iodide (KI) blockade of thyroid irradiation by ^{131}I from radioactive fallout," *Health Physics*, vol. 78, no. 6, pp. 660–667, 2000.

[42] NAS, Committee to Assess the Distribution and Administration of Potassium Iodide in the Event of a Nuclear Incident, National Research Council, *Distribution and Administration of Potassium Iodide in the Event of a Nuclear Incident*, National Academies Press, Washington, DC, USA, 2004.

[43] L. B. Zablotska, E. Ron, A. V. Rozhko et al., "Thyroid cancer risk in Belarus among children and adolescents exposed to radioiodine after the Chornobyl accident," *British Journal of Cancer*, vol. 104, no. 1, pp. 181–187, 2011.

[44] J. Robbins, J. T. Dunn, A. Bouville et al., "Iodine nutrition and the risk from radioactive iodine: a workshop report in the chernobyl long-term follow-up study," *Thyroid*, vol. 11, no. 5, pp. 487–491, 2001.

[45] USFDA, "Potassium Iodide as a Thyroid Blocking Agent in Radiation Emergencies," 2001, http://www.fda.gov/downloads/Drugs/.../Guidances/ucm080542.pdf.

[46] G. Ginsberg, D. Hattis, R. Miller, and B. Sonawane, "Pediatric pharmacokinetic data: implications for environmental risk assessment for children," *Pediatrics*, vol. 113, no. 4, pp. 973–983, 2004.

[47] N. Chen, K. Aleksa, C. Woodland, M. Rieder, and G. Koren, "Ontogeny of drug elimination by the human kidney," *Pediatric Nephrology*, vol. 21, no. 2, pp. 160–168, 2006.

[48] S. N. de Wildt, G. L. Kearns, J. S. Leeder, and J. N. van den Anker, "Cytochrome P450 3A: ontogeny and drug disposition," *Clinical Pharmacokinetics*, vol. 37, no. 6, pp. 485–505, 1999.

[49] A. M. Leung, L. E. Braverman, X. He, T. Heeren, and E. N. Pearce, "Breastmilk iodine concentrations following acute dietary iodine intake," *Thyroid*, vol. 22, no. 11, pp. 1176–1180, 2012.

[50] D. A. Fisher, T. H. Oddie, and D. Epperson, "Effect of increased dietary iodide on thyroid accumulation and secretion in euthyroid Arkansas subjects," *The Journal of Clinical Endocrinology & Metabolism*, vol. 25, no. 12, pp. 1580–1590, 1965.

[51] B. S. Arant Jr., "Developmental patterns of renal functional maturation compared in the human neonate," *Journal of Pediatrics*, vol. 92, no. 5, pp. 705–712, 1978.

[52] R. Čukuranović; and S. Vlajković, "Age related anatomical and functional characteristics of human kidney," *Facta Universitatis*, vol. 12, no. 2, pp. 61–69, 2005.

[53] T. H. Oddie, J. H. Meade Jr., J. Myhill, and D. A. Fisher, "Dependence of renal clearance of radioiodide on sex, age and thyroidal status," *The Journal of Clinical Endocrinology & Metabolism*, vol. 26, no. 12, pp. 1293–1296, 1966.

[54] IOM, "Dietary reference intakes for vitamin A, vitamin K, arsenic, boron, chromium, copper, iodine, iron, manganese, molybdenum, nickel, silicon, vanadium, and zinc," A Report of the Panel on Micronutrients, Subcommittees on Upper Reference Levels of Nutrients and of Interpretation and Uses of Dietary Reference Intakes, and the Standing Committee on the Scientific Evaluation of Dietary Reference Intakes. Food and Nutrition Board, Institute of Medicine, National Academy Press, Washington, DC, USA, 2001.

[55] C. W. Murray, S. K. Egan, H. Kim, N. Beru, and P. M. Bolger, "US food and drug administration's total diet study: dietary intake of perchlorate and iodine," *Journal of Exposure Science & Environmental Epidemiology*, vol. 18, no. 6, pp. 571–580, 2008.

[56] B. C. Blount, D. Q. Rich, L. Valentin-Blasini et al., "Perinatal exposure to perchlorate, thiocyanate, and nitrate in New Jersey mothers and newborns," *Environmental Science & Technology*, vol. 43, no. 19, pp. 7543–7549, 2009.

[57] T. Zhang, Q. Wu, H. W. Sun, J. Rao, and K. Kannan, "Perchlorate and iodide in whole blood samples from infants, children, and adults in Nanchang, China," *Environmental Science & Technology*, vol. 44, no. 18, pp. 6947–6953, 2010.

[58] D. A. Fisher and T. H. Oddie, "Neonatal thyroidal hyperactivity. Response to cooling," *The American Journal of Diseases of Children*, vol. 107, no. 6, pp. 574–581, 1964.

[59] L. Spallek, L. Krille, C. Reiners, R. Schneider, S. Yamashita, and H. Zeeb, "Adverse effects of iodine thyroid blocking: a systematic review," *Radiation Protection Dosimetry*, vol. 150, no. 3, pp. 267–277, 2012.

[60] P. Verger, A. Aurengo, B. Geoffroy, and B. le Guen, "Iodine kinetics and effectiveness of stable iodine prophylaxis after intake of radioactive iodine: a review," *Thyroid*, vol. 11, no. 4, pp. 353–360, 2001.

[61] R. J. Kuczmarski, C. L. Ogden, S. S. Guo et al., "2000 CDC Growth Charts for the United States: methods and development," *Vital and Health Statistics. Series 11*, no. 246, pp. 1–190, 2002.

[62] I. Sharkey, A. V. Boddy, H. Wallace, J. Mycroft, R. Hollis, and S. Picton, "Body surface area estimation in children using weight alone: application in paediatric oncology," *British Journal of Cancer*, vol. 85, no. 1, pp. 23–28, 2001.

[63] J. L. Noteboom et al., "Protection of the infant thyroid from radioactive contamination by the administration of stable iodide. An experimental evaluation in chimpanzees," *Radiation Research*, vol. 147, no. 6, pp. 698–706, 1997.

[64] Y. Hamada, T. Udono, M. Teramoto, and T. Sugawara, "The growth pattern of chimpanzees: somatic growth and reproductive maturation in *Pan troglodytes*," *Primates*, vol. 37, no. 3, pp. 279–295, 1996.

[65] J. Nauman and J. Wolff, "Iodide prophylaxis in Poland after the chernobyl reactor accident: benefits and risks," *The American Journal of Medicine*, vol. 94, no. 5, pp. 524–532, 1993.

[66] G. A. Thomas, J. A. Bethel, A. Galpine, W. Mathieson, M. Krznaric, and K. Unger, "Integrating research on thyroid cancer after chernobyl—the chernobyl tissue bank," *Clinical Oncology*, vol. 23, no. 4, pp. 276–281, 2011.

[67] E. Cardis, A. Kesminiene, V. Ivanov et al., "Risk of thyroid cancer after exposure to ^{131}I in childhood," *Journal of the National Cancer Institute*, vol. 97, no. 10, pp. 724–732, 2005.

[68] D. S. Riggs, "Quantitative aspects of iodine metabolism in man," *Pharmacological reviews*, vol. 4, no. 3, pp. 284–370, 1952.

[69] P. B. Zanzonico, "Age-dependent thyroid absorbed doses for radiobiologically significant radioisotopes of iodine," *Health Physics*, vol. 78, no. 1, pp. 60–67, 2000.

[70] M. Jang, H. K. Kim, C. W. Choi, and C. S. Kang, "Age-dependent potassium iodide effect on the thyroid irradiation by ^{131}I and ^{133}I in the nuclear emergency," *Radiation Protection Dosimetry*, vol. 130, no. 4, pp. 499–502, 2008.

[71] A. Lumen, D. R. Mattie, and J. W. Fisher, "Evaluation of perturbations in serum thyroid hormones during human pregnancy due to dietary iodide and perchlorate exposure using a biologically based dose-response model," *Toxicological Sciences*, vol. 133, no. 2, pp. 320–341, 2013.

[72] A. Gutmann, "Safeguarding children—pediatric research on medical countermeasures," *The New England Journal of Medicine*, vol. 368, no. 13, pp. 1171–1173, 2013.

[73] E. A. Merrill, R. A. Clewell, P. J. Robinson et al., "PBPK model for radioactive iodide and perchlorate kinetics and perchlorate-induced inhibition of iodide uptake in humans," *Toxicological Sciences*, vol. 83, no. 1, pp. 25–43, 2005.

[74] E. D. McLanahan, P. White, L. Flowers, and P. M. Schlosser, "The use of PBPK models to inform human health risk assessment: case study on perchlorate and radioiodide human lifestage models," *Risk Analysis*, vol. 34, no. 2, pp. 356–366, 2014.

[75] E. D. McLanahan, M. E. Andersen, J. L. Campbell Jr., and J. W. Fisher, "Competitive inhibition of thyroidal uptake of dietary iodide by perchlorate does not describe perturbations in rat serum total T4 and TSH," *Environmental Health Perspectives*, vol. 117, no. 5, pp. 731–738, 2009.

[76] P. Ekerot, D. Ferguson, E.-L. Glämsta et al., "Systems pharmacology modeling of drug-induced modulation of thyroid hormones in dogs and translation to human," *Pharmaceutical Research*, vol. 30, no. 6, pp. 1513–1524, 2013.

[77] A. Kleensang, A. Maertens, M. Rosenberg et al., "t4 workshop report: pathways of toxicity," *ALTEX*, vol. 31, no. 1, pp. 53–61, 2014.

20

Extralaryngeal Terminal Division of the Inferior Laryngeal Nerve: Anatomical Classification by a Surgical Point of View

Emin Gurleyik

Department of Surgery, Duzce University, Medical Faculty, 81650 Duzce, Turkey

Correspondence should be addressed to Emin Gurleyik; egurleyik@yahoo.com

Academic Editor: Gary L. Francis

Background. Complete anatomic knowledge including all variations of the inferior laryngeal nerve (ILN) is mandatory for thyroid surgeon. Extralaryngeal terminal division (ETD) of the ILN has significant importance for the safety of thyroidectomy. *Material and Methods.* Surgical dissection of 200 ILNs was performed on 100 cases. The presence of ETD of the nerve was determined intraoperatively. We propose by a surgical point of view a regional (segmental) classification of ETD of the ILN along its cervical course. *Results.* ETD has been observed in 54/200 nerves (27%). Great majority are bifurcated nerves (trifurcation 2%). Four types of ETD are classified. In type 1 (arterial; 46.3%), ETD has occurred near inferior thyroid artery (ITA). In type 2 (postarterial; 31.5%), division has been found on postarterial segment. In type 3 (prelaryngeal; 11%), division has been located very close to laryngeal entry point. In type 4 (prearterial; 11%), ETD has occurred before the nerve crossing the ITA. *Conclusions.* ETD of the ILN is a common anatomical variation. The bifurcation occurs in the ILN at various distances from laryngeal entry point. The classification increasing surgeons' awareness may help to simplify identification and exposure of terminal branches. Preservation of both extralaryngeal terminal branches of the ILN has paramount importance for the safety of thyroid operations.

1. Introduction

The safety of thyroid operations mainly depends on complete anatomic knowledge of the inferior laryngeal nerve (ILN) including all its variations. The nerve has many anatomic variations along its expected and unexpected cervical course. The important one is cervical (extralaryngeal) branching of the nerve. The presence of many branches and sensory innervations of adjacent tissues by thin branches of ILN has been reported up to 90%. These branches have been established by anatomical studies under direct or microscopic observation [1, 2]. These thin neural structures are not generally perceived during surgery of the thyroid. Therefore, these branches are important scientific knowledge by anatomical point of view but not by surgical point. On the other hand, extralaryngeal terminal division (bifurcation) of the ILN is

an anatomic variation macroscopically discovered during operations along cervical course of the nerve. The terminally bifurcated nerve has usually two larger branches which have same or closer size as diameter. Larger branches of the nerve may have significant effect on function of laryngeal musculature. The thyroid surgeon must carefully expose and preserve the integrity of both terminal branches if present. Therefore, macroscopic terminal division of the nerve seems to carry great importance by surgical point of view.

In this study, we aim to establish the rate of anatomical features and location of division along cervical course of the nerve and surgical importance of extralaryngeal terminal bifurcation of the ILN in series of thyroidectomy cases. We try to classify anatomical location of division point on the cervical course of the nerve.

2. Patients and Methods

A prospective study on surgical anatomy of the ILN was conducted on 100 patients with surgical diseases of the thyroid gland between May 2009 and September 2012. Patients with reoperative surgery for treatment of recurrent diseases were not included. Total thyroidectomy is the surgical procedure in all these 100 patients. All operations were performed by a single surgeon in order to provide a standard dissection. Main subjects of this study are the presence and incidence of extralaryngeal terminal division of the nerve which are macroscopically observed. Location of this division along cervical course of the ILN is determined. Lateral sides (unilaterally right or left, or bilateral) of the terminal division are also noted during thyroid operations.

2.1. The Dissection Technique of ILN. After freeing and medially mobilizing lateral lobes of the thyroid gland at both sides with classical surgical approach, the inferior thyroid arteries (ITA) were identified, isolated, and a loop of silk suture was placed around arteries for traction. With usual lateral approach, ILNs were identified below the artery and fully isolated at both sides. The nerve is carefully exposed in the trachea-esophageal groove until its laryngeal entry point. The dissection is performed using binocular loupe. If macroscopically and clearly delineated terminal divisions of the nerve are identified along its cervical course, we study anatomical features of these branches.

2.2. Extralaryngeal Terminal Division of the ILN. Division of the ILN occurs along its cervical course prior to laryngeal entry. The branches are macroscopically observed during thyroid operations, and they enter separately into the larynx by different points.

2.3. Classification of Terminal Division of the Nerve. We propose a regional (segmental) classification of extralaryngeal terminal division of the ILN along its cervical course. The classification is based on surgical exposition steps of the entire nerve and on the rate of different location of the bifurcation point. Risk regions for injury to the nerve are also taken into account for classification of extralaryngeal bifurcation of the ILN by surgical point of view. Regions and anatomical location of terminal division is classified basing on two relatively constant landmarks; the neurovascular (ILN and ITA) crossing point and laryngeal entry point of the nerve (Table 1; Figure 1).

3. Results

Results were obtained from surgical dissection of 100 consecutive total thyroidectomy cases. Two hundred ILNs were identified, isolated, and entirely exposed along their cervical courses until the laryngeal entry. Seventy-seven percent of our patients are females. The incidence and anatomic features of extralaryngeal terminal division of the ILN are the main subject of the study.

TABLE 1: Classification of anatomical location of terminal division point of the ILN*.

Type	Region	Definition
1	Arterial	Division occurs at or closely adjacent (± 5 mm) to neurovascular crossing of the ILN and the ITA*.
2	Postarterial	Division occurs in the first (proximal) half of the distance between neurovascular crossing and laryngeal entry point of the ILN.
3	Prelaryngeal	Division occurs in the second (distal) half of the distance between neurovascular crossing and laryngeal entry point of the ILN.
4	Prearterial	Division occurs before (proximal to) neurovascular crossing of the ILN and the ITA.

*ILN: inferior laryngeal nerve. ITA: inferior thyroid artery.

Extralaryngeal terminal divisions of ILNs were determined in 43 (43%) patients. We observed bilateral division in 11 (11%) patients. Extralaryngeal terminal division has been macroscopically observed in 54/200 nerves (27%). The rate of division of the ILN is 19% and 35% at right and left sides, respectively (Table 2).

The ILNs have been terminally trifurcated (divided by 3 branches) along their cervical courses in 4 (4%) patients unilaterally, 2 trifurcations at right or left sides each. This result reflects an incidence of trifurcation as 2% of exposed ILNs (Table 2; Figure 2).

The location of terminal division along cervical course of the nerve is another remarkable finding of the present study. The cervical course of the nerve is divided by four segments in which the neuro-vascular crossing (the ILN and the ITA) and laryngeal entry points are found as important landmarks for regional classification and location of terminal division of the nerve. Approximately half (46.3%) of the terminal division of the ILN has occurred in arterial region. Type 1 is a more common location of division point followed by Type 2. Type 3 (prelaryngeal) and Type 4 (prearterial) have seldom observed as location of terminal division of the ILN (Table 3). Intraoperative photos of various locations of terminal division point of the ILN show in vivo anatomic variations of the nerves (Figures 3, 4, 5, and 6).

4. Discussion

Microanatomic studies have shown that the ILN divides intralaryngeal branches to anastomose with branches of the internal laryngeal nerve. Size of these branches has been reported 0.6 mm as diameter [3]. When a surgeon macroscopically observes a single trunk nerve in its cervical course, it has intralaryngeal branches for connections of laryngeal nerves. Sometimes these branches have been exposed prior to laryngeal entry. Therefore, we can comment that extralaryngeal terminal division of the ILN is a premature branching of the nerve. By a surgical point of view, the awareness about

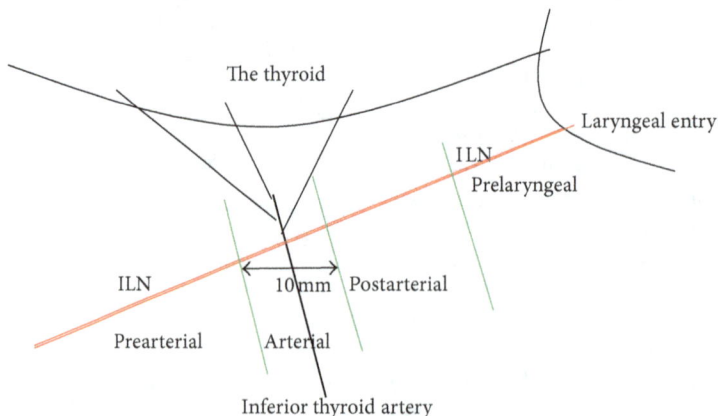

FIGURE 1: Segments in cervical course of the inferior laryngeal nerve (ILN).

TABLE 2: The rate and lateral site of terminal division (bifurcation) of the inferior laryngeal nerve.

	Cases	Division	Bilateral division	Division at right side	Division at left side
Total thyroidectomy	100	43 (43)*	11	8	24
Inferior laryngeal nerve Trifurcation	200	54 (27) 4 (2)		19 (19) 2 (2)	35 (35) 2 (2)
Sex (Female/male)	77/23	33/10		15/4	27/8

*Numbers in parentheses are percentages.

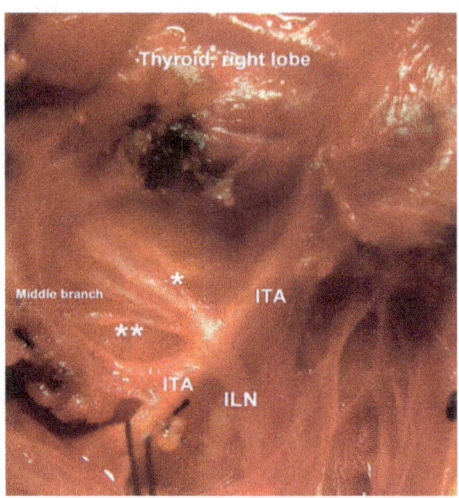

FIGURE 2: Extralaryngeal terminal *trifurcation* of the right ILN. Division of the nerve occurs at neurovascular crossing. *Anterior branch, **Posterior branch.

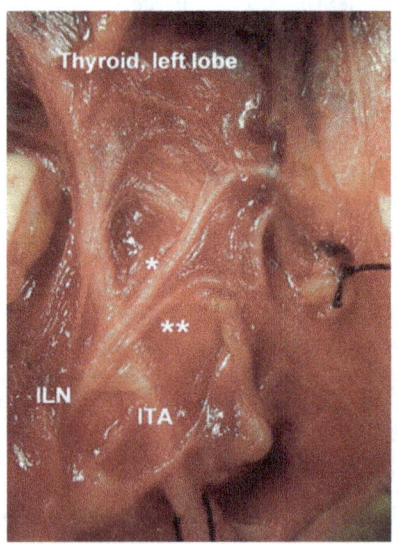

FIGURE 3: Terminal division of the left inferior laryngeal nerve (ILN) occurs at arterial segment (Type 1). *Anterior branch. **Posterior branch. ITA: inferior thyroid artery.

the occurrence of premature terminal division is important that exposing bifurcation and larger branches of the nerve separately prevent nerve injury during thyroid operations. In this study, we try to increase surgeons' awareness about this anatomic variation of the ILN by anatomically classifying the distribution of branching in its cervical course.

Complete exposure of ILN is mandatory to avoid nerve injury and laryngeal muscle palsy. Its anatomic variations threaten nerve integrity even in experienced hands. Our

rates (27% of ILNs) of macroscopically discovered extralaryngeal terminal division show that this is a common anatomic variation. Therefore, surgeons frequently encounter bifurcated nerve during thyroidectomy operations. Previous manuscripts have also reported the usualness of this variation [1, 2, 4, 5]. The incidence of bifurcated nerve has been reported between 18% and 43% [6–11]. Sometimes, we can

TABLE 3: The incidence of terminal division of the ILN according to anatomical classification.

Type	Regions	Definition	Right	Left	Total
1	Arterial	Division occurs at or closely adjacent to neurovascular crossing.	9 (47.4)*	16 (45.7)	25 (46.3)
2	Postarterial	Division occurs in the first (proximal) half of the distance between neurovascular crossing and laryngeal entry.	7 (36.8)	10 (28.6)	17 (31.5)
3	Prelaryngeal	Division occurs in the second (distal) half of the distance between neurovascular crossing and laryngeal entry.	2 (10.5)	4 (11.4)	6 (11.1)
4	Prearterial	Division occurs before (proximal to) neurovascular crossing.	1 (5.3)	5 (14.3)	6 (11.1)
			19 (100)	35 (100)	54 (100)

*Numbers in parentheses are percentages.

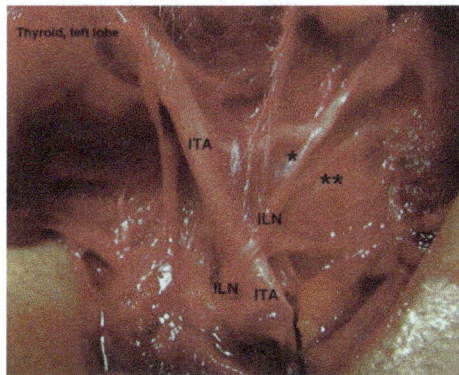

FIGURE 4: Terminal division of the left inferior laryngeal nerve (ILN) occurs at post-arterial segment (Type 2). *Anterior branch. **Posterior branch. ITA: inferior thyroid artery.

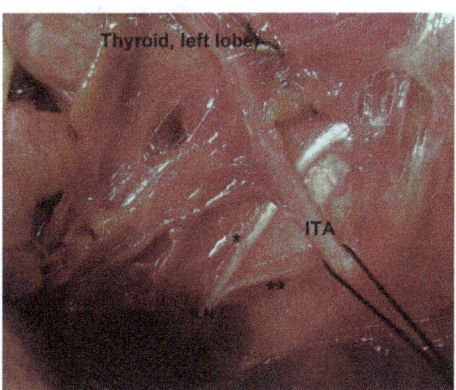

FIGURE 6: Terminal division of the left inferior laryngeal nerve (ILN) occurs at pre-arterial segment (Type 4). *Anterior branch. **Posterior branch. ITA: inferior thyroid artery.

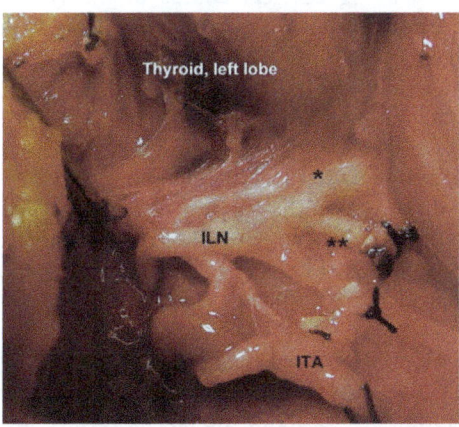

FIGURE 5: Terminal division of the left inferior laryngeal nerve (ILN) occurs at pre-laryngeal segment (Type 3). *Anterior branch. **Posterior branch. ITA: inferior thyroid artery.

unusually find three terminal branches of the ILN in its cervical course. Our incidence (2% of ILNs) of trifurcated nerve shows that ILN is rarely divided three terminal branches prior to its laryngeal entry. The mean incidence of terminal trifurcation of the ILN has also been reported approximately 2% (between 1% and 3.8%) in previous studies [6, 8, 10, 12]. The incidence of extralaryngeal terminal division of the ILN is high in which surgeons must strongly take into account the presence of this variation and be cautious exposing the ILN.

Terminal division of the nerve may occur unilaterally or bilaterally at both sides. We generally observed unilateral bifurcation of the ILN in which 75% of our patients have got unilateral variation. Bilateral terminal division of the ILN is relatively uncommon. Bilaterality of this variation has been observed in 11% of our thyroidectomy cases and in 25% of patients with bifurcated nerves. Extralaryngeal bilateral division of the nerve has been reported in a large range of incidence between 3, to 33% [6, 7, 9–11, 13]. In our series, the left ILN (35%) is more commonly bifurcated than the right one (19%). The report of Makay et al. [12] confirms this finding of higher rate at the left side. Based on anatomical knowledge, this is an expected result. The left nerve recurrent under aortic arch is longer than the right one which is recurrent under right subclavian artery. Therefore, extralaryngeal division of the longer nerve is more commonly expected than the shorter one. On the other hand, the majority of previous studies have reported equal or slightly higher incidence at the right side. The rate has been found as 23, to 59% at the right and 10, to 49% at the left side [6, 7, 9–11, 13]. Branched ILNs may represent a risk factor for nerve palsy. Knowledge of this anatomical variation and its routine investigation are essential. Surgeon's awareness of bifurcated ILN at both sides is required for the safety of thyroid operations.

In case of bifurcated ILN, anatomical location of division point along its cervical course is crucial in order to securely identify, to properly expose all branches of the nerve, and to protect nerve integrity without inadvertent injury to neural structures. In our study, we determined various locations of division point along the cervical course of the exposed ILN. Approximately in half (25/54) of the bifurcated nerves, the division occurs at or very close to nerve-artery crossing point. Bifurcation of the nerve just adjacent to neuro-vascular (the ILN and the ITA) crossing is the most common location of the division point of the ILN. The division of the nerve occurs distal to the ITA (after nerve-artery crossing) in approximately 1/3 of our cases in which this is found as the second common location along the cervical course of the nerve. Beside these two common findings, we also determined two other locations of the division point. The bifurcation of the nerve seldom occurs proximal to the ITA (before nerve-artery crossing). The division point is uncommonly observed very close to the laryngeal entry of the nerve.

We try to classify anatomic location of division point of the ILN along its cervical course aiming to increase surgeon's awareness. In order to establish an understandable classification some anatomic structures and surgical variables are taken into account.

(1) *Landmarks to delineate cervical segments along cervical course of the ILN*: two relatively constant landmarks (inferior thyroid artery and laryngeal entry point) help to divide cervical course of the nerve by four segments; pre-arterial, arterial, post-arterial, and pre-laryngeal.

(2) *Surgical technique to identify and expose the ILN*: the ILN is identified at close proximity of ITA by standard lateral approach technique. The nerve dissection begins in arterial region, and is proximally and distally advanced towards laryngeal entry in order to expose the entire nerve.

(3) *Rates of division of the nerve in various locations*: approximately half of nerve bifurcation occurs near ITA.

Therefore, anatomic landmarks, surgical technique of nerve identification and exposition, and location rates of division point contribute to the classification of extralaryngeal bifurcation. Extralaryngeal bifurcation of the ILN is a common variation which carries great importance for preservation of its motor function. We think that to be familiar with location of division point of the nerve in its cervical course is significantly helpful to avoid nerve injury. We propose an anatomical classification of extralaryngeal terminal division of the ILN. Terminal division of the nerve is classified by four types.

Type 1. The bifurcation occurs at or very close (−/+ 5 mm) to nerve-artery crossing point. The identification and dissection of the nerve generally begins at this point by standard lateral approach. In experienced hands, the nerve is easily found adjacent to the artery. Therefore, this type of bifurcation is also easily identifiable with careful dissection. This location is the most common type of nerve division in our series.

Both branches are individually followed until their separated laryngeal entry.

Type 2. After identification of the nerve trunk, the dissection is advanced in both distal and proximal direction in order to display entire cervical course of the ILN. In some patients, nerve bifurcation occurs distally to the artery, near Berry ligament. In our series, the rate of post-arterial (Type 2) division of the nerve is found approximately in one third of our patients with bifurcated nerve.

Type 3. During distal dissection of the ILN trunk, another type of bifurcation is discovered at the most distal part of the extralaryngeal ILN. Pre-laryngeal (Type 3) bifurcation occurs most distally just before laryngeal entry of the nerve. This distal part is generally covered by ligament of Berry and thyroidal tissue. This region where the nerve is more superficial is reported as the most dangerous site for nerve injury. If the bifurcation is not identified proximally (Types 1 and 2), surgeons are faced with a dangerous situation. Surgeons must be aware of this distal division of the ILN. If surgeons identify single trunk of the nerve at arterial region, the dissection is carefully advanced to distal part for possible pre-laryngeal bifurcation. This type of most distal bifurcation must take a strong place in surgeons mind in order to avoid a disaster after the operation. Fortunately, pre-laryngeal (Type 3) division of the nerve seldom occurs as 11% of our patients with bifurcated nerve.

Type 4. The dissection of the nerve is also advanced proximal to the artery along cervical course of the ILN. In some patients, bifurcation of the nerve is found at proximal segment of the nerve before artery crossing. Pre-arterial (Type 4) bifurcation which is found in 11% of our patients, is a relatively uncommon variation according to Types 1 and 2 division.

In case of bifurcation of the ILN, the location of motor fibers in nerve branches has extreme importance for preservation motor function. The motor fibers are located exclusively in the anterior branch, and the posterior branch is sensory in function [4, 7, 9, 11]. In some cases. posterior cricoarytenoid (PCA) muscles receive any kind of nerve fibers from posterior division of the ILN. These fibers contribute innervations of PCA muscle [14, 15]. On the other hand, Maranillo et al. [16] have reported that PCA muscles, the only abductor muscle of the larynx receive motor fiber from anterior division of the ILN.

Extralaryngeal terminal branches of the ILN can be a potential cause of nerve injury due to visual misidentification. This anatomical variation cannot be predicted preoperatively and might be associated with higher rate of nerve injury [17]. Extralaryngeal bifurcation of the ILN increases the risk of vocal cord palsy by two folds [18]. Recognition of bifurcation is crucial. Preservation of all branches is required for prevention of vocal cord palsy. We think that the most dangerous situation is misidentification and misinterpretation of relatively larger posterior branch as the main trunk of the nerve. In this situation, the anterior branch is under the greatest risk. Inadvertent division of motor fibers may lead to laryngeal muscles palsy despite the surgeon believing the nerve was preserved. In recent years intraoperative neural monitoring (IONM) assessing motor function of the nerve, helps surgeons to identify securely the ILN during thyroid surgery. IONM has gained widespread acceptance as an adjunct to visual nerve identification. Visual identification and a standard and uniform use of IONM facilitate to establish motor fibers of the nerve especially in high risk patients [19, 20]. Anatomical variations of the nerve including extralaryngeal division might be considered as high risk situations. Therefore, visual identification of the ILN and IONM may be extremely helpful for preserving motor function and preventing vocal cord palsy in case of bifurcated ILN.

5. Conclusion

Extralaryngeal terminal division of the ILN is a common anatomical variation.

The bifurcation occurs in different segment of the ILN along its cervical course at various distances from cricothyroid membrane (laryngeal entry point). In the majority of such cases, the point of division is located near arterial junction (ILN and ITA crossing point). On the other hand, surgeons must take into account that there are also uncommon locations of the bifurcation.

The anatomic classification of division point may increase surgeons' awareness of this variation. The classification may also lead to simplify identification and exposure of terminal branches.

The ILN must be macroscopically identified and preserved during thyroidectomy in order to prevent vocal cord palsy. Identification, exposure, and preservation of both extralaryngeal terminal branches of the ILN possess paramount importance in order to prevent nerve injury. Misidentification and misinterpretation of the posterior branch as the main trunk of the ILN put the anterior branch and motor fibers under the greatest risk. Inadvertent division of motor fibers may lead to laryngeal muscles palsy despite the surgeon believing the nerve was preserved.

References

[1] W. J. Tang, S. Q. Sun, X. L. Wang, Y. X. Sun, and H. X. Huang, "An applied anatomical study on the recurrent laryngeal nerve and inferior thyroid artery," *Surgical and Radiologic Anatomy*, vol. 34, no. 4, pp. 325–332, 2012.

[2] B. Yalçin, H. Tuğcu, N. Cantürk, and H. Ozan, "Laryngeal branching pattern of the inferior laryngeal nerve, before entering the larynx," *Surgical and Radiologic Anatomy*, vol. 28, no. 4, pp. 339–342, 2006.

[3] L. Naidu, L. Ramsaroop, P. Partab, and K. S. Satyapal, "Galen's "Anastomosis" revisited," *Clinical Anatomy*, vol. 25, no. 6, pp. 722–728, 2012.

[4] C. R. Cernea, F. V. C. Hojaij, D. de Carlucci Jr. et al., "Recurrent laryngeal nerve: a plexus rather than a nerve?" *Archives of Otolaryngology*, vol. 135, no. 11, pp. 1098–1102, 2009.

[5] T. Shao, W. Yang, T. Zhang et al., "A newly identified variation at the entry of the recurrent laryngeal nerve into the larynx," *Journal of Investigative Surgery*, vol. 23, no. 6, pp. 314–320, 2010.

[6] C. Casella, G. Pata, R. Nascimbeni, F. Mittempergher, and B. Salerni, "Does extralaryngeal branching have an impact on the rate of postoperative transient or permanent recurrent laryngeal nerve palsy?" *World Journal of Surgery*, vol. 33, no. 2, pp. 261–265, 2009.

[7] J. W. Serpell, M. J. Yeung, and S. Grodski, "The motor fibers of the recurrent laryngeal nerve are located in the anterior extralaryngeal branch," *Annals of Surgery*, vol. 249, no. 4, pp. 648–652, 2009.

[8] P. V. Pradeep, B. Jayashree, and S. S. Harshita, "A closer look at laryngeal nerves during thyroid surgery: a descriptive study of 584 nerves," *Anatomy Research International*, vol. 2012, Article ID 490390, 6 pages, 2012.

[9] E. Kandil, M. Abdel Khalek, R. Aslam, P. Friedlander, C. F. Bellows, and D. Slakey, "Recurrent laryngeal nerve: significance of the anterior extralaryngeal branch," *Surgery*, vol. 149, no. 6, pp. 820–824, 2011.

[10] T. Beneragama and J. W. Serpell, "Extralaryngeal bifurcation of the recurrent laryngeal nerve: a common variation," *ANZ Journal of Surgery*, vol. 76, no. 10, pp. 928–931, 2006.

[11] E. Kandil, S. Abdelghani, P. Friedlander et al., "Motor and sensory branching of the recurrent laryngeal nerve in thyroid surgery," *Surgery*, vol. 150, no. 6, pp. 1222–1227, 2011.

[12] O. Makay, G. Icoz, M. Yilmaz, M. Akyildiz, and E. Yetkin, "The recurrent laryngeal nerve and the inferior thyroid artery—anatomical variations during surgery," *Langenbeck's Archives of Surgery*, vol. 393, no. 5, pp. 681–685, 2008.

[13] C. Page, P. Foulon, and V. Strunski, "The inferior laryngeal nerve: surgical and anatomic considerations. Report of 251 thyroidectomies," *Surgical and Radiologic Anatomy*, vol. 25, no. 3-4, pp. 188–191, 2003.

[14] R. L. Eller, M. Miller, J. Weinstein, and R. T. Sataloff, "The innervation of the posterior cricoarytenoid muscle: exploring clinical possibilities," *Journal of Voice*, vol. 23, no. 2, pp. 229–234, 2009.

[15] E. Kruse, A. Olthoff, and R. Schiel, "Functional anatomy of the recurrent and superior laryngeal nerve," *Langenbeck's Archives of Surgery*, vol. 391, no. 1, pp. 4–8, 2006.

[16] E. Maranillo, X. Leon, C. Orus, M. Quer, and J. R. Sanudo, "Variability in nerve patterns of the adductor muscle group supplied by the recurrent laryngeal nerve," *Laryngoscope*, vol. 115, no. 2, pp. 358–362, 2005.

[17] F. Y. Chiang, I. C. Lu, H. C. Chen et al., "Anatomical variations of recurrent laryngeal nerve during thyroid surgery: how to identify and handle the variations with intraoperative neuromonitoring," *Kaohsiung Journal of Medical Sciences*, vol. 26, no. 11, pp. 575–583, 2010.

[18] J. J. Sancho, M. Pascual-Damieta, J. A. Pereira, M. J. Carrera, J. Fontané, and A. Sitges-Serra, "Risk factors for transient vocal cord palsy after thyroidectomy," *British Journal of Surgery*, vol. 95, no. 8, pp. 961–967, 2008.

[19] G. W. Randolph, H. Dralle, and International Intraoperative Monitoring Study Group, "Electrophysiologic recurrent laryngeal nerve monitoring during thyroid and parathyroid surgery: international standards guideline statement," *Laryngoscope*, vol. 121, no. 1, supplement, pp. S1–S16, 2011.

[20] M. Barczyński, A. Konturek, and S. Cichoń, "Randomized clinical trial of visualization wersus neuromonitoring of recurrent laryngeal nerves during thyroidectomy," *British Journal of Surgery*, vol. 96, no. 3, pp. 240–246, 2009.

21

Short Course High Dose Radiotherapy in the Treatment of Anaplastic Thyroid Carcinoma

Mark J. Stavas,[1,2] **Eric T. Shinohara,**[1] **Albert Attia,**[1] **Matthew S. Ning,**[1]
Jeffrey M. Friedman,[1] **and Anthony J. Cmelak**[1]

[1] *Department of Radiation Oncology, Vanderbilt University Medical Center, Nashville, TN 37232, USA*
[2] *Department of Radiation Oncology, Vanderbilt University School of Medicine, 1301 Medical Center Drive, B913/TVC,*
  Nashville, TN 37232, USA

Correspondence should be addressed to Mark J. Stavas; mark.j.stavas@vanderbilt.edu

Academic Editor: B. C. Stack Jr.

Purpose. Anaplastic thyroid carcinoma (ATC) is a rare but aggressive tumor with limited survival. To date, the ideal radiation treatment schedule, one that balances limited survival with treatment efficacy, remains undefined. In this retrospective series we investigate the effectiveness and tolerability of hypofractionated radiation therapy in the treatment of ATC. *Methods.* 17 patients with biopsy proven ATC treated between 2004 and 2012 were reviewed for outcomes and toxicity. All patients received short course radiation. *Results.* The most commonly prescribed dose was 54 Gy in 18 fractions. Median survival was 9.3 months. 47% of patients were metastatic at diagnosis and the majority of patients (88%) went on to develop metastasis. Death from local progression was seen in 3 patients (18%), 41% experienced grade 3 toxicity, and there were no grade 4 toxicities. *Conclusions.* Here we demonstrated the safety and feasibility of hypofractionated radiotherapy in the treatment of ATC. This approach offers shorter treatment courses (3-4 weeks) compared to traditional fractionation schedules (6-7 weeks), comparable toxicity, local control, and the ability to transition to palliative care sooner. Local control was dependent on the degree of surgical debulking, even in the metastatic setting.

1. Introduction

Anaplastic thyroid carcinoma (ATC) is a rare but deadly tumor with a median survival of 5-6 months and less than 20% survival at one year [1, 2]. ATC occurs with a slight female predominance (1.5 : 1 ratio) with a peak incidence in the sixth and seventh decades of life [3]. The majority of patients (>75%) develop distant metastasis either at the time of diagnosis or shortly thereafter, with the lungs being the most commonly affected organ [4]. Despite its low incidence, ATC accounts for up to 39% of thyroid cancer deaths [2] with disease-specific mortality approaching 100% [5].

In addition to its poor prognosis, ATC causes significant site-specific morbidity. Commonly, individuals present with a rapidly enlarging neck mass causing symptoms of dysphagia, odynophagia, dyspnea, anxiety, and vocal cord paralysis. Unless aggressive treatments are applied, such as surgical resection and external beam radiation therapy (EBRT), patients die from uncontrolled local progression causing suffocation and massive bleeding [6, 7]. Furthermore, rapid airway obstruction remains a major cause of death even in patients undergoing tracheostomy [8, 9]. Therefore, treatment approaches should emphasize the importance of local control even in the metastatic setting.

Given the morbidity and poor prognosis of ATC, palliative and supportive care remain an essential part in the management of these patients [5, 10]. Owing to disappointing results with current treatments strategies, there have been many attempts to improve clinical outcomes. The most promising one, in terms of local control, has been with trimodality therapy combining surgery with chemotherapy and radiation [11]. Various altered fractionation schedules have been proposed such as twice daily treatments or protracted once daily courses, but these schedules do not consider the challenges posed upon patients with limited survival. Two of the main concerns with twice daily treatments are the burden of transportation and association with significant acute toxicities. Furthermore, even with the use of standard fraction sizes and traditional 30-day treatment courses, treatment related side effects tend to be serious, requiring hospitalizations, parenteral nutrition, and delays in supportive care [12].

To date, an optimal radiation approach to ATC (one that considers both outcomes and quality of life) has not been defined. Because of the significant toxicities and logistical challenges related to prolonged or twice daily treatment schedules, our institution has shifted to treat ATC with maximum surgical debulking followed by short course high dose (hypofractionated) radiotherapy with or without chemotherapy. From our experience, shorter treatment courses minimize the challenges associated with transportation and on-treatment toxicity. In addition, shorter courses may lessen the burden of care in this population, especially when the concern for long-term radiation effects is less critical. Most importantly, the quality of life in patients with limited survival should be of highest priority. Here we retrospectively review our use of hypofractionated radiotherapy in the treatment of ATC.

2. Methods

2.1. Patients. Following institutional review board approval, patients with pathologically proven ATC referred to the department of radiation oncology between 2004 and 2012 were retrospectively reviewed for outcomes and treatment toxicity. All patients received ≥2.5 Gy dose per fraction (median dose 3 Gy (range 2.5–4 Gy)). Patients with metastases at the time of diagnosis were included because local control of the primary site was a major issue in this population.

2.2. Treatment. All patients underwent a computed tomography simulation for treatment planning. They were placed in a long thermoplastic mask for immobilization with their neck in maximum extension. The treatment volumes were constructed using presurgical cranial/caudal margins and the postsurgical axial margins including the entire thyroid bed. Typical fields for the primary tumor extended from just below the hyoid bone to the level VI cervical and upper mediastinal lymph nodes (Figure 1). Only the involved and at risk nodal levels were treated. Megavoltage external beam radiation was delivered using intensity modulated radiation therapy (IMRT) and Eclipse planning software. Avoidance structures such as the trachea, esophagus, and spinal cord were contoured and well-defined dose constraints were applied. The maximum spinal cord dose was ≤36 Gy in 3 Gy fractions. Patients were treated once daily Monday through Friday. Treatment toxicity and follow-up images were reviewed in the medical record.

2.3. Follow-Up and Endpoints. Patients were assessed during treatment and subsequently every 2–4 weeks after treatment

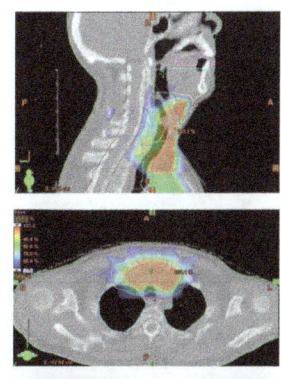
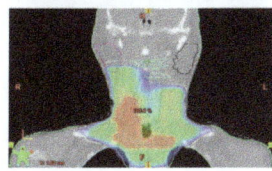

FIGURE 1: Radiation dose distribution for a 65-year-old male with ATC, status post gross total resection with involved cervical nodes. 51 Gy delivered in 17 fractions.

for both response and toxicity. Local control and treatment response were retrospectively evaluated for this analysis based on physical exam and radiographic assessment. Clinically, local control was defined as the absence of physical progression of disease or radiological progression. Physical progression was defined as disease progression requiring any intervention after radiation to protect the airway such as tracheostomy, surgical debulking, or death from upper airway compression. Radiographically, local control was defined as no increase in size greater than 25% posttreatment. At the time of this analysis, two patients had died during radiotherapy with not enough time to assess treatment response. Both of these patients had unresectable disease and received two fractions of radiation before death. These patients were not included in the outcomes measures. Toxicity was measured according to the National Cancer Institute Common Toxicity Criteria for Adverse Events version 4.0. Toxicity was scored weekly using CTC criteria during the radiation on treatment visit. After completion of treatment, patients were followed up approximately every 4 weeks at Vanderbilt University Medical Center.

2.4. Statistics. All patients who survived treatment were considered eligible for assessment. Outcomes and survival were assessed for all patients. Continuous features were described using means, medians, and ranges whereas categorical features were summarized with frequency counts and percentages. All data were calculated from the time of pathological diagnosis. All patients were followed up until death or last documented follow-up.

3. Results

3.1. Patient Characteristics. Seventeen patients were diagnosed with anaplastic thyroid carcinoma and completed

TABLE 1: Patient demographics.

Patient	Gender	Age	Date of diagnosis	KPS	Size (cm)	PEG post-XRT	First site of metastasis
1	F	70	1/16/04	80	2.6	No	Pulmonary
2	M	58	6/30/05	80	3.2	No	Pulmonary
3	F	84	4/6/06	60	5.7	No	Pulmonary
4	F	60	4/25/06	70	4.0	Yes	Pulmonary
5	F	77	5/18/06	50	5.2	No	None
6	F	72	9/8/06	60	5.0	No	None
7	F	68	1/2/08	80	3	No	Pulmonary
8	M	78	12/19/07	70	5.9	Yes	Skin and chest
9	F	68	12/7/07	80	4	Yes	Pulmonary
10	M	77	12/15/08	70	5.3	No	Pulmonary
11	M	63	4/21/10	70	16	No	Pulmonary
12	M	80	9/15/10	70	6.0	No	Pulmonary
13	F	76	9/15/10	60	6.0	No	Pulmonary
14	M	62	7/21/11	80	2.5	No	Pulmonary
15	M	74	8/31/11	70	8.0	No	Pulmonary
16	M	70	6/11/12	70	2.5	Yes	Pulmonary
17	F	66	6/21/11	80	2.2	No	Pulmonary

TABLE 2: Tumor characteristics.

Patient	TNM stage	Margin	Surgery	Nodal dissection	Survival (months)
1	T4aN0M1	Negative	Total thyroidectomy	Yes	21.9
2	T4aN0M0	Positive	Total thyroidectomy	Yes	23.6
3	T4aN0M0	N/A	None	No	14.2
4	T4aN1aM1	Gross residual disease	Partial thyroidectomy	No	4.7
5	T4aN1bM0	Gross residual disease	Partial thyroidectomy	Yes	2.3
6	T4bN0M0	Negative	Total thyroidectomy	Yes	24.0
7	T4aN1bM1	Gross residual disease	Partial thyroidectomy	No	9.3
8	T4bN1bM1	Positive	Total thyroidectomy	Yes	5.8
9	T4aN1bM0	Positive	Total thyroidectomy	Yes	10.0
10	T4aN1bM1	Positive	Total thyroidectomy	Yes	6.5
11	T4aN1bM0	Positive	Partial thyroidectomy	Yes	23.3
12	T4aN1aM1	N/A	None	No	6.2
13	T4aN0M0	Negative	Total thyroidectomy	No	17.8*
14	T4aN1bM0	Positive	Total thyroidectomy	Yes	4.4
15	T4bN0M0	Positive	Total thyroidectomy	Yes	7.9
16	T4aN1aM1	N/A	None	No	3.8*
17	T4aN0M1	Negative	Total thyroidectomy	Yes	16.1*

*Date of last follow-up.

treatment with hypofractionated radiotherapy between 2004 and 2012. Nine patients were female and 8 were male (M : F ratio, 1 : 1.1). The median age of diagnosis was 70 years (range, 58–84 years). The median Karnofsky performance status was 70 (range, 50–80). Patient and tumor characteristics are described in Tables 1, 2, and 3. All 17 patients had ATC confirmed by pathological review at our institution. The majority of patients (88%) received concurrent chemotherapy, which consisted of weekly paclitaxel (135 mg/m^2) or weekly carboplatin (AUC 1-2) and paclitaxel (135 mg/m^2).

3.2. Treatment. Fourteen patients underwent surgical resection prior to radiation (82.3%): ten patients underwent a total thyroidectomy and 4 patients underwent a partial thyroidectomy. Three patients were deemed inoperable at the time of diagnosis: 1 patient due to medical comorbidities and 2 patients due to unresectable disease. The most frequently used fraction size was 3.0 Gy, and the most frequently prescribed dose was 54 Gy in 18 daily fractions (35.3%) with a range of 40–62.5 Gy (Table 3). The median number of fractions was 18 (range, 10–25).

TABLE 3: Treatment characteristics.

Patient	Elapsed days	Completed treatment	Dose	Fraction	Concurrent chemotherapy	Local control
1	29	Yes with delay	5100	17	Yes	Yes
2	23	Yes	5100	17	Yes	Yes
3	37	Yes	6250	25	No	No
4	36	Yes with delay	5700	19	Yes	No
5	27	Yes with delay	5700	19	Yes	Yes
6	29	Yes	5500	22	Yes	Yes
7	23	Yes	5400	18	Yes	Yes
8	24	Yes	5400	18	Yes	Yes
9	24	Yes	5400	18	Yes	Yes
10	13	Yes	4000	10	No	Yes
11	23	Yes	4950	18	Yes	Yes
12	23	Yes	5400	18	Yes	Yes
13	36	Yes	6250	25	Yes	Yes
14	26	Yes	5400	18	Yes	Yes
15	22	Yes	5100	17	Yes	Yes
16	25	Yes	5400	18	Yes	No
17	21	Yes	4500	15	Yes	Yes

TABLE 4: Toxicity.

Grade	Toxicity/number of patients (%)			
	Dysphagia	Esophagitis	Dermatitis	Total (N)
1	7 (45)	9 (53)	7 (45)	17 (100)
2	6 (35)	5 (29)	6 (35)	17 (100)
3	4 (24)	3 (18)	4 (24)	7 (41)
4	0	0	0	0

3.3. *Local Control and Survival.* The median survival was 9.3 months. For those with metastatic disease at diagnosis, the median survival was 6.4 months; for those without initial metastases, median survival was 14.2 months. Seven of the 17 patients (41%) were alive one year after initial diagnosis. Two of the 8 patients with metastatic disease at diagnosis were alive after one year, while 5 of the 9 patients (56%) without initial metastases were alive after one year.

Eight patients (47%) had metastatic disease at the time of diagnosis. The median time from diagnosis to metastasis was 2.1 months, and 88% of irradiated patients developed metastatic disease. The lungs were the first site of metastasis in 93% of patients. Fourteen patients had died at the time of analysis. Three patients were lost to follow-up after a mean of 12.5 months. These patients were assumed dead with survival calculated from the last date of follow-up.

Fourteen of the 17 patients (82%) maintained local control of disease at the time of death. Two patients required palliative tracheostomies and one patient required surgical debulking after irradiation. In the patients who experienced local progression, 2 had unresectable disease at diagnosis and 1 received a partial thyroidectomy. Four patients required percutaneous gastrostomy tube placement following radiation. Radiation induced esophagitis was the reason for gastrostomy tube placement in 2 of 4 patients.

3.4. *Toxicity and Feasibility.* Treatment related toxicities were graded using the National Cancer Institute Common Toxicity Criteria for Adverse Events version 4.0. Specifically, dysphagia, esophagitis, and radiation dermatitis were analyzed as documented in the medical record. The incidences of grades 1–4 toxicities are listed in Table 4. All patients experienced grade 1 or 2 toxicities. There were no grade 4 toxicities. However, 7 out of 17 patients (41%) experienced at least one grade 3 toxicity. Moreover, patients with grade 3 toxicity in one category were more likely to have grade 3 toxicity in another category (HR = 1.33). Frequently, this was the result of symptomatic overlap between esophagitis and dysphagia. Patients who were deemed unresectable at diagnosis or underwent a partial resection prior to radiation were more likely to develop grade 3 dysphagia during treatment. This appeared to be related to local tumor progression resulting in mechanical obstruction as opposed to radiation induced esophagitis. Patients who underwent a complete resection prior to the start of radiation experienced the fewest toxicities and treatment delays.

All patients completed their radiation course as prescribed. A treatment delay was defined as an interruption between two radiation fractions greater than 5 days or a total treatment time 10 days greater than expected. Three out of 17 patients experienced treatment delays (18%). All three patients required inpatient admission with a mean hospitalization time of 3.6 days. Reasons for a treatment delay were local progression requiring tracheostomy or poor nutritional intake requiring gastrostomy tube placement.

4. Discussion

Given the poor prognosis and rapid progression of this disease, early integration of palliative and supportive care is essential when managing these patients. Knowing when and what type of radiation treatment to deliver can be a clinical challenge and requires a comprehensive understanding of the disease's natural history, sequelae of symptoms, treatment effectiveness, and goals of care. Unfortunately, patients with ATC are confronted with an aggressive disease that affects critical respiratory organs and local control remains a primary determinant of quality of life even in the metastatic setting. Results from the present study appear similar to prior studies with regard to local control and survival (Table 5).

Similar to other reports, our data underline the importance of surgical debulking in the management of ATC. Junor et al. reported that patients who underwent a total or partial thyroidectomy had prolonged survival times compared with patients for whom only a biopsy was feasible [7]. Surgical debulking can prevent distressing symptoms such as airway compression and it is recommended even in the presence of metastasis [16, 17]. Furthermore, reducing the burden of local disease may improve the efficacy of adjuvant therapy. However, surgery alone cannot alter the course of this disease [18]. The combination of surgery and radiotherapy is an independent predictor of reduced cause-specific mortality in patients with ATC [19], though the ideal adjuvant radiation regimen remains unclear.

The low incidence and poor survival rates of patients with ATC limit the ability to conduct large Phase III trials. Most of the available evidence for radiotherapy is derived from single institutional retrospective series. Wang et al. reported on 47 patients with ATC who received radiotherapy as either once or twice daily fractionation escalating up to 66 Gy. Median survival was 5.6 months, but patients receiving higher doses of radiation (45–66 Gy) had significantly longer survival times compared to those receiving doses less than 40 Gy (11.1 versus 3.2 months; $P < 0.001$) [13]. In our series, delivering larger doses in a shorter period of time maintained the concept of dose escalation, yielding an average biologically equivalent dose of 70.2 Gy.

Several common treatment schedules are used in radiation oncology including once daily treatments for ~25–35 days, twice daily treatments for ~15–25 days, and hypofractionated treatments for ~1–20 days. Typically, radiation oncologists attempt to achieve the same total effective dose; therefore, if the number of treatments decreases, the total dose per treatment must increase or the dose is delivered twice daily. One of the major challenges with twice daily treatments is the 6-hour break between fractions. The patient spends most of the day in the clinic or arranging transportation to and from it. The second challenge is increased acute

toxicity, which is an important consideration when treating the head and neck region.

Toxicity is divided into acute and late-responding effects depending on whether the tissue is more likely to manifest radiation damage around the time of treatment or in the future. Larger radiation doses per day correspond to greater risk of damage in late-responding tissues (such as the spinal cord) as compared to smaller doses given over a protracted course. However, in patients with limited survival, shorter treatment courses are practical because the patient will not live long enough to face the increased risk of long-term side effects, which classically occur many months to years later.

In the pursuit of better outcomes, several studies have examined the use of twice daily accelerated radiotherapy. De Crevoisier demonstrated treatment effectiveness, but 33% of their patients experienced grade III or IV acute mucositis with a significant amount of chemotherapy induced hematologic toxicity [14]. Dandekar et al. reported that greater than 70% of their patients experienced grade III or IV acute dysphagia and esophagitis and many of these patients discontinued treatment, with less than 10% survival at one year [20].

In our series, toxicity with hypofractionated radiotherapy continued to be an issue with 41% of patients experiencing grade 3 toxicities, but no grade 4 toxicities. The important difference between this regimen and others was that acute toxicities were seen near the end of treatment or after the patient had finished their radiation, thereby limiting the number of treatment related breaks and total treatment time. This allowed patients to continue forward with adjuvant systemic therapy or palliative and supportive care as needed. From the perspective of patient comfort, shorter treatment courses are preferable to longer courses, especially in the setting of limited survival.

Local recurrence in this disease can have devastating consequences and patients have a median survival of 66 days after local progression (McIver et al. anaplastic thyroid carcinoma: a 50-year experience at a single institution, 2001). This study also demonstrated that radiation after complete or near complete resection did not improve local control but did delay the time to local progression (5 versus 3 months). However, radiation or surgery did appear to improve survival over palliative care alone. In previous studies by Tennvall et al. and Werner et al., death from local failure was seen in 36% and 24% of patients, respectively. These studies used twice daily treatment schedules of varying doses and chemotherapy regimens [11, 21]. In our study, death attributed to local failure was seen in 18% of patients, though the patients who developed local failure were inoperable at the time of diagnosis or only received a partial resection or biopsy. Similarly, Foote et al. achieved local control in 30% of patients with variable radiation schedules and dual chemotherapy; however, patients with metastatic disease at diagnosis were excluded from their study [22]. These patients account for a significant portion of patients with ATC and were included in our series. Results from the present study suggest that a hypofractionated regimen is as effective as hyperfractionated regimens and while treatment courses were slightly longer, patients were only treated once per day.

TABLE 5: Major radiation series comparing outcomes of anaplastic thyroid carcinoma.

Author	Intent	Median radiation dose	Resection	Fractionation	Local control	Chemotherapy	Radiation duration	Median survival
Wang et al. [13]	Definitive	60 Gy (45–66)	61%	Once daily or bid	94% (6 months)	No	4–6 weeks	11.1 months
	Palliative	40 Gy (split course)	50%	Once daily	65% (6 months)	16% (prior to or during)	4–6 weeks	3.2 months
de Crevoisier et al. [14]	Definitive	40 Gy (later boost to 50–55 Gy)	71%	Bid	68% (45 median FU)	Prior to and after	3–4 weeks	10 months (both arms)
	Palliative	40 Gy (later boost to 50–55 Gy)	50%	Bid	68% (45 median FU)	Prior to and after	3–4 weeks	
Dumke et al. [15]	Both	50 Gy (6–60.4)	80%	Daily or bid	Unknown	15%	Unknown	5 months; if >50 Gy 10.5 months
Stavas et al.	Definitive	54 Gy (49.5–62.5)	89%	Daily	89% (at time of death)	88% (concurrent)	23.5 days (13–36)	14.2 months
	Palliative	54 Gy (40–57)	75%	Daily	75% (at time of death)		26 days (22–37)	6.4 months

There were multiple limitations in this study including the single institutional retrospective nature, small patient numbers, and variable radiation doses. Most patients received upfront resection possibly because of smaller tumors. Therefore, selection bias may have influenced the overall survival. Despite these issues, this treatment approach is unreported in the literature. Results from the present study suggest that a hypofractionated regimen with concurrent chemotherapy is well tolerated with a favorable toxicity profile and rates of local control when compared with previously used fractionation schemes. While there was no formal assessment of quality of life, given the favorable toxicity as well as the convenience of a shorter, once a day treatment regimen, we believe that this regimen may improve the quality of life in these patients with a generally poor outcome. Based on our results, short course hypofractionated radiation therapy appears to be a viable and safe option in the treatment of ATC and remains a sensible approach given the poor prognosis and symptomatic needs of this patient population. Specifically, this protocol may be useful in patients who have difficulty with a twice daily regimen due to either travel or concerns about their ability to tolerate the acute effects of a twice daily regimen.

References

[1] F. D. Gilliland, W. C. Hunt, D. M. Morris, and C. R. Key, "Prognostic factors for thyroid carcinoma. A population-based study of 15, 698 cases from the Surveillance, Epidemiology and End Results (SEER) program 1973–1991," *Cancer*, vol. 79, pp. 564–573, 1997.

[2] S. A. Hundahl, I. D. Fleming, A. M. Fremgen, and H. R. Menck, "A National Cancer Data Base report on 53, 856 cases of thyroid carcinoma treated in the U.S., 1985–1995," *Cancer*, vol. 83, pp. 2638–2648, 1998.

[3] K. B. Ain, "Anaplastic thyroid carcinoma: behavior, biology, and therapeutic approaches," *Thyroid*, vol. 8, no. 8, pp. 715–726, 1998.

[4] C. Are and A. R. Shaha, "Anaplastic thyroid carcinoma: biology, pathogenesis, prognostic factors, and treatment approaches," *Annals of Surgical Oncology*, vol. 13, no. 4, pp. 453–464, 2006.

[5] R. L. Neff, W. B. Farrar, R. T. Kloos, and K. D. Burman, "Anaplastic thyroid cancer," *Endocrinology and Metabolism Clinics of North America*, vol. 37, no. 2, pp. 525–538, 2008.

[6] B. Jereb, J. Stjernsward, and T. Lowhagen, "Anaplastic giant cell carcinoma of the thyroid. A study of treatment and prognosis," *Cancer*, vol. 35, no. 5, pp. 1293–1295, 1975.

[7] E. J. Junor, J. Paul, and N. S. Reed, "Anaplastic thyroid carcinoma: 91 patients treated by surgery and radiotherapy," *European Journal of Surgical Oncology*, vol. 18, no. 2, pp. 83–88, 1992.

[8] R. K. Tan, R. K. Finley III, D. Driscoll, V. Bakamjian, W. L. Hicks Jr., and D. P. Shedd, "Anaplastic carcinoma of the thyroid: a 24-year experience," *Head and Neck*, vol. 17, no. 1, pp. 41–48, 1995.

[9] E. Tallroth, G. Wallin, G. Lundell, T. Löwhagen, and J. Einhorn, "Multimodality treatment in anaplastic giant cell thyroid carcinoma," *Cancer*, vol. 60, no. 7, pp. 1428–1431, 1987.

[10] R. C. Smallridge, K. B. Ain, S. L. Asa et al., "American Thyroid Association guidelines for management of patients with anaplastic thyroid cancer," *Thyroid*, vol. 22, pp. 1104–1139, 2012.

[11] J. Tennvall, G. Lundell, P. Wahlberg et al., "Anaplastic thyroid carcinoma: three protocols combining doxorubicin, hyperfractionated radiotherapy and surgery," *British Journal of Cancer*, vol. 86, no. 12, pp. 1848–1853, 2002.

[12] M. Troch, O. Koperek, C. Scheuba et al., "High efficacy of concomitant treatment of undifferentiated (anaplastic) thyroid cancer with radiation and docetaxel," *The Journal of Clinical Endocrinology and Metabolism*, vol. 95, no. 9, pp. E54–E57, 2010.

[13] Y. Wang, R. Tsang, S. Asa, B. Dickson, T. Arenovich, and J. Brierley, "Clinical outcome of anaplastic thyroid carcinoma treated with radiotherapy of once- and twice-daily fractionation regimens," *Cancer*, vol. 107, no. 8, pp. 1786–1792, 2006.

[14] R. de Crevoisier, E. Baudin, A. Bachelot et al., "Combined treatment of anaplastic thyroid carcinoma with surgery, chemotherapy, and hyperfractionated accelerated external radiotherapy," *International Journal of Radiation Oncology Biology Physics*, vol. 60, no. 4, pp. 1137–1143, 2004.

[15] A.-K. Dumke, T. Pelz, and D. Vordermark, "Long-term results of radiotherapy in anaplastic thyroid cancer," *Radiation Oncology*, vol. 9, no. 1, article 90, 2014.

[16] P. I. Haigh, P. H. Ituarte, H. S. Wu et al., "Completely resected anaplastic thyroid carcinoma combined with adjuvant chemotherapy and irradiation is associated with prolonged survival," *Cancer*, vol. 91, pp. 2335–2342, 2001.

[17] O. Nilsson, J. Lindeberg, J. Zedenius et al., "Anaplastic giant cell carcinoma of the thyroid gland: treatment and survival over a 25-year period," *World Journal of Surgery*, vol. 22, no. 7, pp. 725–730, 1998.

[18] B. McIver, I. D. Hay, D. F. Giuffrida et al., "Anaplastic thyroid carcinoma: a 50-year experience at a single institution," *Surgery*, vol. 130, no. 6, pp. 1028–1034, 2001.

[19] E. Kebebew, F. S. Greenspan, O. H. Clark, K. A. Woeber, and A. McMillan, "Anaplastic thyroid carcinoma: treatment outcome and prognostic factors," *Cancer*, vol. 103, no. 7, pp. 1330–1335, 2005.

[20] P. Dandekar, C. Harmer, Y. Barbachano et al., "Hyperfractionated Accelerated Radiotherapy (HART) for anaplastic thyroid carcinoma: toxicity and survival analysis," *International Journal of Radiation Oncology Biology Physics*, vol. 74, no. 2, pp. 518–521, 2009.

[21] B. Werner, J. Abele, A. Alveryd et al., "Multimodal therapy in anaplastic giant cell thyroid carcinoma," *World Journal of Surgery*, vol. 8, no. 1, pp. 64–68, 1984.

[22] R. L. Foote, J. R. Molina, J. L. Kasperbauer et al., "Enhanced survival in locoregionally confined anaplastic thyroid carcinoma: a single-institution experience using aggressive multimodal therapy," *Thyroid*, vol. 21, no. 1, pp. 25–30, 2011.

22

Papillary Thyroid Cancer, Macrofollicular Variant: The Follow-Up and Analysis of Prognosis of 5 Patients

Varlık Erol,[1] Özer Makay,[1] Yeşim Ertan,[2] Gökhan İçöz,[1] Mahir Akyıldız,[1] and Mustafa Yılmaz[1]

[1] Division of Endocrine Surgery, Department of General Surgery, School of Medicine, Ege University, Bornova, 35100 Izmir, Turkey
[2] Department of Pathology, School of Medicine, Ege University, Bornova, 35100 Izmir, Turkey

Correspondence should be addressed to Özer Makay; ozer.makay@ege.edu.tr

Academic Editor: Giovanni Tallini

Objective. The main aim of this study was to comparatively analyze the recurrence and prognosis of this rare variant with the literature by analyzing the follow-up data of 5 patients diagnosed with papillary cancer macrofollicular variant. *Methods.* The demographic data, radiological and pathological data, and prognostic data of 5 patients who underwent surgery for thyroid cancer and were diagnosed with papillary cancer macrofollicular variant pathologically were retrospectively analyzed. *Results.* The mean age of patients whose mean follow-up period was determined as 7.2 years was 41, and the male/female ratio was 4/1. All patients underwent total thyroidectomy. The pathology report of 2 patients (40%) revealed macrofollicular variant of papillary microcancer, and 3 patients papillary cancer macrofollicular variant. Central dissection was performed in one patient (20%) due to macroscopic pathologic lymph node and 4 metastatic lymph nodes were reported. Also, locoregional recurrence was present in 3 out of 5 patients (60%). *Conclusions.* Although an impression of earlier and increased risk of recurrence in papillary carcinoma with macrofollicular variant has been documented, more studies with extensive follow-up times and large populations are required.

1. Introduction

Thyroid cancer is the most common endocrine malignancy, it accounts for less than 1% of all cancers, and the tumors usually progress slowly [1]. Papillary thyroid cancer is the most common of all thyroid cancers. It makes up 80% of all thyroid cancers [2]. Despite high survival rates, local recurrence and metastasis occur in some patients and this may require more aggressive surgical treatment. It is more common in women; the incidence varies according to different reports. Male : female ratio varies from 1 : 2 to 1 : 10. They often appear in the third and fifth decades of life [3, 4]. Papillary thyroid carcinoma exhibits a morphologically wide spectrum. Follicular variant of papillary thyroid cancer subtypes is characterized by follicles lined by cells with nuclear features of papillary carcinoma. Follicles are usually associated with small, dense colloids [5]. Macrofollicular variant of papillary carcinoma (MVPC) is a rare subtype of follicle variant, and it was first defined by Albores-Saavedra et al. in 1991 [6] and was described as encapsulated follicular variant that includes more than 50% macrofollicular in each section. Macrofollicle was defined as a follicle that is of a diameter greater than 250 μm. In this study, the aim was to examine the prognostic features of MVPC by analyzing the follow-up results of 5 patients diagnosed with MVPC.

2. Materials and Methods

Demographic data, preoperative data, postoperative treatment methods (hormone replacement, radioactive iodine ablation therapy), locoregional recurrence rates, and prognostic factors of patients who underwent surgery due to thyroid cancer in Ege University Hospital, Department of General Surgery, Division of Endocrine Surgery, and were diagnosed with MVPC between January 2000 and January 2006 were retrospectively analyzed.

All treatment decisions were taken by an endocrine council consisting of general surgeons, endocrinologists, nuclear medicine specialists, pathologists, and radiologists, by adopting a multidisciplinary approach. In our clinic, we applied total thyroidectomy for patients diagnosed with thyroid cancer, in a way that no visible tissue would be left behind.

Locoregional recurrence was described as cases having pathological lymph nodes on ultrasonography and/or cytology and/or a new determination of a previously nonexisting tissue or presence of increased levels of thyroglobulin.

3. Results

The mean age of the patients included in the study was 41 (38–48). Four of them were females (80%) and 1 was male (20%). The mean follow-up duration was 7.2 years (5.3–11.2). While the reason for one patient's admission was symptoms of hyperthyroidism, no symptoms were detected in other patients. On physical examination, one of the patients had palpable thyroid nodules on right upper lobe, and another had bilateral palpable nodules. No palpable lymph nodes were detected in any of the patients. All patients had euthyroid thyroid function tests. None of the patients had thyroid cancer history in their families. None of the patients were detected to have pathological lymph nodes after ultrasonographic evaluation. All patients underwent a total thyroidectomy.

In the histological examination of tumors that were observed in thyroidectomy materials, macrofollicular structures were determined in most areas and microfollicular in some others. These cells lining the follicles were of clear nuclei and showed obvious deformity of the nuclear membrane, notch structure, and sparse pseudoinclusion. It was remarkable that a portion of the cells lining macrofollicles had hyperchromatic nuclei. Also, vacuolization was spotted in colloid in the periphery of the follicle structures. With these histological findings, the tumor found in all patients was reported to be MVPC (Figures 1 and 2). More than 50% of the cross-sectional area of the tumor was composed of macrofollicles (follicles 250 μm in diameter) in all patients. Pathological tumor sizes were reported as <1 cm in 2 patients, 1.1–2 cm in another two, and 2.1–3 cm in the last one. Multifocal tumors were reported in one patient. There was no tumor invasion (soft tissue, capsules, and vessels) in any of the patients. Upon detecting lymph nodes in intraoperative macroscopic pathology, one patient (20%) was applied ipsilateral central (6th level) lymph node dissection and 4 metastatic lymph nodes were reported histologically out of 11 dissected lymph nodes.

While four of the patients (80%) were applied radioactive iodine ablation (RIA) in the postoperative period, 1 (20%) was not. The patient, who was detected to have lymph node metastases, received RIA at a dose of 225 mCi, and the other three received <150 mCi. Locoregional recurrence was detected in three patients. One patient was operated due to recurrence, and others were controlled by RIA. Mortality was observed in none of the patients (Table 1).

4. Discussion

Papillary thyroid carcinoma is the most common malignant tumor of the thyroid gland, and it is in the group of well-differentiated tumors thanks to good prognosis. It is also the type of thyroid cancer which has the widest histological

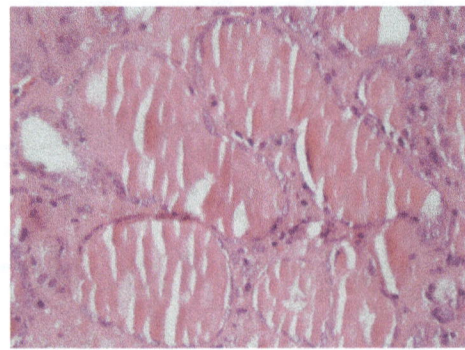

FIGURE 1: MVPC histological image (hematoxylin and eosin, ×20).

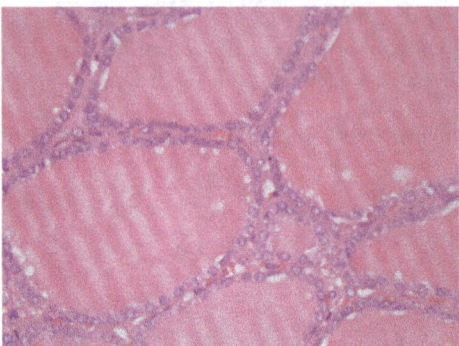

FIGURE 2: Follicular structures lined by tumor cells that include papillary carcinoma nuclear features.

spectrum. MVPC histologically consists of follicles and cells of papillary cancer nuclear characteristics which line these follicles. While macrofollicles can also be encountered in classical papillary cancer and follicular variant, more than 50% of the tumor in macrofollicular variant consists of macrofollicles. Defining this variant is important as it can easily be mistaken with benign thyroid lesions, such as nodular goiter and follicular adenoma. Macrofollicles in MVPC are lined by tumor cells with nuclei that are large, overlapping, clear, and notched and that sometimes have cores containing pseudoinclusion [7]. Minor nuclear irregularities can also be seen in benign lesions, but this histological finding is not enough for a cancer diagnosis alone [7]. In addition, unlike benign thyroid lesions, there is a remarkable nuclear deformity in the shapes of cells. Histological diagnosis is made according to nuclear properties of tumor cells paving the macrofollicles because macrofollicles are lined by squamous cells in some MVPCs [8].

Definitions as case presentations exist in the literature, the largest series of which is the one made by Albores-Saavedra et al. in 1991 with 29 patients to define MVPC and republished the results in 1997 with the adding up new cases [9]. There are no large series of patients, but it can be said that it is more common in females than males [6]. Similarly, male/female ratio was 4/1. MVPC was reported to have a very good prognosis with its lower rate of lymph node metastasis compared to classical papillary cancer [9, 10]. Clinically, they are usually included in nonaggressive tumors, and in the study of Albores-Saavedra et al. rate of lymph node metastasis was

TABLE 1: General characteristics of patients.

	n (%)
Age	
≤45	4 (80%)
>45	1 (20%)
Gender	
Female	4 (80%)
Male	1 (20%)
Ultrasonographic nodule size	
≤1 cm	0
1.1–2 cm	3 (60%)
2.1–3 cm	2 (40%)
>3 cm	0
Histopathological tumor size	
≤1 cm	2 (40%)
1.1–2 cm	2 (40%)
2.1–3 cm	1 (20%)
3.1–4 cm	0
>4 cm	0
Surgical technique	
Total thyroidectomy	5 (100%)
Histopathology	
MVPC	5 (100%)
Lymph node metastasis	1 (20%)
Tumor invasion	0
Postoperative treatment	
Radioiodine ablation	4 (80%)
≤150 mCi	3 (75%)
>150 mCi	1 (25%)
Locoregional recurrence	3 (60%)
Radioiodine ablation (>150 mCi)	1 (33.3%)
Radioiodine ablation (≤150 mCi)	2 (66.6%)
Mortality	0

reported as 11.8%, in their second study as 20.6%, and in another study by Evans as 7.1% (1 metastasis in 14 patients) [6, 9, 11]. In this study, lymph node metastasis rate was determined as 20%. MVPC lymph node metastases rate's being lower while it is higher in general papillary cancer is associated with the fact that it is a well-limited capsulated and having low proliferative activity [6, 9].

Contrary to the abovementioned good prognostic data, 2 out of 29 patients were reported to have capsular invasion, vascular invasion, and lung metastasis in the study of Albores-Saavedra et al. [9]. Also, in the study by Cardenas et al. 2 cases with aggressive behaviour (extrathyroid extension, lymph nodes, and bone and lung metastases) were reported [12]. In this study, distant metastasis and death were not detected in a mean follow-up period of 7.2 years, and locoregional recurrence rate was observed to be high (60%). In a study we conducted in our clinic but not yet published, 5

out of 181 patients (2.7%) diagnosed with well-differentiated thyroid cancer were detected to have MVPC. In a mean follow-up period of 7.1 years, locoregional recurrence rate of 181 patients was determined to be 22.6% (41 patients), and the locoregional recurrence rate of MVPC group in this group of patients was found to be higher (60%). In this small series, we describe two cases of microcarcinoma exhibiting macrofollicular architecture: these are two aspects generally correlated with an excellent prognosis. Regarding the clinical behavior of these cases in this series, one of the recurrent patients had a microcarcinoma. This patient, as well as the rest in this series, had no invasion reported on histopathological review. The other microcarcinoma patient had no recurrence during follow-up.

Although MVPC is said to be a variant that has a perfect prognosis and less rate of lymph node metastasis than those of classical papillary cancer, in this study the rate of lymph node metastasis was found to be 20% and locoregional recurrence rate 60%. It can be argued that the number of patients included is not enough to make definite statements about prognosis, but studies including such large groups do not exist in the literature. Special care should be given especially because one can encounter other benign thyroid diseases in fine-needle aspiration biopsy and histological evaluation.

As its histological subtypes and the clinical behaviour of these subtypes are highly variable, this definition has started to prove insufficient though papillary cancer is one of the diseases with best prognosis. For this reason, we are of the opinion that prospective prognostic studies that evaluate all papillary cancer subtypes together with higher number of patients are a need today.

References

[1] G. H. Sakorafas, J. Giotakis, and V. Stafyla, "Papillary thyroid microcarcinoma: a surgical perspective," *Cancer Treatment Reviews*, vol. 31, no. 6, pp. 423–438, 2005.

[2] G. P. Sadler and O. H. Clark, "Thyroid and parathyroid," in *Schwartz's Principles of Surgery*, vol. 36, pp. 1661–1687, McGraw-Hill, New York, NY, USA, 7th edition, 1999.

[3] C. A. Muro-Cacho and N. N. K. Ku, "Tumors of the thyroid gland: histologic and cytologic features—part 1," *Cancer Control*, vol. 7, no. 3, pp. 276–287, 2000.

[4] S. A. Hundahl, I. D. Fleming, A. M. Fremgen, and H. R. Menck, "A national cancer data base report on 53,856 cases of thyroid carcinoma treated in the US, 1985–1995," *Cancer*, vol. 82, pp. 2638–2648, 1998.

[5] D. Chung, R. A. Ghossein, and O. Lin, "Macrofollicular variant of papillary carcinoma: a potential thyroid FNA pitfall," *Diagnostic Cytopathology*, vol. 35, no. 9, pp. 560–564, 2007.

[6] J. Albores-Saavedra, E. Gould, C. Vardaman, and F. Vuitch, "The macrofollicular variant of papillary thyroid carcinoma: a study of 17 cases," *Human Pathology*, vol. 22, no. 12, pp. 1195–1205, 1991.

[7] V. A. LiVolsi, "Papillary neoplasms of the thyroid: pathologic and prognostic features," *The American Journal of Clinical Pathology*, vol. 97, no. 3, pp. 426–434, 1992.

[8] R. A. De Lellis, R. V. Lloyd, P. U. Heitz, and C. Eng, *World Health Organization Classification of Tumors. Pathology and Genetics of Tumors of Endocrine Organs*, IARC Pres, Lyon, France, 2004.

[9] J. Albores-Saavedra, I. Housini, F. Vuitch, and W. H. Snyder, "Macrofollicular variant of papillary thyroid carcinoma with minor insular component," *Cancer*, vol. 80, pp. 1110–1116, 1997.

[10] M. L. Carcangiu, G. Zampi, A. Pupi, A. Castagnoli, and J. Rosai, "Papillary carcinoma of the thyroid. A clinicopathologic study of 241 cases treated at the University of Florence, Italy," *Cancer*, vol. 55, no. 4, pp. 805–828, 1985.

[11] H. L. Evans, "Encapsulated papillary neoplasms of the thyroid: a study of 14 cases followed for a minimum of 10 years," *The American Journal of Surgical Pathology*, vol. 11, no. 8, pp. 592–597, 1987.

[12] M. G. Cardenas, S. Kini, and M. Wisgerhof, "Two patients with highly aggressive macrofollicular variant of papillary thyroid carcinoma," *Thyroid*, vol. 19, no. 4, pp. 413–416, 2009.

23

New Molecular Targeted Therapy and Redifferentiation Therapy for Radioiodine-Refractory Advanced Papillary Thyroid Carcinoma

Kai-Pun Wong and Brian Hung-Hin Lang

Division of Endocrine Surgery, Department of Surgery, The University of Hong Kong, Queen Mary Hospital, Pokfulam Road, Hong Kong, Hong Kong

Correspondence should be addressed to Brian Hung-Hin Lang, blang@hku.hk

Academic Editor: Katsuhiro Tanaka

Although the majority of papillary thyroid carcinoma could be successfully managed by complete surgical resection alone or resection followed by radioiodine ablation, a small proportion of patients may develop radioiodine-refractory progressive disease which is not amenable to surgery, local ablative treatment or other treatment modalities. The use of FDG-PET/CT scan for persistent/recurrent disease has improved the accuracy of restaging as well as cancer prognostication. Given that patients with RAI-refractory disease tend to do significantly worse than those with radioiodine-avid or non-progressive disease, an increasing number of phase I and II studies have been conducted to evaluate the efficacy of new molecular targeted drugs such as the tyrosine kinase inhibitors and redifferentiation drugs. The overall response rate of these drugs ranged between 0–53%, depending on whether the patients had been previously treated with these drugs, performance status and extent of disease. However, drug toxicity remains a major concern in administration of target therapies. Nevertheless, there are also ongoing phase III studies evaluating the efficacy of these new drugs. The aim of the review was to summarize and discuss the results of these targeted drugs and redifferentiation agents for patients with progressive, radioiodine-refractory papillary thyroid carcinoma.

1. Introduction

Papillary thyroid carcinoma (PTC) is the most common type of differentiated thyroid carcinoma (DTC) and its age-adjusted incidence has doubled in the last 25 years [1]. Despite its relatively good prognosis with a 10-year cancer-specific survival above 90%, locoregional recurrences and distant metastasis do occur not infrequently [2]. Of the 5–20% patients who may develop locoregional recurrences, approximately two-thirds of these recurrences involved the cervical lymph nodes. On the other hand, up to 10–15% patients would either present with distant metastasis at diagnosis or develop distant metastasis some time after initial treatment [3]. It is not uncommon to encounter patients with initial persistent locoregional recurrence who also later develop distant metastasis. Perhaps, this is a sign of disease progression. Since most patients would have had a total thyroidectomy and radioiodine (RAI) ablation as their initial therapy, disease monitoring or surveillance often relies on regular measurement of thyroglobulin (Tg) and high resolution neck ultrasound (USG) [4]. FDG-PET/CT scan is now often used as a staging tool in patients with suspected disease recurrence.

In terms of treating locoregional recurrence, a formal selective neck dissection for lymph node recurrence is usually preferred but at times when certain compartments has been previously dissected, a focused neck dissection or completion compartmental neck dissection might be preferred [2]. However, despite the best surgical effort, only approximately one-third of patients would become biochemically cured of the disease (i.e., athyroglobulinemia) and therefore, the American Thyroid Association (ATA) only recommended surgical removal of clinically significant metastatic lymph nodes to prevent future locoregional complications [2, 5, 6].

Other options include percutaneous ethanol injection and radiofrequency ablation (RFA) as their efficacy have been shown in several studies [7–9]. The decision for further adjuvant RAI therapy after reoperative neck dissection depends on the completeness of the dissection [5]. After that, local external beam radiation therapy (EBRT) might be considered in patients with gross unresectable, residual recurrence in the thyroid bed or lateral neck area. Adjuvant external beam radiation in patients with residual microscopic disease could achieve a higher 10-year local relapse-free rate (93% versus 78%) and disease free survival (100% versus 95%) compared with nonradiated patients [10].

In terms of treating patients with distant metastasis, surgical resection is often not the first treatment modality unless a patient has a solitary metastasis which is located near to or in a vital area such as the brain or vertebra. EBRT might be considered in patients with unresectable painful bone metastasis or metastatic lesion which might develop future debilitating complication, for example, fracture, neurological symptoms, compressing or invading of vital structures. In patient with brain metastasis not amendable to surgical resection, whole brain irradiation for multiple lesion or gamma knife radiosurgery for selected patients are acceptable options [5, 11]. RAI is often used as the first-line treatment for patients with distant metastases because it is highly effective in the treatment of small sized distant metastases. Although pulmonary pneumonitis and fibrosis are potential complications which could arise from repeated high-dose RAI treatment, it is recommended that pulmonary micrometastases should be treated with RAI (100–200 mCi) therapy and repeated every 6–12 months so long as the disease continues to concentrate RAI (i.e., RAI-avid) and responds clinically. RAI is generally recommended in patients with nonpulmonary RAI-avid distant metastases, although it might be less effective than pulmonary RAI-avid metastases [2, 5].

As a result, one of the most controversial and difficult issues in treating advanced PTC is how to manage non-RAI-avid disease or RAI-refractory. A patient is defined as having RAI-refractory disease if there is at least one lesion without RAI uptake or a lesion has progressed within a year following RAI treatment or persisted after the administration of a cumulative activity of more than 600 mCi. The current evidence suggests that RAI is of little benefit in patients with RAI-refractory disease [12, 13]. Furthermore, repeated dosage of RAI is associated with dose related complications like salivary gland damage, dental caries, nasolacrimal duct obstruction, and secondary malignancy [5, 14]. Although in the setting of a negative diagnostic RAI scan, small metastases may demonstrate a small measurable benefit to RAI (in terms of decreased Tg), it is of no use at all in large-sized metastases [12, 13]. Therefore, RAI is generally not recommended in RAI-refractory disease and the current treatment options are mainly restricted to conservative treatment, metastectomy, symptomatic control (e.g., drainage of effusions), endobronchial laser ablation, and/or external beam radiation in locally advanced carcinoma. Although age and patient performance status are important considerations when deciding on which treatment option

might be preferred, with better understanding and advances in the molecular biology that underlies the development and progression of advanced PTC, many new molecular targeted drugs have been examined or are being examined in the setting of a clinical trial. To date, the available drugs have been targeting two specific molecular pathways in thyroid oncogenesis, namely the mitogen-activated protein kinase (MAPK) pathway and the phosphatidyl-inositol-tri-phosphate kinase (PI3K) pathway. Figure 1 shows the main signaling pathways involved in thyroid oncogenesis. Redifferentiation therapy is a potential alternative for RAI-refractory disease. Redifferentiating agents could potentially reactivate the RAI uptake ability of DTC. The aim of the present paper is to evaluate the efficacy of these new molecular targeted drugs as well as redifferentiation therapy in the treatment of RAI-refractory advanced or metastatic PTC by reviewing the current literature.

2. Approach to Patients with RAI-Refractory Advanced PTC

Before starting novel therapy, patients with RAI refractory disease should be accurately characterized in terms of age, performance status, histology, disease extent and location, and progression rate [16]. Diagnostic procedures should consist of neck ultrasonography to look for possible concomitant locoregional disease, thin-cut CT neck, thorax, and abdomen to look for other distant metastases and MRI brain for small brain metastases. FDG-PET may also be employed because it helps to localize disease and prognosticate patient risk [36]. For patients with neoplastic foci and high FDG uptakes, local therapy such as radical resection, RFA might be considered as these high FDG-uptake foci are likely to be more aggressive, less differentiated and have higher growth rate [37]. In terms of measuring treatment response, the response evaluation criteria in solid tumors (RECIST) criteria are often used. This is carried out by repeating standardized imaging (usually CT or MRI) every 6 months. Interestingly, there is no evidence to suggest that novel treatment such as targeted therapy should be better given at an early stage than a later stage when the tumor might be larger in size. As most patients with RAI-refractory disease might be asymptomatic for a long period of time, the benefits of targeted therapy must not be outweighed by the drug toxicities and side effects. Therefore, targeted drug is usually commenced when there is documented disease progression by standardized imaging.

3. Potential Molecular Targets

Figure 1 shows the main signaling pathways involved in thyroid oncogenesis [15]. Since rearrangements of RET (or RET/PTC) and point mutations of RAS and BRAF are now believed to be initiating events in the carcinogenesis of PTC, most new targeted drugs have the ability of inhibiting the MAPK pathway and angiogenesis. RET/PTC rearrangements are found more frequently in classical PTC whereas RAS point mutations are mostly found in the follicular variant of PTC. BRAF mutations are mostly found in less differentiated

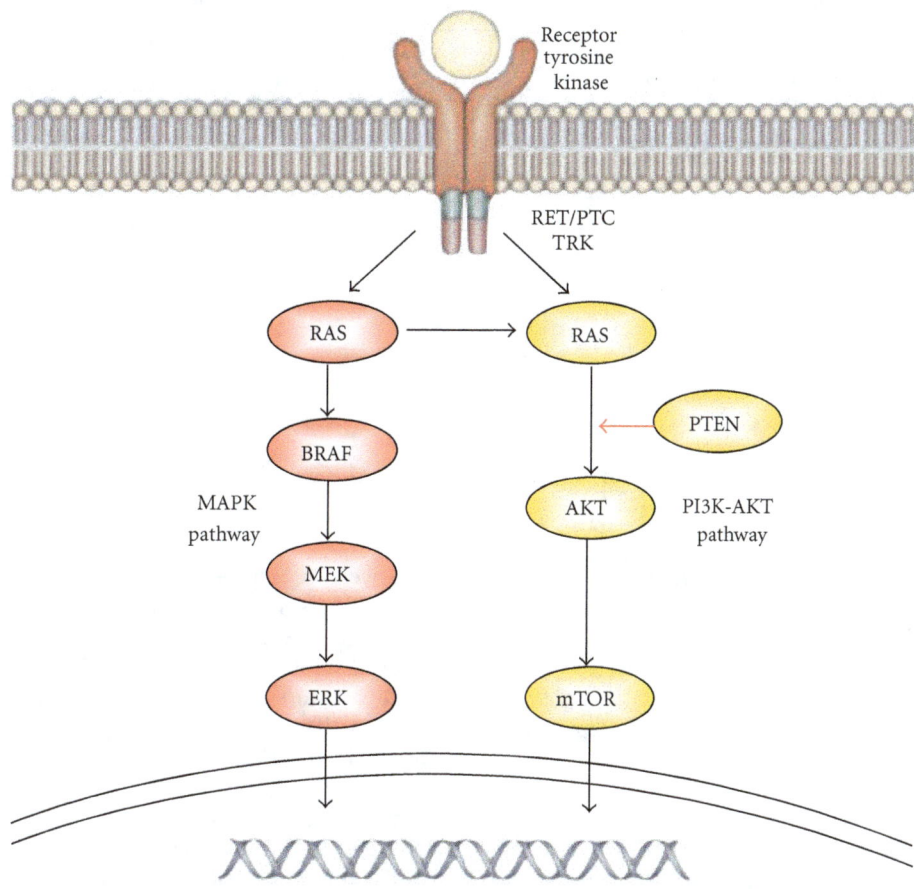

FIGURE 1: The main signaling pathways involved in thyroid carcinogenesis are the MAPK and PI3K-AKT pathway (reproduced with permission) [15].

or tall-cell variant of PTC. The PI3 K pathway may also be activated in some PTC. Other potential targets would be the angiogenic factors like various vascular endothelial growth factors (VEGF 1 and 2), fibroblast growth factor (FGF), and platelet-derived growth factor (PDGF). In vitro studies showed that anti-VEGF therapy could delay DTC growth [35]. Table 1 shows the relationship between various targeted drugs and their molecular targets.

4. New Molecular Targeted Therapy

Table 2 lists the results of various published trials for new targeted therapy in RAI-refractory thyroid carcinoma. Sorafenib was one of the first agents studied in RAI refractory PTC. It is an oral multi-tyrosine kinase inhibitor with multiple targets, including *VEGF-R* 1 to 3, *PDGF-R*, *RET/PTCs*, and *BRAF*. Two American studies have published the results of using sorafenib 400 mg twice daily in advanced PTC [19, 20]. Gupta-Abramson et al. reported the first phase II study in advanced PTC. Of the 18 patients with advanced PTC who received treatment for a minimum of 16 weeks, 4 out of 18 patients had partial response and 10 had stable disease. In this study, the median progression-free survival

was 84 weeks [19]. Kloos et al. reported another phase II study on 41 patients with metastatic papillary thyroid cancer. Of these patients, 15% had partial response and 56% had stable disease lasting for more than 6 months. The median progressive free survival was 15 months [20]. Adverse events were common, most frequent being fatigue (60–74%), hand foot syndrome (58–83%), diarrhea (68–73%), and muscle pain (28–57%) [19, 20]. Most of them were grade 1 or 2, and could be managed with dose reduction or drug holiday. It is interesting to note that about half the patients had to have dose reduction to improve compliance and control toxicity. Total withdrawal of treatment due to grade 3 or worse adverse events were not uncommon (about 16.6%) [19]. Since then, 3 other studies from Europe were published. In a Netherland's study of 30 patients with DTC, 25% of patients achieved partial response. The response rate did not appear to be influenced by gender, age, initial stage, or presence of *BRAF* mutation. However, the radiological response was worse in patients with bone metastases [21]. The authors also studied the possibility of reinduction of RAI uptake after starting the drug but no reinduction was observed [21]. A UK study evaluated 19 patients with DTC treated with sorafenib 400 mg twice daily and the partial

TABLE 1: Kinase inhibitor activities of target therapies on thyroid cancer [16–18].

Drug	Inhibitory concentration 50 [IC_{50}] (nmol/L)							
	VEGFR-1	VEGFR-2	VEGFR-3	RET	$BRAF^{V600E}$	PDGFR-β	Kit	Others
Sorafenib	26	90	20	49	25	57	68	
Axitinib	1.2	0.25	0.29			2	1.7	
Motesanib	2	3	6	59		84	8	
Sunitinib	2	9	17	41		39	1–10	
Pazopanib	10	30	47			84	74	
Lenvatinib (E7080)	22	4	5	35		39		FGFR1 (46)
Cabozantinib (XL-184)		0.035		4				cMET (1.8)
Vandetanib	1600	40	110	130				EGFR (500)
Gefitinib		>10000		3700				EGFR (33)
Selumetinib								MEK1 (14)
Dabrafenib					0.8			

response was 18% at 12 months [23]. Another multicenter study conducted in Spain on metastatic DTC reported the response rate in DTC and PTC were 19% (3 out of 16 patients) and 14% (1 out of 7 patients), respectively. The median progression free survival was 13.5 months in patients [24]. These results appeared comparable to those reported in the two US studies.

In view of the drug toxicities, some authors attempted to reduce the standard dose and evaluated its efficacy. Chen et al. evaluated the efficacy of low dose sorafenib (200 mg twice daily) on 9 patients with RAI refractory pulmonary metastases. After three months of treatment, the partial response (by RECIST criteria) was 33% and stable disease was achieved in 44% of patients. All adverse events were grade 1 or 2. From this study, it appeared that low dose sorafenib could equally achieve satisfactory response in RAI-refractory PTC [22]. Based on initial success in sorafenib, a phase III international randomized controlled trial is currently underway to evaluate it in progressive RAI-refractory metastatic DTC. In this trial, patients are randomized into the placebo arm and drug arm and the primary endpoint is progression-free survival. The final results are awaiting. (NCT00984282).

Axitinib is an oral, potent selective inhibitor of *VEGFRs* 1, 2, and 3. It is selectively less potent in inhibiting platelet derived growth factor receptor beta and *c-KIT*. Cohen et al. published a phase II study on 60 patients with advanced thyroid cancer. Thirty patients with PTC received axitinib 5 mg twice daily oral. Eight patients (26.7%) had partial response. Stable disease lasting for more than 16 weeks was observed in 12 patients (40%). Overall, the median progression-free survival was 18.1 months. Thirty-two patients discontinued axitinib treatment either because of lack of efficacy (10 patients), or adverse effect (8 patients). Hypertension, proteinuria, and fatigue were most common grade 3 or worse events [25].

Motesanib (AMG-706) is a novel oral inhibitor of multiple tyrosine kinases, including *VEGF* receptors, *PDGF* and *KIT*. In an open label phase 2 trials, 93 patients with progressive, locally advanced, or metastatic, RAI-refractory

DTC were prescribed with 125 mg motesanib once daily orally. Fifty-seven (61%) patients had PTC. The objective radiological response assessed was 14%. Of these, 67% achieved stable disease while 35% maintained stable disease for 24 or more weeks. In 75 patients whom had Tg assay, 61 (81%) had reduction in Tg levels. The authors found a significant correlation between the drop in baseline Tg and radiological response rate. Similar to other drugs, adverse effects were a major concern. 94% of all patients experienced adverse events, and 62% had grade 3 or above adverse events. The most common adverse events were hypertension (25%) or diarrhea (13%) There were 2 treatment-related deaths; both were due to pulmonary hemorrhage [26].

Sunitinib is a multitargeted tyrosine kinase inhibitor of *VEGFR* type 1 and 2, *PDGFR* ∂, and β, *c-Kit*, *FLTF*, and *RET*. In a phase II study, 37.5 mg daily sunitinib was prescribed continuously to 35 patients with FDG-avid, RAI-refractory DTC or medullary thyroid carcinoma (MTC). 28% of patients with DTC achieved a RECIST response assessed by 3 monthly CT scan. The median time to progress was 12.8 months in this series. The functional response was also analyzed in this study. In 19 patients with DTC who underwent PET/CT scan before and after 7 days of sunitinib therapy, the percentage change of SUV were −13.5%, 17.5%, and 9.0% for patients with RECIST response, with stable disease and with progressive disease respectively. There was a significant correlation between SUV changes and changes in RECIST criteria ($P = 0.005$). Despite satisfactory functional and RECIST response, hematological and other treatment-related adverse events were also common. Upto 34% of patients suffered grade 3 or worse hematological side effects including leukopenia, neutropenia. Other common adverse effects (≥grade 3) including diarrhea (17%), hand foot syndrome (17%), and fatigue (11%) [27]. Cohen et al. reported another series of 43 patients with either DTC or MTC. In 37 patients with DTC, response rate was 13% and 68% had stable disease. Grade 3/4 haematological adverse effect were comparably common [28].

Pazopanib (Votrient) is a tyrosine kinase inhibitor targeting *VEGFR*, *PDGF*, and *c-KIT*. It has an antiangiogenic effect

TABLE 2: Study on target therapy in radioiodine-refractory papillary thyroid cancer.

Author	Study	Agent	Number of patients [type]	Result			
				Response rate (%)	Stabilization (%)	Progression-free survival (months)	Discontinuation due to adverse effect
Gupta-Abramson et al. [19]	Phase II	Sorafenib	30 [DTC and MTC] (i) DTC: 27/30 (ii) PTC: 18/30	23% 25.9% 22.2%	53% 55.6% 61.1%	18.2 (79 weeks) 19.3 (84 weeks)	16.7%
Kloos et al. [20]	Phase II	Sorafenib	41 [PTC]	15%	56% ($\geq$6 months)	15	—
Hoftijzer et al. [21]	Phase II	Sorafenib	31 [DTC] PTC: 14/31	25%	34% (26 weeks)	13.3 (58 weeks)	19.4%
Chen et al. [22]	Phase II	Sorafenib	9 [PTC]	33%	44%	9.6 (42 weeks)	0
Ahmed et al. [23]	Phase II	Sorafenib	34 [MTC and DTC] PTC: 19/34	15% 18%	74% (6 months)	—	5.9%
Capdevila et al. [24]	Phase II	Sorafenib	34** (i) DTC: 16/34 (ii) PTC: 7/34	32% 19% 14%	41% (6 months) 50% 43%	13.5	—
Cohen et al. [25]	Phase II	Axitinib	60 [DTC] PTC: 30/60	30% 26.7%	38% ($\geq$16 weeks) 40%	18.1	13%
Sherman et al. [26]	Phase II	Motesanib	93 [DTC] PTC: 57/93	14%	35% (24 weeks)	9.3	13%
Carr et al. [27]	Phase II	Sunitinib	35 [DTC and MTC] (i) DTC: 28/35 (ii) PTC: 18/35	31% 28%	46% 68%	12.8	11.4%
Cohen et al. [28]	Phase II	Sunitinib	31 [DTC]	13%	68%	—	—
Bible et al. [29]	Phase II	Pazopanib	37 [DTC] PTC: 15/37	49% 33%	—	11.7	5.4%
Sherman et al. [30]	Phase II	Lenvatinib	58 [DTC] PTC: 43/58	50%	36%	13.3	23%
Cabanillas et al. [31]	Phase II	Cabozantinib	15 [DTC]	53%	40%	—	—
Leboulleux et al. [32]	RCT, phase II	Vandetanib	72 versus 73 [DTC] PTC: 25 versus 24	8.3% versus 5.5%	56% versus 36%*	11.1 versus 5.8* 16.2 versus 5.9	33% versus 6%
Pennell et al. [33]	Phase II	Gefitinib	27** PTC: 11/27	0%	24% (6 months)	3.7	7.4%
Hayes et al. [34]	Phase II	Selumetinib	32 [PTC]	3%	36% (24 weeks)	7.4	—
Falchook et al. [35]	Phase I	Dabrafenib	14 [PTC]	21.4%	—	—	0

DTC: differentiated thyroid cancer, PTC: papillary thyroid cancer, MTC: medullary thyroid cancer; RCT: randomized controlled trial.
*$P < 0.05$.
**Included differentiated, medullary, and anaplastic thyroid carcinoma.

on RAI-refractory DTC. In a phase II study on 37 patients with progressive radioiodine refractory DTC over previous 6 months, partial response was achieved in 18 patients. Response rate was 49% and 33% (5 out of 15%) in patients with DTC and PTC, respectively. 66% of patients were likely to respond lasting for more than 1 year. The response rate was highest among reports of different agent. Adverse effects were common but generally well tolerate. Grade 3 or worse adverse effect was not common, and the commonest was deranged liver function tests (4 patients had raised ALT concentration). Two patients had serious hemorrhagic events (grade 3 lower gastro-intestinal bleeding, and grade 4 intracranial bleeding in the absence of brain metastasis or hypertension) and so had to discontinue treatment [29].

Lenvatinib (E7080) is an oral tyrosine kinase inhibitor targeting VEGFR 1–3, FGFR 1–4, RET, KIT, and PDGFR β. In an international phase II study, 58 patients with advanced progressive DTC were enrolled. Half of them achieved partial response on assessment. For the subgroup which had prior VEGFR inhibitors, 41% had a response whereas those without prior treatment, 54% had a response. However, because adverse effect was common, 23% of patients had to withdraw and 35% had to have a dose reduction [30].

Cabozantinib (XL84) is an oral potent inhibitor of cMET (MET is a membrane receptor that is essential for embryonic development and wound healing), VEGFR2, and RET and is currently undergoing a clinical trial. The results of the phase I trial of this drug appeared promising with 8/15 (53%)

patients having confirmed partial response and 6 (40%) had stable disease [31]. It is worth noting that the majority of these patients had prior *VEGFR* inhibitors. Grades 3, and 4 adverse effects were comparable to other *VEGFR* inhibitors and included diarrhea (20%), hypertension (13%), and hand foot syndrome (13%) [31].

Vandetanib, a tyrosine kinase inhibitor of *RET*, *VEGFR*, and *EGFR* signaling, was the first targeted therapy subjected to large scale multicenter randomized clinical trial [32]. 145 patients with radioiodine refractory differentiated thyroid cancer were enrolled into the trial. Seventy-two patients, including 25 with PTC, were allocated to vandetanib 300 mg per day group and 73 patients, including 24 with PTC were allocated to placebo group. Patients in vandetanib group (median: 11.1 months (95% CI 7.7–14.0)) had longer progression-free survival than placebo group [median: 5.9 months (95% CI 4.0–8.9) ($P = 0.017$). For patient with PTC, median progression-free survival was 16.2 months (95% CI 8.4–22.6) in vandetanib group and 5.9 months (95% CI 3.0–11.5) in placebo group. Although it was not statistically significant, there was a tendency for clinical benefit (Hazard ratio: 0.52, 95% CI 0.26–1.02, $P = 0.056$). However, there was no difference in overall survival (Hazard ratio: 0.83, 95% CI 0.52–1.33, $P = 0.42$). Most frequent adverse events were diarrhea (74%) and hypertension (34%). The incidence of grade 3 or worse adverse events were higher in vandetanib group (53%, 39/73 patients) than placebo group (19%, 14/72 patients), while the commonest were QTc prolongation (14%) and diarrhea (10%) [32].

Since *EGFR* mutations were found in some PTC, Gefitinib, an inhibitor of *EGFR* tyrosine kinase, had been evaluated in a phase II study for advanced PTC. Pennell et al. reported the results of 27 patients with 11 of them suffering from PTC. There was no objective response observed. 24% had stable disease after 6 months of treatment. Five patients with stable disease had significant drop in thyroglobulin (>90% drop) maintained over 3 months. However, no patient achieved partial response by criteria. The authors concluded that this drug had limited biological activity of around 12% only [33].

Other than antiangiogenic therapies, drugs targeting specific molecular pathway, namely MAPK and PI3K, were studied in phase I, and II studies. Selumetinib is a selective oral non-ATP competitive small molecule inhibitor of *MAPK* kinases, *MEK* 1/2. In in vitro studies, Selumetinib was potent in PTC cell line with V600E *BRAF* mutation. It had been recently evaluated in a multicenter phase II study in patient with radioiodine refractory papillary thyroid carcinoma. Selumetinib 100 mg twice daily was prescribed to patients with document progression in the last 12 months. Only 1 patient (3%) achieved partial response and 21 (54%) had stable disease. Common grade 3 to 4 toxicities included rash (18%), fatigue (8%), diarrhea (5%), and peripheral edema (5%). In *BRAF* evaluated patient, *BRAF* mutant had a longer median progression free survival than *BRAF* wide-type tumor, though it was not statistically significant (33 versus 11 weeks, $P = 0.3$) [34].

In a recent published phase I trial, Dabrafenib, inhibitor of *BRAF* kinase for *BRAF* mutant, had showed its anti-tumor activity in 14 patients with *BRAF* mutant PTC. Three of nine assessable patients achieved partial response. Its adverse effect was less common and more tolerable. The most common grade 2 or worse adverse effects were cutaneous squamous cell carcinoma (11%), fatigue (8%), and pyrexia (6%) [35].

In addition to agents which target MAPK and PI3 K-AKT pathways, *mTOR* inhibitors have been widely studied recently. In vitro studies, *mTOR* pathway activation have been found in aggressive and *BRAF* mutated PTC [38, 39]. Phase I study of daily everolimus plus low dose weekly cisplatin reported 1 out of 4 patients achieved prolong stable disease for 6 months [40]. Sherman et al. reported phase II study on use of combination of sorafenib and temsirolimus in 37 patients radioiodine refractory thyroid carcinoma. 21.6% patients had partial response and 56.7% had stable after median time on treatment of 206 days [41].

Studies on combination of target therapy like everolimus/lenalidomide, pazopanib/GSK1120212 (*MEK* inhibitor), and pimasertib (*MEK* inhibitor)/SAR245409 (PI3K/*mTOR* inhibitors) are ongoing and hopefully, results would become available in the near future [42–44].

Majority of studies focused on patients with PTC or small subgroup of follicular thyroid carcinoma (FTC) patients (Table 2); current evidences on treatment specific on FTC were limited. Applicability and efficacy of target therapies on patient with follicular thyroid carcinoma have to be further evaluated.

5. Redifferentiation of RAI-Refractory Thyroid Carcinoma

Redifferentiation remains an ongoing area of research in RAI-refractory thyroid carcinoma because development of de-differentiated phenotype of DTC leads to loss or absence of radioiodine uptake ability. Redifferentiating agents could potentially reactivate the RAI uptake ability of thyroid carcinoma. Retinoids, chemically related to Vitamin A, were the first widely studied agents for potential application on redifferentiation in radioiodine refractory thyroid cancer.

Early in vitro studies showed that decreased expression of retinoic acid receptor in thyroid cancer cell [45]. Treatment with retinoids could upgrade the sodium-iodine symporter (NIS) and thus induce redifferentiation and iodine uptake by tumor cell. Grüning et al. reported their series on 14 RAI-refractory patients and showed that 2/14 showed slightly increased uptake [46]. Similar results have been found by other authors. Short et al. reported the results of 16 patients with RAI uptake negative DTC. Patients were prescribed oral isotretinoid 1.5 mg/kg/day for 8 weeks. RAI scan repeated 2 weeks later reviewed only 1/16 (6.25%) patient had increased radio-iodine uptake [47]. Simon et al. reported a more promising result of using 13-cis-retinoic acid as a sole treatment. Fifty patients with RAI-refractory DTC were treated with 13-cis-retinoic acid at dosage of 1.5 mg/kg daily over 5 weeks. Thirteen (26%) showed marked increase in RAI uptake while 8 patients (16%) showed mild increased in RAI uptake in the post-therapy scan. Tumor size was assessed in 37 patients and of these, 6 had tumor regression while 22 had static disease. As a whole, 19 (38%) patients showed either response or stable in clinical response. However, further analysis reviewed that increased RAI uptake did not always correlate with clinical response [48]. More recently, Oh et al. incorporated retinoic acid into RAI ablation to treat RAI refractory PTC. Oral isotretinoid was prescribed for 6 weeks at 1–1.5 mg/kg daily and then followed by single dose of RAI. At 6-month follow up, 1 patient showed completed response, 9 had partial response, 9 had stable and 28 had progressive disease. Overall response rate was 21.3% [49].

Due to the limited benefits, routine use of retinoic acid alone is not recommended. Preliminary study showed enlightening clinical response in refractory cancer results only in combination therapy. Therefore, further studies are indicated to evaluate its clinical application, dosage, duration, and combination regimen.

Thiazolidinedione, an antidiabetic medication, is another potential redifferentiation agent. It acts as a peroxisome proliferator-activated receptor gamma agonist. It was shown to have both redifferentiation and anti-proliferative effects in in vitro study of thyroid cancer cells [50]. In an open phase II trial of 20 patients with Tg-positive RAI-refractory DTC, 25% (5/20) regained RAI uptake. 60% (12/20) had stable disease and 15% (3/20) had reduction in tumor marker. Overall, 5 patients had a partial response in terms of decreased Tg or positive RAI uptake on scan. However, no complete or partial response was noted in any patients according to RECIST criteria [51]. Other agents, including histone deacetylase inhibitor, (e.g., valproic acid, trichostatin, and depsipeptide), DNA demethylating agents, (e.g., 5-azacytidine), and arsenic trioxide, had shown differentiation inducing properties in thyroid cancer cells in in vitro studies [52–55]. Potential clinical application had to be further validated by future studies.

6. Conclusion

Managing RAI-refractory advanced or metastatic PTC remains challenging. Given the fact that RAI is of little benefit in this group of patients, various treatment options such as observation, symptomatic control, surgery, local ablative therapy, metastectomy, and EBRT might be considered. New molecular targeted drugs including tyrosine kinase inhibitors and redifferentiation drugs are new promising therapeutic options for this specific group of patients.

References

[1] Hong Kong Cancer Registry, "Cancer incidence and mortality in Hong Kong 1983–2006," Hong Kong Cancer Registry, Hong Kong, 2012, http://www3.ha.org.hk/cancereg/.

[2] B. H. Lang, K. P. Wong, and K. Y. Wan, "Postablation stimulated thyroglobulin level is an important predictor of biochemical complete remission after reoperative cervical neck dissection in persistent/recurrent papillary thyroid Carcinoma," Annals of Surgical Oncology. In press.

[3] H. Tala and R. M. Tuttle, "Contemporary post surgical management of differentiated thyroid carcinoma," Clinical Oncology, vol. 22, no. 6, pp. 419–429, 2010.

[4] H. Wong, K. P. Wong, T. Yau et al., "Is there a role for unstimulated thyroglobulin velocity in predicting recurrence in papillary thyroid carcinoma patients with detectable thyroglobulin after radioiodine ablation?" Annals of Surgical Oncology, vol. 19, no. 11, pp. 3479–3485, 2012.

[5] D. S. Cooper, G. M. Doherty, B. R. Haugen et al., "Revised American thyroid association management guidelines for patients with thyroid nodules and differentiated thyroid cancer," Thyroid, vol. 19, no. 11, pp. 1167–1214, 2009.

[6] D. T. Hughes, A. M. Laird, B. S. Miller et al., "Reoperative lymph node dissection for recurrent papillary thyroid cancer and effect on serum thyroglobulin," Annals of Surgical Oncology, vol. 19, no. 9, pp. 2951–2957, 2012.

[7] D. E. Dupuy, J. M. Monchik, C. Decrea, and L. Pisharodi, "Radiofrequency ablation of regional recurrence from well-differentiated thyroid malignancy," Surgery, vol. 130, no. 6, pp. 971–977, 2001.

[8] B. D. Lewis, I. D. Hay, J. W. Charboneau, B. McIver, C. C. Reading, and J. R. Goellner, "Percutaneous ethanol injection for treatment of cervical lymph node metastases in patients with papillary thyroid carcinoma," American Journal of Roentgenology, vol. 178, no. 3, pp. 699–704, 2002.

[9] K. Nakada, K. Kasai, Y. Watanabe et al., "Treatment of radioiodine-negative bone metastasis from papillary thyroid carcinoma with percutaneous ethanol injection therapy," Annals of Nuclear Medicine, vol. 10, no. 4, pp. 441–444, 1996.

[10] R. W. Tsang, J. D. Brierley, W. J. Simpson et al., "The effects of surgery, radioiodine, and external radiation therapy on the clinical outcome of patients with differentiated thyroid carcinoma," Cancer, vol. 82, no. 2, pp. 375–388, 1998.

[11] M. Luster, F. Lippi, B. Jarzab et al., "rhTSH-aided radioiodine ablation and treatment of differentiated thyroid carcinoma: a comprehensive review," Endocrine-Related Cancer, vol. 12, no. 1, pp. 49–64, 2005.

[12] F. Pacini, L. Agate, R. Elisei et al., "Outcome of differentiated thyroid cancer with detectable serum Tg and negative diagnostic ^{131}I whole body scan: comparison of patients treated with high ^{131}I activities versus untreated patients," The Journal of Clinical Endocrinology & Metabolism, vol. 86, no. 9, pp. 4092–4097, 2001.

[13] V. Fatourechi, I. D. Hay, H. Javedan, G. A. Wiseman, B. P. Mullan, and C. A. Gorman, "Lack of impact of radioiodine therapy in tg-positive, diagnostic whole-body scan-negative patients with follicular cell-derived thyroid cancer," The Journal of Clinical Endocrinology & Metabolism, vol. 87, no. 4, pp. 1521–1526, 2002.

[14] B. H. Lang, I. O. L. Wong, K. P. Wong et al., "Risk of second primary malignancy in differentiated thyroid carcinoma treated with radioactive iodine therapy," Surgery, vol. 151, no. 6, pp. 844–850, 2012.

[15] Y. E. Nikiforov and M. N. Nikiforova, "Molecular genetics and diagnosis of thyroid cancer," Nature Reviews Endocrinology, vol. 7, no. 10, pp. 56–80, 2011.

[16] M. Schlumberger and S. I. Sherman, "Approach to the patient with advanced differentiated thyroid cancer," European Journal of Endocrinology, vol. 166, no. 1, pp. 5–11, 2012.

[17] F. Pacini, L. Brilli, and S. Marchisotta, "Targeted therapy in radioiodine refractory thyroid cancer," Quarterly Journal of Nuclear Medicine and Molecular Imaging, vol. 53, no. 5, pp. 520–525, 2009.

[18] E. Grande, J. José Díez, C. Zafon et al., "Thyroid cancer: molecular aspects and new therapeutic strategies," *Journal of Thyroid Research*, vol. 2012, Article ID 847108, 10 pages, 2012.

[19] V. Gupta-Abramson, A. B. Troxel, A. Nellore et al., "Phase II trial of sorafenib in advanced thyroid cancer," *Journal of Clinical Oncology*, vol. 26, no. 29, pp. 4714–4719, 2008.

[20] R. T. Kloos, M. H. Shah, M. D. Ringel et al., "Phase II trial of sorafenib in metastatic thyroid cancer," *Journal of Clinical Oncology*, vol. 27, no. 10, pp. 1675–1684, 2009.

[21] H. Hoftijzer, K. A. Heemstra, H. Morreau et al., "Beneficial effects of sorafenib on tumor progression, but not on radioiodine uptake, in patients with differentiated thyroid carcinoma," *European Journal of Endocrinology*, vol. 161, no. 6, pp. 923–931, 2009.

[22] L. Chen, Y. Shen, Q. Luo, Y. Yu, H. Lu, and R. Zhu, "Response to sorafenib at a low dose in patients with radioiodine-refractory pulmonary metastases from papillary thyroid carcinoma," *Thyroid*, vol. 21, no. 2, pp. 119–124, 2011.

[23] M. Ahmed, Y. Barbachano, A. Riddell et al., "Analysis of the efficacy and toxicity of sorafenib in thyroid cancer: a phase II study in a UK based population," *European Journal of Endocrinology*, vol. 165, no. 2, pp. 315–322, 2011.

[24] J. Capdevila, L. Iglesias, I. Halperin et al., "Sorafenib in metastatic thyroid cancer," *Endocrine-Related Cancer*, vol. 19, no. 2, pp. 209–216, 2012.

[25] E. E. W. Cohen, L. S. Rosen, E. E. Vokes et al., "Axitinib is an active treatment for all histologic subtypes of advanced thyroid cancer: results from a phase II study," *Journal of Clinical Oncology*, vol. 26, no. 29, pp. 4708–4713, 2008.

[26] S. I. Sherman, L. J. Wirth, J. P. Droz et al., "Motesanib diphosphate in progressive differentiated thyroid cancer," *The New England Journal of Medicine*, vol. 359, no. 1, pp. 31–42, 2008.

[27] L. L. Carr, D. A. Mankoff, B. H. Goulart et al., "Phase II study of daily sunitinib in FDG-PET-positive, iodine-refractory differentiated thyroid cancer and metastatic medullary carcinoma of the thyroid with functional imaging correlation," *Clinical Cancer Research*, vol. 16, no. 21, pp. 5260–5268, 2010.

[28] E. E. Cohen, B. M. Needles, K. J. Cullen et al., "Phase 2 study of sunitinib in refractory thyroid cancer," *Journal of Clinical Oncology*, vol. 26, no. 15, supplement, ASCO Meeting Abstracts 6025, 2008.

[29] K. C. Bible, V. J. Suman, J. R. Molina et al., "Efficacy of pazopanib in progressive, radioiodine-refractory, metastatic differentiated thyroid cancers: results of a phase 2 consortium study," *The Lancet Oncology*, vol. 11, no. 10, pp. 962–972, 2010.

[30] S. I. Sherman, B. Jarzab, M. E. Cabanillas et al., "A phase II trial of the multitargeted kinase inhibitor E7080 in advanced radioiodine (RAI)-refractory differentiated thyroid cancer (DTC)," *Journal of Clinical Oncology*, vol. 29, no. 15, supplement, ASCO Meeting Abstracts 5503, 2011.

[31] M. E. Cabanillas, M. S. Brose, D. A. Ramies et al., "Antitumor activity of cabozantinib (XL184) in a cohort of patients (pts) with differentiated thyroid cancer (DTC)," *Journal of Clinical Oncology*, vol. 30, no. 15, supplement, ASCO Meeting Abstracts 5547, 2012.

[32] S. Leboulleux, L. Bastholt, T. Krause et al., "Vandetanib in locally advanced or metastatic differentiated thyroid cancer: a randomised, double-blind, phase 2 trial," *The Lancet Oncology*, vol. 13, no. 9, pp. 897–905, 2012.

[33] N. A. Pennell, G. H. Daniels, R. I. Haddad et al., "A phase II study of gefitinib in patients with advanced thyroid cancer," *Thyroid*, vol. 18, no. 3, pp. 317–323, 2008.

[34] D. N. Hayes, A. S. Lucas, T. Tanvetyanon et al., "Phase II efficacy and pharmacogenomic study of Selumetinib (AZD6244, ARRY-142886) in iodine-131 refractory papillary thyroid carcinoma with or without follicular elements," *Clinical Cancer Research*, vol. 18, no. 7, pp. 2056–2065, 2012.

[35] G. S. Falchook, G. V. Long, R. Kurzrock et al., "Dabrafenib in patients with melanoma, untreated brain metastases, and other solid tumours: a phase 1 dose-escalation trial," *The Lancet*, vol. 379, no. 9829, pp. 1893–1901, 2012.

[36] B. H. H. Lang and T. T. Law, "The role of 18F-fluorodeoxyglucose positron emission tomography in thyroid neoplasms," *Oncologist*, vol. 16, no. 4, pp. 458–466, 2011.

[37] W. Wang, S. M. Larson, M. Fazzari et al., "Prognostic value of [18F]fluorodeoxyglucose positron emission tomographic scanning in patients with thyroid cancer," *The Journal of Clinical Endocrinology & Metabolism*, vol. 85, no. 3, pp. 1107–1113, 2000.

[38] A. Faustino, J. P. Couto, H. Pópulo et al., "mTOR pathway overactivation in BRAF mutated papillary thyroid carcinoma," *The Journal of Clinical Endocrinology & Metabolism*, vol. 97, no. 7, pp. E1139–E1149, 2012.

[39] M. A. Kouvaraki, C. Liakou, A. Paraschi et al., "Activation of mTOR signaling in medullary and aggressive papillary thyroid carcinomas," *Surgery*, vol. 150, no. 6, pp. 1258–1265, 2011.

[40] M. G. Fury, E. Sherman, S. Haque et al., "A phase I study of daily everolimus plus low-dose weekly cisplatin for patients with advanced solid tumors," *Cancer Chemotherapy and Pharmacology*, vol. 69, no. 3, pp. 591–598, 2012.

[41] E. J. Sherman, A. L. Ho, M. G. Fury et al., "A phase II study of temsirolimus/sorafenib in patients with radioactive iodine (RAI)-refractory thyroid carcinoma," *Journal of Clinical Oncology*, vol. 30, no. 15, supplement, ASCO Meeting Abstracts 5514, 2012.

[42] T. K. Owonikoko, R. D. Harvey, J. S. Kauh et al., "A phase I study of the safety and pharmacodynamic effects of everolimus in combination with lenalidomide in patients with advanced solid malignancies," *Journal of Clinical Oncology*, vol. 30, no. 15, supplement, ASCO Meeting Abstracts 2576, 2012.

[43] S. R. Ahmed, N. S. Azad, D. Wilmot Ball et al., "A phase I study determining the safety and tolerability of combination therapy with pazopanib, a VEGFR/PDGFR/raf inhibitor, and GSK1120212, a MEK inhibitor, in advanced solid tumors enriched with patients with advanced differentiated thyroid cancer," *Journal of Clinical Oncology*, vol. 30, no. 15, supplement, ASCO Meeting Abstracts TPS3117, 2012.

[44] J. R. Infante, L. Gandhi, G. Shapiro et al., "Phase Ib combination trial of a MEK inhibitor, pimasertib (MSC1936369B), and a PI3K/mTOR inhibitor, SAR245409, in patients with locally advanced or metastatic solid tumors," *Journal of Clinical Oncology*, vol. 30, no. 15, supplement, ASCO Meeting Abstracts TPS3118, 2012.

[45] L. A. Hansen, C. C. Sigman, F. Andreola, S. A. Ross, G. J. Kelloff, and L. M. De Luca, "Retinoids in chemoprevention and differentiation therapy," *Carcinogenesis*, vol. 21, no. 7, pp. 1271–1279, 2000.

[46] T. Grüning, C. Tiepolt, K. Zöphel, J. Bredow, J. Kropp, and W. G. Franke, "Retinoic acid for redifferentiation of thyroid cancer—does it hold its promise?" *European Journal of Endocrinology*, vol. 148, no. 4, pp. 395–402, 2003.

[47] S. C. Short, A. Suovuori, G. Cook, G. Vivian, and C. Harmer, "A phase II study using retinoids as redifferentiation agents to increase iodine uptake in metastatic thyroid cancer," *Clinical Oncology*, vol. 16, no. 8, pp. 569–574, 2004.

[48] D. Simon, C. Körber, M. Krausch et al., "Clinical impact of retinoids in redifferentiation therapy of advanced thyroid cancer: final results of a pilot study," *European Journal of Nuclear Medicine and Molecular Imaging*, vol. 29, no. 6, pp. 775–782, 2002.

[49] S. W. Oh, S. H. Moon, B. Y. Cho et al., "Combined therapy with ^{131}I and retinoic acid in Korean patients with radioiodine-refractory papillary thyroid cancer," *European Journal of Nuclear Medicine and Molecular Imaging*, vol. 38, no. 10, pp. 1798–1805, 2011.

[50] M. L. Martelli, R. Iuliano, I. Le Pera et al., "Inhibitory effects of peroxisome poliferator-activated receptor gamma on thyroid carcinoma cell growth," *The Journal of Clinical Endocrinology & Metabolism*, vol. 87, no. 10, pp. 4728–4735, 2002.

[51] E. Kebebew, S. Lindsay, O. H. Clark, K. A. Woeber, R. Hawkins, and F. S. Greenspan, "Results of rosiglitazone therapy in patients with thyroglobulin-positive and radioiodine-negative advanced differentiated thyroid cancer," *Thyroid*, vol. 19, no. 9, pp. 953–956, 2009.

[52] N. Fortunati, M. G. Catalano, K. Arena, E. Brignardello, A. Piovesan, and G. Boccuzzi, "Valproic acid induces the expression of the Na+/I- symporter and Iodine uptake in poorly differentiated thyroid cancer cells," *The Journal of Clinical Endocrinology & Metabolism*, vol. 89, no. 2, pp. 1006–1009, 2004.

[53] W. T. Shen and W. Y. Chung, "Treatment of thyroid cancer with histone deacetylase inhibitors and peroxisome proliferator-activated receptor-γ agonists," *Thyroid*, vol. 15, no. 6, pp. 594–599, 2005.

[54] T. Kondo, T. Nakazawa, D. Ma et al., "Epigenetic silencing of TTF-1/NKX2-1 through DNA hypermethylation and histone H3 modulation in thyroid carcinomas," *Laboratory Investigation*, vol. 89, no. 7, pp. 791–799, 2009.

[55] E. Fröhlich, B. Czarnocka, P. Brossart, and R. Wahl, "Antitumor effects of arsenic trioxide in transformed human thyroid cells," *Thyroid*, vol. 18, no. 11, pp. 1183–1193, 2008.

24

Leptin: A Correlated Peptide to Papillary Thyroid Carcinoma?

Mehdi Hedayati,[1] Parichehr Yaghmaei,[2] Zahra Pooyamanesh,[2] Marjan Zarif Yeganeh,[1] and Laleh Hoghooghi Rad[1]

[1] Obesity Research Center, Research Institute for Endocrine Sciences, Shahid Beheshti University of Medical Sciences, 1985717413 Tehran, Iran
[2] Department of Biology, Faculty of Basic Sciences, Science Research Campus of Islamic Azad University, 1939614484 Tehran, Iran

Correspondence should be addressed to Mehdi Hedayati, hedayati@endocrine.ac.ir

Academic Editor: Oliver Gimm

Introduction. Leptin as an adipose-tissue-related peptide hormone contributes to the control of food intake, energy expenditure, and other activities such as cell proliferation. Therefore, association of leptin level with thyroid cancer has been suggested recently. Considering that thyroid cancer is the most common endocrine cancer, the aim of this study was evaluation of leptin levels in thyroid cancer. *Materials and Methods.* 83 patients with papillary thyroid cancer (35 males and 48 females) with 90 healthy persons as control group (40 male and 50 females) were selected. serum thyroxine, thyrotropin, and leptin levels were determined in both groups. As a body fat tissue affects leptin level, so height and weight were measured and body mass index was calculated too. *Results.* There was no statistically significant difference in age, serum Thyroxine, and Thyrotropin levels. BMI in women was more than in men in both groups. Serum leptin levels in thyroid cancer group were significantly higher than control group ($P < 0.05$). *Conclusion.* The results of this study showed an acceptable association between the hormone Leptin levels with papillary thyroid cancer, so it may be considerad as a correlated peptide which may help in the diagnosis or confirmation of thyroid cancer beside in other specific tumor markers.

1. Introduction

leptin with 16 kDa molecular weight mainly produces by white adipose tissue cells [1]. So its level is proportional to the adipose tissue mass [2]. leptin as a neuroendocrine hormone has effects on the glucose metabolism, sexual maturation, reproduction, pituitary-adrenal axis, immune system, thyroid, and growth hormones level [3–6]. The association between this neuroendocrine hormone with obesity and some cancers has been proposed. Probably this hormone is an important risk factor in carcinogenesis, because obesity itself can promote tumorgenesis and is a risk factor for cancer over time [7, 8]. On the other hand, leptin plays an important role in the oxidation reactions such as fatty acid oxidation [9] and angiogenesis [10]. There are many reports concerning the effect of leptin on stimulation of cell mitosis and its involvement in carcinogenic stages of breast, clone, prostate, lung, kidney, and ovary cells [11–16]. Studies have shown that leptin by increase of cell proliferation and inhibition of apoptosis is involved in creating certain types of tumors [17–19].

leptin acts through its receptor on the cell surface and its receptor expression also increases following the activity of PI3K/AKT pathway and increases the activity of antiapoptosis molecules such as Bcl-XL and XIAP [20]. In some cancer cells, expression of leptin receptor levels and stimulation by leptin will lead to increase of cell proliferation [21]. leptin stimulates expression of some molecules such as CyclinD1, CDK2 and c-Myc that result in cell cycle progression and cell proliferation [21, 22].

The Important molecular pathways, such as JAK/STAT3, PI3K/AKT, ERK/MAPK, in many cancer cells can be activated by leptin/leptin receptors [21–24]. Furthermore, leptin with the induction of VEGF and VEGF-R2 molecules expression plays an important role in the tumorigenesis [25]. These molecules are involved in many malignancies such as colon, stomach, endometrial, ovarian, and breast cancer [26–30]. Additionally, increased serum levels of leptin and its receptor have been associated with distant metastases, disease recurrence, and lower survival in patients with breast cancer [31]. Increased expression of leptin and its receptor in papillary thyroid cancer has been proved. This hormone probably through its receptor and activation of the PI3K/AKT pathway plays an important role in papillary thyroid cancer pathogenesis. It also seems that the oncogenic effects of leptin on papillary thyroid carcinoma cells are related to the stimulating cell proliferation and apoptosis inhibition. Involvement of thyroid hormones on basal metabolism and regulating appetite and weight control in many scientific reports is given explicitly [10, 32–34]. The most common endocrine malignancy is thyroid cancer, and papillary form of thyroid cancer is the most common type of thyroid cancer (80–90%) [32]. The aim of this study was determining the serum leptin levels in patients with papillary thyroid cancer and its comparison with healthy subjects.

2. Materials and Methods

2.1. Subjects

Patients. The case population consisted of 83 individuals, including 35 males and 48 females, 14 to 62 years (mean age 38.6 years) with papillary thyroid cancer (PTC). They were referred to Research Institute for Endocrine Sciences, Shahid Beheshti University of Medical Science. Also, 90 persons were selected as control group (40 male and 50 females) from referred to the laboratory with normal thyroid function tests (TSH: 0.3 = 3.5 mIU/L, T4: 4.5 = 12.5 μg/dL, T = Up: 25 = 35% and T3: 75 = 210 ng/mL) with age, sex, BMI matched with case group. Both groups were also matched for age and sex. The participants were included in the survey after obtaining an informed consent. Also, the clinical examination was performed by endocrinologist. The diagnosis of PTC was confirmed by histopathologic documents. This study has been approved by Institutional Review Board and Ethics Committee of Obesity Research Center, Research Institute for Endocrine Sciences, Shahid Beheshti University of Medical Sciences.

2.2. Methods. Blood sampling was performed in both studied groups. For preparation of serum, 3 mL of whole blood was collected from antecubital vein in sitting position and was incubated 10 min in RT for coagulation. Then sera separated by 10 min centrifugation at 3000 rpm and the obtained sera were aliquoted in three 0.5 mL microtubes. The isolated serum samples from each individual were stored in 1 mL Eppendorf microtubes at −80°C (Japan's Sanyo C Company).

Anthropometric characteristics, including height and weight of patients and control group, were measured by height measuring scaled balance (Seca, German company); height with 0.5 cm and weight with 250 g sensitivity were reported. These data were used to calculate the body mass index (kg/m^2). Demographic profiles, including age, and sex were also recorded. Those individuals, who were using drugs affecting thyroid function and obesity drugs, were excluded.

In groups thyroxine, thyrotropin, and leptin hormones were measured by ELISA method. The used kits were prepared from the Canadian company (DBC Company, Ontario, Canada). The ELISA reader was from Tecan Austrian Company and Sunrise Model. Human thyrotropin and leptin hormones were determined based on sandwich ELISA method, whereas a thyroxin hormone was measured according to the competitive EIA method. The sensitivity of thyroxine, thyrotropin, and leptin kits was 0.6 μg/dL, 0.1 mU/L, and 0.4 ng/mL, respectively. Additionally, the coefficients of variation for these assays were 6.2%, 7.1%, and 6.5%, respectively.

2.2.1. Statistical Analysis. According to the normal distribution of data obtained by testing Kolmogorov-Smirnov (KS) ($P = 0.68$ for case group and $P = 0.52$ for control group), the frequency, mean and standard deviation were used to describe characteristics. All the data were in normal distribution (except leptin after normalization). The independent t-test was used to compare mean (except leptin with geometric mean and CI 95%) of variables between two groups. Comparison of qualitative data was done with Chi-square test. Further, data was analyzed using statistical software (SPSS 15), and significant level was considered at 0.05.

3. Results

Demographic profiles and anthropometric characteristics of participants are provided in Table 1. The results of thyroid hormones test, including thyroxine and thyrotropin in both control and patients groups, are given in Table 2. Since the leptin hormone secreted from adipose tissue is different in male and female, therefore the different levels of measured leptin hormone in two groups are shown in Table 3 (gender based). Height, weight, and body mass index between males and females of both groups were significant ($P < 0.05$). In addition, a significant difference ($P < 0.05$) was observed between the leptin hormone levels in males and females in both healthy and cancer groups. The amount of leptin hormone in cancer patients was higher than that in normal individuals, significantly ($P < 0.05$).

4. Discussion

Our data showed that the serum leptin levels of Iranian patients with papillary thyroid carcinoma were significantly higher than those in control group subjects. This increased level was observed in both males and females with papillary thyroid carcinoma. As this increased level was observed in both gender and different ages, so it could be related to thyroid carcinoma and it is independent of sex and age. Even though in this study the leptin level was higher in females than males in both groups, this is probably related to more adipose tissue mass in women. Both leptin and thyroid hormones cause thermogenesis and reduce body weight therefore maybe it is considered as a first association between the two hormones. The hunger reduces the leptin

TABLE 1: Anthropometric characteristics of participants.

Group	Sex	Height (cm)	Weight (kg)	BMI (kg/m²)	Mean age (year)
Control	Female (50)	159.5 ± 12.1	61.9 ± 0.3	24.5 ± 2.3	38.1 ± 12.5
	Male (40)	169.2 ± 10.5	66.3 ± 0.2	23.2 ± 2.0	37.9 ± 15.8
Case	Female (48)	160.2 ± 11.6	63.7 ± 0.3	24.9 ± 2.7	39.1 ± 13.7
	Male (35)	170.4 ± 11.3	68.4 ± 0.2	23.7 ± 2.4	37.5 ± 17.0

TABLE 2: Serum levels of thyroxin and thyrotropin hormones in participants.

Group	Thyroxin (μg/dL)	Thyrotropin (mU/L)
Control	9.1 ± 2.9	2.4 ± 1.2
Case	8.9 ± 3.0	2.6 ± 1.0

TABLE 3: Serum leptin levels in participants.

Group	Females serum leptin level (ng/mL)	Males serum leptin level (ng/mL)
Control	4.3 ± 6.9	2.2 ± 5.6
Case	19.6 ± 23.3 ($P < 0.05$)	10.4 ± 17.3 ($P < 0.05$)

and thyroid hormones levels [35]. High levels of thyroid hormones decrease leptin expression in adipose tissue. But the most studies have not shown significant changes in leptin levels in hypothyroidism and hyperthyroidism disorders [36, 37]. However, increased leptin level in postpartum thyroiditis has been reported [38]. Akinci et al. reported that leptin levels increased in papillary thyroid carcinoma in Turkish population [39]. But in their study only 34 cases were investigated, the status of thyroid function in patients and healthy group was not evaluated, and age-matching was not considered [39]. In our study, 83 persons were matched for age, sex, and BMI. Assessing thyroid function in patients and healthy individuals was performed, and no significant difference was observed in both groups.

In both above studies, BMI in women was higher than in men, which was quite predictable. In both studies leptin levels in women were higher than those in men that is because of increased fat mass in women. In one study Cheng et al. showed that expression of leptin and/or leptin receptor in papillary thyroid cancer was associated with neoplasm aggressiveness, including tumor size and lymph node metastasis [40]. Interestingly, in another study, Uddin et al. demonstrated that leptin plays an important role in papillary thyroid cancer pathogenesis through PI3K/AKT pathway via its receptor (Ob-R) and is a potential prognostic marker associated with an aggressive phenotype and poor survival [32].

One of the limitations of our study was inability to followup the patients after surgery. Therefore, reduction or normalization of high leptin levels in thyroid cancer patients was not assessed. However, a significant increase of serum leptin levels in Iranian patients with papillary thyroid carcinoma maybe used as a reliable marker to diagnose or confirm papillary thyroid cancer. In addition if the leptin levels in cancer patients decrease after thyroidectomy, it will be used for the followup treatment, possibly. So a before-after study is recommended for future investigations instead of case control study. Thus, leptin level measurement can be used to followup the treatment of patients.

Strongly high leptin level in papillary thyroid cancer patients in comparison with health subject potentially suggests leptin as a peptide marker of papillary thyroid cancer. It means that adipose tissue secreted hormones, proteins, and peptides potentially may have application in diagnosis, confirmation, and/or treatment followup.

Acknowledgments

This study was supported by a research grant from Endocrine Research Center, Shahid Beheshti University of Medical Sciences. The authors are indebted to kind collaboration of several endocrinology specialists. They express their gratitude to the staffs of Laboratory at Endocrine Research Center, for their skillful technical assistance.

References

[1] C. Liu, X. J. Liu, G. Barry, N. Ling, R. A. Maki, and E. B. De Souza, "Expression and characterization of a putative high affinity human soluble leptin receptor," *Endocrinology*, vol. 138, no. 8, pp. 3548–3554, 1997.

[2] M. Wauters, R. V. Considine, and L. F. Van Gaal, "Human leptin: from an adipocyte hormone to an endocrine mediator," *European Journal of Endocrinology*, vol. 143, no. 3, pp. 293–311, 2000.

[3] M. W. Schwartz, R. J. Seeley, L. A. Campfield, P. Burn, and D. G. Baskin, "Identification of targets of leptin action in rat hypothalamus," *Journal of Clinical Investigation*, vol. 98, no. 5, pp. 1101–1106, 1996.

[4] R. S. Ahlma, D. Prabakaran, C. Mantzoros et al., "Role of leptin in the neuroendocrine response to fasting," *Nature*, vol. 382, no. 6588, pp. 250–252, 1996.

[5] H. F. Escobar-Morreale, F. E. Del Rey, and G. M. De Escobar, "Thyroid hormones influence serum leptin concentrations in the rat," *Endocrinology*, vol. 138, no. 10, pp. 4485–4488, 1997.

[6] M. J. M. Diekman, J. A. Romijn, E. Endert, H. Sauerwein, and W. M. Wiersinga, "Thyroid hormones modulate serum leptin levels: observations in thyrotoxic and hypothyroid women," *Thyroid*, vol. 8, no. 12, pp. 1081–1086, 1998.

[7] L. Vona-Davis and D. P. Rose, "Adipokines as endocrine, paracrine, and autocrine factors in breast cancer risk and progression," *Endocrine-Related Cancer*, vol. 14, no. 2, pp. 189–206, 2007.

[8] D. D. Deo, A. P. Rao, S. S. Bose et al., "Differential effects of leptin on the invasive potential of androgen-dependent and -independent prostate carcinoma cells," *Journal of Biomedicine and Biotechnology*, vol. 2008, no. 1, Article ID 163902, 2008.

[9] J. H. Pinkney, S. J. Goodrick, J. Katz et al., "Leptin and the pituitary-thyroid axis: a comparative study in lean, obese, hypothyroid and hyperthyroid subjects," University of Bristol, Department of Medicine, Bristol Royal Infirmary, Bristol, UK.

[10] H. Y. Park, H. M. Kwon, H. J. Lim et al., "Potential role of leptin in angiogenesis: leptin induces endothelial cell proliferation and expression of matrix metalloproteinases in vivo and in vitro," *Experimental and Molecular Medicine*, vol. 33, no. 2, pp. 95–102, 2001.

[11] Z. Liu, T. Uesaka, H. Watanabe, and N. Kato, "High fat diet enhances colonic cell proliferation and carcinogenesis in rats by elevating serum leptin," *International Journal of Oncology*, vol. 19, no. 5, pp. 1009–1014, 2001.

[12] R. Brauner, C. Trivin, M. Zerah et al., "Diencephalic syndrome due to hypothalamic tumour: a model of the relationship between weight and puberty onset," *Journal of Clinical Endocrinology and Metabolism*, vol. 91, pp. 2467–2473, 2006.

[13] T. Jaffe and B. Schwartz, "Leptin promotes motility and invasiveness in human colon cancer cells by activating multiple signal-transduction pathways," *International Journal of Cancer*, vol. 123, no. 11, pp. 2543–2556, 2008.

[14] S. N. O'Brien, B. H. Welter, and T. M. Price, "Presence of leptin in breast cell lines and breast tumors," *Biochemical and Biophysical Research Communications*, vol. 259, no. 3, pp. 695–698, 1999.

[15] L. Li, Y. Gao, L. L. Zhang, and D. L. He, "Concomitant activation of the JAK/STAT3 and ERK1/2 signaling is involved in leptin-mediated proliferation of renal cell carcinoma Caki-2 cells," *Cancer Biology and Therapy*, vol. 7, no. 11, pp. 1787–1792, 2008.

[16] R. Ribeiro, A. Araújo, C. Lopes, and R. Medeiros, "Immunoinflammatory mechanisms in lung cancer development: is leptin a mediator?" *Journal of Thoracic Oncology*, vol. 2, no. 2, pp. 105–108, 2007.

[17] C. Garofalo and E. Surmacz, "Leptin and cancer," *Journal of Cellular Physiology*, vol. 207, no. 1, pp. 12–22, 2006.

[18] M. R. Hoda, S. J. Keely, L. S. Bertelsen, W. G. Junger, D. Dharmasena, and K. E. Barrett, "Leptin acts as a mitogenic and antiapoptotic factor for colonic cancer cells," *British Journal of Surgery*, vol. 94, no. 3, pp. 346–354, 2007.

[19] O. O. Ogunwobi and I. L. P. Beales, "The anti-apoptotic and growth stimulatory actions of leptin in human colon cancer cells involves activation of JNK mitogen activated protein kinase, JAK2 and PI3 kinase/Akt," *International Journal of Colorectal Disease*, vol. 22, no. 4, pp. 401–409, 2007.

[20] S. Uddin, R. Bu, M. Ahmed et al., "Overexpression of leptin receptor predicts an unfavorable outcome in Middle Eastern ovarian cancer," *Molecular Cancer*, vol. 8, p. 74, 2009.

[21] Q. L. K. Lam, S. Wang, O. K. H. Ko, P. W. Kincade, and L. Lu, "Leptin signaling maintains B-cell homeostasis via induction of Bcl-2 and cyclin D1," *Proceedings of the National Academy of Sciences of the United States of America*, vol. 107, no. 31, pp. 13812–13817, 2010.

[22] M. Okumura, M. Yamamoto, H. Sakuma et al., "Leptin and high glucose stimulate cell proliferation in MCF-7 human breast cancer cells: reciprocal involvement of PKC-α and PPAR expression," *Biochimica et Biophysica Acta—Molecular Cell Research*, vol. 1592, no. 2, pp. 107–116, 2002.

[23] D. L. Morris and L. Rui, "Recent advances in understanding leptin signaling and leptin resistance," *American Journal of Physiology—Endocrinology and Metabolism*, vol. 297, no. 6, pp. E1247–E1259, 2009.

[24] Y. Wang, K. K. Kuropatwinski, D. W. White et al., "Leptin receptor action in hepatic cells," *Journal of Biological Chemistry*, vol. 272, no. 26, pp. 16216–16223, 1997.

[25] R. R. Gonzalez, S. Cherfils, M. Escobar et al., "Leptin signaling promotes the growth of mammary tumors and increases the expression of vascular endothelial growth factor (VEGF) and its receptor type two (VEGF-R2)," *Journal of Biological Chemistry*, vol. 281, no. 36, pp. 26320–26328, 2006.

[26] M. Koda, M. Sulkowska, L. Kanczuga-Koda, E. Surmacz, and S. Sulkowski, "Overexpression of the obesity hormone leptin in human colorectal cancer," *Journal of Clinical Pathology*, vol. 60, no. 8, pp. 902–906, 2007.

[27] S. J. Hong, K. W. Kwon, S. G. Kim et al., "Variation in expression of gastric leptin according to differentiation and growth pattern in gastric adenocarcinoma," *Cytokine*, vol. 33, no. 2, pp. 66–71, 2006.

[28] M. Koda, M. Sulkowska, A. Wincewicz et al., "Expression of leptin, leptin receptor, and hypoxia-inducible factor 1α in human endometrial cancer," *Annals of the New York Academy of Sciences*, vol. 1095, pp. 90–98, 2007.

[29] M. Ishikawa, J. Kitayama, and H. Nagawa, "Enhanced expression of leptin and leptin receptor (OB-R) in human breast cancer," *Clinical Cancer Research*, vol. 10, no. 13, pp. 4325–4331, 2004.

[30] X. Hu, S. C. Juneja, N. J. Maihle, and M. P. Cleary, "Leptin—A growth factor in normal and malignant breast cells and for normal mammary gland development," *Journal of the National Cancer Institute*, vol. 94, no. 22, pp. 1704–1711, 2002.

[31] N. K. Saxena, D. Sharma, X. Ding et al., "Concomitant activation of the JAK/STAT, PI3K/AKT, and ERK signaling is involved in leptin-mediated promotion of invasion and migration of hepatocellular carcinoma cells," *Cancer Research*, vol. 67, no. 6, pp. 2497–2507, 2007.

[32] S. Uddin, P. Bavi, A. K. Siraj et al., "Leptin-R and its association with PI3K/AKT signaling pathway in papillary thyroid carcinoma," *Endocrine-Related Cancer*, vol. 17, no. 1, pp. 191–202, 2010.

[33] R. Valcavi, M. Zini, R. Peino, F. F. Casanueva, and C. Dieguez, "Influence of thyroid status on serum immunoreactive leptin levels," *Journal of Clinical Endocrinology and Metabolism*, vol. 82, no. 5, pp. 1632–1634, 1997.

[34] C. S. Mantzoros, H. N. Rosen, S. L. Greenspan, J. S. Flier, and A. C. Moses, "Short-term hyperthyroidism has no effect on leptin levels in man," *Journal of Clinical Endocrinology and Metabolism*, vol. 82, no. 2, pp. 497–499, 1997.

[35] G. Légràdi, C. H. Emerson, R. S. Ahima, J. S. Flier, and R. M. Lechan, "Leptin prevents fasting-induced suppression of prothyrotropin-releasing hormone messenger ribonucleic acid in neurons of the hypothalamic paraventricular nucleus," *Endocrinology*, vol. 138, no. 6, pp. 2569–2576, 1997.

[36] S. Sreenan, J. F. Caro, and S. Refetoff, "Thyroid dysfunction is not associated with alterations in serum leptin levels," *Thyroid*, vol. 7, no. 3, pp. 407–409, 1997.

[37] R. Seven, "Thyroid status and leptin in Basedow-Graves and multinodular goiter patients," *Journal of Toxicology and Environmental Health—Part A*, vol. 63, no. 8, pp. 575–581, 2001.

[38] G. Mazziotti, A. B. Parkes, M. Lage, L. D. K. E. Premawardhana, F. F. Casanueva, and J. H. Lazarus, "High leptin

levels in women developing postpartum thyroiditis," *Clinical Endocrinology*, vol. 60, no. 2, pp. 208–213, 2004.

[39] M. Akinci, F. Kosova, B. Cetin, S. Aslan, Z. Ari, and A. Cetin, "Leptin levels in thyroid cancer," *Asian Journal of Surgery*, vol. 32, no. 4, pp. 216–223, 2009.

[40] S.-P. Cheng, C.-W. Chi, C.-Y. Tzen et al., "Clinicopathologic significance of leptin and leptin receptor expressions in papillary thyroid carcinoma," *Surgery*, vol. 147, no. 6, pp. 847–853, 2010.

25

Thyroid Carcinoma in Children and Adolescents

Fernanda Vaisman,[1, 2] Rossana Corbo,[1, 2] and Mario Vaisman[1]

[1] Endocrinology Service, Universidade Federal do Rio de Janeiro, Rio de Janiro, RJ, Brazil
[2] Endocrinology Service, Instituto Nacional do Cancer, Rio de Janeiro, Rio de Janeiro, RJ, Brazil

Correspondence should be addressed to Fernanda Vaisman, fevaisman@globo.com

Academic Editor: Ana O. Hoff

Thyroid cancer in children and adolescents is usually a major concern for physicians, patients, and parents. Controversies regarding the aggressiveness of the clinical presentation and the ideal therapeutic approach remain among the scientific community. The current recommendations and staging systems are based on data generated by studies in adults, and this might lead to overtreating in some cases as well as undertreating in others. Understanding the differences in the biology, clinical course, and outcomes in this population is crucial for therapeutic decisions. This paper evaluates the biology, clinical presentation, recurrences, and overall survival as well as the staging systems in children and adolescents with differentiated thyroid cancer.

1. Introduction

Palpable thyroid nodules can be diagnosed in 4 to 7% of the adult population. The high-resolution ultrasounds are able to detect nodules around 19% of the adult population, reaching up to 67% in populations at higher risk such as women and elderly individuals [1]. Considering autopsy series, this prevalence can reach 50%. Although common, only 5% are malignant [2].

Thyroid cancer is a rare pathology in childhood and adolescence being responsible for 1.5–3% of all carcinomas in this age group in the USA and Europe [3]. Such as the adults, the differentiated thyroid carcinoma is the most commonly found, especially the papillary carcinoma. In this population, age, family history of thyroid disease and radiation exposure are very important factors as already shown in various ser-ies [4–6], especially after the Chernobyl accident, when a substantial increase in the incidence of thyroid carcinoma in children exposed to radiation was documented [7].

Staging thyroid carcinoma in children and adolescents is still a controversial issue. To avoid overtreating, a risk classification system, with the highest accuracy as possible, should be used to identify patients who should be treated in a more conservative or more aggressive way.

The current treatment recommendation is the total thyroidectomy followed by radioiodine therapy, based on good response and high disease-free survival rate for this age group. However, many authors question the aggressiveness of this treatment given the long lifespan of these patients and long-term complications of high doses of radioiodine.

This revision aims to evaluate the initial therapeutic approach for children and adolescents with DTC regarding surgery, adjuvant therapy, and staging.

2. Epidemiology of the Disease

The incidence of clinically palpable thyroid nodules in children is estimated to be around 1–1.5%. However, in teenagers, this prevalence may reach 13% [8]. When compared to adults, children have four times greater risk of malignancy when a thyroid nodule is diagnosed. In the US, around 350 individuals aged less than 20 years receive the diagnosis of thyroid carcinoma annually [9]. In Brazil, the incidence can reach 2% of all pediatric cancers according to the National Cancer Institute database [10].

Besides being a rare disease, the differentiated thyroid carcinoma accounts for about 0.5–3% of all malignancies in the pediatric population [8]. In addition, the thyroid is one of the most common sites of a second primary tumor in children who received external beam radiotherapy to the neck for the treatment of other neoplasms.

The occurrence of thyroid carcinoma in early childhood is very rare. In the literature, there are isolated cases of differentiated thyroid carcinoma in neonates and infants aged less than 1 year old [11, 12].

Furthermore, the incidence of thyroid cancer seems to increase with age. In a series with 235 children and adolescents who followed Maria Skłodowska Memorial Cancer Center and Institute of Oncology for thyroid cancer, 5% were diagnosed under 6 years old, 10% with 7–9 years, increasing substantially after 10 years old. The difference between boys and girls was seen more clearly after 13-14 years old [13]. Also the latest records of SEER cohort (Surveillance, Epidemiology and End Results) from a group of 1753 patients aged less than 20 years confirm the greater incidence in girls (0.89 cases/100,000 for girls versus 0.2 cases/100,000 for boys) [14].

3. Risk Factors

In the past 60 years, the incidence of thyroid carcinoma in the pediatric age group presented two distinct peaks. The first occurred around 1950 due to the use of radiation for the treatment of common childhood conditions such as *Tinea capitis*, acne, chronic tonsillitis, and thymus hyperplasia [15, 16]. In these cases, the thyroid carcinoma was diagnosed on average 10–20 years after exposure, but with risk persisting until 40 years later. When the causal relationship between neck irradiation and thyroid carcinoma was established, such practices were abandoned leading to a decreasing incidence in this population [11]. These data led to acceptance of ionizing radiation, a risk factor for the development of thyroid cancer [17]. Similarly, external beam radiotherapy for the treatment of other childhood malignancies would also be associated with an increased incidence of thyroid carcinoma in this population [18–20].

A second peak incidence occurred in the mid-1990s in some regions of Eastern Europe on behalf of the nuclear accident that occurred in Chernobyl in 1986 [4–6]. The first cases were diagnosed approximately 4-5 years later, especially in children under 5 years old at the time of exposure [4, 21]. About 75% of these cases were exposed to the radioactive fallout between birth and 14 years of age, with most of the other 25% being from 14 to 17 years old at the time of exposure [21]. The Chernobyl accident confirmed the high-er sensitivity of the pediatric population, to the effects of radiation when compared to adults [22].

The effects of ionizing radiation on thyroid remain of great interest of the scientific community. The British Childhood Cancer Survivor Study (BCCSS) is a cohort of 17,980 patients who were followed on average for 17.4 years, so far, whose main objective is to determine the occurrence of a second primary tumor. Eighty-eight percent of thyroid carcinomas were found in patients undergoing radiotherapy covering the cervical region. The risk of thyroid carcinoma was higher in patients treated for Hodgkin's disease (RR 3.3—IC: 1.1–10.1) and non-Hodgkin Lymphoma (RR 3.4—IC: 1.1–10.7) [23].

4. Presentation in Childhood

Regarding the clinical presentation, some characteristics are markedly different in pediatric population.

First, the tumor volume tends to be larger in patients with less than 20 years old when compared to patients diagnosed between 20 and 50 years [24]. Zimmerman et al. already showed, in 1988 [25], that newly diagnosed tumors were greater than 4 cm in 36% of children as opposed to 15% of adults and had less than 1 cm in 9% of children as opposed to 22% of adults. In series contemplating only patients with papillary carcinoma, only 1.5–3% of tumors had less than 1 cm size at diagnosis [26, 27].

Furthermore, probably due to the fact that thyroid volume is smaller in children, an early involvement of thyroid capule and surrounding tissue is seen [28]. Thus, the category of microcarcinoma (including tumors with less than 1 cm), commonly used in adults, should be avoided in children, since a 1 cm tumor constitutes a very important finding in this age group.

Secondly, the multicentricity also occurs more frequently in the pediatric age group, especially in the subtype papillary carcinoma [29, 30]. Such outbreaks have been considered as polyclonal in most cases [31]. This becomes especially important as it can be used as an argument in favor of total thyroidectomy as primary surgical approach for these patients.

Third, pediatric patients have a higher probability of cervical lymph node metastasis as well as distant metastasis [21, 32]. In a series done at the Mayo Clinic with 1039 patients with papillary thyroid carcinoma, cervical lymph node invol-vement was detected in 90% and metastasis distance in approximately 7% of children versus 35% of cervical lymph node involvement and 2% of distance metastasis in adults [25]. In a study performed by our group with 65 children and adolescents, the occurrence lymph node metastasis at diagnosis was 61.5%, local invasion 39.5%, and distant metastases 29.2%, all of them being in the lungs [33]. As the diagnostic methods improved, clinical presentation of differentiated thyroid carcinoma in the pediatric age group has changed over time. A review held at the University of Michigan comparing patients diagnosed between 1936–1970 with those diagnosed between 1971 and 1990 showed that the patients diagnosed more recently had a lower in-cidence of lymph node involvement (36% versus 63%), less local invasion (6% versus 31%), and lower incidence of lung metastases (6% versus 19%), reflecting a precocity in diagnosis over the decades, with a consequent better pro-gnosis, particularly if older than 10 years of age [34].

The most common site of distant metastasis in children is the lung with just a few cases described of bone metastases [12, 35] and of central nervous system metastases [12, 36].

The histological subtype follows a distribution similar to adults: 90–95% papillary carcinomas and 5% follicular [9, 37, 38]. Poorly differentiated tumors as insular and anaplastic are extremely rare [38].

5. Prevalence of Mutations and Expression of NIS

An important difference between thyroid carcinoma in pediatric and adult age is related to the high prevalence of expression of sodium-iodide transporter (NIS) in metastatic focus found in children [39–41]. In the absence of stimulation of TSH, the expression of NIS is undetectable in 65% of papillary tumors and 56% of follicular in patients with less than 20 years [39]. In contrast, the expression of NIS is absent or negligible in 90% of differentiated carcinomas in adults, either when searched by PCR with reverse transcription [40] or by Immunohistochemistry [42].

The greater expression of NIS in the pediatric population results in greater responsiveness to radioiodine treatment and better prognosis. In young patients, the recurrence risk increases in those who do not express the protein NIS when compared to those who have it [39]. Thus, the degree of NIS expression correlates with radioiodine avidity by metastases [43] and lower clinical recurrence rates [44].

Regarding the molecular biology of these tumors, apparently RET-PTC rearrangements occur in childhood more frequently than in adults, especially in the radiation-related tumors. Initial studies of Chernobyl-associated PTC identified RET/PTC-3 as the most common form of RET rearrangement in radiation-induced childhood PTC [45–49]. However, Pisarchik et al. found that 29% of adult and childhood PTC in Belarus actually contained RET/PTC-1 rearrangements [45]. It was hypothesized that the increase in frequency of the RET/PTC-1 rearrangements in those adults could be related to a longer latency period in those cases. In addition, patients who had RET/PTC-3 rearrangements were diagnosed much earlier after the Chernobyl incident [45]. Motomura et al. reported that 71% of sporadic PTC from children in the United States and 87% of PTC from children living in radiation-contaminated areas of Belarus contain rearrangements of the RET oncogene [50, 51].

Besides RET/PTC rearrangements, other groups suggested the immunohistochemical overexpression of MET associated with high recurrence rate in children and adolescents [51], in addition to the immunohistochemical overexpression of growth factors of vascular endothelium [52] and telomerase, however, without definitive findings [53].

In the case of follicular carcinomas, the two most frequently involved genes would be RAS and PPAR gamma, and their rearrangement might serve as a trigger to the transformation from adenoma to carcinoma [54]. However, little is known about its role in the prognosis of such neoplasms.

6. Prognosis

The prognosis of these tumors in childhood is a very interesting issue. Despite having a greater recurrence rate when compared to adults, survival seems to be better [55]. Mazzaferri and Kloos in a series with 16.6 years of followup, found a recurrence rate, in patients with less than 20 years old, around 40%, while those with more than 20 years of age had 20% recurrence rates [24]. In contrast, survival is greater than in adults. In a study done in Minsk with a large cohort of 741 patients, the survival rate was 99.3% in 5 years and 98.5% in 10 years in a pediatric population [56].

Age seems to be a very important prognostic factor in thyroid cancer. Children and adolescents are usually classified as having a better prognosis and they are classified together with all patients under 45 years old. However, Lazar et al. showed that patients with less than 10 years, mainly prepubertal, had a worse prognosis than the older and more advanced pubertal stages patients [34].

7. Treatment

Regardless, the biology of papillary and follicular tumors, the therapeutic approach is very similar for both subtypes of tumors [12, 55]. As well as in adults, the treatment of differentiated thyroid carcinoma is based on the combination of three therapeutic modalities: surgery, hormone replacement with levothyroxine, and radioiodine treatment. The surgery can vary from lobectomy to total thyroidectomy accompanied by cervical lymphadenectomy in various ways. Latest guidelines recommend total thyroidectomy, mainly for larger tumors, 1 cm [24, 57, 58] associated with cervical dissection of central or lateral compartment block if lymph node metastases are seen in preoperative imaging or during the surgery. The main surgical complications include persistent hypoparathyroidism and laryngeal nerve damage that may cause a wide spectrum of clinical consequences: from hoarseness to total vocal cord paralysis, with need for definitive tracheotomy [59].

After a total or near-total thyroidectomy, the volume of remaining gland should be less than 2 g seen in the cervical ultrasound performed around one month after surgery [55].

Even after total thyroidectomy, some radioiodine uptake is seen in the thyroid bed. Generally, this phenomenon is assigned to the remaining normal thyroid cells left by the surgeon to protect the nerve and around Berry's ligament. However, because multicentricity and metastatic disease are more common in the pediatric age group, the possibility of such outbreaks being malignant cells cannot be ruled out. Thus, most societies recommend radioiodine ablation in the vast majority of patients under 45 years old but none of them make specific recommendations for children and adolescents [55, 58–60]. However, the radioiodine treatment should be used to complement, not replace, the total thyroidectomy. The success of ablation is significantly lower in patients who have undergone less extensive surgery, such as near-total thyroidectomy [24, 61]. In most cases, one dose of radioiodine treatment is capable of achieving complete ablation; however, the procedure may have to be repeated usually 6–12 months after the first [62]. Some variables seem to influence the success of thyroid remnant ablation and the most important one seems to be the presence of lymph node metastases in low risk patients [33]. However, little is known about the prognostic significance of achieving a successful ablation with the first dosage of I-131 in patients with differentiated thyroid cancer. Mazzaferri and Jhiang have shown that adult patients with a successful ablation had a better prognosis than those who failed: disease-free survival was 87% versus 49% after 10 years; additionally, thyroid-cancer related survival was 93% versus 78% [63]. On the other hand, the Mayo Clinic studies did not show a major impact in the overall survival and in the recurrence rates [25, 64].

The third treatment modality is thyroid hormone replacement. This suppressive therapy with thyroid hormone is believed to reduce the risk of growth or tumor proliferation induced by TSH [65]. In children and adolescents still undergoing growth, there are several studies that guarantee the efficacy and safety of this approach, particularly with regard to their final height, as long as they are carefully controlled [55].

Possible side effects of long-term suppressive therapy include osteoporosis and cardiovascular disease, especially of left ventricular hypertrophy [65, 66]; such are effects documented in adults.

8. Radioiodine in Childhood and Its Side Effects

The radioiodine treatment in pediatric age should be preferably administered in capsule form, in association with an antiemetic medication, in an attempt to ensure that the activity administered has been fully ingested.

Iodine 131 therapy can lead to a temporary loss of salivary flow and change of taste in up to 30% of the cases [59]. However, permanent xerostomia is rare. The most serious side effect from radioiodine treatment is radiation-induced leukemia that happen in 1 out of 26 treated patients in a study held in Netherlands with children and adolescents [59]. Another concern is pulmonary fibrosis that may occur in up to 1% of cases, mostly in those with diffuse lung metastases. Both effects are dose dependent and usually are seen in patients that underwent multiple treatments with a total dose above 600 mCi [59].

The actinic sialoadenitis is common but usually is reversible [67]. This complication is more frequent in the absence of iodine-avid metastases and discrete thyroid remnant, situations with greater availability of radioiodine to the salivary glands [34, 67]. A transitional impairment of spermatogenesis [34, 67, 68] is observed after ablation thera-py with high doses of iodine 131. Permanent infertility is possible with accumulated high doses [69]. Usually the production of testosterone is preserved [68, 69], although an elevation of LH can occur [69]. In women, an increment of FSH and reversible menstrual changes [68, 69] and even infertility and early menopause [69] may occur after high doses of radioiodine.

Whereas the maximum dose absorbed by the gonads is 5 mGy/mCi, Maxon inferred that permanent infertility does not occur in women with doses up to 300 mCi iodine-131 and happen in less than 10% of men with this same dose. With doses of 800 mCi or more, infertility would go up to 60% of women and more than 90% of men [69, 70].

In adolescent boys, radioiodine can also cause a decrease in quantity and affect sperm quality leading to infertility that may be transient or permanent [71].

9. Controversies

Even with all knowledge acquired today, the controversies on the ideal approach of these patients remain. The lack of studies demonstrating real benefit in overall survival of these patients comparing the different therapeutic modalities contributes to this discussion. Groups like the Mayo Clinic advocate a conservative treatment (considering the possibility of partial thyroidectomy without adjuvant radioiodine therapy) using as argument the observation of 1.7% mortality after 28 years of monitoring and 3.4% recurrence in 30 years in 58 patients under 17 years at diagnosis, in which only 38% underwent total thyroidectomy and 17% radioiodine treatment adjuvant, that is, a good evolution even without the traditionally recommended intensive treatment [25].

The main arguments of those who prefer a more aggressive approach are based on studies with long follow-up period analyzing disease-free survival and recurrence rate. For example, Chow et al., in this univariate analysis, showed that the local recurrence rate in children was reduced from 42% to 6.3% when radioiodine adjuvant treatment was per-formed ($P = .0001$) [72].

The application of the current staging system created by the International Union against Cancer (AJCC/UICC) based on the TNM and age is recommended for all types of tumors including thyroid [73], in an attempt to standardize the tumoral extension description [73]. However, in thyroid carcinoma, TNM staging does not take into consideration several additional factors that influence the evolution and prognosis and so has a limited capacity of predicting outcome in some cases. Thus, several other staging systems are being proposed in the attempt to achieve a better accuracy, among them: CAEORTC, AGES, AMES, MACE, and ATA. [58, 74–77]. These systems take into account factors identified as predictor of outcomes in retrospective studies, usually taking into consideration the presence of metastases, the age of the patient, and the extent of the tumor site. However, most of them were developed to predict cancer-specific mortality not to predict recurrence [76]. Because the mortality is low, there is not an ideal standing system for thyroid cancer yet, especially when it comes to the pediatric population. These patients are usually grouped with minors 45 years which may be responsible for the low accuracy of all existing systems for patients under 20 years of age, that clearly have a different clinical presentations and biology when compared to older patients. In a recent study performed with 65 patients under 20 years old, the staging system proposed by ATA in 2009 seems to be better than the others for predicting disease-free survival [33]. More studies with this specific population are needed to develop a specific risk assessment for this age group.

10. Conclusion

Although children with DTC typically present with locoregional metastases and a high rate of distant metastatic disease, overall survival is very good. Treatment should be based on their increased risk for recurrence instead of overall mortality, and lifelong followup is required because recurrence and death may not occur for decades after diagnosis. Initial treatment will generally include total thyroidectomy and central compartment lymph node dissection especially if lymph node disease is found in the preoperative evaluation. Radioiodine ablation should be individualized and given to those with a higher risk of recurrence.

Large multicenter studies are needed to better understand optimal treatment approaches to this unique population. All care of pediatric DTC should be delivered by multidisciplinary specialized teams which include both pediatricians and thyroid cancer specialists to minimize possible complications and ensure competent followup.

References

[1] G. H. Tan and H. Gharib, "Thyroid incidentalomas: management approaches to nonpalpable nodules discovered incidentally on thyroid imaging," *Annals of Internal Medicine*, vol. 126, no. 3, pp. 226–231, 1997.

[2] L. Hegedus, "Clinical practice. The thyroid nodule," *The New England Journal of Medicine*, vol. 351, pp. 1764–1771, 2004.

[3] R. T. Greenlee, M. B. Hill-Harmon, T. Murray, and M. Thun, "Cancer statistics, 2001," *Cancer Journal for Clinicians*, vol. 51, no. 1, pp. 15–36, 2001.

[4] M. C. Mahoney, S. Lawvere, K. L. Falkner et al., "Thyroid cancer incidence trends in Belarus: examining the impact of Chernobyl," *International Journal of Epidemiology*, vol. 33, no. 5, pp. 1025–1033, 2004.

[5] S. Murbeth, M. Rousarova, H. Scherb, and E. Lengfelder, "Thyroid cancer has increased in the adult populations of countries moderately affected by Chernobyl fallout," *Medical Science Monitor*, vol. 10, no. 7, pp. CR300–CR306, 2004.

[6] T. Parfitt, "Chernobyl's legacy. 20 years after the power station exploded, new cases of thyroid cancer are still rising, say experts," *The Lancet*, vol. 363, no. 9420, p. 1534, 2004.

[7] E. D. Williams, "Cancer after nuclear fallout: lessons from Chernobyl accident," *Nature Reviews*, vol. 2, no. 7, pp. 543–549, 2002.

[8] J. Josefson and D. Zimmerman, "Thyroid nodules and cancers in children," *Pediatric Endocrinology Reviews*, vol. 6, no. 1, pp. 14–23, 2008.

[9] L. Bernstein and J. Gurney, "Carcinomas and other malignant epithelial neoplasms," in *Cancer Incidence and Survival among Children and Adolescents: United States SEER Program 1975–1995*, pp. 139–148, Cancer Statistics Branch, National Cancer Institute, Bethesda, Md, USA, 1999.

[10] *Childhood and Adolescent Cancer in Brazil: Data from Mortality and Population- Based Registries*, National Cancer Institute, Brazilian Society of Pediatric Oncology, Rio de Janeiro, Brazil, 2009, http://www.inca.gov.br.

[11] J. K. Harness, N. W. Thompson, M. K. McLeod, J. L. Pasieka, A. Fukuuchi, and P. L. Gerfo, "Differentiated thyroid carcinoma in children and adolescents," *World Journal of Surgery*, vol. 16, no. 4, pp. 547–554, 1992.

[12] K. D. Newman, T. Black, G. Heller et al., "Differentiated thyroid cancer: determinants of disease progression in patients <21 years of age at diagnosis: a report from the surgical discipline committee of the children's cancer group," *Annals of Surgery*, vol. 227, no. 4, pp. 533–541, 1998.

[13] M. Niedziela, E. Korman, D. Breborowicz et al., "A prospective study of thyroid nodular disease in children and adolescents in western Poland from 1996 to 2000 and the incidence of thyroid carcinoma relative to iodine deficiency and the Chernobyl disaster," *Pediatric Blood and Cancer*, vol. 42, no. 1, pp. 84–92, 2004.

[14] A. R. Hogan, Y. Zhuge, E. A. Perez, L. G. Koniaris, J. I. Lew, and J. E. Sola, "The incidence of pediatric thyroid cancer is increasing and is higher in girls than in boys and may have an adverse outcome," *Journal of Surgery Research*, vol. 156, pp. 167–172, 2009.

[15] E. Ron, J. H. Lubin, R. E. Shore et al., "Thyroid cancer after exposure to external radiation: a pooled analysis of seven studies," *Radiation Research*, vol. 141, pp. 259–277, 1995.

[16] J. H. Lubin, D. W. Schafer, E. Ron, M. Stovall, and R. J. Carroll, "A reanalysis of thyroid neoplasms in the Israeli tinea capitis study accounting for dose uncertainties," *Radiation Research*, vol. 161, no. 3, pp. 359–368, 2004.

[17] O. Catelinois, P. Verger, M. Colonna, A. Rogel, D. Hemon, and M. Tirmarche, "Projecting the time trend of thyroid cancers: its impact on assessment of radiation-induced cancer risks," *Health Physics*, vol. 87, no. 6, pp. 606–614, 2004.

[18] J. Blatt, A. Olshan, M. J. Gula, P. S. Dickman, and B. Zaranek, "Second malignancies in very-long-term survivors of childhood cancer," *American Journal of Medicine*, vol. 93, no. 1, pp. 57–60, 1992.

[19] P. Black, A. Straaten, and P. Gutjahr, "Secondary thyroid carcinoma after treatment for childhood cancer," *Medical and Pediatric Oncology*, vol. 31, pp. 91–95, 1998.

[20] S. Acharya, K. Sarafoglou, M. LaQuaglia et al., "Thyroid neoplasms after therapeutic radiation for malignancies during childhood or adolescence," *Cancer*, vol. 97, no. 10, pp. 2397–2403, 2003.

[21] R. M. Tuttle, F. Vaisman, and M. D. Tronko, "Clinical presentation and clinical outcomes in chernobyl-related paediatric thyroid cancers: what do we know now? What can we expect in the future?" *Clinical Oncology (Royal College of Radiologists)*, vol. 23, no. 4, pp. 268–275, 2011.

[22] L. A. Michel and J. E. Donckier, "Thyroid cancer 15 years after Chernobyl," *The Lancet*, vol. 359, no. 9321, p. 1947, 2002.

[23] A. J. Taylor, A. P. Croft, A. M. Palace et al., "Risk of thyroid cancer in survivors of childhood cancer: results from the British childhood cancer survivor study," *International Journal of Cancer*, vol. 125, no. 10, pp. 2400–2405, 2009.

[24] E. L. Mazzaferri and R. T. Kloos, "Clinical review 128: current approaches to primary therapy for papillary and follicular thyroid cancer," *Journal of Clinical Endocrinology and Metabolism*, vol. 86, pp. 1447–1463, 2001.

[25] D. Zimmerman, I. D. Hay, I. R. Gough et al., "Papillary thyroid carcinoma in children and adults: long-term follow-up of 1039 patients conservatively treated at one institution during three decades," *Surgery*, vol. 104, no. 6, pp. 1157–1166, 1988.

[26] M. E. Dottorini, A. Vignati, L. Mazzucchelli, G. Lomuscio, and L. Colombo, "Differentiated thyroid carcinoma in children and adolescents: a 37-year experience in 85 patients," *Journal of Nuclear Medicine*, vol. 38, pp. 669–675, 1997.

[27] S. M. Chow, S. C. Law, W. M. Mendenhall et al., "Differentiated thyroid carcinoma in childhood and adolescence—clinical course and role of radioiodine," *Pediatric Blood and Cancer*, vol. 42, no. 2, pp. 176–183, 2004.

[28] J. Farahati, E. P. Demidchik, J. Biko, and C. Reiners, "Inverse association between age at the time of radiation exposure and extent of disease in cases of radiation-induced childhood thyroid carcinoma in Belarus," *Cancer*, vol. 88, no. 6, pp. 1470–1476, 2000.

[29] R. Katoh, J. Sasaki, H. Kurihara, K. Suzuki, Y. Iida, and A. Kawaoi, "Multiple thyroid involvement (intraglandular metastasis) in papillary thyroid carcinoma. A clinicopathologic study of 105 consecutive patients," *Cancer*, vol. 70, no. 6, pp. 1585–1590, 1992.

[30] J. L. Pasieka, N. W. Thompson, M. K. McLeod, R. E. Burney, M. Macha, and T. S. Reeve, "The incidence of bilateral well differentiated thyroid cancer found at completion thyroidectomy," *World Journal of Surgery*, vol. 16, no. 4, pp. 711–716, 1992.

[31] S. L. Sugg, L. Zheng, I. B. Rosen, J. L. Freeman, S. Ezzat, and S. L. Asa, "ret/PTC-1, -2, and -3 oncogene rearrangements in human thyroid carcinomas: implications for metastatic potential?" *Journal of Clinical Endocrinology and Metabolism*, vol. 81, no. 9, pp. 3360–3365, 1996.

[32] D. K. Robie, C. W. Dinauer, R. M. Tuttle et al., "The impact of initial surgical management on outcome in young patients with differentiated thyroid cancer," *Journal of Pediatric Surgery*, vol. 33, no. 7, pp. 1134–1140, 1998.

[33] F. Visman, D. A. Bulzico, C. H. C. N. Pessoa et al., "Prognostic factors of a good response to initial therapy in children and adolescents with differentiated thyroid cancer," *Clinics*, vol. 66, no. 2, pp. 1–6, 2011.

[34] L. Lazar, Y. Lebenthal, A. Steinmetz, M. Yackobovitch-Gavan, and M. Phillip, "Differentiated thyroid carcinoma in pediatric patients: comparison of presentation and course between prepubertal children and adolescents," *Journal of Pediatrics*, vol. 154, no. 5, pp. 708–714, 2009.

[35] M. Schlumberger, F. De Vathaire, J. P. Travagli et al., "Differentiated thyroid carcinoma in childhood: long term follow-up of 72 patients," *Journal of Clinical Endocrinology and Metabolism*, vol. 65, no. 6, pp. 1088–1094, 1987.

[36] I. D. Hay, "Brain metastases from papillary thyroid carcinoma," *Archives of Internal Medicine*, vol. 147, no. 3, pp. 607–611, 1987.

[37] H. R. Harach and E. D. Williams, "Childhood thyroid cancer in England and Wales," *British Journal of Cancer*, vol. 72, no. 3, pp. 777–783, 1995.

[38] A. A. Hassoun, I. D. Hay, J. R. Goellner, and D. Zimmerman, "Insular thyroid carcinoma in adolescents: a potentially lethal endocrine malignancy," *Cancer*, vol. 79, no. 5, pp. 1044–1048, 1997.

[39] A. Patel, S. Jhiang, S. Dogra et al., "Differentiated thyroid carcinoma that express sodium-iodide symporter have a lower risk of recurrence for children and adolescents," *Pediatric Research*, vol. 52, no. 5, pp. 737–744, 2002.

[40] M. D. Ringel, J. Anderson, S. L. Souza et al., "Expression of the sodium iodide symporter and thyroglobulin genes are reduced in papillary thyroid cancer," *Modern Pathology*, vol. 14, no. 4, pp. 289–296, 2001.

[41] A. Faggiano, J. Coulot, N. Bellon et al., "Age dependent variation of follicular size and expression of iodine transporters in human thyroid tissue," *Journal of Nuclear Medicine*, vol. 45, no. 2, pp. 232–237, 2004.

[42] C. Mian, L. Lacroix, L. Alzieu et al., "Sodium iodide symporter and pendrin expression in human thyroid tissues," *Thyroid*, vol. 11, no. 9, pp. 825–830, 2001.

[43] M. R. Castro, E. R. Bergert, J. R. Goellner, I. D. Hay, and J. C. Morris, "Immunohistochemical analysis of sodium iodide symporter expression in metastatic differentiated thyroid cancer: correlation with radioiodine uptake," *Journal of Clinical Endocrinology and Metabolism*, vol. 86, no. 11, pp. 5627–5632, 2001.

[44] J. J. Min, J. K. Chung, Y. Lee et al., "Relationship between expression of the sodium/iodide symporter and 131I uptake in recurrent lesions of differentiated thyroid carcinoma," *European Journal of Nuclear Medicine*, vol. 28, no. 5, pp. 639–645, 2001.

[45] A. V. Pisarchik, G. Ermak, E. P. Demidchik, L. S. Mikhalevich, N. A. Kartel, and J. Figge, "Low prevalence of the ret/PTC3r1 rearrangement in a series of papillary thyroid carcinomas presenting in Belarus ten years post-chernobyl," *Thyroid*, vol. 8, no. 11, pp. 1003–1008, 1998.

[46] C. A. W. Welch Dinauer, R. M. Tuttle, D. K. Robie et al., "Clinical features associated with metastasis and recurrence of differentiated thyroid cancer in children," *Clinical Endocrinology*, vol. 49, no. 5, pp. 619–628, 1998.

[47] S. Klugbauer, E. Lengfelder, E. P. Demidchik, and H. M. Rabes, "High prevalence of RET rearrangement in thyroid tumors of children after the Chernobyl reactor accident," *Oncogene*, vol. 11, no. 12, pp. 2459–2467, 1995.

[48] L. DeGroot, E. Kaplan, M. McCormick, and F. Strauss, "Natural history, treatment, and course of papillary thyroid carcinoma," *Journal of Clinical Endocrinology and Metabolism*, vol. 71, pp. 414–424, 1990.

[49] I. Bongarzone, L. Fugazzola, P. Vigneri et al., "Age-related activation of the tyrosine kinase receptor protooncogenes RET and NTRK1 in papillary thyroid carcinoma," *Journal of Clinical Endocrinology and Metabolism*, vol. 81, no. 5, pp. 2006–2009, 1996.

[50] T. Motomura, Y. E. Nikiforov, H. Namba et al., "ret rearrangements in Japanese pediatric and adult papillary thyroid cancers," *Thyroid*, vol. 8, no. 6, pp. 485–489, 1998.

[51] R. Ramirez, D. Hsu, A. Patel et al., "Over-expression of hepatocyte growth factor/scatter factor (HGF/SF) and the HGF/SFreceptor (cMET) are associated with a high risk of metastasis and recurrence for children and young adults with papillary thyroid carcinoma," *Clinical Endocrinology*, vol. 53, no. 5, pp. 635–644, 2000.

[52] C. Fenton, A. Patel, C. Dinauer, D. K. Robie, R. M. Tuttle, and G. L. Francis, "The expression of vascular endothelial growth factor and the type 1 vascular endothelial growth factor receptor correlate with the size of papillary thyroid carcinoma in children and young adults," *Thyroid*, vol. 10, no. 4, pp. 349–357, 2000.

[53] A. M. Straight, A. Patel, C. Fenton, C. Dinauer, R. M. Tuttle, and G. L. Francis, "Thyroid carcinomas that express telomerase follow a more aggressive clinical course in children and adolescents," *Journal of Endocrinological Investigation*, vol. 25, no. 4, pp. 302–308, 2002.

[54] M. N. Nikiforova, R. A. Lynch, P. W. Biddinger et al., "RAS point mutations and PAX8-PPAR gamma rearrangement in thyroid tumors: evidence for distinct molecular pathways in thyroid follicular carcinoma," *Journal of Clinical Endocrinology and Metabolism*, vol. 88, no. 5, pp. 2318–2326, 2003.

[55] E. L. Mazzaferri and N. Massoll, "Management of papillary and follicular (differentiated) thyroid cancer: new paradigms using recombinant human thyrotropin," *Endocrine Related Cancer*, vol. 9, no. 4, pp. 227–247, 2002.

[56] Y. E. Demidchik, E. P. Demidchik, and C. Reiners, "Comprehensive clinical assessment of 741 operated pediatric thyroid cancer cases in Belarus," *Annals of Surgery*, vol. 243, pp. 525–532, 2006.

[57] A. L. Maia, L. S. Ward, G. A. Carvalho et al., "Nódulos de tireóide e câncer diferenciado de tireóide: consenso Brasileiro," *Arquivos Brasileiros de Endocrinologia e Metabologia*, vol. 51, no. 5, pp. 867–893, 2007.

[58] D. S. Cooper, G. M. Doherty, B. R. Haugen et al., "Revised American thyroid association management guidelines for patients with thyroid nodules and differentiated thyroid cancer," *Thyroid*, vol. 19, no. 11, pp. 1167–1214, 2009.

[59] H. M. van Santen, D. C. Aronson, T. Vulsma et al., "Frequent adverse events after treatment for childhood onset differentiated thyroid carcinoma: a single institute experience," *European Journal of Cancer*, vol. 40, no. 11, pp. 1743–1751, 2004.

[60] B. Jarzab, D. Handkiewicz-Junak, and J. Włoch, "Juvenile differentiated thyroid carcinoma and the role of radioiodine in its treatment: a qualitative review," *Endocrine Related Cancer*, vol. 12, no. 4, pp. 773–803, 2005.

[61] F. Pacini, M. Schlumberger, H. Dralle et al., "European consensus for the management of patients with differentiated thyroid carcinoma of the follicular epithelium," *European Journal of Endocrinology*, vol. 154, no. 6, pp. 787–803, 2006.

[62] F. A. Verburg, B. Keizer, C. J. M Lips et al., "Prognostic significance of good response to initial therapy with radioiodine of differentiated thyroid cancer patients," *European Journal of Endocrinology*, vol. 152, pp. 33–37, 2005.

[63] E. L. Mazzaferri and S. M. Jhiang, "Long-term impact of initial surgical and medical therapy on papillary and follicular thyroid cancer," *American Journal of Medicine*, vol. 97, no. 5, pp. 418–428, 1994.

[64] I. D. Hay, T. Gonzalez-Lousada, M. S. Reunalda, J. A. Honetschalger, and M. L. Richards, "Thompson GB. Long-term outcome in 215 children and adolescents with papillary thyroid cancer treated during 1940 though 2008," *World Journal of Surgery*, vol. 34, pp. 1192–202, 2010.

[65] G. Matuszewska, J. Roskosz, J. Włoch et al., "Evaluation of effects of L-thyroxine therapy in differentiated thyroid carcinoma on the cardiovascular system—prospective study," *Wiadomosci Lekarskie*, vol. 54, supplement 1, pp. 373–377, 2001.

[66] B. Biondi, S. Fazio, C. Carella et al., "Cardiac effects of long term thyrotropin-suppressive therapy with levothyroxine," *Journal of Clinical Endocrinology and Metabolism*, vol. 77, no. 2, pp. 334–338, 1993.

[67] C. Dinauer and G. L. Francis, "Thyroid cancer in children," *Endocrinology and Metabolism Clinics of North America*, vol. 36, no. 3, pp. 779–806, 2007.

[68] F. Pacini, M. Gasperi, L. Fugazzola et al., "Testicular function in patients with differentiated thyroid carcinoma treated with radioiodine," *Journal of Nuclear Medicine*, vol. 35, no. 9, pp. 1418–1422, 1994.

[69] J. P. Raymond, M. Izembart, V. Marliac et al., "Temporary ovarian failure in thyroid cancer patients after thyroid remnant ablation with radioactive iodine," *Journal of Clinical Endocrinology and Metabolism*, vol. 69, no. 1, pp. 186–190, 1989.

[70] L. Vini, S. Hyer, A. Al-Saadi, B. Pratt, and C. Harmer, "Prognostic for fertility and ovarian function after treatment with radioiodine for thyroid cancer," *Postgraduate Medical Journal*, vol. 78, no. 916, pp. 92–93, 2002.

[71] G. E. Krassas and N. Pontikides, "Gonadal effect of radiation from 131I in male patients with thyroid carcinoma," *Archives of Andrology*, vol. 51, no. 3, pp. 171–175, 2005.

[72] S. M. Chow, S. Yau, S. H. Lee, W. M. Leung, and S. C. K. Law, "Pregnancy outcome after diagnosis of differentiated thyroid carcinoma: no deleterious effect after radioactive iodine treatment," *International Journal of Radiation Oncology Biology Physics*, vol. 59, no. 4, pp. 992–1000, 2004.

[73] International Union Against Cancer (UICC), *TNM Classification of Malignant Tumors*, Wiley, New York, NY, USA, 7th edition, 2009.

[74] C. Wittekind, C. C. Compton, F. L. Greene, and L. H. Sobin, "TNM residual tumor classification revisited," *Cancer*, vol. 94, no. 9, pp. 2511–2516, 2002.

[75] A. R. Shaha, T. R. Loree, J. P. Shah et al., "Prognostic factors and risk group analysis in follicular carcinoma of the thyroid," *Surgery*, vol. 118, no. 6, pp. 1131–1138, 1995.

[76] I. D. Hay, E. J. Bergstralh, J. R. Goellner et al., "Predicting outcome in papillary thyroid carcinoma: development of a reliable prognostic scoring system in a cohort of 1779 patients surgically treated at one institution during 1940 through 1989," *Surgery*, vol. 114, no. 6, pp. 1050–1058, 1993.

[77] S. I. Sherman, J. D. Brierley, M. Sperling et al., "Prospective multicenter study of thyroid carcinoma treatment: initial analysis of staging and outcome. National thyroid cancer treatment cooperative study registry group," *Cancer*, vol. 83, pp. 1012–1021, 1998.

26

Weight Gain and Serum TSH Increase within the Reference Range after Hemithyroidectomy Indicate Lowered Thyroid Function

Tina Toft Kristensen,[1] Jacob Larsen,[2] Palle Lyngsie Pedersen,[3] Anne-Dorthe Feldthusen,[4] Christina Ellervik,[3] Søren Jelstrup,[1] and Jan Kvetny[5,6]

[1] *Department of Otorhinolaryngology-Head and Neck Surgery, Koege Hospital, Region Zealand, 4600 Koege, Denmark*
[2] *Department of Clinical Pathology, Naestved Hospital, Region Zealand, 4700 Naestved, Denmark*
[3] *Department of Clinical Biochemistry, Naestved Hospital, Region Zealand, 4700 Naestved, Denmark*
[4] *Department of Gynecology and Obstetrics, Naestved Hospital, Region Zealand, 4700 Naestved, Denmark*
[5] *Department of Internal Medicine, Naestved Hospital, Region Zealand, 4700 Naestved, Denmark*
[6] *University of Southern Denmark, 5230 Odense, Denmark*

Correspondence should be addressed to Tina Toft Kristensen; tikr@regionsjaelland.dk

Academic Editor: Massimo Tonacchera

Background. Weight gain is frequently reported after hemithyroidectomy but the significance is recently discussed. Therefore, the aim of the study was to examine changes in body weight of hemithyroidectomized patients and to evaluate if TSH increase within the reference range could be related to weight gain. *Methods*. In a controlled follow-up study, two years after hemithyroidectomy for benign euthyroid goiter, postoperative TSH and body weight of 28 patients were compared to preoperative values and further compared to the results in 47 matched control persons, after a comparable follow-up period. *Results*. Two years after hemithyroidectomy, median serum TSH was increased over preoperative levels (1.23 versus 2.08 mIU/L, $P < 0.01$) and patients had gained weight (75.0 versus 77.3 kg, $P = 0.02$). Matched healthy controls had unchanged median serum TSH (1.70 versus 1.60 mIU/L, $P = 0.13$) and weight (69.3 versus 69.3 kg, $P = 0.71$). Patients on thyroxin treatment did not gain weight. TSH increase was significantly correlated with weight gain ($r = 0.43$, $P < 0.01$). *Conclusion*. Two years after hemithyroidectomy for benign euthyroid goiter, thyroid function is lowered within the laboratory reference range. Weight gain of patients who are biochemically euthyroid after hemithyroidectomy may be a clinical manifestation of a permanently decreased metabolic rate.

1. Background

Hemithyroidectomy is recommended as a treatment for a symptomatic unilateral benign nontoxic thyroid nodule or as a diagnostic surgical procedure in case of an indeterminate solitary thyroid nodule [1]. Whereas hypothyroidism is a recognized consequence of hemithyroidectomy with incidence rates ranging from 11% to 49% [2–4], only a single study has addressed the subject if lowered thyroid function within the laboratory reference range of the euthyroid majority of hemithyroidectomized patients may have clinical consequences [5]. It is the authors' experience that euthyroid patients, undergoing thyroidectomy, in spite of euthyroidism, report weight gain. However, studies concerning weight changes in euthyroid individuals after thyroidectomy are sparse. In 2011, it was reported that individuals after near total thyroidectomy, even if kept euthyroid by thyroxin supplement, gained more weight than euthyroid controls [6].

The aim of the present study was to examine if lowered metabolic rate, reflected by changes in TSH, could explain the weight gain, frequently reported by patients who remain within the euthyroid normal range of thyroid function after hemithyroidectomy for benign euthyroid goiter.

2. Materials and Methods

2.1. Hemithyroidectomy Group. This study was designed as a controlled follow-up study with a matched control group. The study group and control group have been described in detail previously [7]. We reviewed the hospital charts of all patients (n = 74) who underwent hemithyroidectomy in the time period from September 2008 to July 2009 at the Department of Otorhinolaryngology-Head and Neck Surgery, Slagelse Hospital, Hospital South, Region Zealand, Denmark. Criteria of inclusion were (1) no previous goiter surgery, (2) no previous radioiodine treatment for goiter, (3) no previous radiation therapy to the cervical region, (4) no previous or present medical treatment of hyperthyroidism or thyroid hormone substitution therapy, (5) preoperative value of TSH in the laboratory reference range (0.4–3.77 mIU/L), (6) benign pathologic diagnosis of resected tissue, (7) preoperative body mass index (BMI) between 20 and 35 kg/m^2, and (8) age older than 18 years. Exclusion criteria were disease or medical treatment known to affect body weight.

Baseline (preoperative) measures of weight, height, and serum TSH were obtained from hospital charts. At the routine preoperative examination, patients' weight had been measured to the nearest 0.5 kg and height to the nearest 0.5 cm wearing indoor clothes and without shoes. A nonfasting venous blood sample had been drawn and analysed for serum concentrations of TSH.

Hemithyroidectomy was performed by one of four surgeons, who all used identical technique which involved total left or right thyroid lobectomy and isthmusectomy and, if present, resection of the pyramidal lobe with preservation of the contralateral thyroid lobe. The weight and morphology of the resected thyroid lobe were recorded.

Forty-six patients (11 men and 35 women) aged 32–74 years fulfilled the inclusion criteria and were invited to the study. Twenty-eight patients responded to the invitation (6 men and 22 women), resulting in a 61% participation rate. At the follow-up visit, patients reported medical history and current medication and were weighed to the nearest 0.5 kg wearing indoor clothes and without shoes, and a nonfasting venous blood sample was collected and analyzed for serum concentrations of TSH and antibodies against thyroid peroxidase (TPO-ab).

2.2. Control Group. The control persons were recruited from participants in the Danish General Suburban Population Study (GESUS) [8], which is conducted in the area of Denmark (with previous mild iodine deficiency) from which we also had recruited the hemithyroidectomy group. Control persons' criteria of inclusion were (1) reported absence of previous or present thyroid disease, (2) reported absence of previous or present medical treatment for thyroid disease, and (3) values of TSH and thyroid hormones within the laboratory reference ranges. Exclusion criteria were disease or

medical treatment known to affect body weight. The control persons were matched for sex, age, BMI, smoking status, and presence of TPO-abs to the hemithyroidectomized patients. Ages were matched within 5-year age groups. BMI was matched to groups of BMI between 20 and 24.9, 25 and 29.9, and 30 and 35 kg/m^2. Smoking status was matched to either current smoking status or no-smoking status, and presence of TPO-ab was matched to either TPO-ab positivity (TPO-ab > 60 kU/L) or TPO-ab negativity (TPO-ab < 60 kU/L). Baseline values of weight (to the nearest 0.5 kg), height (to the nearest 0.5 cm), and serum TSH were obtained from the GESUS database. Twenty months after the participation in the GESUS, we invited 80 controls (18 men, 62 women) to the study with the intention to include two controls for every hemithyroidectomized patient. Fifty-three persons responded to the invitation, resulting in a 66% participation rate. Six of these were excluded: two due to other ethnicity than Caucasian, two due to subsequent endocrine disease, and two due to antipsychotic medical treatment known to cause weight gain. Control persons reported medical history and current medication, they were weighed to the nearest 0.5 kg wearing indoor clothes and without shoes, and a nonfasting venous blood sample was collected and analyzed for serum concentrations of TSH. In total, the control group included 47 persons (9 men, 38 women). The heights obtained at the baseline examination of both study groups were used in the calculation of BMI at baseline and at follow-up. BMI was calculated as body weight (kg) divided by the square of the height (m).

2.3. Biochemical Variables. Measurements of TSH and of thyroid hormones free thyroxin (fT$_4$) and total triiodothyronine (T$_3$) were performed using an electrochemical luminescent immunoassay (Roche Cobas 6000, Basel, Switzerland). Reference range for TSH is 0.30–3.77 mIU/L (CV < 7%), fT$_4$ is 10.0–26.0 pmol/L (CV < 5%), and T$_3$ is 1.20–2.80 nmol/L (CV < 4%). Thyroid peroxidase antibody (TPO-ab) was measured by KRYPTOR anti-TPOn (BRAHMS, Hennigsdorf, Germany), with a detection limit of 10 kU/L.

2.4. Statistical Analysis. An a priori power calculation based on a TSH alteration of 0.1 mIU/L, alpha = 0.05, and power of 0.95, indicated a sample size of 27 patients in each group. Comparison between baseline values of responders and of nonresponders in both study groups was performed using the chi-square test for categorical variables, and as Shapiro-Wilk's test demonstrated absent normality of the measured parameters, the Mann-Whitney U test was used for continuous variables. Likewise, for the baseline comparison between the hemithyroidectomy and the control group, we used the chi-square test for categorical variables and the Mann-Whitney U test for continuous variables. The Wilcoxon signed-rank test was used to compare the change in medians of body weight and serum TSH of the hemithyroidectomy and the control group at baseline and at follow-up. The Spearman correlation coefficient was used to evaluate the correlation of the variables. Significant difference was defined as a P value < 0.05.

TABLE 1: Comparison between responders and nonresponders of the study groups.

Responders	Control group			Hemithyroidectomy group		
	Yes ($n = 47$)	No ($n = 27$)	P value	Yes ($n = 28$)	No ($n = 18$)	P value
Males (%)	19.1	33.3	0.17[*]	21.4	50.0	0.37[*]
Age (years)	53 (43–62)	47 (40–58)	0.22	51.5 (43–60)	53.5 (45–58)	0.81
Weight (kg)	69.3 (62.2–81.4)	78.5 (67.5–92.0)	0.16	75.0 (63.5–85.0)	87.0 (65.0–98.0)	0.87
BMI (kg/m^2)	25.0 (22.7–29.0)	27.7 (23.6–29.9)	0.24	26.1 (23.1–28.3)	29.1 (23.9–32.3)	0.17
TSH (mIU/L)	1.70 (1.10–2.20)	1.70 (1.10–2.20)	0.85	1.23 (0.91–1.59)	1.02 (0.68–1.57)	0.17

The Mann-Whitney U test for continuous variables (median and interquartile range are presented). [*]Chi-square test was for categorical variables. Significant difference was defined as a P value < 0.05. BMI: body mass index; TSH: thyroid stimulating hormone.

The match procedure and all analyses of results were evaluated using the STATA statistical package software programme (Statacorp, V. 12.0, College Station, TX, USA).

2.5. Ethical Considerations. The study was approved by the Regional Ethics Committee of Zealand, Denmark (SJ-10 and SJ-245), and by the Danish Data Protection Agency and registered in ClinicalTrials.gov (NCT01358136). The study conformed to the principles of the Declaration of Helsinki. Informed consent was obtained from all hemithyroidectomized patients prior to inclusion in the study. Informed consent was obtained from all control persons prior to participation in the GESUS as well as prior to inclusion in the current study.

3. Results

The indications of hemithyroidectomy (14 right and 14 left hemithyroidectomies) were suspicion of malignancy in 19 cases (67.9%) (cold areas in scintiscan or susceptible FNAB) and compressive symptoms in 9 cases (32.1%). The 28 hemithyroidectomized patients suffered no surgical complications such as secondary haemorrhage, infection, and temporary or permanent recurrent laryngeal nerve paresis. No patients were diagnosed histologically with Hashimoto's thyroiditis, although four patients showed increased TPO-ab > 60 kU/L (14.3%).

The participation rates were 61% in the hemithyroidectomy group and 66% in the control group. Table 1 provides data that the nonresponders in both study groups did not differ from the responders regarding age, sex and baseline weight, BMI, or serum TSH.

Table 2 provides baseline data of the responders of the study groups, indicating that there were no statistically significant differences in sex, age, BMI, smoking status, and presence of TPO-abs. The baseline median TSH was significantly lower in the hemithyroidectomy group as previously reported [7] than in the control group (1.23, 0.91–1.51 versus 1.70, 1.10–2.20, $P = 0.01$), and the median duration of follow-up in the hemithyroidectomy group was significantly longer than in the control group (25, 23–30 versus 20, 19–21 months, $P < 0.01$).

Two years after hemithyroidectomy, 8 of 28 patients (28.6%) received thyroid hormone replacement therapy.

TABLE 2: Comparison between study groups at baseline.

Variables	Control group ($n = 47$)	Hemithyroidectomy group ($n = 28$)	P value
Males (%)	19.2%	21.4%	0.81[*]
Age (years)	53 (43–62)	51.5 (43–60)	0.59
Weight (kg)	69.3 (62.2–81.4)	75.0 (63.5–85.0)	0.43
BMI (kg/m^2)	25.0 (22.7–29.0)	26.1 (23.1–28.3)	0.65
Smokers (%)	8.5	14.3	0.43[*]
TPO-ab positivity (%)	12.8	14.3	0.85[*]

The Mann-Whitney U test was used for continuous variables (median and interquartile range are presented). [*]Chi-square test for categorical variables. Significant difference was defined as a P value < 0.05. BMI: body mass index; TPO-ab: thyroid peroxidase antibody.

Three patients (10.7%) demonstrated biochemical subclinical hypothyroidism with raised serum TSH values (>3.77 mIU/L) and values of fT_4 and tT_3 in the normal range, and they were referred to further evaluation by an endocrinologist. The remaining 17 patients (60.7%) were clinically euthyroid as was the case with those with subclinical hypothyroidism.

3.1. Postoperative Thyroid Function. In total, 26 of the 28 patients (92.9%) showed increased levels of TSH over preoperative levels, compared to the control group in which 19 of 47 (40.4%) presented increased levels of TSH over baseline levels ($P < 0.001$). Figure 1 presents the values of serum TSH of the hemithyroidectomy group and of the control group, measured at baseline and after follow-up. The figure demonstrates a significant TSH increase within the reference range of the hemithyroidectomy group two years after hemithyroidectomy, compared to the healthy control group.

3.2. Postoperative Body Weight. Two years after hemithyroidectomy, 18 of 28 patients (64.3%) had gained weight and 10 of 28 had lost weight compared to the control group where 22 of 47 (46.8%) had gained weight and 25 of 47 had lost weight ($P = 0.02$). Figure 2 presents the values of body weight of the hemithyroidectomy group and of the control group,

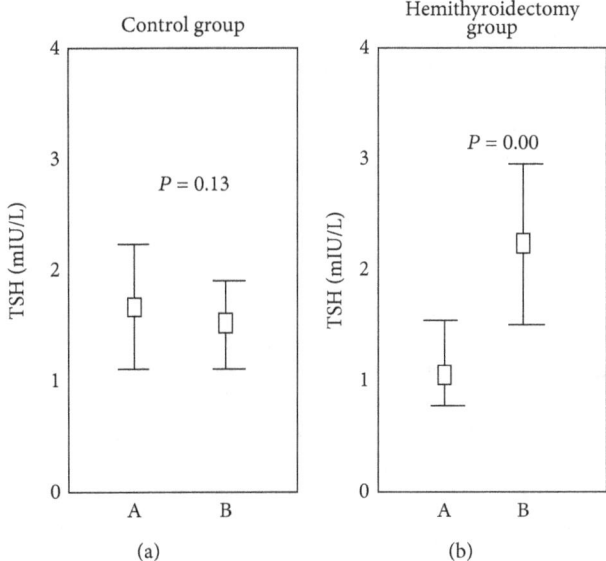

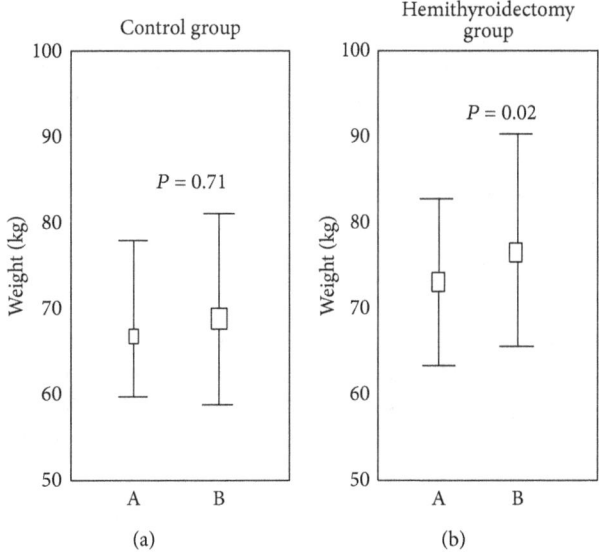

FIGURE 1: TSH changes between baseline and follow-up. TSH changes of the hemithyroidectomy group ($n = 28$) and of the control group ($n = 47$) after a two-year follow-up period. The median, upper, and lower quartiles are presented. Outliers are excluded. The Wilcoxon signed-rank test was used. Statistical significance was demonstrated whenever $P < 0.05$.

FIGURE 2: Weight changes between baseline and follow-up. Weight changes of the hemithyroidectomy group ($n = 28$) and of the control group ($n = 47$). The median, upper, and lower quartiles are presented. Outliers are excluded. The Wilcoxon signed-rank test was used. Statistical significance was demonstrated whenever $P < 0.05$.

measured at baseline and after follow-up. Two years postoperatively, the median body weight of the hemithyroidectomized group had increased significantly with an annual weight gain of 1.1 kg. In comparison, the median body weight of the healthy control group was unchanged after a 20-month follow-up.

In the 8 persons treated with thyroxin, the weight did not change. Weight before operation was 66 kg (59–76) versus weight after operation 66 kg (57–78, $P = 0.75$) (median and quartiles) in contrast to weight changes in the group without thyroxin treatment (Figure 2). Although the preoperative weight appears lower in the postoperative thyroxin treated group, the difference was not statistical significant ($P = 0.06$).

We examined the relation between changes in TSH and weight in the participants of both study groups, who had gained weight during follow-up, and we observed a significant correlation between the relative change in TSH and weight gain (Figure 3). We then examined the possibility of a factor to predict weight gain in the hemithyroidectomized group. Forward multiple logistic regression analysis with weight gain as dependent and preoperative weight, preoperative TSH, weight of resected thyroid tissue, and smoking status as independent variables did not, however, reveal a significant contributor.

4. Discussion

The major finding was a 1.1 kg annual weight increase in hemithyroidectomized person without thyroxin treatment compared to matched controls, who did not gain weight. Our

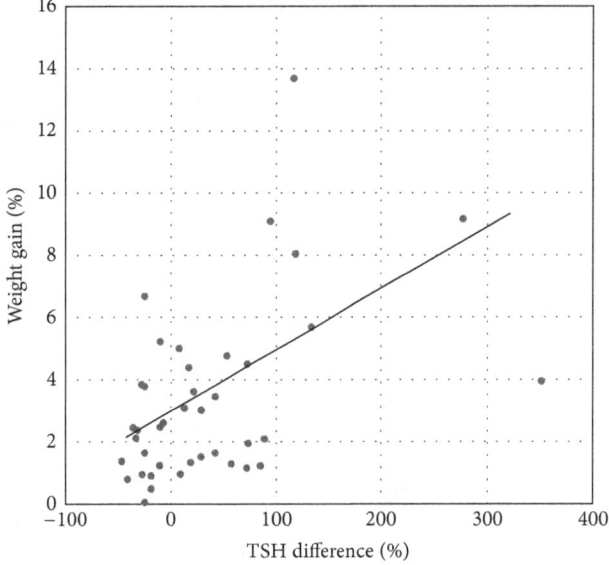

FIGURE 3: Correlation between relative changes in weight and serum TSH. Correlation between percent increase in weight and percent change in serum TSH of the hemithyroidectomy group ($n = 18$) and the control group ($n = 22$) during the follow-up period ($r = 0.43$, $P < 0.01$).

result regarding postoperative TSH is in coherence with previous studies' reports of increased TSH within the laboratory reference range 1 and 3 years after hemithyroidectomy [2, 5, 9, 10]. The clinical significance of a posthemithyroidectomy TSH increase has not, however, previously been addressed. In the present study, 28.6% received levothyroxine two years after hemithyroidectomy, which is comparable to the post-hemithyroidectomy hypothyroidism rates reported in the literature [2–4] and it is noteworthy that these patients did not gain weight. The exact clinical consequences of having a permanently increased TSH after hemithyroidectomy still need to be studied.

Serum TSH levels within the laboratory reference range have been associated with BMI in cross-sectional population-based studies [11] and, in a longitudinal design, increase in TSH over time, but within the euthyroid range they were associated with weight gain [12, 13]. Moreover, it has been demonstrated that small variations in thyroid function, with serum TSH variations within the normal laboratory range, resulted in decreased resting energy expenditure of patients on T_4 substitution [14]. These studies indicate that the well-known association between low thyroid function and weight gain extends into the euthyroid states and propose the hypothesis that an increase in TSH reflects decreased metabolic rate causing weight gain and not the other way around [15, 16]. In support of this hypothesis speaks the present study, where TSH increase, induced by hemithyroidectomy for benign unilateral goiter, is significantly related to weight gain and the fact that thyroxine treated patients did not gain weight. Weight loss prior to operation may have contributed as a possible malignancy would cause concern in some and hence induce weight loss.

The pituitary gland is sensitive to small changes in serums T_4 and T_3 and, before and after thyroid surgery, measurement of serum TSH is used routinely to screen for thyroid dysfunction. Each individual has a unique level of thyroid function, and the individual normal ranges for thyroid function are much narrower than the population-based reference ranges [17]. Postoperative test results that are abnormal for the individual can therefore be unnoticed in the wide population-based reference range if the preoperative thyroid function is not taken into consideration. In this setting, the 1.1 kg annual weight gain of the hemithyroidectomy group might be a clinical reflection of a permanently increased TSH to a level that is outside the normal range of the individual.

The annual weight gain of 1.1 kg of the hemithyroidectomy group is relatively modest. However, it is still concerning and could over time become clinically significant. In a previous study, total thyroidectomy for hyperthyroidism resulted in continuous weight gain during a 4-year follow-up period [18], suggesting that weight gain after thyroid surgery is more likely a reflection of a permanently changed thyroid function than it is a regain of previously lost weight. We did not find a factor that could predict weight gain after hemithyroidectomy, which might be explained by the limited number of participating patients.

The study is limited by its follow-up design and the 61% participation rate, although this rate is comparable to (and even in the higher spectrum of) that reported in population studies. Reasons for nonresponse may be due to long distance to the outpatient clinic and the fact that the hemithyroidectomized patients are generally healthy and employed. The major concern with the participation rates of the study group is the potential for nonresponse bias. However, the nonresponding hemithyroidectomized patients and controls did not differ from the responding ones regarding preoperative weight, BMI, or thyroid function (Table 1), and we find it unlikely that postoperative and follow-up thyroid function and body weight of nonresponders should be different from the responders'. Another limitation is the heterogeneity of collection of preoperative body weight data of the hemithyroidectomy group, since they have been weighed by different health care providers at the routine preoperative examination. The follow-up study design may have had an advantage since engagement in life style changes of the hemithyroidectomy group due to higher awareness of the risk of weight gain could not have had any confounding effect on the results and it is important to notice that the 1.1 kg annual weight gain of the hemithyroidectomy group is considerably greater than the reported annual weight increase of 0.4 kg of westernized populations [19].

5. Conclusion

Two years postoperatively, serum TSH of hemithyroidectomized patients was significantly increased within the reference range and patients had gained weight significantly. Our study confirms the patient-reported weight gain after hemithyroidectomy and proposes the hypothesis that weight gain of patients who are biochemically euthyroid after hemithyroidectomy for benign euthyroid goiter may be a clinical manifestation of a permanently decreased metabolic rate.

References

[1] R. Paschke, L. Hegedüs, E. Alexander, R. Valcavi, E. Papini, and H. Gharib, "Thyroid nodule guidelines: agreement, disagreement and need for future research," *Nature Reviews Endocrinology*, vol. 7, no. 6, pp. 354–361, 2011.

[2] E. A. Farkas, T. A. King, J. S. Bolton, and G. M. Fuhrman, "A comparison of total thyroidectomy and lobectomy in the treatment of dominant thyroid nodules," *American Surgeon*, vol. 68, no. 8, pp. 678–682, 2002.

[3] S. Y. Su, S. Grodski, and J. W. Serpell, "Hypothyroidism following hemithyroidectomy: a retrospective review," *Annals of Surgery*, vol. 250, no. 6, pp. 991–994, 2009.

[4] M. Vaiman, A. Nagibin, P. Hagag, A. Kessler, and H. Gavriel, "Hypothyroidism following partial thyroidectomy," *Otolaryngology—Head and Neck Surgery*, vol. 138, no. 1, pp. 98–100, 2008.

[5] P. Cheung, J. Boey, and J. Wong, "Thyroid function after hemithyroidectomy for benign nodules," *World Journal of Surgery*, vol. 10, no. 4, pp. 718–723, 1986.

[6] J. Jonklaas and H. Nsouli-Maktabi, "Weight changes in euthyroid patients undergoing thyroidectomy," *Thyroid*, vol. 21, no. 12, pp. 1343–1351, 2011.

[7] T. Toft Kristensen, J. Larsen, P. Lyngsie Pedersen et al., "Persistent cellular metabolic changes after hemithyroidectomy for benign euthyroid goiter," *European Thyroid Journal*, vol. 3, no. 1, pp. 10–16, 2014.

[8] H. Bergholdt, L. Bathum, J. Kvetny, D. Rasmussen, B. Moldow, G. Jemec et al., "Study design, participation and characteristics

of the Danish General Suburban Population Study," *Danish Medical Bulletin*, vol. 60, article A4669, 2013.

[9] A. Johner, O. L. Griffith, B. Walker et al., "Detection and management of hypothyroidism following thyroid lobectomy: evaluation of a clinical algorithm," *Annals of Surgical Oncology*, vol. 18, no. 9, pp. 2548–2554, 2011.

[10] P. Lindblom, S. Valdemarsson, B. Lindergård, J. Westerdahl, and A. Bergenfelz, "Decreased levels of ionized calcium one year after hemithyroidectomy: importance of reduced thyroid hormones," *Hormone Research*, vol. 55, no. 2, pp. 81–87, 2001.

[11] N. Knudsen, P. Laurberg, L. B. Rasmussen et al., "Small differences in thyroid function may be important for body mass index and the occurrence of obesity in the population," *The Journal of Clinical Endocrinology and Metabolism*, vol. 90, no. 7, pp. 4019–4024, 2005.

[12] C. S. Fox, M. J. Pencina, R. B. D'Agostino et al., "Relations of thyroid function to body weight: cross-sectional and longitudinal observations in a community-based sample," *Archives of Internal Medicine*, vol. 168, no. 6, pp. 587–592, 2008.

[13] A. Nyrnes, R. Jorde, and J. Sundsfjord, "Serum TSH is positively associated with BMI," *International Journal of Obesity*, vol. 30, no. 1, pp. 100–105, 2006.

[14] H. Al-Adsani, L. J. Hoffer, and J. E. Silva, "Resting energy expenditure is sensitive to small dose changes in patients on chronic thyroid hormone replacement," *The Journal of Clinical Endocrinology and Metabolism*, vol. 82, no. 4, pp. 1118–1125, 1997.

[15] B. Biondi, "Thyroid and obesity: an intriguing relationship," *The Journal of Clinical Endocrinology and Metabolism*, vol. 95, no. 8, pp. 3614–3617, 2010.

[16] T. Reinehr, "Obesity and thyroid function," *Molecular and Cellular Endocrinology*, vol. 316, no. 2, pp. 165–171, 2010.

[17] S. Andersen, K. M. Pedersen, N. H. Bruun, and P. Laurberg, "Narrow individual variations in serum T(4) and T(3) in normal subjects: a clue to the understanding of subclinical thyroid disease," *The Journal of Clinical Endocrinology and Metabolism*, vol. 87, no. 3, pp. 1068–1072, 2002.

[18] S. Tigas, J. Idiculla, G. Beckett, and A. Toft, "Is excessive weight gain after ablative treatment of hyperthyroidism due to inadequate thyroid hormone therapy?" *Thyroid*, vol. 10, no. 12, pp. 1107–1111, 2000.

[19] M. Rosell, P. Appleby, E. Spencer, and T. Key, "Weight gain over 5 years in 21 966 meat-eating, fish-eating, vegetarian, and vegan men and women in EPIC-Oxford," *International Journal of Obesity*, vol. 30, no. 9, pp. 1389–1396, 2006.

27

Free Thyroxine Level in the High Normal Reference Range Prescribed for Nonpregnant Women may Reduce the Preterm Delivery Rate in Multiparous

P. Torremante,[1] F. Flock,[2] and W. Kirschner[3]

[1] *Praxis für Gynäkologie und Geburtshilfe, Marktplatz 29, 88416 Ochsenhausen, Germany*
[2] *Frauenklinik des Klinikums Memmingen, Klinikum Memmingen, Bismarckstraße 23, 87700 Memmingen, Germany*
[3] *Institut Forschung, Beratung und Evaluation, FB+E Forschung, Beratung Evaluation GmbH, Postfach 10 03 35, 10563 Berlin, Germany*

Correspondence should be addressed to P. Torremante, dr.torremante@onlinemed.de

Academic Editor: Noriyuki Koibuchi

Preterm birth is the most common reason for perinatal morbidity and mortality in the western world. It has been shown that in euthyreotic pregnant women with thyroid autoimmune antibodies, L-Thyroxine replacement reduces preterm delivery rate in singleton pregnancies. We investigated in a nonrandomized retrospective observational study whether L-Thyroxine replacement, maintaining maternal free thyroxine serum level in the high normal reference range prescribed for nonpregnant women also influences the rate of preterm delivery in women without thyroid autoimmune antibodies. As control group for preterm delivery rate, data from perinatal statistics of the State of Baden-Württemberg from 2006 were used. The preterm delivery rate in the study group was significantly reduced. The subgroup analysis shows no difference in primiparous but a decline in multiparous by approximately 61% with L-Thyroxine replacement. Maintaining free thyroxine serum level in the high normal reference range prescribed for nonpregnant women may reduce the preterm delivery rate.

1. Introduction

The prevalence of preterm birth, defined as delivery before 37 completed weeks' gestation, varies from 6% to 15%, depending on geographical and demographic features of the population studied. Preterm births account for 75% of perinatal deaths, with over two-thirds of these arising in preterm infants delivered before 32 weeks' gestation. In 2002, this was the most frequent cause of neonatal deaths in the USA. 65%–75% of preterm births are defined as spontaneous preterm births caused by spontaneous preterm labor or preterm premature rupture of the membranes and 30%–35% of preterm deliveries are medically indicated due to maternal or fetal complications in pregnancy. About one-quarter of preterm births occur in multiple pregnancies [1–5].

Various epidemiological risk factors were identified. These encompass advanced age or teenage pregnancy, parity, race, history of cervical cone biopsy, low body mass index, tobacco use, assisted conception with in vitro fertilisation, and gamete intrafallopian transfer, especially for singleton gesta-

tions, systemic and genital-tract infection, and low parental socioeconomic status, this being the most important factor [1–4, 6]. Thanks to advances in neonatal medicine, the outcome for preterm infants born at or after 32 weeks' gestation is similar to that of full-term infants. Limits of viability have been lowered to a gestational age (GA) as low as 23 weeks at the expense of physical disabilities and long-term neurodevelopmental consequences [2, 4, 5, 7].

Thyroid hormones are essential for differentiation and maturation of the fetus and placenta and are especially important for the development of the fetal central nervous system. Epidemiological studies have demonstrated that the intelligence quotient (IQ) of the offspring correlates with maternal free thyroxine (fT4) serum level. The higher maternal fT4, the higher the IQ of the offspring [8–13]. In a study with euthyroid thyroid peroxidase antibody (TPOAb) positive pregnant women receiving substitution with L-Thyroxine (L-T4) it proved possible to decrease their preterm birth rate [14–16]. Thyroid hormones may also provide protection against preterm delivery in women without TPOAb.

The aim of this study is to investigate whether L-T4 replacement therapy by maintaining maternal fT4 in the high normal reference range prescribed for nonpregnant women can also lower the preterm birth rate in pregnant women who do not have thyroid autoimmune antibodies. For this purpose, a group of pregnant women, who had been treated with L-T4 with the goal of elevating maternal fT4 serum level to the high normal reference range prescribed for nonpregnant women to achieve an optimal fetal supply with thyroxine, were retrospectively examined.

2. Subjects and Methods

This clinical trial is a retrospective nonrandomized observational study with prospectively designed data. From April 2001 to March 2010, all pregnant women below 12 weeks' gestation presenting for their first medical consultation for prenatal care in a medical office were offered a serological thyroid scan. This included basal TSH, free triiodothyronine (fT3), free thyroxine (fT4), thyroglobulin antibody test (TgAb), thyroid peroxidase antibody test (TPOAb), and TSH receptor antibody test (TSH-R-Ab).

The primary object was to elevate maternal fT4 to the high normal reference range for nonpregnant adults in order to optimise fetal brain development. For this purpose, and for better interpretation, the normal reference range for nonpregnant adults (fT4 12.14–19.62 pmol/L) was divided into thirds. The division was made as follows: the lower third ranged from 12.14–14.72 pmol/L, the middle third ranged from 14.72–17.17 pmol/L, and the upper third ranged from 17.17–19.62 pmol/L. All women with an fT4 serum level in the lower and middle third of the reference range for nonpregnant adults at the first consultation were given a variable dose of L-T4, usually starting with 25 μg–50 μg L-T4 per day, after informed consent, to raise the fT4 serum level in the high normal reference range (upper third) for nonpregnant adults. All women with a physiological fT4 serum level in the high normal reference range (upper third) for nonpregnant adults at the first consultation were only serological assessed and L-T4 therapy was started later when serum fT4 declined to the middle or lower third. Additionally, each woman received supplements containing 200 μg iodide and 400 μg folic acid.

Maternal fT4 serum levels were regularly assessed after an interval of 24 hours from the last L-T4 intake every 4 weeks during routinely performed serological scans for pregnancy care and if necessary, the L-T4 dose was adjusted. For adjustment, a variable dosage for example, between 25–50 μg/die L-T4 was usually applied. If the increased dose was not tolerated, it was recommended to continue with the last tolerated dose and to increase it one week later. TSH was not further assessed because the goal was to avoid a low maternal fT4 serum level in pregnancy for optimal fetal brain development, and a decline of the fT4 serum level is not automatically accompanied by an increase of the TSH level. Furthermore, maternal TSH is not related to the cognitive competence of the offspring [12]. Moreover, in pregnancy, TSH shows dependencies with other pregnancy-associated hormonal fluctuations and the interval between two blood samples of 4 weeks is too short for precise TSH readings [17]. Thyroid function control was handled by determining fT4 and not TSH as is the case when assessing central hypothyroidism [18–20].

Prenatal care included measurement of body weight, blood pressure, urinary test for protein, glucose, blood, and nitrite. Check intervals were as follows: every 4 weeks until the 30 weeks' gestation, thereafter every 3 weeks, weekly after the 35 weeks' gestation, and after term every 2 days. Beginning at 20 weeks' gestation a digital vaginal examination was performed, and if necessary an ultrasound scan of the cervix length was done.

Ultrasound scans were performed between gestation weeks 9–12, 19–22, and 29–32. If required, color Doppler sonography and special ultrasound scan to rule out fetal malformation were undergone. A cardiotocographic survey of the fetus was routinely started at 28 weeks' gestation and thereafter at each visit.

Women who developed preterm labor were treated with orally applied magnesium. In case of hospitalisation, treatment of preterm labor was performed according to hospital guidelines, for example, bed rest, intravenous fluids, tocolytic therapy, and steroid administration, if clinically indicated. Administration of L-T4 was continued during treatment for preterm labor.

All pregnant women were delivered in an obstetric unit in different hospitals in the vicinity. Routinely, the newborns were medically examined by the gynaecologist who had assisted parturition immediately after birth. Apgar score and arterial blood gas analysis from the umbilical cord were measured. A further examination of the newborn was performed by a paediatrician between the 3rd–7th day of life. After discharge, all children in Germany have regular medical checkups performed by a paediatrician or family physician in private office in regular intervals beginning at 4–6 weeks after birth until adolescence. 6–8 weeks postpartum all women had a medical check for controlling uterine involution and after establishing normal serum fT4 levels, L-T4 substitution was discontinued.

The study group included all women who fulfilled the following criteria: women with singleton pregnancies who had their first antenatal check before the 12 weeks' gestation, determined by ultrasound (crown-rump length). The women presented regularly for inspection until birth. Since this clinical trial was designed as a retrospective nonrandomized observational study, we chose a surrogate as control group. The study was performed in the State of Baden-Württemberg, so we used as control group the preterm delivery rate from all 87.897 singleton pregnancies of the State of Baden-Württemberg, Germany, in the year 2006, collected in central database (GeQiK) with unknown thyroid status. The processed data, provided to us by the database GeQik of the perinatal statistics of the State of Baden-Württemberg were related to preterm birth rate, maternal age and parity status. A further comparison of more obstetrical details and perinatal outcomes was not possible to realize. Preterm delivery was defined as parturition before completion of the 37 weeks' gestation.

3. Laboratory Analysis

Serum basal TSH and fT4 were measured using a third generation electrochemiluminescence immunoassay (Elecsys 1010/2010–MODULAR ANALYTICS E170 from Roche Diagnostics GmbH–Mannheim, Germany). Reference values for TSH were 0.27–4.2 μIU/mL and for fT4 12.14–19.62 pmol/L. Intra- and interassay coefficients of variation were 3.0% and 7.2% for TSH, and 1.4% and 3.5% for fT4. Thyroid antibodies were also determined using the abovementioned analytic test. Thyroid antibody titers were considered positive for TPO-Ab titers above 34 U/mL, for Tg-Ab titers above 115 U/mL, and for the anti-TSH receptor-Ab titers above 2.0 U/L.

4. Statistical Analysis

Basis for data of the control group are population parameters statistical analysis took place by calculating the 99% confidence intervals (99%-CI) of the values in the study group.

5. Results

Between April 2001 and March 2010, 771 pregnant women presented for medical care. Among these, 96 (13%) had a first trimester abortion, 12 (2%) moved away to other regions, 18 (2%) had multiple pregnancy, 87 (11%) presented after 12 weeks' gestation. 558 (72%) women met the study inclusion criteria, being under 12 weeks' gestation with singleton pregnancy.

Among these 558 women there were 108 (19%) women with autoimmune thyroid antibodies, 43 primiparous, and 65 multiparous. By taking away these 108 women, there remained 450 women without autoimmune thyroid antibodies defining the study group.

Regarding the distribution of maternal age and parity status (primiparous versus multiparous), the study group and control group were almost identical. In the study group, 39.8% were primiparous versus 39.2% in control group, and 60.2% were multiparous in study group versus 60.8% in control group. Dictated by body mass index (BMI), 61% of the primiparous group had normal weight at first consultation, and 39% were overweight or obese. Of the multiparous group, 60% had normal weight at first consultation and 40% were overweight or obese. There was a similar mean weight gain of 10–15 kg for primiparous and multiparous in pregnancy.

Peripartum outcome and fetal outcome resulted as follows: 68% of primiparous and 73% of multiparous had vaginal delivery within the study group. Cesarean section occurred in 34% of the primiparous (15% were elective, and 19% were emergency cesarean section) and in 28% of the multiparous (17% were elective, and 11% were emergency cesarean section). Pregnancy-induced hypertension occurred in 9 (2%) women of the study group (5 primiparous and 4 multiparous). Data from 2 women (1 primiparous and 1 multiparous) are missing. In the study group 22 (4.8%) women had breech presentation at term (11 were primiparous and 11 were multiparous).

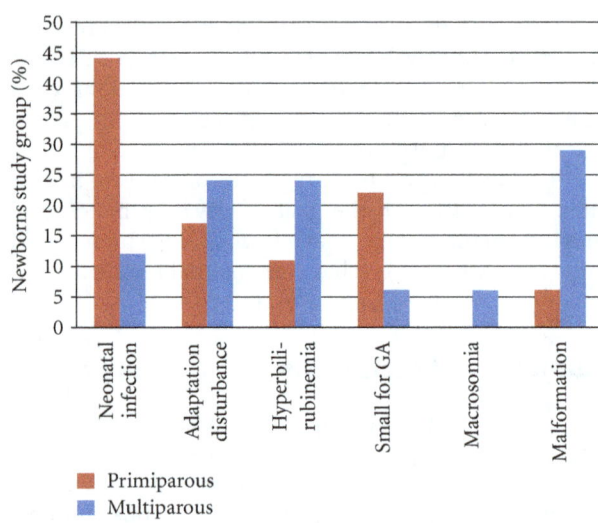

FIGURE 1: Percentage distribution of the reasons for referral of newborns in a paediatric hospital ($n = 35$). Preterm births are not shown.

Data for Apgar score and arterial umbilical cord pH were almost complete. There is data missing for 2 Apgar scores and 8 arterial umbilical cord pHs. An Apgar score below 3, as a sign of impaired vitality was not registered at all and only 2 (0.5%) newborns had an arterial umbilical cord pH below 7.00, demonstrating asphyxia.

Apart from preterm births that were all referred to a pediatric hospital, further 35 newborns were referred to a pediatric hospital, 18 (11%) born by primiparous, and 17 (6%) born by multiparous.

Reasons for newborn referral to a pediatric hospital are listed in Figure 1.

Thyroid status of the study group is presented as shown in Figure 2. Only 16% of primiparous and 18% of multiparous had fT4 serum level in the high normal reference range prescribed for nonpregnant women at first consultation.

Preterm birth rate was first evaluated for the whole study group and separately depending on parity status, primiparous versus multiparous.

In the study group there were 20 preterm births (4.4%), 13 in primiparous (7.3%) and 7 in multiparous (2.6%). The gestational age of the preterm deliveries is shown in Table 1.

70% of preterm births from the study group were spontaneous preterm births caused by spontaneous preterm labor or preterm premature rupture of the membranes and 30% of preterm births were medically indicated by pregnancy-induced hypertension, HELLP syndrome, ovarian tumor, and acute pancreatitis concurring with obesity.

Preterm birth rate in the study group was 4.4% (99%-CI 1.9%–6.9%) versus 7.1% in the control group corresponding to a reduction of 38%. The subgroup analysis, according to parity status showed a preterm birth rate for primiparous in the study group of 7.3% versus 7.6% in the control group, and for multiparous a preterm birth rate of 2.6% in study group (99%-CI 0.1%–5.1%) versus 6.7% in the control group, respectively (Table 2).

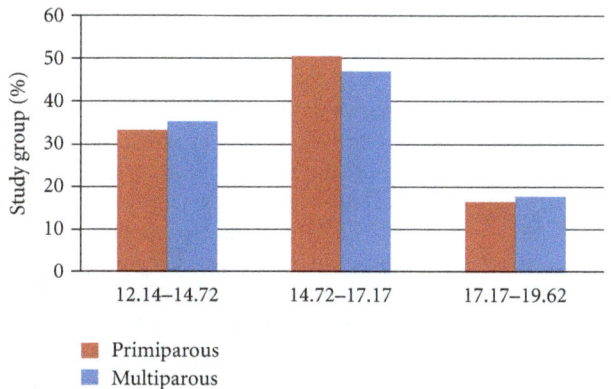

FIGURE 2: Percentage distribution of maternal fT4 serum level at first consultation subdivided into lower third, middle third and upper third of the reference range for nonpregnant women (n = 450).

TABLE 1: Numbers of preterm births plotted on gestational week and parity status in the study group (n = 450).

Weeks' GA	<31 + 6	32 + 0 − 33 + 6	34 + 0 − 37 + 0
Primiparous	1	3	9
Multiparous	2	1	4

TABLE 2: Percentage of preterm birth rates plotted on parity status in the study group and control group.

	Total	Primiparous	Multiparous
Study group	4.4%	7.3%	2.6%
Control group	7.1%	7.6%	6.7%

Thus, the reduction of preterm birth rate by maintaining maternal fT4 serum level in pregnancy in the high normal reference range prescribed for nonpregnant women is effective in multiparous but not in primiparous. The preterm birth rate dropped by approximately 61% in the multiparous of the study group.

Since there was no fixed dosage for L-T4 therapy and patients were advised to maintain the dosage unchanged in case of intolerance when dose augmentation had to occur, side effects were rarely noted. Nevertheless, if patients experienced adverse reactions, the L-T4 dose was reduced. Moreover, undesirable side effects for the fetus and newborn such as tachycardia or other signs of induced hyperthyroidism did not occur at all and were not recorded during cardiotocographic controls. Due to the variable L-T4 dose and the intake regime, L-T4 was well tolerated by pregnant women and complaints such as palpitations, tachycardia, and other undesirable clinical signs of hyperthyroidism were very rare and transient. However, pregnancy-associated nausea was more pronounced, predominantly in the first trimester.

6. Discussion

To our knowledge this is the first study presenting an essential benefit for reducing preterm birth rate in euthyroid multiparous women without thyroid autoimmune antibodies by keeping maternal fT4 serum level in the high normal reference range prescribed for nonpregnant women with L-T4 substitution. The preterm birth rate for multiparous in the study group declined by 61%. Primiparous did not benefit from L-T4 therapy. Possibly, the pathomechanism of preterm birth is essentially different among primiparous compared to multiparous, which would imply the necessity of different therapeutic strategies.

These results are in contrast to two other studies. Casey et al. found no mentionable risk for pregnancy outcome if the fT4 serum level was found to be in the lowest third of the gestational age specific reference range. Clearly, Goldman et al. recently compared pregnancy outcome in women with subclinical hypothyroidism and in women with hypothyroxinaemia defined as fT4 serum level below the 2.5th percentile. They failed to determine a link between subclinical hypothyroidism and adverse pregnancy outcome and hypothyroxinemia was not associated with the majority of pregnancy complications [21, 22].

In this study, a high maternal fT4 serum level decreased preterm birth rate in multiparous by yet unknown mechanisms. In some studies, it has been shown that human chorionic gonadotropin (hCG) plays a part in maintenance of uterine quiescence in the third trimester, and hence could be an endogenous tocolytic agent. HCG exerts a potent myometrial relaxant effect in human myometrium in the third trimester and inhibits preterm delivery in animals. Thyroid hormone stimulates the synthesis of hCG and the level of serum thyroid hormone is a positive regulator of serum thyrotropin bioactivity. Due to the fact that TSH and hCG share a certain similarity, being members of the same glucoprotein family, it appears possible that serum thyroid hormones can also positively regulate hCG bioactivity, which in turn increases the biological effects on the myometrium until parturition [1, 4, 14, 23].

The study group received L-T4 substitution to avoid a low maternal fT4 serum level for an optimal fetal brain development. The prevalence of low maternal fT4 levels is probably 150–200 times more common than congenital hypothyroidism [24, 25]. It was demonstrated that if maternal serum fT4 is low, fetal T3 levels in the brain will be low even in the presence of normal maternal and fetal serum fT3, suggesting that both T3 and T4 in the fetal brain are dependant on maternal fT4. Low maternal fT4 serum levels could have detrimental effects on fetal brain development. In animal experiments, it was demonstrated that even a modest and transient decrease in maternal fT4 resulted in altered brain histogenesis and cytoarchitecture of the fetal cerebral cortex [26, 27]. Various observational studies have shown that maternal subclinical hypothyroidism and low fT4 serum levels caused a significant decrease in IQ scores of the progeny. [8–11, 28–36]. In contrast to these findings, only one study failed to find an association between maternal thyroid function and cognitive test scores in children [37].

Handling thyroid function control by assessing only fT4 for a goal-oriented value as was done in this study and which is similar to controlling central hypothyroidism carries the risk to over dosage L-T4 and to provoke potentially metabolic hyperthyroidism. The usual assessment of an adequate L-T4 dose in replacement therapy is done by determining TSH and fT4 levels, preferably in a blood sample taken before ingestion of the subsequent L-T4 dose [38]. In nonpregnant states it takes 6–9 weeks and more to normalize a suppressed TSH value typically found when initiating L-T4 administration. As a consequence, it has been shown that patients taking 100 to 150 μg/d of L-T4 have a nearly 50% probability that serum TSH will be undetectable [39]. Determining TSH below an interval of 6–9 weeks would be likely to result in a suppressed TSH level but would not necessarily be accompanied by an fT4 serum level in the upper third of the reference range [40].

Furthermore, L-T4 replacement therapy is commonly associated with supraphysiologically high fT4 and low fT3 serum levels, in general without hyperthyroid symptoms. Since fT3 serum level is maintained within normal limits by decreased peripheral conversion of the prohormone L-T4, supraphysiological fT4 serum levels are not considered to be harmful. Therefore, supraphysiological serum fT4 levels in patients taking L-T4 are not necessarily accompanied by clinical consequences, if there are no signs or symptoms of clinical toxicity. Clinical experience with pregnant women on TSH suppressive thyroid therapy after thyroid cancer treatment does not appear to indicate any complications [41, 42]. Silva and Larson have shown that T4 is preferentially converted to T3 in the pituitary gland to a greater degree than in other tissues, so that its TSH suppressive effect is greater than its metabolic effect. In other words, exogenously administered L-T4 suppresses both the pituitary gland and the thyroid gland as well [43].

In contrast to supraphysiological fT4 serum concentration seen in L-T4 replacement therapy, hyperthyroidism is defined as an excessive thyroid hormone production due to thyroid overactivity. The vast majority of cases of hyperthyroidism in pregnancy are induced by Graves' disease, toxic adenoma, or thyroid hormone resistance, where the negative feedback mechanism no longer functions. In these pathological conditions the overactive thyroid gland secretes both the metabolically inactive prohormone T4 and the metabolically highly active hormone T3 causing multiple symptoms. In Graves' disease, the intrathyroidal type-II deiodinase (D2), which activates thyroid hormone, has a 50 to 150 fold higher activity than in placenta and contributes significantly to the intrathyroidal T3 production and secretion [44]. Hyperthyroidism caused by Graves' disease and toxic multinodular goiter, high T3 concentrations are the result of excessive production and release from the thyroid gland and not of peripheral deiodination [45]. This explains why patients with Graves' disease or with toxic adenoma present symptoms of hyperthyroidism in contrast to patients taking L-T4 in a TSH suppressive dose. Additionally, in replacement therapy with a TSH suppressive L-T4 dose, T3 is derived completely from peripheral monodeiodination in the liver, kidney, or muscle because the thyroid gland is also suppressed. To achieve physiological levels of T3 in humans treated with L-T4, it is necessary to maintain fT4 levels at the higher end of the normal range [46, 47]. Only under pathological conditions, such as massive metastatic follicular thyroid cancer has T3 thyrotoxicosis by increased conversion of administered L-T4 been described [48]. L-T4 replacement

therapy is associated with supraphysiologically high fT4 and low fT3 serum levels without hyperthyroid symptoms, since the fT3 serum level is maintained within normal limits by decreased peripheral conversion of the prohormone L-T4. This metabolic variance constitutes a fundamental difference between endogenously produced thyroid hormones T4 and especially T3 and exogenously administered thyroid hormone like L-T4. L-T4 has a safe latitude in dosage and even after massive acute ingestion only minimal symptoms are seen as the peak T3 level does not exceed the upper reference range limit, while fT4 and the metabolically inactive rT3 show very high serum levels [41, 43, 45, 47, 49–56].

Thyroid hormones are the most prescribed drugs worldwide and are considered to be safe. Relevant adverse effects are usually manifested in older patients. Disputable side effects are the risk of atrial fibrillation in patients with intrinsic heart disease and increased bone loss in postmenopausal women [57, 58].

Since there was no fixed dose regimen for L-T4 therapy in the study group, patients were advised to maintain their dosage unchanged in case of intolerance, and when dose augmentation proved necessary, side effects rarely occurred and in none L-T4 had to be discontinued. Nevertheless, if patients experienced adverse reactions the L-T4 dose was reduced. Moreover, undesirable side effects for the fetus and newborn such as tachycardia or other signs of induced hyperthyroidism did not occur at all and were not recorded during cardiotocographic controls. However, pregnancy-associated nausea was more pronounced, predominantly in the first trimester in only a few women. By reducing the L-T4 dosage, pregnancy-associated nausea resolved.

7. Conclusion

In summary, thyroid hormone replacement therapy aiming at holding maternal fT4 serum levels in the upper third of the reference range prescribed for nonpregnant women and controlling this therapy by determining fT4 seems to be safe and to have beneficial effects for both mother and fetus. In all probability it will reduce preterm birth rates in multiparous. These results have yet to be confirmed by further prospective randomized studies.

Acknowledgment

The authors want to thank Professor S. Kunz Chairman of the Advisory Board "Obstetrics and Gynecology" and Miss Susanne Rode from the Federal Office for Quality Assurance in Hospitals (GeQiK (R)) in Baden-Württemberg for providing us with data from the Perinatal Survey Baden-Württemberg. We would like to thank John M. Lindquist, Surgeon and General Practitioner, for language correction and proof-reading as native speaker.

References

[1] R. L. Goldenberg, J. F. Culhane, J. D. Iams, and R. Romero, "Epidemiology and causes of preterm birth," *The Lancet*, vol. 371, no. 9606, pp. 75–84, 2008.

[2] J. Tucker and W. McGuire, "Epidemiology of preterm birth," *British Medical Journal*, vol. 329, no. 7467, pp. 675–678, 2004.

[3] J. Langhoff-Roos, U. Kesmodel, B. Jacobsson, S. Rasmussen, and I. Vogel, "Spontaneous preterm delivery in primiparous women at low risk in Denmark: population based study," *British Medical Journal*, vol. 332, no. 7547, pp. 937–939, 2006.

[4] M. M. Slattery and J. J. Morrison, "Preterm delivery," *Lancet*, vol. 360, no. 9344, pp. 1489–1497, 2002.

[5] W. M. Callaghan, M. F. MacDorman, S. A. Rasmussen, C. Qin, and E. M. Lackritz, "The contribution of preterm birth to infant mortality rates in the United States," *Pediatrics*, vol. 118, no. 4, pp. 1566–1573, 2006.

[6] J. P. Menard, C. Mazouni, I. Salem-Cherif et al., "High vaginal concentrations of atopobium vaginae and gardnerella vaginalis in women undergoing preterm labor," *Obstetrics and Gynecology*, vol. 115, no. 1, pp. 134–140, 2010.

[7] R. E. Hoekstra, T. B. Ferrara, R. J. Couser, N. R. Payne, and J. E. Connett, "Survival and long-term neurodevelopmental outcome of extremely premature infants born at 23–26 weeks' gestational age at a tertiary center," *Pediatrics*, vol. 113, no. 1, pp. E1–E6, 2004.

[8] A. L. Den Ouden, J. H. Kok, P. H. Verkerk, R. Brand, and S. P. Verloove-Vanhorick, "The relation between neonatal thyroxine levels and neurodevelopmental outcome at age 5 and 9 years in a national cohort of very preterm and/or very low birth weight infants," *Pediatric Research*, vol. 39, no. 1, pp. 142–145, 1996.

[9] R. Z. Klein, J. D. Sargent, P. R. Larsen, S. E. Waisbren, J. E. Haddow, and M. L. Mitchell, "Relation of severity of maternal hypothyroidism to cognitive development of offspring," *Journal of Medical Screening*, vol. 8, no. 1, pp. 18–20, 2001.

[10] E. P. Kasatkina, L. N. Samsonova, V. N. Ivakhnenko et al., "Gestational hypothyroxinemia and cognitive function in offspring," *Neuroscience and Behavioral Physiology*, vol. 36, no. 6, pp. 619–624, 2006.

[11] P. O. D. Pharoah, K. J. Connolly, R. P. Ekins, and A. G. Harding, "Maternal thyroid hormone levels in pregnancy and the subsequent cognitive and motor performance of the children," *Clinical Endocrinology*, vol. 21, no. 3, pp. 265–270, 1984.

[12] J. Henrichs, J. J. Bongers-Schokking, J. J. Schenk et al., "Maternal thyroid function during early pregnancy and cognitive functioning in early childhood: the generation R study," *Journal of Clinical Endocrinology and Metabolism*, vol. 95, no. 9, pp. 4227–4234, 2010.

[13] M. J. Costeira, P. Oliveira, N. C. Santos et al., "Psychomotor development of children from an iodine-deficient region," *Journal of Pediatrics*, vol. 159, no. 3, pp. 447–453, 2011.

[14] N. Ohara, T. Tsujino, and T. Maruo, "The role of thyroid hormone in trophoblast function, early pregnancy maintenance, and fetal neurodevelopment," *Journal of Obstetrics and Gynaecology Canada*, vol. 26, no. 11, pp. 982–990, 2004.

[15] R. Negro, G. Formoso, T. Mangieri, A. Pezzarossa, D. Dazzi, and H. Hassan, "Levothyroxine treatment in euthyroid pregnant women with autoimmune thyroid disease: effects on obstetrical complications," *Journal of Clinical Endocrinology and Metabolism*, vol. 91, no. 7, pp. 2587–2591, 2006.

[16] E. Ausó, R. Lavado-Autric, E. Cuevas, F. Escobar Del Rey, G. Morreale De Escobar, and P. Berbel, "A moderate and transient deficiency of maternal thyroid function at the beginning of fetal neocorticogenesis alters neuronal migration," *Endocrinology*, vol. 145, no. 9, pp. 4037–4047, 2004.

[17] B. M. Casey and K. J. Leveno, "Thyroid disease in pregnancy," *Obstetrics and Gynecology*, vol. 108, no. 5, pp. 1283–1292, 2006.

[18] E. Ferretti, L. Persani, M. L. Jaffrain-Rea, S. Giambona, G. Tamburrano, and P. Beck-Peccoz, "Evaluation of the adequacy of levothyroxine replacement therapy in patients with central hypothyroidism," *Journal of Clinical Endocrinology and Metabolism*, vol. 84, no. 3, pp. 924–929, 1999.

[19] M. Slawik, B. Klawitter, E. Meiser et al., "Thyroid hormone replacement for central hypothyroidism: a randomized controlled trial comparing two doses of thyroxine (T4) with a combination of T4 and triiodothyronine," *Journal of Clinical Endocrinology and Metabolism*, vol. 92, no. 11, pp. 4115–4122, 2007.

[20] A. Lania, L. Persani, and P. Beck-Peccoz, "Central hypothyroidism," *Pituitary*, vol. 11, no. 2, pp. 181–186, 2008.

[21] B. M. Casey, J. S. Dashe, C. Y. Spong, D. D. McIntire, K. J. Leveno, and G. F. Cunningham, "Perinatal significance of isolated maternal hypothyroxinemia identified in the first half of pregnancy," *Obstetrics and Gynecology*, vol. 109, no. 5, pp. 1129–1135, 2007.

[22] J. Cleary-Goldman, F. D. Malone, G. Lambert-Messerlian et al., "Maternal thyroid hypofunction and pregnancy outcome," *Obstetrics and Gynecology*, vol. 112, no. 1, pp. 85–92, 2008.

[23] J. H. A. Oliveira, E. R. Barbosa, T. Kasamatsu, and J. Abucham, "Evidence for thyroid hormone as a positive regulator of serum thyrotropin bioactivity," *Journal of Clinical Endocrinology and Metabolism*, vol. 92, no. 8, pp. 3108–3113, 2007.

[24] G. M. de Escobar, M. J. Obregon, and F. E. del Rey, "Clinical perspective: is neuropsychological development related to maternal hypothyroidism or to maternal hypothyroxinemia?" *Journal of Clinical Endocrinology and Metabolism*, vol. 85, no. 11, pp. 3975–3987, 2000.

[25] G. M. de Escobar, M. J. Obregón, and F. Escobar del Rey, "Maternal thyroid hormones early in prenancy and fetal brain development," *Best Practice and Research: Clinical Endocrinology and Metabolism*, vol. 18, no. 2, pp. 225–248, 2004.

[26] J. H. Goodman and M. E. Gilbert, "Modest thyroid hormone insufficiency during development induces a cellular malformation in the corpus callosum: a model of cortical dysplasia," *Endocrinology*, vol. 148, no. 6, pp. 2593–2597, 2007.

[27] R. Lavado-Autric, E. Ausó, J. V. García-Velasco et al., "Early maternal hypothyroxinemia alters histogenesis and cerebral cortex cytoarchitecture of the progeny," *Journal of Clinical Investigation*, vol. 111, no. 7, pp. 1073–1082, 2003.

[28] C. Gyamfi, R. J. Wapner, and M. E. D'Alton, "Thyroid dysfunction in pregnancy: the basic science and clinical evidence surrounding the controversy in management," *Obstetrics and Gynecology*, vol. 113, no. 3, pp. 702–707, 2009.

[29] Y. Li, Z. Shan, W. Teng et al., "Abnormalities of maternal thyroid function during pregnancy affect neuropsychological development of their children at 25–30 months," *Clinical Endocrinology*, vol. 72, no. 6, pp. 825–829, 2010.

[30] B. J. Smit, J. H. Kok, T. Vulsma, J. M. Briet, K. Boer, and W. M. Wiersinga, "Neurologic development of the newborn and young child in relation to maternal thyroid function," *Acta Paediatrica*, vol. 89, no. 3, pp. 291–295, 2000.

[31] A. K. Sinha, M. R. Pickard, and R. P. Ekins, "Maternal hypothyroxinemia and brain development: I. A hypothetical control system governing fetal exposure to maternal thyroid hormones," *Acta Medica Austriaca*, vol. 19, supplement 1, pp. 40–48, 1992.

[32] L. Kooistra, S. Crawford, A. L. Van Baar, E. P. Brouwers, and V. J. Pop, "Neonatal effects of maternal hypothyroxinemia during early pregnancy," *Pediatrics*, vol. 117, no. 1, pp. 161–167, 2006.

[33] V. J. Pop, E. P. Brouwers, H. L. Vader, T. Vulsma, A. L. Van Baar, and J. J. De Vijlder, "Maternal hypothyroxinaemia during early pregnancy and subsequent child development: a 3-year follow-up study," *Clinical Endocrinology*, vol. 59, no. 3, pp. 282–288, 2003.

[34] V. J. Pop, J. L. Kuijpens, A. L. Van Baar et al., "Low maternal free thyroxine concentrations during early pregnancy are associated with impaired psychomotor development in infancy," *Clinical Endocrinology*, vol. 50, no. 2, pp. 149–155, 1999.

[35] H. A. Wijnen, L. Kooistra, H. L. Vader, G. G. Essed, B. W. Mol, and V. J. Pop, "Maternal thyroid hormone concentration during late gestation is associated with foetal position at birth," *Clinical Endocrinology*, vol. 71, no. 5, pp. 746–751, 2009.

[36] M. Obregon, R. Calvo, F. E. del Rey, and G. M. de Escobar, "Ontogenesis of thyroid function and interactions with maternal function," *Endocrine Development*, vol. 10, pp. 86–98, 2007.

[37] E. Oken, L. E. Braverman, D. Platek, M. L. Mitchell, S. L. Lee, and E. N. Pearce, "Neonatal thyroxine, maternal thyroid function, and child cognition," *Journal of Clinical Endocrinology and Metabolism*, vol. 94, no. 2, pp. 497–503, 2009.

[38] W. M. Wiersinga, "Thyroid hormone replacement therapy," *Hormone Research*, vol. 56, no. 1, pp. 74–81, 2001.

[39] M. Helfand and L. M. Crapo, "Monitoring therapy in patients taking levothyroxine," *Annals of Internal Medicine*, vol. 113, no. 6, pp. 450–454, 1990.

[40] B. Bakker, M. J. E. Kempers, J. J. M. De Vijlder et al., "Dynamics of the plasma concentrations of TSH, FT4 and T3 following thyroxine supplementation in congenital hypothyroidism," *Clinical Endocrinology*, vol. 57, no. 4, pp. 529–537, 2002.

[41] J. H. Metsman, "Hyperthyroidism in pregnancy," *Best Practice and Research: Clinical Endocrinology and Metabolism*, vol. 18, no. 2, pp. 267–288, 2004.

[42] F. Pacini, M. Schlumberger, H. Dralle et al., "European consensus for the management of patients with differentiated thyroid carcinoma of the follicular epithelium," *European Journal of Endocrinology*, vol. 154, no. 6, pp. 787–803, 2006.

[43] A. Mortoglou and Candiloros H, "The serum triiodothyronine to thyroxine (T3/T4) ratio in various thyroid disorders and after Levothyroxine replacement therapy," *Hormones*, vol. 3, pp. 120–126, 2004.

[44] D. Salvatore, H. Tu, J. W. Harney, and P. R. Larsen, "Type 2 iodothyronine deiodinase is highly expressed in human thyroid," *Journal of Clinical Investigation*, vol. 98, no. 4, pp. 962–968, 1996.

[45] P. Laurberg, H. Vestergaard, S. Nielsen et al., "Sources of circulating 3,5,3'-triiodothyronine in hyperthyroidism estimated after blocking of type 1 and type 2 iodothyronine deiodinases," *Journal of Clinical Endocrinology and Metabolism*, vol. 92, no. 6, pp. 2149–2156, 2007.

[46] W. M. Wiersinga, "Thyroid hormone replacement therapy," *Hormone Research*, vol. 56, no. 1, pp. 74–81, 2001.

[47] J. Jonklaas, B. Davidson, S. Bhagat, and S. J. Soldin, "Triiodothyronine levels in athyreotic individuals during levothyroxine therapy," *Journal of the American Medical Association*, vol. 299, no. 7, pp. 769–777, 2008.

[48] A. Miyauchi, Y. Takamura, Y. Ito et al., "3,5,3′-Triiodothyronine thyrotoxicosis due to increased conversion of administered levothyroxine in patients with massive metastatic follicular thyroid carcinoma," *Journal of Clinical Endocrinology and Metabolism*, vol. 93, no. 6, pp. 2239–2242, 2008.

[49] V. V. Fadeyev, T. B. Morgunova, J. P. Sytch, and G. A. Melnichenko, "TSH and thyroid hormones concentrations in patients with hypothyroidism receiving replacement therapy with L-thyroxine alone or in combination with L-triiodothyronine," *Hormones*, vol. 4, no. 2, pp. 101–107, 2005.

[50] K. A. Woeber, "Levothyroxine therapy and serum free thyroxine and free triiodothyronine concentrations," *Journal of Endocrinological Investigation*, vol. 25, no. 2, pp. 106–109, 2002.

[51] C. J. Pearce and R. L. Himsworth, "Total and free thyroid hormone concentrations in patients receiving maintenance replacement treatment with thyroxine," *British Medical Journal*, vol. 288, no. 6418, pp. 693–695, 1984.

[52] K. Liewendahl, T. Helenius, B. A. Lamberg, H. Mahonen, and G. Wagar, "Free thyroxine, free triiodothyronine, and thyrotropin concentrations in hypothyroid and thyroid carcinoma patients receiving thyroxine therapy," *Acta Endocrinologica*, vol. 116, no. 3, pp. 418–424, 1987.

[53] J. F. Iverson and C. N. Mariash, "Optimal free thyroxine levels for thyroid hormone replacement in hypothyroidism," *Endocrine Practice*, vol. 14, no. 5, pp. 550–555, 2008.

[54] P. Laurberg, C. Bournaud, J. Karmisholt, and J. Orgiazzi, "Management of Graves' hyperthyroidism in pregnancy: focus on both maternal and foetal thyroid function, and caution against surgical thyroidectomy in pregnancy," *European Journal of Endocrinology*, vol. 160, no. 1, pp. 1–8, 2009.

[55] T. Ishihara, M. Nishikawa, K. Ikekubo et al., "Thyroxine (T4) metabolism in an athyreotic patient who had taken a large amount of T4 at one time," *Endocrine Journal*, vol. 45, no. 3, pp. 371–375, 1998.

[56] S. H. Mandel, A. R. Magnusson, B. T. Burton, J. R. Swanson, and S. H. LaFranchi, "Massive levothyroxine ingestion. Conservative management," *Clinical Pediatrics*, vol. 28, no. 8, pp. 374–376, 1989.

[57] J. B. Williams, "Adverse effects of thyroid hormones," *Drugs and Aging*, vol. 11, no. 6, pp. 460–469, 1997.

[58] A. L. Mitchell, B. Hickey, J. L. Hickey, and S. H. S. Pearce, "Trends in thyroid hormone prescribing and consumption in the UK," *BMC Public Health*, vol. 9, article 132, 2009.

28

Local Reference Ranges of Thyroid Volume in Sudanese Normal Subjects using Ultrasound

Mohamed Yousef,[1] Abdelmoneim Sulieman,[1] Bushra Ahmed,[2] Alsafi Abdella,[1] and Khaled Eltom[3]

[1] College of Medical Radiologic Science, Sudan University of Science and Technology, Baladya Street, P.O. Box 1908, Khartoum 11111, Sudan
[2] College of Radiology and Nuclear Medicine, The National Ribat University, Nile Street, Burri, P.O. Box 55, Khartoum 11111, Sudan
[3] Radiation and Isotope Center, Khartoum (RICK), Algaser Street, P.O. Box 846, Khartoum 11111, Sudan

Correspondence should be addressed to Mohamed Yousef, mohnajwan@yahoo.com

Academic Editor: Fausto Bogazzi

This study aimed to establish a local reference of thyroid volume in Sudanese normal subjects using ultrasound. A total of 103 healthy subjects were studied, 28 (27.18%) females and 75 (72.82%) males. Thyroid volume was estimated using *ellipsoid formula*. The mean age and range of the subjects was 21.8 (19–29) years; the mean body mass index (BMI) was 22.3 (16.46–26.07) kg/m^2. The overall mean volume ± SD volume of the thyroid gland for both lobes in all the patients studied was 6.44 ± 2.44 mL. The mean volume for both lobes in females and males were 5.78 ± 1.96 mL and 6.69 ± 2.56 mL, respectively. The males' thyroid volume was greater than the females'. The mean volume of the right and left lobes of the thyroid gland in males and females were 3.38 ± 1.37 mL and 3.09 ± 1.24 mL, respectively. The right thyroid lobe volume was greater than the left. The values obtained in this study were lower than those reported from previous studies.

1. Introduction

Ultrasound has become one of the primary imaging modalities for the assessment of the major glands of internal secretion within the cervical region. The thyroid gland is among the most commonly imaged glands using ultrasound due to the limitation of clinical examination [1]. Computed tomography (CT) and magnetic resonance imaging (MRI) provide structural information of the thyroid gland just like ultrasound but are relatively more expensive. Thyroid ultrasound appears suitable in tropical Africa [2, 3] where more sophisticated modern imaging techniques may not be readily available or are very expensive.

Anatomically, the normal thyroid gland consists of two lobes which lie on the anterolateral surface of the trachea extending from the thyroid cartilage superiorly to the sixth tracheal ring inferiorly. They are asymmetrical with the right lobe being larger than the left, and the thyroid gland is larger

in males [4, 5]. In recent decades, sonography has become the gold standard for assessment of the thyroid gland [6].

Sonography has improved with the development of high-frequency transducers, which allow a more detailed study of the thyroid gland [7]. As a result, the World Health Organization (WHO) and the International Council for the Control of Iodine Deficiency Disorders (ICCIDD) now consider sonography the diagnostic method for assessment of goiter [8]. It is most often used in assessing the incidence of goiter in Third World populations, especially in children [9]. Intra- and interobserver variation can lead to differences in volume calculation, irrespective of the correction factor. Nevertheless, a more optimal correction factor will give a more realistic measurement of thyroid volume.

Volumetric evaluation of the thyroid gland is based on the use of an ellipsoid model. Hence, a value is obtained that replaces clinical evaluation of volume. With the ellipsoid model, the height, the width, and the depth of each lobe are measured and multiplied. The obtained result is then multiplied by a correction factor [10].

The work of Brunn et al. [11] in 1981 was based on volume measurement of cadaver glands subsequently immersed in water.

Brunn et al. [11] concluded that a modified correction factor of 0.479 resulted in a more accurate assessment of thyroid volume compared with the previously accepted correction factor of $\pi/6$ or 0.524.

In Sudan, there is absence of domestic reference for thyroid volumes; in Sudan, as for as we know, no study was published in the open literature, regarding the thyroid volume.

This study aimed to establish a local reference of thyroid volume in Sudanese normal subjects using ultrasound.

2. Materials and Methods

This study was done in the Sudan University of Science and Technology, College of Medical Radiological Science during the period from 2007 up to 2010.

2.1. Ultrasound Machines. The ultrasound system used is general electric (GE) medical system, made by Yokogawa medical system, Ltd., 7-127 Asahigaoka 4-chome, Hino-shi Tokyo, Japan. Model 2302650 with serial of 1028924YM7 and manufacturing date of April 2005, a grey scale real-time ultrasound machine, fitted with a 10 MHz transducer was used for the study.

2.2. Volunteers. A total of 103 healthy students from the Sudan University of Science and Technology, College of Medical Radiologic Sciences were involved in this study. The ethics and research committee approved the study, and consents were obtained from all volunteers prior to the examination.

2.3. Exclusion Criteria. Subjects with anterior neck swelling or clinical evidence of thyroid disease were excluded. Furthermore, women during menstruation, pregnant, women who have delivered within the last 12 months, were excluded from the study because this may affect the thyroid size. The data was collected and analyzed using SPSS for windows version 17.

2.4. Measurement Technique for Thyroid Volume. With the ellipsoid model, the height, the width, and the depth of each lobe are measured and multiplied. The obtained result was then multiplied by a correction factor, which is $\pi/6$ or 0.524 [12]. The subjects were examined in supine position, with pillow placed under their shoulders to hyperextend the neck. US gel was applied over the thyroid area. The transducer was directly placed on the skin over the thyroid gland, and an image of each lobe was obtained in transverse and longitudinal planes. The craniocaudal and the sagittal dimensions of both lobes were measured on the longitudinal image. The transverse dimension was measured on the transverse image.

TABLE 1: Volume of the thyroid gland.

Gender	Thyroid volume	Right lobe volume	Left lobe volume
Female			
Mean	5.78	3.03	2.75
N	28	28	28
Std. deviation	1.96	1.02	1.05
Male			
Mean	6.69	3.51	3.21
N	75	75	75
Std. deviation	2.56	1.46	1.28
Total			
Mean	6.44	3.38	3.09
N	103	103	103
Std. deviation	2.44	1.37	1.24

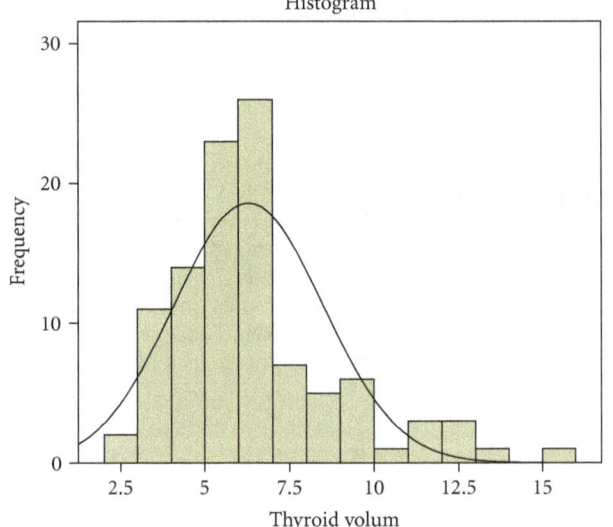

Mean = 6.44
N = 103
Std. deviation = 2.436

FIGURE 1

3. Results

The 103 subjects studied consist of 28 (27.18 %) females and 75 (72.82%) males. The mean age of the subjects was 21.79 years with a range of 19–29 years. The overall mean volume of the thyroid gland for both lobes in all the patients studied was 6.44 ± 2.44 (Table 1 and Figure 1). The mean volume for both lobes in females and males was 5.78 ± 2 (1.96) mL and 6.69 (2.56) mL, respectively. The mean volume of the right and left lobes of the thyroid gland in all the patients studied were 3.38 ± 2 (1.37) mL and 3.09 ± 2 (1.24) mL, respectively (Table 1). The right thyroid lobe volume was greater than the left.

TABLE 2: Comparison of thyroid volume studies.

Author	Gender	Age range (years)	Number of subjects	Thyroid volume (mL) ± SD	Country
Current study	75 M 28 F	19–29	103	6.44 ± 2.44	Sudan
Ivanac et al. [23]		20–38	51	10.68 ± 2.83	Croatia
Ahidjo et al. [24]	71 M 72 F	23–69	143	8.55 ± 1.82	Nigeria
Chanoine et al. [25]		17–20	256	11.6 ± 4.4	Belgium
Adibi et al. [26]	123 M 77 F	37.27 ± 11.80	200	9.53 ± 3.68	Iran

The mean thyroid volume of the right lobe among the females studied was 3.03 mL, and the left was 2.75 mL (Table 1). The values were greater for the right than the left lobe. In males, the right and the left lobes of the thyroid gland volumes were 3.51 mL and 3.21 mL, respectively, (Table 1). The values were greater for the right than the left lobe and more than that of the females.

4. Discussion

In recent decades, the WHO has changed the diagnostic criteria for goiter. The diagnosis of goiter used to be based on palpation, but now it is based on volume measurement using sonography. Volume measurement of the thyroid gland is especially easy to obtain because the gland has a different echogenicity compared with adjacent soft tissues [11]. Due to its conical morphology, a thyroid lobe is assumed to resemble an ellipsoid, and its volume is approximated using height × width × depth × a correction factor. Other methods such as the 3D sonography and the automated transverse surface area method have been proposed to evaluate thyroid volume [13, 14].

Thyroid lobes, however, show variations in shape as is evident in anatomic and imaging studies [15, 16]. Failure of the thyroid gland to descend from foramen caecum along the thyroglossal duct to the anterior aspect of the neck accounts for the rare ectopic location of the thyroid tissue at the base of the tongue (lingual thyroid) as well as the presence of thyroglossal duct cyst along this developmental tract [12]. The thyroid size was found to increase during pregnancy and decreases up to 12 months postpartum period [17, 18]. The menstrual cycle also seems to associate with cyclical alteration of thyroid size in healthy women [19], and, for that reasons, these subjects were excluded from this study.

The overall mean thyroid gland volume combined for both lobes and sexes obtained from this study was 6.44 cm³. There was no previous local study for comparison to the best of our knowledge. But in Africa, Anele [3] studied the thyroid gland volume among Nigerians. This value showed the thyroid dimensions to be slightly lower than the Western values [5, 20].

This study has shown that the right thyroid lobe volume (3.38 mL) was greater than the left (3.09 mL) with significant statistical difference between the right and the left lobe volumes in both sexes. This finding is in agreement with

previous studies done among the Caucasians and the Chinese [5, 20, 21].

The total mean values for the females (5.78 mL) and the males (6.69 mL) have shown the thyroid gland to be greater in males compared to females. Anele [3] found no significant difference in the thyroid volume between males and females. This finding differs from our study and most of the previous studies [5, 20–22].

In conclusion, the thyroid volume obtained in this study was in the lower range of the values reported in previous studies (Table 2). The volume of the right lobe of the gland was greater than the left in both sexes. The mean thyroid volume in the males is greater than that in the females, a local reference of thyroid volume was established, and further studies are required to establish national references thyroid volume in Sudan.

References

[1] A. Archie and M. Alexander, "The thyroid, the parathyroid, the salivary glands and the cervical lymphnodes," in *The NICER Year Book 1996*, B. Goldberg and H. Petterson, Eds., pp. 399–429, The NICER Institute, Oslo, Norway, 1996.

[2] B. O. Iko, "Grey scale ultrasonography of the thyroid gland, Nigeria," *Tropical and Geographical Medicine*, vol. 38, no. 1, pp. 21–27, 1986.

[3] T. Anele, "Ultrasound volumetric measurement of normal thyroid in Nigerians," *The West African Journal of Ultrasound*, vol. 2, no. 1, pp. 10–12, 2001.

[4] S. P. Ryan and N. M. J. Nicholas, "The thyroid and parathyroid glands," in *Anatomy for Diagnostic Imaging*, S. P. Ryan and N. M. J. Nicholas, Eds., pp. 35–37, WB Saunders, Philadelphia, Pa, USA, 1994.

[5] A. Tahir, A. Ahidjo, and H. Yusuph, "Ultrasonic assessment of thyroid gland size in Maiduguri, Nigeria," *The West African Journal of Ultrasound*, vol. 3, no. 1, pp. 26–31, 2001.

[6] J. Massol, L. Pazart, S. Aho, G. Strauch, J. Leclere, and P. Durieux, "Management of thyroid nodules: preliminary results of a practice survey with 685 general and specialist practitioners," *Annales d'Endocrinologie*, vol. 54, no. 4, pp. 220–225, 1993.

[7] J. N. Bruneton, C. Balu-Maestro, P. Y. Marcy, P. Melia, and M. Y. Mourou, "Very high frequency (13 MHz) ultrasonographic examination of the normal neck: detection of normal lymph nodes and thyroid nodules," *Journal of Ultrasound in Medicine*, vol. 13, no. 2, pp. 87–90, 1994.

[8] World Health Organization, "Indicators for assessing iodine deficiency disorders and their control through salt iodization," World Health Organization, Geneva, Switzerland, 1994, [Document no. WHO/NUT94.6].

[9] "Recommended normative values for thyroid volume in children aged 6–15 years: World Health Organization and International Council for Control of Iodine Deficiency Disorders," *Bulletin of the World Health Organization*, vol. 75, pp. 95–97, 1997.

[10] M. C. Brown and R. Spencer, "Thyroid gland volume estimated by use of ultrasound in addition to scintigraphy," *Acta Radiologica: Oncology, Radiation, Therapy Physics and Biology*, vol. 17, no. 4, pp. 337–341, 1978.

[11] J. Brunn, U. Block, G. Ruf, I. Bos, W. P. Kunze, and P. C. Scriba, "Volumetric analysis of thyroid lobes by real-time ultrasound," *Deutsche Medizinische Wochenschrift*, vol. 106, no. 41, pp. 1338–1340, 1981.

[12] J. L. Jamesone and A. P. Weetman, "Disorders of the thyroid gland," in *Harrison's Principles of Internal Medicine*, E. Braunwald, A. S. Fauci, D. L. Kasper, S. L. Hauser, D. L. Longo, and J. L. Jameson, Eds., pp. 2060–2061, McGraw-Hill, New York, NY, USA, 15th edition, 2001.

[13] S. Schlögl, E. Werner, M. Lassmann et al., "The use of three-dimensional ultrasound for thyroid volumetry," *Thyroid*, vol. 11, no. 6, pp. 569–574, 2001.

[14] W. Shabana, E. Peeters, P. Verbeek, and M. M. Osteaux, "Reducing inter-observer variation in thyroid volume calculation using a new formula and technique," *The European Journal of Ultrasound*, vol. 16, no. 3, pp. 207–210, 2003.

[15] T. Robbins et al., "Thyroid anatomy," in *Otolaryngology—Head and Neck Surgery*, C. W. Cummings, J. M. Fredrickson, L. A. Harker, C. J. Krause, and D. E. Schuller, Eds., pp. 2445–2449, Mosby, St. Louis, Mo, USA, 3rd edition, 1998.

[16] "Endocrinal system: thyroid," in *Gray's Anatomy*, R. Warwick and P. L. Williams, Eds., pp. 1373–1375, Longman Group, Edinburgh, UK, 35th edition, 1973.

[17] N. G. Rasmussen, P. J. Hornnes, and L. Hegedus, "Ultrasonographically determined thyroid size in pregnancy and post partum: the goitrogenic effect of pregnancy," *The American Journal of Obstetrics and Gynecology*, vol. 160, no. 5, pp. 1216–1220, 1989.

[18] M. Nelson, G. G. Wickus, R. H. Caplan, and E. A. Beguin, "Thyroid gland size in pregnancy. An ultrasound and clinical study," *Journal of Reproductive Medicine*, vol. 32, no. 12, pp. 888–890, 1987.

[19] L. Hegedus, S. Karstrup, and N. G. Rasmussen, "Evidence of cyclic alterations of thyroid size during the menstrual cycle in healthy women," *The American Journal of Obstetrics and Gynecology*, vol. 155, no. 1, pp. 142–145, 1986.

[20] Y. L. Hsiao and T. C. Chang, "Ultrasound evaluation of thyroid abnormalities and volume in Chinese adults without palpable thyroid glands," *Journal of the Formosan Medical Association*, vol. 93, no. 2, pp. 140–144, 1994.

[21] P. Langer, "Normal thyroid size versus goiter—postmortem thyroid weight and ultrasonographic volumetry versus physical examination," *Endocrinologia Experimentalis*, vol. 23, no. 2, pp. 67–76, 1989.

[22] F. Azizi, M. Malik, E. Bebars, H. Delshad, and A. Bakir, "Thyroid volumes in school children of the Emirates," *Journal of Endocrinological Investigation*, vol. 26, no. 1, pp. 56–60, 2003.

[23] G. Ivanac, B. Rožman, F. Škreb, B. Brkljačić, and L. Pavić, "Ultrasonographic measurement of the thyroid volume," *Collegium Antropologicum*, vol. 28, no. 1, pp. 287–291, 2004.

[24] A. Ahidjo, A. Tahir, and M. Tukur, "Ultrasound determination of thyroid gland volume among adult Nigerians," *The Internet Journal of Radiology*, vol. 4, no. 2, 2006.

[25] J. P. Chanoine, V. Toppet, R. Lagasse, M. Spehl, and F. Delange, "Determination of thyroid volume by ultrasound from the neonatal period to late adolescence," *The European Journal of Pediatrics*, vol. 150, no. 6, pp. 395–399, 1991.

[26] A. Adibi, M. Sirous, A. Aminorroaya et al., "Normal values of thyroid gland in Isfahan, an iodine replete area," *Journal of Research in Medical Sciences*, vol. 13, no. 2, pp. 55–60, 2008.

29

Rap2A is Upregulated in Invasive Cells Dissected from Follicular Thyroid Cancer

Indira Prabakaran,[1] **Jillian R. Grau,**[2] **Robert Lewis,**[1]
Douglas L. Fraker,[1] **and Marina A. Guvakova**[1]

[1] *Department of Surgery, School of Medicine, University of Pennsylvania, Philadelphia, PA 19104, USA*
[2] *Department of Pathology and Laboratory Medicine, School of Medicine, University of Pennsylvania, Philadelphia, PA 19104, USA*

Correspondence should be addressed to Marina A. Guvakova, guvakova@mail.med.upenn.edu

Academic Editor: Maria Domenica Castellone

The development of molecular biomarkers (BMs) of follicular thyroid carcinoma is aimed at advancing diagnosis of follicular neoplasm, as histological examination of those tumors does not lend itself to definitive diagnosis of carcinoma. We assessed the relative levels of expression of 6 genes: *CCND2, PCSK2, PLAB, RAP2A, TSHR,* and *IGF-1R* in archived thyroid tissue. The quantitative real-time PCR analysis revealed a significant change in 3 genes: *PSCK2* (a 22.4-fold decrease, $P = 2.81E - 2$), *PLAB* (an 8.3-fold increase, $P = 9.81E - 12$), and *RAP2A* (a 6.3-fold increase, $P = 9.13E - 10$) in carcinoma compared with adenoma. Expression of *PCSK2* was equally low, *PLAB* was equally high, whereas *RAP2A* expression was significantly higher (25.9-fold, $P = 0.039$) in microdissected carcinoma cells that have invaded through the thyroid capsule and entered blood vessels than in thyroid tumor cells growing under the capsule. Thus, *RAP2A* appeared as a unique and worthy of further evaluation candidate BM associated with invasion of thyroid follicular cells.

1. Introduction

Differentiated thyroid carcinomas originating from the follicular epithelium have a papillary (range, 65–88%) and a follicular (range, 9–23%) histotype [1]. Although follicular thyroid carcinomas (FTCs) are the second most common differentiated thyroid cancers, they are more aggressive than papillary thyroid carcinomas (PTCs) and invade into the capsule (minimally invasive) and veins (angioinvasive) within the thyroid gland. Importantly, mortality is related to the degree of invasion [2]. Furthermore, FTC has a greater rate of recurrence and is frequently associated with distant metastasis to the lung, bone, brain, and liver [3, 4]. Total thyroidectomy represents the dominant method of surgical treatment for follicular neoplasms diagnosed preoperatively by fine needle aspirates (FNAs). Distinguishing follicular adenoma from minimally invasive or encapsulated angioinvasive carcinoma in FNA can be extremely challenging [3, 5]. Gene and micro-RNA (miRNA) expression profiling are being investigated to identify potential BMs differentiating benign from malignant follicular tumors [6, 7]. Such BMs might be clinically useful to help predicting follicular thyroid malignancy and reduce the frequency of surgical procedures by identifying those patients with benign lesions who do not require surgical excision. So far, however, global genetic screens have not improved preoperative diagnosis of FTC. Hence, novel approaches are necessary to identify potential preoperative molecular BMs to facilitate the diagnosis of FTC. One of the approaches could be discovering specific molecular BMs associated with invasion of thyroid follicular cells.

2. Materials and Methods

2.1. Thyroid Tissue. Cases of follicular-patterned thyroid cancer are quite rare; even lesser is the number of remaining samples available for research. For this study, a unique cohort of patients diagnosed with follicular-patterned thyroid cancer was identified on review of medical records from the Hospital of University of Pennsylvania between 1992 and 2007.

After reexamination of 16 available formalin-fixed, paraffin-embedded (FFPE) tissues (for histological presence of vascular and/or capsular invasion) and initial determination of integrity of total RNA in the tissue scrapes, we found that two samples had degraded RNA, one sample had too little RNA to be amplified by *in vitro* transcription (IVT), in two samples the areas of invasion had already been cut through, and 10 specimens fully met study's criteria. Subsequently, the study was performed in specimens from 8 patients diagnosed with FTC, 1 patient diagnosed with FTC-Hürthle cell carcinoma (HCC), 1 patient diagnosed with HCC, and 10 patients diagnosed with follicular thyroid adenoma (FTA). Groups of patients with FTA (mean age, 52.4 ± 16.2 SD years) and follicular thyroid malignancy (mean age, 50.8 ± 13.1 SD, years) were age matched (Table 1). Ten normal FFPE thyroid samples were from patients who underwent surgery after diagnosis of larynx squamous cell carcinoma (mean age, 62.4 ± 7.0 SD, years). Histopathological analysis of all tissues was performed by a surgical pathology fellow (JG) and confirmed by a thyroid pathologist (Dr. Virginia LiVolsi). The study protocol was approved by the University of Pennsylvania Institutional Review Board committee.

2.2. Thyroid Tissue Analysis: RNA Extraction, cDNA Synthesis, and Quantitative Real-Time PCR (Q-RT-PCR). RNA was extracted from the normal, adenoma, and cancer tissue scrapes using the Absolutely RNA FFPE kit (Stratagene, La Jolla, CA). In addition, RNA was extracted from a snap frozen thyroid carcinoma using the High Pure RNA Tissue kit (Roche Diagnostics, Indianapolis, IN) to use as a positive control and generate a standard curve for all subsequent PCR reactions. Integrity of RNA from a snap frozen tissue was determined by 260 to 280 nm ratio using a DU 640 spectrophotometer (Beckman Coulter, Fullerton, CA). Integrity of the scraped tissue RNA was assessed by Q-RT-PCR using $3'ACTB$ and $5'ACTB$ primers (Table 2) and the Paradise Sample Quality Assessment Kit (Molecular Devices, Sunnyvale, CA). 10–100 ng of the scraped tissue RNA or 500 ng of a positive control RNA were reverse-transcribed into single-stranded cDNA using the first-strand cDNA synthesis kit (Roche Diagnostics, Indianapolis, IN). cDNA synthesis was carried out in a $20\,\mu L$ reaction mix containing $5\,mM$ $MgCl_2$, $1\,mM$ dNTPs, 0.04 units of random primers $p(dN)_6$, 50 units of RNase inhibitor, and 20 units of Avian Myeloblastosis Virus (AMV) reverse transcriptase. Q-RT-PCR was performed using $3\,\mu L$ of the first-strand cDNA with $1\,\mu M$ of the housekeeping gene, *ACTB*, or target gene-specific primers (Table 2) using the LightCycler 2.0 (Roche Molecular Biochemicals, Mannheim, Germany) instrument and the LightCycler Fast Start DNA Master[PLUS] SYBR Green 1 kit (Roche Diagnostics, Indianapolis, IN) according to the manufacturer's instructions. PCR parameters were a 10 min preincubation time at 95°C followed by 45 cycles of denaturation (10 sec at 95°C), annealing (10 sec at 55°C), and extension (25 sec at 72°C). A standard curve for each of the target and housekeeping gene was generated for every PCR run to determine levels of gene expression. All reactions were performed in duplicates with at least three repeats.

Relative expression of each target gene in all samples was determined as a ratio of mRNA of target gene to mRNA of the housekeeping gene as described in [8].

2.3. Laser-Capture Microdissection (LCM). LCM was performed as in the frozen thyroid tissue samples [9] with modifications. Briefly, FFPE blocks of FTC were cut into $7\,\mu m$ thick sections, mounted on RNase-free membrane slides (MMI, Manchester, NH), deparaffinated with d-limonene, rehydrated with sequential washes of 100%, 95%, and 75% ethanol, and then washed in nuclease-free water. Next, slides were stained with Paradise staining solution (Arcturus Engineering Inc., Mountain View, CA), dehydrated in Xylene for a minimum of 5 min, and air dried. Cells from areas of angioinvasion, capsular invasion, and tumor under the capsule were dissected onto Capsure HS LCM Caps (MMI, Manchester, NH) using a Laser Capture Micro-dissection microscope Nikon ECLIPSE TE 2000-S and MMI Cell Tools software (MMI, Manchester, NH).

2.4. Dissected Thyroid Cancer Cell Analysis: RNA Extraction and Amplification, cDNA Synthesis, and Q-RT-PCR. RNA was extracted from laser-captured microdissected cancer cells using the Absolutely RNA FFPE kit (Stratagene, La Jolla, CA). Assessment of the integrity of cellular RNA was performed by Q-RT-PCR using $3'ACTB$ and $5'ACTB$ primers. Amplification of RNA from laser-captured microdissected cells was performed using the Ambion MessageAmp II aRNA kit (Ambion, Austin, TX). We used the IVT method which is based on the linear amplification protocol developed and validated previously [10, 11]. The advantage of such a technique is that the product of the reaction is unable to act as template and the yield of any individual species within a mixed population is for the most part determined by the template concentration that is not changed. Amplification was linear when at least 1ng of LCM RNA was used as the input for IVT. Two rounds of linear amplification of the mRNA fraction of at least 1 ng total cellular RNA were performed. First-strand cDNA synthesis yielded cDNA incorporating a T-7 promoter sequence. This cDNA was converted to a double-stranded transcription template by a second-strand synthesis reaction utilizing exogenous primers that yielded double-stranded cDNA. Double-stranded cDNA was then used as a template for IVT with T7 RNA polymerase to generate amplified antisense RNA (aRNA). Integrity of aRNA samples was determined as described above. aRNA samples with a $3'ACTB$ to $5'ACTB$ ratio of ≤20 or a 260 to 280 nm ratio between 1.8 and 2.2 were used for further experiments. 10–100 ng of aRNA was converted to cDNA using $1\,\mu M$ target gene-specific primers and the first-strand cDNA synthesis kit (Roche Diagnostics, Indianapolis, IN). Q-RT-PCR was then performed for the housekeeping gene, *ACTB*, and target genes as described above. After all the reactions were performed in duplicates with at least three repeats, relative expression of target genes was determined.

2.5. Statistical Analysis. Data were reported as mean ± standard error of the mean (SEM). Comparisons between

TABLE 1: Clinical data of patients from whom follicular thyroid tumor tissue samples were collected.

Gender	Age, years	FNA diagnosis	Nodule size, cm	Final diagnosis	Invasion vascular/capsular
F	48	Follicular neoplasm	5.6 × 4.0 × 2.4	FTC	+/+
M	64	NA	NA	FTC	+/+
F	51	Follicular neoplasm	2.0 × 1.5 × 1.0	FTC	+/+
F	48	Follicular neoplasm	3.6 × 3.0 × 2.2	FTC	+/+
F	56	NA	NA	FTC	+/+
M	25	NA	NA	FTC	+/+
F	40	Follicular neoplasm	3.0 × 2.5 × 1.5	FTC	+/+
F	59	Follicular neoplasm	3.8 ×1.8 × 1.7	HCC, angioinvasive	+/+
M	45	Follicular neoplasm	3.8 × 3.1 × 2.5	FTC	+/+
M	72	Benign goiter	7.0 × 5.3 × 4.3	FTC and HCC	−/+
M	45	Follicular neoplasm	3.2 × 3.0 × 3.0	FTA	−/−
M	76	Follicular neoplasm	3.1 × 5.3 × 2.6	FTA	−/−
M	41	Follicular neoplasm	3.1 × 2.1 × 1.7	FTA	−/−
F	76	Follicular neoplasm	3.1 × 2.0 × 1.5	FTA	−/−
M	64	Follicular neoplasm	4.5 × 4.4 × 3.3	FTA	−/−
M	60	NA	3.8 × 3.0 × 5.0	FTA	−/−
F	28	Follicular neoplasm	2.5 × 2.2 × 2.0	FTA	−/−
F	52	Follicular neoplasm	5.0 × 4.0 × 3.5	FTA	−/−
F	44	Follicular neoplasm	4.5 × 3.5 × 2.9	FTA	−/−
F	38	Follicular neoplasm	3.1 × 1.9 × 1.5	FTA	−/−

N/A: records were not available.

TABLE 2: A list of tested genes and encoded by them proteins, including the gene and protein accession numbers and corresponding intron-spanning primers used for Q-RT-PCR.

Gene	GenBank	Primer sequence	Protein	Swiss-Prot
CCND-2	AY888219	S_CAC TTG TGA TGC CCT GAC TG AS_ACG GTA CTG CTG CAG GCT AT	G1/S-specific cyclin-D2	P30279
PCSK2	BC040546	S_AGC ATA CAA CTC CAA GGT TGC AS_GCT GTA GAT GTC AAT CAG CTG TG	Proprotein convertase subtilisin/kexin type 2	Q8IWA8
PLAB	BC008962	S_CAA CCA GAG CTG GGA AGA TT AS_AGA GAT ACG CAG GTG CAG GT	Placental bone morphogenetic protein	Q99988
RAP2A	NM 021033	S_AGA TCA TCC GCG TGA AGC AS_CCC CAC TCT TCA GCA AGG	Ras-related protein-2a	P10114
TSHR	BC024205	S_GGA TAT GCT TTC AAT GGG ACA AS_GCA TCT TTG TCA ATA ACT GTC AGG	Thyroid-stimulating hormone receptor	P16473
IGF1R	NM000875	S_GTG AAA GTG ACG TCC TGC ATT TC AS_CCT TGT AGT AAA CGG TGA AGC TGA	Insulin-like growth factor I receptor	P08069
3′ACTB	NP001092	S_TCC CCC AAC TTG AGA TGT ATG AAG AS_AAC TGG TCT CAA GTC AGT GTA CAG G	Actin, cytoplasmic 1	P60709
5′ACTB	NP001092	S_ATC CCC CAA AGT TCA CAA TG AS_GTG GCT TTT AGG ATG GCA AG	Actin, cytoplasmic 1	P60709

S: sense, forward primer 5′ to 3′; AS: antisense, backword primer 3′ to 5′.

normal, benign, and cancer groups were made by using one-way analysis of variance (ANOVA). A value of $P < .05$ was considered as statistically significant.

3. Results and Discussion

In this exploratory study, we investigated the expression of the potential thyroid cancer-discriminating genes: *CCND2, PCSK2, PLAB, RAP2A, TSHR,* and *IGF-1R* (Table 2) by comparing their expression at the mRNA levels in the normal thyroid tissue, benign follicular lesions, and follicular carcinomas. The target genes have been chosen based on importance of abnormal expression and activities of the thyroid-stimulating hormone receptor (TSHR) and insulin- like growth factor type I receptor (IGF-IR) in thyroid tumorigenesis [12, 13] and the results of gene micro-array analysis showing differential expression of *CCND2, PCSK2, PLAB, RAP2A* in FTC [14, 15]. We found no statistically significant difference in *CCND2, TSHR,* and *IGF-1R* mRNA expression between the groups of normal thyroid, benign and malignant thyroid cancer (Figure 1(a)). There was no difference between the levels of mRNA expression of *PCSK2, PLAB,* and *RAP2A* between normal thyroid and FTA (Figure 1(b)). Interestingly, however, in the Q-RT-PCR analysis of FTA and cancer, *PSCK2* was markedly downregulated (22.4-fold), whereas *PLAB* and *RAP2A* were notably upregulated (8.3- and 6.3-fold, resp.) in cancer. Furthermore, a comparative mRNA expression analysis revealed a statistically significant difference in *PCSK2* ($P = 2.81E - 2$), *PLAB* ($P = 9.81E - 12$) and *RAP2A* ($P = 9.13E - 10$) expression between groups of benign and malignant thyroid tumors (Figure 1(b)). Thus, in tested age-matched cohort of 20 patients diagnosed with follicular-patterned thyroid neoplasm, the levels of *CCND2, TSHR,* and *IGF-1R* were not significantly different; *PLAB* and *RAP2A* were significantly increased, whereas *PCSK2* was significantly decreased in cancer compared with adenoma. Overexpression of *PLAB* and *PCSK2* as well as down-regulation of *CCND2* has been found in frozen sections of FTC [15]. Weber et al. proposed that a combination of those three genes allowed the accurate molecular classification of FTC versus FTA with a high specificity and sensitivity. However, Shibru et al. were unable to confirm the diagnostic accuracy of the 3-gene assay either in frozen tissue or in FNAs [16]. The difference is likely attributed to the difference in types of analyzed tissue, as Shibru et al. compared a benign group represented by hyperplastic nodule, FTA, Hürthle cell adenomas (HCAs) with a collective group of thyroid malignancies, including FTC, PTC, follicular variant of PTC, HCC. Although FTC and HCC may carry similar molecular alterations [17], PTC has distinct genetic features (somatic alterations such as *RET/PTC* translocation and *BRAF* mutations) that distinguish them from FTC [6]. Our data are in close agreement with the findings reported by Weber et al. except that the observed down-regulation of *CCND2* in cancer has not reached statistical significance.

Intratumoral heterogeneity is well-recognized phenomenon [5, 18, 19], so it is plausible that within areas of invasion tumor cells are genetically different from the rest of tumor.

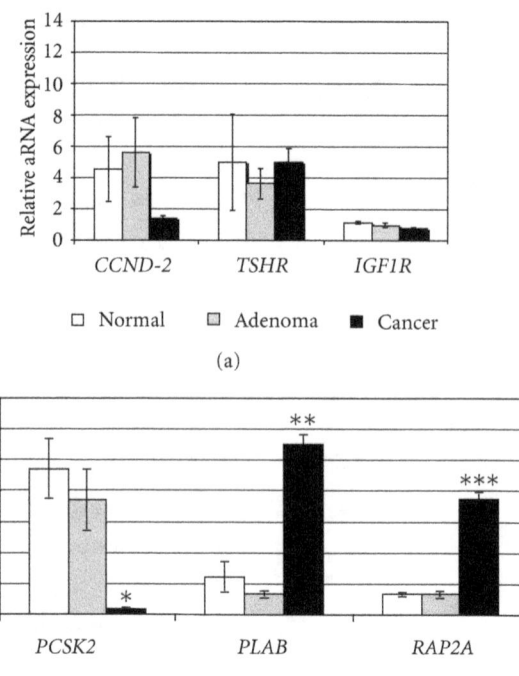

FIGURE 1: Evaluation of *CCND2, TSHR, IGF-1R* (a) and *PCSK2, PLAB, RAP2A* (b) mRNA expression by Q-RT-PCR in tissue samples from the human thyroid (normal, benign, cancer). All PCR reactions were performed in duplicates with at least three repeats. Mean of normalized expression level of mRNA in each analyzed group ($n = 10$) are shown. Bar, SEM. $^*P = 2.81E - 2$, $^{**}P = 9.81E - 12$, and $^{***}P = 9.13E - 10$.

Here, we tested the hypothesis that in thyroid malignancy differential expression of molecular BMs may be detected in thyroid follicular cancer cells invaded through the tumor capsule and entered into vasculature. The three genes (*PCSK2, PLAB,* and *RAP2A*) were selected for in-depth analysis because of their significantly different expression in cancers compared with adenomas (Figure 1(b)). To ensure the presence of invasion in freshly cut 7μm thick sections of cancer tissue, a thyroid pathologist reviewed slides stained with hematoxylin and eosin and marked the areas of invasion using diagnostic criteria adopted in our institution [3]. Nine angioinvasive samples of thyroid cancers had both capsular and vascular invasion; one minimally invasive specimen had only capsular invasion. Eight out of ten specimens had more than one invasive focus. To selectively isolate population of thyroid carcinoma cells that have invaded the capsule to enter blood vessels and to compare them to the cells remained in the main tumor mass, we applied an LCM method as illustrated in Figure 2(a). After dissecting multiple areas, the captured cells from each of the cancer specimens were pooled in to two matched groups: (i) remained under the tumor capsule ("noninvasive" group) and (ii) invaded the capsule and/or entered blood vessels ("invasive" group). The total RNA was assessed in the captured tumor cells, and samples with an adequate amount of input RNA (>1.0 ng)

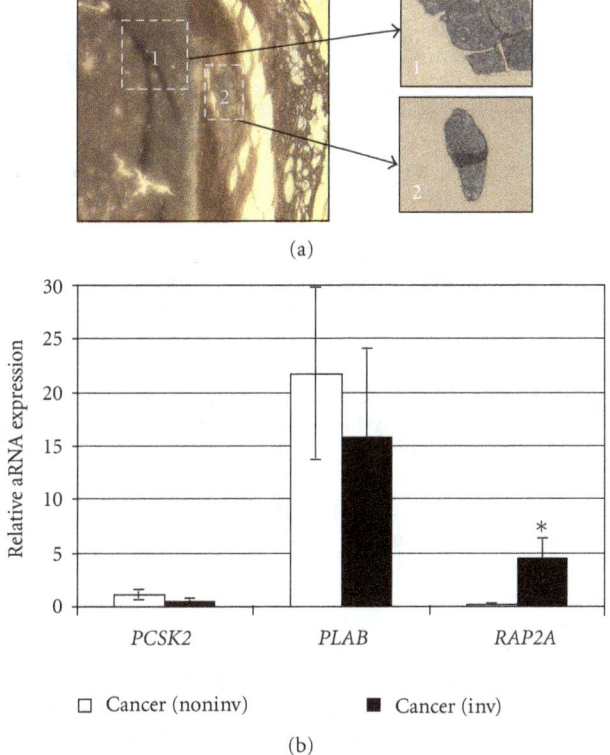

(a)

(b)

FIGURE 2: An example of laser-capture micro-dissection in follicular thyroid carcinoma. (a) FTC tissue before (left) and after collecting the groups of cells from the main tumor mass (inset 1) and angioinvasive area (inset 2). Original magnification, 200x. (b) Histogram, relative expression of PCSK2, PLAB, RAP2A in the cells collected from matched noninvasive and invasive areas of the same specimens ($n = 4$). Mean of normalized expression levels of aRNA in each group is shown. Bar, SEM. *$P = 0.039$.

were subjected to two rounds of linear amplification by *in vitro* transcription to further increase the amount of RNA. Twice-amplified aRNA of high quality only was used for a cDNA preparation and Q-RT-PCR with specific primers for target genes. As expected from the analysis of tissue scrapes, PSCK2 expression was low in the cells from the main tumor mass; it was insignificantly different ($P = 0.322$) in invasive cells dissected from the same specimens (Figure 2(b)). Likewise, PLAB expression was equally high in both types of dissected cells ($P = 0.698$). The results of the Q-RT-PCR analysis for RAP2A aRNA were intriguing, as the relative level of RAP2A expression was 25.9-fold higher ($P = 0.039$) in the cells dissected from areas of invasion. RAP2A encodes Ras-related protein 2a (Rap-2a), a member of the Ras family of small GTPases (Rap1a/b and Rap2a/b/c) that has been reported to induce cytoskeleton rearrangements promoting cell rounding and cell migration [20, 21]. Although activating mutations of Rap have not been reported, up regulation of Rap activating guanine nucleotide exchange factors [22, 23] and down regulation of Rap GTPase-activating proteins promoting Rap inactivation [24, 25] have been found in human tumors including thyroid carcinomas [26]. High levels of expression of Rap2, but not

Rap1, have been detected in human thyroid cancer cell lines. Importantly, Rap2 protein expression was several fold higher in anaplastic than in well-differentiated papillary thyroid cancer cells [27]. Furthermore, increased Rap activity has been shown to promote carcinoma cells invasion *in vitro* and *in vivo* [28, 29]. We found up regulation of human gene encoding Rap-2a in follicular thyroid cancer tissue, particularly in the regions enriched with invasive cancer cells. It could be speculated that thyroid tumor cells "require" the genetic changes in RAP2A, in addition to PSCK2 and PLAB, to allow them to invade and/or "maintain and flourish" in the nonnative areas of the tumor capsule and blood vessels.

4. Conclusions

We demonstrated the feasibility of combining LCM and Q-RT-PCR for analysis of gene expression in microscopic clusters dissected from FFPE thyroid tissue. Our study is a first and important step in the assessment of novel molecular BMs associated with invasion of follicular thyroid carcinoma cells, despite the relatively small sample size. Validation of diagnostic applicability of RAP2A requires a follow-up work in larger tissue sample sets.

Acknowledgments

The authors are extremely grateful to Dr. Virginia LiVolsi for reviewing clinical samples of follicular thyroid tumors and providing critical comments on the paper. They also thank members of the Eastern Division of the Cooperative Human Tissue Network for providing frozen samples of the thyroid and members of the Gastrointestinal Morphology Core at the University of Pennsylvania for sharing with us a laser-capture micro-dissection work station. Special thanks to Theresa Pasha for excellent technical support. J. R. Grau, current address: Lehigh Valley Health Network, Department of Pathology and Laboratory Medicine, Cedar Crest & I-78, P.O. Box 689, Allentown, Pennsylvania 18105-1556.

References

[1] L. Enewold, K. Zhu, E. Ron et al., "Rising thyroid cancer incidence in the United States by demographic and tumor characteristics, 1980–2005," *Cancer Epidemiology Biomarkers and Prevention*, vol. 18, no. 3, pp. 784–791, 2009.

[2] C. Y. Lo, W. F. Chan, K. Y. Lam, and K. Y. Wan, "Follicular thyroid carcinoma: the role of histology and staging systems in predicting survival," *Annals of Surgery*, vol. 242, no. 5, pp. 708–715, 2005.

[3] Z. W. Baloch and V. A. LiVolsi, "Our approach to follicular-patterned lesions of the thyroid," *Journal of Clinical Pathology*, vol. 60, no. 3, pp. 244–250, 2007.

[4] R. L. Witt, "Initial surgical management of thyroid cancer," *Surgical Oncology Clinics of North America*, vol. 17, no. 1, pp. 71–91, 2008.

[5] J. L. Hunt, V. A. Livolsi, Z. W. Baloch et al., "A novel microdissection and genotyping of follicular-derived thyroid tumors to predict aggressiveness," *Human Pathology*, vol. 34, no. 4, pp. 375–380, 2003.

[6] M. Eszlinger, K. Krohn, S. Hauptmann, H. Dralle, T. J. Giordano, and R. Paschke, "Perspectives for improved and more accurate classification of thyroid epithelial tumors," *Journal of Clinical Endocrinology and Metabolism*, vol. 93, no. 9, pp. 3286–3294, 2008.

[7] F. Weber, R. E. Teresi, C. E. Broelsch, A. Frilling, and C. Eng, "A limited set of human MicroRNA Is deregulated in follicular thyroid carcinoma," *Journal of Clinical Endocrinology and Metabolism*, vol. 91, no. 9, pp. 3584–3591, 2006.

[8] J. Becker, P. Schmidt, F. Musshoff, M. Fitzenreiter, and B. Madea, "MOR1 receptor mRNA expression in human brains of drug-related fatalities—a real-time PCR quantification," *Forensic Science International*, vol. 140, no. 1, pp. 13–20, 2004.

[9] K. Kaserer, V. Knezevic, B. Pichlhöfer et al., "Construction of cDNA libraries from microdissected benign and malignant thyroid tissue," *Laboratory Investigation*, vol. 82, no. 12, pp. 1707–1714, 2002.

[10] R. N. Van Gelder, M. E. Von Zastrow, A. Yool, W. C. Dement, J. D. Barchas, and J. H. Eberwine, "Amplified RNA synthesized from limited quantities of heterogeneous cDNA," *Proceedings of the National Academy of Sciences of the United States of America*, vol. 87, no. 5, pp. 1663–1667, 1990.

[11] H. Zhao, T. Hastie, M. L. Whitfield, A. L. Børresen-Dale, and S. S. Jeffrey, "Optimization and evaluation of T7 based RNA linear amplification protocols for cDNA microarray analysis," *BMC Genomics*, vol. 3, article 31, 2002.

[12] A. Ciampolillo, C. De Tullio, E. Perlino, and E. Maiorano, "The IGF-I axis in thyroid carcinoma," *Current Pharmaceutical Design*, vol. 13, no. 7, pp. 729–735, 2007.

[13] C. García-Jiménez and P. Santisteban, "TSH signalling and cancer," *Arquivos Brasileiros de Endocrinologia e Metabologia*, vol. 51, no. 5, pp. 654–671, 2007.

[14] S. Chevillard, N. Ugolin, P. Vielh et al., "Gene expression profiling of differentiated thyroid neoplasms: diagnostic and clinical implications," *Clinical Cancer Research*, vol. 10, no. 19, pp. 6586–6597, 2004.

[15] F. Weber, L. Shen, M. A. Aldred et al., "Genetic classification of benign and malignant thyroid follicular neoplasia based on a three-gene combination," *Journal of Clinical Endocrinology and Metabolism*, vol. 90, no. 5, pp. 2512–2521, 2005.

[16] D. Shibru, J. Hwang, E. Khanafshar, Q. Y. Duh, O. H. Clark, and E. Kebebew, "Does the 3-gene diagnostic assay accurately distinguish benign from malignant thyroid neoplasms?" *Cancer*, vol. 113, no. 5, pp. 930–935, 2008.

[17] F. Weber, M. A. Aldred, C. D. Morrison et al., "Silencing of the maternally imprinted tumor suppressor ARHI contributes to follicular thyroid carcinogenesis," *Journal of Clinical Endocrinology and Metabolism*, vol. 90, no. 2, pp. 1149–1155, 2005.

[18] S. Glöckner, H. Buurman, W. Kleeberger, U. Lehmann, and H. Kreipe, "Marked intratumoral heterogeneity of c-myc and cyclinD1 but not of c-erbB2 amplification in breast cancer," *Laboratory Investigation*, vol. 82, no. 10, pp. 1419–1426, 2002.

[19] S. M. Wiseman, T. R. Loree, W. L. Hicks et al., "Anaplastic thyroid cancer evolved from papillary carcinoma: demonstration of anaplastic transformation by means of the inter-simple sequence repeat polymerase chain reaction," *Archives of Otolaryngology—Head and Neck Surgery*, vol. 129, no. 1, pp. 96–100, 2003.

[20] S. J. McLeod, A. H. Y. Li, R. L. Lee, A. E. Burgess, and M. R. Gold, "The Rap GTPases regulate B cell migration toward the chemokine stromal cell-derived factor-1 (CXCL12): potential role for Rap2 in promoting B cell migration," *Journal of Immunology*, vol. 169, no. 3, pp. 1365–1371, 2002.

[21] K. Taira, M. Umikawa, K. Takei et al., "The traf2- and nck-interacting kinase as a putative effector of Rap2 to regulate actin cytoskeleton," *The Journal of Biological Chemistry*, vol. 279, no. 47, pp. 49488–49496, 2004.

[22] T. Hirata, H. Nagai, K. Koizumi et al., "Amplification, up-regulation and over-expression of C3G (CRK SH3 domain-binding guanine nucleotide-releasing factor) in non-small cell lung cancers," *Journal of Human Genetics*, vol. 49, no. 6, pp. 290–295, 2004.

[23] V. Yajnik, C. Paulding, R. Sordella et al., "DOCK4, a GTPase activator, is disrupted during tumorigenesis," *Cell*, vol. 112, no. 5, pp. 673–684, 2003.

[24] D. H. Gutmann, S. Saporito-Irwin, J. E. DeClue, R. Wienecke, and A. Guha, "Alterations in the rap1 signaling pathway are common in human gliomas," *Oncogene*, vol. 15, no. 13, pp. 1611–1616, 1997.

[25] L. Zhang, L. Chenwei, R. Mahmood et al., "Identification of a putative tumor suppressor gene Rap1GAP in pancreatic cancer," *Cancer Research*, vol. 66, no. 2, pp. 898–906, 2006.

[26] A. Nellore, K. Paziana, C. Ma et al., "Loss of rap1GAP in papillary thyroid cancer," *Journal of Clinical Endocrinology and Metabolism*, vol. 94, no. 3, pp. 1026–1032, 2009.

[27] X. Dong, C. Korch, and J. L. Meinkoth, "Histone deacetylase inhibitors upregulate Rap1GAP and inhibit Rap activity in thyroid tumor cells," *Endocrine-Related Cancer*, vol. 18, no. 3, pp. 301–310, 2011.

[28] C. L. Bailey, P. Kelly, and P. J. Casey, "Activation of Rap1 promotes prostate cancer metastasis," *Cancer Research*, vol. 69, no. 12, pp. 4962–4968, 2009.

[29] M. Itoh, C. M. Nelson, C. A. Myers, and M. J. Bissell, "Rap1 integrates tissue polarity, lumen formation, and tumorigenic potential in human breast epithelial cells," *Cancer Research*, vol. 67, no. 10, pp. 4759–4766, 2007.

30

Hypothyroidism in Pancreatic Cancer: Role of Exogenous Thyroid Hormone in Tumor Invasion—Preliminary Observations

Konrad Sarosiek,[1] Ankit V. Gandhi,[1] Shivam Saxena,[1] Christopher Y. Kang,[1] Galina I. Chipitsyna,[2] Charles J. Yeo,[1] and Hwyda A. Arafat[2]

[1]Departments of Surgery, Jefferson Pancreatic, Biliary and Related Cancer Center, Thomas Jefferson University, Philadelphia, PA 19107, USA
[2]Department of Biomedical Sciences, University of New England, Biddeford, ME 04005, USA

Correspondence should be addressed to Galina I. Chipitsyna; galina727@gmail.com

Academic Editor: Noriyuki Koibuchi

According to the epidemiological studies, about 4.4% of American general elderly population has a pronounced hypothyroidism and relies on thyroid hormone supplements daily. The prevalence of hypothyroidism in our patients with pancreatic cancer was much higher, 14.1%. A retrospective analysis was performed on patients who underwent pancreaticoduodenectomy (Whipple procedure) or distal pancreatectomy and splenectomy (DPS) at Thomas Jefferson University Hospital, Philadelphia, from 2005 to 2012. The diagnosis of hypothyroidism was correlated with clinicopathologic parameters including tumor stage, grade, and survival. To further understand how thyroid hormone affects pancreatic cancer behavior, functional studies including wound-induced cell migration, proliferation, and invasion were performed on pancreatic cancer cell lines, MiaPaCa-2 and AsPC-1. We found that hypothyroid patients taking exogenous thyroid hormone were more than three times likely to have perineural invasion, and about twice as likely to have higher T stage, nodal spread, and overall poorer prognostic stage ($P < 0.05$). Pancreatic cancer cell line studies demonstrated that exogenous thyroid hormone treatment increased cell proliferation, migration, and invasion ($P < 0.05$). We conclude that exogenous thyroid hormone may contribute to the progression of pancreatic cancer.

1. Introduction

Invasive pancreatic cancer is the fourth leading cause of cancer death in the United States. Most patients with pancreatic cancer have a dismal prognosis and a median survival rate of less than 6 months [1, 2]. At the time of diagnosis, the disease is often discovered to be in its late stages, as more than 85% of patients have tumors that have metastasized [2]. Currently, surgery remains one of the few options to decrease pancreatic cancer mortality. Despite many advances in cancer biology over the past years, pancreatic cancer remains an elusive disease process that requires further studies to understand its molecular biology and investigate possible therapeutic targets.

Thyroid hormones (T_3 and T_4) are steroid hormones that regulate body growth, brain maturation, and metabolism. Although the major product of the thyroid is T_4, most of it is converted to more biologically active T_3 that binds to nuclear thyroid receptors and modulates the expression of proteins traditionally known to increase basal metabolic rate and enhance growth [3]. Disorders of the thyroid that result in either a deficiency or excess of thyroid hormones are extremely common and can have various effects on the human body. According to the NHANES national 1999–2002 survey, the prevalence of hypothyroidism in the general US population was 3.7% [4]. Of note, the prevalence of thyroid disorders increases with age (up to 4.4% for 60 years and older) and is consistent with females having higher rates of hypothyroidism than men [5–8].

Due to the established effect of thyroid hormone on growth and development, many have hypothesized a connection between thyroid hormone and cancer. One of the first reports linking these two comes from a 1976 article that examines the relationship between supplemental thyroid hormone intake and breast cancer. In a study with 5,000 female patients, it was calculated that the rate of breast cancer in patients taking thyroid supplements for hypothyroidism was 12.1% versus 6.2% in a control group [9]. Since then, many studies have sparked a debate about a relationship between hypothyroidism and malignancy. A search of the literature reveals that hypothyroidism may be a risk factor for respiratory, colon, breast, and liver cancer [10–14]. Cell line experiments in breast and prostate cancer corroborate these findings by demonstrating that treatment with T_3 enhances cellular proliferation [15, 16].

In this study, a retrospective analysis was performed on patients who underwent pancreaticoduodenectomy (Whipple procedure) or distal pancreatectomy and splenectomy (DPS) at Thomas Jefferson University Hospital, Philadelphia, from 2005 to 2012. The diagnosis of hypothyroidism was correlated with clinicopathologic parameters including tumor stage, grade, and survival. To further understand how thyroid hormone affects pancreatic cancer behavior, functional studies including wound-induced cell migration, proliferation, and invasion were performed on pancreatic cancer cell lines, MiaPaCa-2 and AsPC-1.

2. Materials and Methods

2.1. Data Collection. For this cross-sectional study, a database search was conducted for patients who underwent pancreaticoduodenectomy (Whipple procedure) or distal pancreatectomy and splenectomy (DPS) at Thomas Jefferson University Hospital, Philadelphia, PA, from 2005 to 2012. The eligibility criteria consisted of patients with a diagnosis of invasive pancreatic cancer confirmed by biopsy. Exclusion criteria consisted of patients with a history of noninvasive, benign pancreatic pathology or incomplete medical history. Data collection included patient sex, age, body mass index (BMI), medical history, medications, surgical information, survival, tumor staging, and differentiation by hypothyroid status. The TNM staging system as outlined by the American Joint Committee on Cancer (AJCC) was used to define pancreatic lesions. Patients were defined to be hypothyroid if they had a positive medical hypothyroidism and were taking synthetic or desiccated thyroid hormone. The Institutional Review Board of Thomas Jefferson University Hospital, Philadelphia, PA, approved this study.

MiaPaCa-2 (ATCC CRL-1420) and AsPC-1 (ATCC CRL-1682) were purchased from ATCC. MTT cell growth, migration, and transwell invasion assays were performed as previously described [17].

2.2. Statistical Analyses. Descriptive statistics were calculated on patient clinicopathological features. Differences in gender,

smoking status, venous-lymphatic invasion, perineural invasion, T stage, N stage, prognostic stage, and differentiation by hypothyroid status were determined by Chi-square test. Differences in age and BMI were determined by unpaired Student's t-test. Survival analysis was performed using Kaplan-Meier curves and Mantel-Cox log rank test, where survival was defined as time between date of surgery and date of death or of last follow-up. All functional experiments were performed 3 to 5 times. Functional studies were analyzed for statistical significance by Student's t-test analysis, or two-way ANOVA. Data are presented as mean ± SEM. All tests of significance were two-sided with an alpha value of 0.05. Analyses were performed with the assistance of a computer program (Prism 6.0, GraphPad Software, Inc., La Jolla, CA).

3. Results

3.1. Patient Characteristics. An overview of the clinical patient data is summarized in Table 1. Of 504 patients in the database, 71 patients were found to be hypothyroid (of males, 7.7% and, of females, 20.8% were hypothyroid). As expected, the hypothyroid group had a significantly greater proportion of females than males ($P < 0.001$). The age of patients in the hypothyroid group (67.8) was similar to the age of patients in the euthyroid group (64.6). BMI was not significantly different in the hypothyroid group when compared to the euthyroid group (27.9 versus 26.3, resp.). Lastly, there was no significant difference in smoking status between two groups.

3.2. Pancreatic Pathology. Pancreatic tissue specimens stratified by pathology are shown in Table 2. Majority of the biopsies (85%) were invasive ductal adenocarcinoma. Second most common pathology was invasive IPMN (6%), followed by endocrine, papillary, acinar cell, and mucinous cancers.

3.3. Clinicopathological Parameters by Hypothyroid Status. As shown in Table 3, there were no differences in survival (Figure 1), venous-lymphatic invasion, and differentiation between hypothyroid and euthyroid patients. Compared to euthyroid patients, hypothyroid patients taking exogenous thyroid hormone were more than three times likely to have perineural invasion and about twice as likely to have a higher T stage, nodal spread, and overall poorer prognostic stage.

3.4. T_3 Increases Cell Proliferation, Migration, and Invasion. To evaluate whether T_3 was associated with cell viability, MiaPaCa-2 cells were treated with T_3 (0–5000 nM) and quantified via the MTT assay (Figure 2(a)). The addition of T_3 significantly ($P < 0.05$) increased cell proliferation after 48 and 72 hours across all concentrations of T_3. Additionally, MiaPaCa-2 cells were treated with T_3 to evaluate its role in cell migration (Figure 2(b)). T_3 significantly ($P < 0.05$) increased cell migration at 48- and 72-hour time points at 1 and 10 nM of T_3 compared to the control. Lastly, the role of exogenous thyroid hormone in invasion was evaluated via transwell infiltration assay. Cells were treated with T_3 (0–10 nM), and the extent of invasion was quantified via MTT assay (Figure 2(c)). Adding T_3 significantly ($P < 0.05$)

TABLE 1: Clinical characteristics of patients.

	Hypothyroid ($n = 71$)	Euthyroid ($n = 433$)	Total ($n = 504$)
Male, n (%)	20 (28.2)	239 (55.2)	259 (51.4)
Female, n (%)	51 (71.8)	194 (44.8)	245 (48.6)
Age, mean (SD)	67.8 (12.6)	64.6 (12.1)	65.1 (12.2)
BMI, mean (SD)	27.9 (5.6)	26.3 (5.3)	26.5 (5.4)
Smoking status, n (%), yes	32 (53.3)	200 (54.9)	232 (54.7)
Smoking status, n (%), no	28 (46.7)	164 (45.1)	192 (45.3)

TABLE 2: Pancreatic tissue specimens stratified by pathology.

Pancreatic malignancy	n (%)
Invasive ductal adenocarcinoma	427 (84.7)
Invasive IPMN	31 (6.2)
Endocrine	22 (4.4)
Papillary	17 (3.4)
Acinar cell	4 (0.8)
Mucinous	3 (0.6)
All invasive pancreatic pathologies	504 (100)

increased cell invasion. Similar data ($P < 0.05$) were obtained for AsPC-1 cells (data not shown).

4. Discussion

The objective of this study was to evaluate the prevalence of hypothyroidism and thyroid hormone supplementation in patients with pancreatic cancer and to correlate hypothyroidism diagnosis with various clinicopathologic parameters. Furthermore, functional studies were performed on MiaPaCa-2 and AsPC-1 pancreatic cancer cell lines to study how exogenous thyroid hormone influences cell behavior. To our knowledge, this is the first study to suggest a higher prevalence of thyroid hormone supplementation in patients with pancreatic cancer and to demonstrate the proliferative effects of T_3 in pancreatic cancer cell lines.

The association between hypothyroidism and neoplasia remains controversial. Despite conflicting reports in the literature, studies have shown that hypothyroidism may correlate with many cancers including respiratory, colon, breast, and liver cancer [10–14]. Some studies even suggest that a diagnosis of hypothyroidism may result in poor response to therapy in patients with breast cancer [18]. Other studies argue that high levels of thyroid hormones induce cancer cell proliferation while low levels slow disease progress [19]. A number of prospective case-control studies have indicated that subclinical hyperthyroidism increases risk of certain solid tumors and that spontaneous hypothyroidism may delay onset or reduce aggressiveness of cancers [20–22]. A controlled prospective trial of induced hypothyroidism beneficially affected the course of glioblastoma [20].

In our study, the prevalence of patients with hypothyroidism treated with medication was 14.1% (7.7% in males, 20.8% in females). This percentage is much higher than the prevalence of overt hypothyroidism reported in the elderly

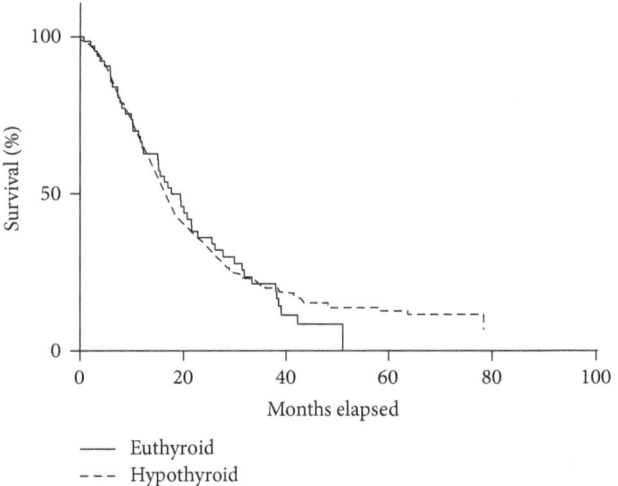

FIGURE 1: Kaplan-Meier curve comparing hypothyroid and euthyroid patients. There was no difference in survival. $P = 0.742$.

(4.4%) and is consistent with females having higher rates of hypothyroidism than men [4–8].

Metastasis is one of the most significant predictors of mortality in patients with pancreatic cancer. When comparing hypothyroid and euthyroid patients with pancreatic cancer, hypothyroid patients on thyroid hormone supplementation were found to have significantly ($P < 0.05$) higher rates of nodal spread and a T stage of T3 or higher, signifying that the tumor has already extended beyond the walls of the pancreas. It was not surprising that these patients were more likely to have a poorer prognostic stage (OR 1.9). Interestingly, patients on thyroid hormone supplementation also had significantly higher rates of perineural invasion (OR 3.4). Perineural invasion is a poorly understood process by which cancer cells metastasize to nerves and their surrounding neural sheaths [23]. Although metastatic spread via neural invasion is often overlooked, PDAC has one of the highest rates of perineural invasion when compared to other malignancies, and it is a substantial cause of pain in pancreatic cancer patients [24]. Despite these poor prognostic factors, there was no significant difference in survival between patients taking thyroid hormone supplementation compared to patients who were not on medication. This might be due to the limitations of this study. One of the limitations was possible selection bias in the patient population. Because surgery was reserved for patients with resectable disease only, our study might not accurately capture patients with advanced diseases. Another limitation was little information available regarding the diagnosis of hypothyroidism. TSH measurement was not used to diagnose or quantify the degree of hypothyroidism. Similarly, the date and duration of hypothyroidism and thyroid hormone implementation were not available at the time of the surgery. Lastly, due to difficulties in patient follow-up after hospital discharge, the survival data were not the most current.

However, because all patients with hypothyroidism were taking exogenous thyroid medication, one may hypothesize that exogenous thyroid hormone may be responsible for

TABLE 3: Clinicopathologic parameters of hypothyroid and euthyroid patients with invasive PDA.

	Hypothyroid	Euthyroid	OR [95% CI]	P value
Median survival (months)	17.7	16.6		0.742
Venous-lymphatic invasion, n (%)			0.91 [0.52–1.58]	0.733
Yes	28 (48)	185 (51)		
No	30 (52)	180 (49)		
Perineural invasion, n (%)			3.38 [1.19–9.58]	0.012*
Yes	62 (94)	335 (82)		
No	4 (6)	73 (18)		
T stage, n (%)			2.10 [1.00–4.37]	0.045*
Low stage (T0–T2)	9	98		
High stage (T3-T4)	61	317		
Nodal status, n (%)			2.05 [1.12–3.75]	0.018*
N0	15 (22)	157 (36)		
N1	54 (78)	276 (64)		
Prognostic stage, n (%)			1.89 [1.03–3.48]	0.037*
Low stage (0–2A)	15 (22)	142 (34)		
High stage (2B-3)	54 (78)	270 (66)		
Differentiation, n (%)				0.612
Well	10 (14)	46 (12)		
Moderate	44 (64)	242 (61)		
Poor	15 (22)	105 (27)		

Hypothyroid patients were found to have higher rates of perineural invasion, nodal spread, and advanced prognostic stage. *$P < 0.05$.

increasing growth and metabolism of pancreatic cancer cells, thus responsible for promoting tumor invasion and spread to nearby structures. Functional assays that were performed demonstrated that treatment of MiaPaCa-2 and AsPC-1 cells with physiologic concentrations of thyroid hormone caused an increase in cell proliferation, migration, and invasion at 48 h and 72 h. These results are consistent with studies that demonstrate proliferative effect of T_3 in breast cancer, prostate cancer, and hepatocellular carcinoma. It was also shown that T_3 contributes to breast cancer cell proliferation through estrogen response elements mediated gene expression, by promoting the effects of estrogens themselves [15] or by upregulating TGF-α mRNA expression [25]. Murine glioma cell lines and human prostatic carcinoma cells also revealed the increased proliferation in response to physiological concentrations of both T_3 and T_4 [16, 26, 27]. T_3 also promotes cell proliferation and invasion in human hepatoma cell lines in cooperation with TGF-β [28, 29]. Thyroid hormones enhance the development of gastric cancer in rats by stimulating the proliferation of gastric cancer cells [14, 30]. Additionally, thyroid hormones act as growth factors in both papillary and follicular human thyroid cancer cell lines [31]. It was shown that both T_3 and T_4 caused proliferation of malignant glioma U-87 MG cells through PI3-kinase, Src kinase, and ERK1/2 signaling cascades [32]. T_3 and T_4 promote both tumor cell division and angiogenesis by activating mitogen-activated protein kinase (MAPK) via binding to a hormone receptor on the $\alpha v \beta 3$ integrin, overexpressed on many human myelomas and other cancer cells [33, 34]. Other in vitro studies of thyroid hormones action in cancer cells implicated many molecular targets,

including TGF-β, hyperphosphorylation of Rb, and MAP kinase pathways [15, 16, 26, 35, 36]. Thyroid hormones have also been shown to promote angiogenesis in cancer cells by upregulating HIF-1α [35, 37].

5. Conclusions

This study demonstrates that there may be an association between thyroid hormone supplementation and pancreatic cancer invasion. Although the use of exogenous thyroid hormone may not necessarily be involved in the initial insult responsible for tumorigenesis, it may contribute to the progression of preexisting tumor. Increased perineural invasion, higher T stage, nodal spread, and advanced prognostic stage in hypothyroid patients may be due to enhanced metabolism of malignant cells via thyroid hormone supplementation. The proliferative effects of T_3 on MiaPaCa-2 and AsPC-1 cells support this hypothesis.

We propose that spontaneous hypothyroidism might develop in cancer patients as a protection mechanism against tumor progress/spread, but thyroid hormone supplementation might abolish this action. Clinical studies have shown [38] that interventional lowering of serum-free T_4 may be associated with extended survival in patients with some terminal cancers, and compassionate medical induction of hypothyroxinemia could be considered for patients with advanced cancers to whom other avenues of treatment are closed [38]. Thus, accumulating clinical evidence may justify new, broadly based controlled studies in cancer patients to determine the possible contribution of thyroid hormone to tumor behavior. Insights into molecular mechanism of this

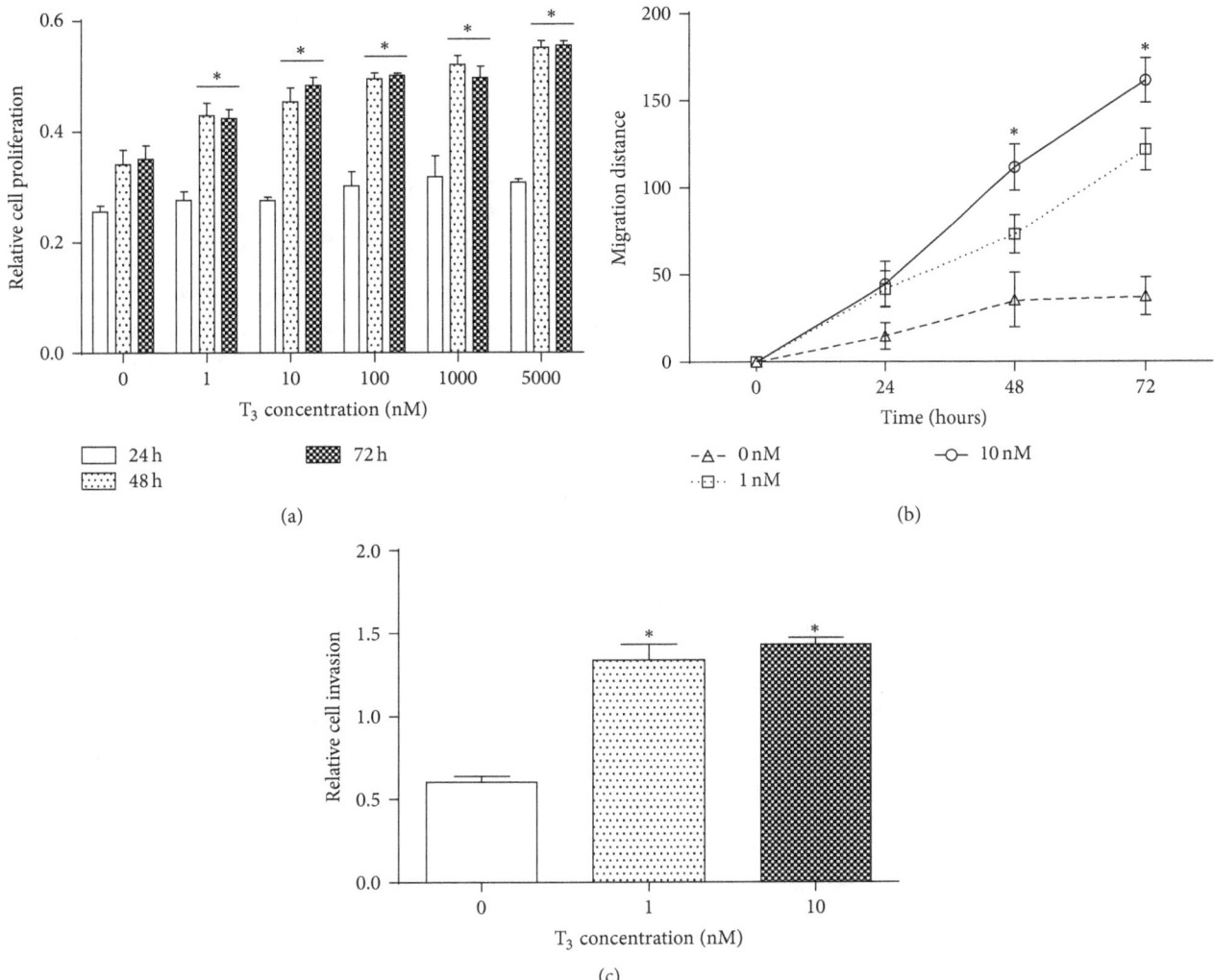

FIGURE 2: Effects of exogenous thyroid hormone treatment on PDAC cells proliferation, migration, and invasion ($P < 0.05$). (a) Proliferation assay of MiaPaCa-2 cells incubated with T_3. Proliferation was increased at all concentrations after 48 and 72 hours. $^*P < 0.05$. (b) Migration assay of MiaPaCa-2 cells incubated with T_3. Cell migration was increased after 48 and 72 hours. $^*P < 0.05$. (c) Transwell infiltration assay of MiaPaCa-2 cells incubated with T_3. Cell invasion was increased by 1 and 10 nM T_3. $^*P < 0.05$.

process might uncover possible targets which would allow thyroid hormone supplementation without promoting cancer progression.

Competing Interests

All named authors have no financial interests in respect of this work and its publication or other interests that might be perceived to influence the results and/or discussion reported in this paper.

Acknowledgments

Authors acknowledge research support and funding they have received from the Department of Surgery, Thomas Jefferson University Hospital, Philadelphia, PA, and Department of Biomedical Sciences, University of New England, Biddeford, ME, relevant to the work described.

References

[1] A. F. Hezel, A. C. Kimmelman, B. Z. Stanger, N. Bardeesy, and R. A. Depinho, "Genetics and biology of pancreatic ductal adenocarcinoma," *Genes and Development*, vol. 20, no. 10, pp. 1218–1249, 2006.

[2] A. Jemal, R. Siegel, E. Ward et al., "Cancer statistics, 2008," *CA: A Cancer Journal for Clinicians*, vol. 58, no. 2, pp. 71–96, 2008.

[3] G. A. Brent, "The molecular basis of thyroid hormone action," *The New England Journal of Medicine*, vol. 331, no. 13, pp. 847–853, 1994.

[4] Y. Aoki, R. M. Belin, R. Clickner, R. Jeffries, L. Phillips, and K. R. Mahaffey, "Serum TSH and total T4 in the United States population and their association with participant characteristics: National Health and Nutrition Examination Survey (NHANES 1999–2002)," *Thyroid*, vol. 17, no. 12, pp. 1211–1223, 2007.

[5] I. M. Bensenor, R. D. Olmos, and P. A. Lotufo, "Hypothyroidism in the elderly: diagnosis and management," *Clinical Interventions in Aging*, vol. 7, pp. 97–111, 2012.

[6] A. R. Cappola, L. P. Fried, A. M. Arnold et al., "Thyroid status, cardiovascular risk, and mortality in older adults," *The Journal of the American Medical Association*, vol. 295, no. 9, pp. 1033–1041, 2006.

[7] J. Gussekloo, E. Van Exel, A. J. M. de Craen, A. E. Meinders, M. Frölich, and R. G. J. Westendorp, "Thyroid status, disability and cognitive function, and survival in old age," *The Journal of the American Medical Association*, vol. 292, no. 21, pp. 2591–2599, 2004.

[8] I. M. Benseñor, A. C. Goulart, P. A. Lotufo, P. R. Menezes, and M. Scazufca, "Prevalence of thyroid disorders among older people: results from the São Paulo Ageing & Health Study," *Cadernos de Saúde Pública*, vol. 27, no. 1, pp. 155–161, 2011.

[9] C. C. Kapdi and J. N. Wolfe, "Breast cancer. Relationship to thyroid supplements for hypothyroidism.," *Journal of the American Medical Association*, vol. 236, no. 10, pp. 1124–1127, 1976.

[10] M. B. Goldman, R. R. Monson, and F. Maloof, "Cancer mortality in women with thyroid disease," *Cancer Research*, vol. 50, no. 8, pp. 2283–2289, 1990.

[11] C. Giani, P. Fierabracci, R. Bonacci et al., "Relationship between breast cancer and thyroid disease: relevance of autoimmune thyroid disorders in breast malignancy," *Journal of Clinical Endocrinology and Metabolism*, vol. 81, no. 3, pp. 990–994, 1996.

[12] J. L. P. Kuijpens, I. Nyklíček, M. W. J. Louwman, T. A. P. Weetman, V. J. M. Pop, and J.-W. W. Coebergh, "Hypothyroidism might be related to breast cancer in post-menopausal women," *Thyroid*, vol. 15, no. 11, pp. 1253–1259, 2005.

[13] G. Rennert, H. S. Rennert, M. Pinchev, and S. B. Gruber, "A case-control study of levothyroxine and the risk of colorectal cancer," *Journal of the National Cancer Institute*, vol. 102, no. 8, pp. 568–572, 2010.

[14] H. Iishi, M. Tatsuta, M. Baba, R. Yamamoto, and H. Taniguchi, "Enhancement by thyroxine of gastric carcinogenesis induced by N-methyl-N′-nitro-N-nitrosoguanidine in Wistar rats," *British Journal of Cancer*, vol. 68, no. 3, pp. 515–518, 1993.

[15] L. C. Hall, E. P. Salazar, S. R. Kane, and N. Liu, "Effects of thyroid hormones on human breast cancer cell proliferation," *Journal of Steroid Biochemistry and Molecular Biology*, vol. 109, no. 1-2, pp. 57–66, 2008.

[16] M.-L. Hsieh and H.-H. Juang, "Cell growth effects of triiodothyronine and expression of thyroid hormone receptor in prostate carcinoma cells," *Journal of Andrology*, vol. 26, no. 3, pp. 422–428, 2005.

[17] K. Sarosiek, E. Jones, G. Chipitsyna et al., "Osteopontin (OPN) isoforms, diabetes, obesity, and cancer; what is one got to do with the other? a new role for opn," *Journal of Gastrointestinal Surgery*, vol. 19, no. 4, pp. 639–650, 2015.

[18] A. Aranda, O. Martínez-Iglesias, L. Ruiz-Llorente, V. García-Carpizo, and A. Zambrano, "Thyroid receptor: roles in cancer," *Trends in Endocrinology and Metabolism*, vol. 20, no. 7, pp. 318–324, 2009.

[19] M. Ellis, K. Cohen, E. S. H. Maman, A. Hercbergs, P. J. Davis, and O. Ashur-Fabian, "THE involvement of thyroid hormones in cancer," *Harefuah*, vol. 154, no. 8, pp. 512–540, 2015.

[20] A. H. Hercbergs, O. Ashur-Fabian, and D. Garfield, "Thyroid hormones and cancer: clinical studies of hypothyroidism in oncology," *Current Opinion in Endocrinology, Diabetes and Obesity*, vol. 17, no. 5, pp. 432–436, 2010.

[21] L. C. Moeller and D. Führer, "Thyroid hormone, thyroid hormone receptors, and cancer: a clinical perspective," *Endocrine-Related Cancer*, vol. 20, no. 2, pp. R19–R29, 2013.

[22] A. M. Mondul, S. J. Weinstein, T. Bosworth, A. T. Remaley, J. Virtamo, and D. Albanes, "Circulating thyroxine, thyroid-stimulating hormone, and hypothyroid status and the risk of prostate cancer," *PLoS ONE*, vol. 7, no. 10, Article ID e47730, 2012.

[23] C. Liebig, G. Ayala, J. A. Wilks, D. H. Berger, and D. J. Albo, "Perineural invasion in cancer: a review of the literature," *Cancer*, vol. 115, no. 15, pp. 3379–3391, 2009.

[24] I. E. Demir, G. O. Ceyhan, F. Liebl, J. G. D'Haese, M. Maak, and H. Friess, "Neural invasion in pancreatic cancer: the past, present and future," *Cancers*, vol. 2, no. 3, pp. 1513–1527, 2010.

[25] S. J. Conde, R. A. M. Luvizotto, M. T. Sibio, M. L. H. Katayama, M. M. Brentani, and C. R. Nogueira, "Tamoxifen inhibits transforming growth factor-α gene expression in human breast carcinoma samples treated with triiodothyronine," *Journal of Endocrinological Investigation*, vol. 31, no. 12, pp. 1047–1051, 2008.

[26] H.-Y. Tang, H.-Y. Lin, S. Zhang, F. B. Davis, and P. J. Davis, "Thyroid hormone causes mitogen-activated protein kinase-dependent phosphorylation of the nuclear estrogen receptor," *Endocrinology*, vol. 145, no. 7, pp. 3265–3272, 2004.

[27] F. B. Davis, H.-Y. Tang, A. Shih et al., "Acting via a cell surface receptor, thyroid hormone is a growth factor for glioma cells," *Cancer Research*, vol. 66, no. 14, pp. 7270–7275, 2006.

[28] K.-H. Tsui, W.-C. Hsieh, M.-H. Lin, P.-L. Chang, and H.-H. Juang, "Triiodothyronine modulates cell proliferation of human prostatic carcinoma cells by downregulation of the B-cell translocation gene 2," *Prostate*, vol. 68, no. 6, pp. 610–619, 2008.

[29] C.-C. Yen, Y.-H. Huang, C.-Y. Liao et al., "Mediation of the inhibitory effect of thyroid hormone on proliferation of hepatoma cells by transforming growth factor-beta," *Journal of Molecular Endocrinology*, vol. 36, no. 1, pp. 9–21, 2006.

[30] R.-N. Chen, Y.-H. Huang, Y.-C. Lin et al., "Thyroid hormone promotes cell invasion through activation of furin expression in human hepatoma cell lines," *Endocrinology*, vol. 149, no. 8, pp. 3817–3831, 2008.

[31] R. Liu, Z. Li, S. Bai et al., "Mechanism of cancer cell adaptation to metabolic stress: proteomics identification of a novel thyroid hormone-mediated gastric carcinogenic signaling pathway," *Molecular and Cellular Proteomics*, vol. 8, no. 1, pp. 70–85, 2009.

[32] H.-Y. Lin, H.-Y. Tang, A. Shih et al., "Thyroid hormone is a MAPK-dependent growth factor for thyroid cancer cells and is anti-apoptotic," *Steroids*, vol. 72, no. 2, pp. 180–187, 2007.

[33] H.-Y. Lin, M. Sun, H.-Y. Tang et al., "L-thyroxine vs. 3,5,3′-triiodo-L-thyronine and cell proliferation: activation of mitogen-activated protein kinase and phosphatidylinositol 3-kinase," *American Journal of Physiology-Cell Physiology*, vol. 296, no. 5, pp. C980–C991, 2009.

[34] K. Cohen, M. Ellis, S. Khoury, P. J. Davis, A. Hercbergs, and O. Ashur-Fabian, "Thyroid hormone is a MAPK-dependent growth factor for human myeloma cells acting via $\alpha v \beta 3$ integrin," *Molecular Cancer Research*, vol. 9, no. 10, pp. 1385–1394, 2011.

[35] M. Pinto, P. Soares, and D. Ribatti, "Thyroid hormone as a regulator of tumor induced angiogenesis," *Cancer Letters*, vol. 301, no. 2, pp. 119–126, 2011.

[36] S. Dinda, A. Sanchez, and V. Moudgil, "Estrogen-like effects of thyroid hormone on the regulation of tumor suppressor proteins, p53 and retinoblastoma, in breast cancer cells," *Oncogene*, vol. 21, no. 5, pp. 761–768, 2002.

[37] T. Otto and J. Fandrey, "Thyroid hormone induces hypoxia-inducible factor 1α gene expression through thyroid hormone receptor β/retinoid X receptor α-dependent activation of hepatic leukemia factor," *Endocrinology*, vol. 149, no. 5, pp. 2241–2250, 2008.

[38] A. Hercbergs, R. E. Johnson, O. Ashur-Jabian et al., "Medically induced euthyroid hypothyroxinemia may extend survival in compassionate need cancer patients: an observational study," *Oncologist*, vol. 20, no. 1, pp. 72–76, 2015.

31

Significance of Interleukin-6 in Papillary Thyroid Carcinoma

Toral P. Kobawala, Trupti I. Trivedi, Kinjal K. Gajjar, Darshita H. Patel, Girish H. Patel, and Nandita R. Ghosh

Division of Molecular Endocrinology, Cancer Biology Department, The Gujarat Cancer & Research Institute, NCH Compound, Asarwa, Ahmedabad, Gujarat 380016, India

Correspondence should be addressed to Nandita R. Ghosh; nandita.ghosh@gcriindia.org

Academic Editor: Noriyuki Koibuchi

This study sought to reveal the significance of IL-6 in papillary thyroid carcinoma by determining its circulating levels, tumoral protein, and mRNA expressions. As compared to the healthy individuals, serum IL-6 was significantly higher in patients with benign thyroid diseases and PTC. Further, its level was significantly higher in PTC patients as compared to patients with benign thyroid diseases. ROC curves also confirmed a good discriminatory efficacy of serum IL-6 between healthy individuals and patients with benign thyroid diseases and PTC. The circulating IL-6 was significantly associated with poor overall survival in PTC patients. IL-6 immunoreactivity was significantly high in PTC patients as compared to the benign thyroid disease patients. Significantly higher IL-6 mRNA expression was also observed in the primary tumour tissues of PTC patients than the adjacent normal tissues. The protein expression of IL-6 at both the circulating and tissue level correlated with disease aggressiveness in PTC patients. Moreover, a significant positive correlation was observed between the IL-6 protein and mRNA expression in the primary tumours of PTC patients. Finally in conclusion, IL-6 has an important role in thyroid cancer progression. Thus targeting IL-6 signalling can help in clinical management of thyroid carcinoma patients.

1. Introduction

IL-6 is apleiotropic cytokine having a central role in the regulation of inflammatory and immune responses [1]. It is secreted by different cell types including macrophages, T and B lymphocytes, fibroblasts, endothelial cells, and cancer cells [2]. It was cloned in 1986 as the B-cell differentiation factor [3].

IL-6 has been known to exert its biological activities through binding to its receptors and further leads to activation of signal transduction via various pathways like: janus kinase/signal transducers and activators of transcription (JAK/STAT), phosphatidylinositol $3'$ kinase/Akt (PI3K/Akt), and mitogen activated protein kinase (MAPK) pathway [4]. Numerous studies indicate that IL-6 and its related signalling pathways have been identified to contribute to proliferation, migration, and invasion of various tumour cells [5–9] and its expression is associated with poor prognosis in many types of cancers [10–12]. Moreover, the physiological role of IL-6 has been shown to promote not only tumour proliferation,

but also metastasis and symptoms of cachexia [6, 13, 14]. Increased expression of IL-6 has been reported in different types of cancers and high serum levels of IL-6 have been associated with metastasis and unfavourable prognosis [2, 15–17]. Further, possible involvement of IL-6 signalling in the resistance to chemotherapy and radiotherapy has been documented in few studies [18–20]. Regarding its therapeutic role, blockade of IL-6 in the various autoimmune and inflammatory diseases, by tocilizumab, a humanized anti-(human IL-6R) monoclonal antibody, has proved to improve symptoms of rheumatoid arthritis, Castleman's disease, and systemic juvenile idiopathic arthritis [21]. IL-6 signalling has also been investigated as a potential target for several types of cancer therapies [22, 23].

Thyroid cancer is the most common and slowly progressing endocrine malignancy, accounting for less than 1% of malignancies diagnosed. Although survival is generally good, the mortality rate is higher than all other endocrine organ cancers. It was estimated that 6 out of every 1 million people die due to thyroid cancer. About 85% of thyroid cancers are papillary thyroid cancer (PTC). Despite high survival rates, local recurrence and metastases may occur in some patients and this may require a more aggressive surgical treatment [24]. Moreover, an association between the thyroid cancer and a history of underlying inflammatory conditions of benign diseases has been evident from the literature. Besides this, very often, a pathologist is confronted with thyroid lesions in which the distinction between benign and malignant can be rather difficult and as a result, the decision supporting one or another has clinical consequences and implies different treatment modalities. Thus, it was hypothesised that IL-6, a proinflammatory cytokine, and one of the chief components of the underlying inflammatory conditions, may help in differential diagnosis of thyroid diseases.

Thus, the goal of this study was to examine the role of IL-6 in benign and papillary thyroid cancer patients and correlate the results with clinicopathological parameters and disease outcome of PTC patients. To achieve this aim, we assessed the circulating levels of IL-6 in both patients with benign thyroid diseases and PTC and compared with healthy individuals. We further studied the protein expression of IL-6 in the primary tumours of PTC patients in relation to the benign tissues and also determined its mRNA expression in the primary tumour as well as adjacent normal tissues of histologically confirmed PTC patients.

2. Materials and Methods

2.1. Patients. Sixty-seven patients with benign thyroid diseases and 83 pathologically confirmed PTC patients were included in this study. This patient group and their clinicopathological features shown in Table 1 are same as mentioned previously [25]. Forty-five out of 67 benign thyroid disease patients underwent surgery at our institute and were included for immunohistochemical analysis. The WHO classification and the AJCC/UICC TNM staging system were used to histopathologically classify the tumours and to stage the thyroid cancer patients, respectively. Accordingly, the patients were grouped into younger (<45 years) and elder (≥45 years) age groups. All patients were followed for a period of 4 years or until death within that period. Complete follow-up details were obtained in 92% (76/83) PTC patients and were included for overall survival (OS) analysis. Nine percent (7/76) patients amongst these had persistent disease and hence were not included for the disease free survival (DFS) analysis. Therefore, 69/76 PTC patients were included for DFS analysis. IL-6 mRNA was determined in the primary tumour and adjacent normal tissues of sixty PTC patients. With respect to IL-6 mRNA expression, DFS was evaluated in 54/60 PTC patients as the rest of six patients had persistent disease and hence were not included for the DFS analysis, while all sixty patients were included for OS analysis.

2.2. Sample Collection. This study has been approved by Institutional Scientific and Ethical Committees and informed consent was obtained from all patients prior to sample collection. To detect the circulating levels of IL-6, pretherapeutic

blood samples were collected from all patients as well as from 67 healthy individuals. Serum was separated after centrifugation and was preserved at −80°C until analysis. Primary tissue samples of patients were collected on ice directly from the operation theatre. Both tumour and adjacent normal tissue were selected by a pathologist and divided into two portions. One portion was submitted for routine histopathological evaluation and the other portion was snap frozen in liquid nitrogen and preserved at −80°C for total RNA extraction. For Immunohistochemistry, paraffin embedded tissue blocks of all the patients (who underwent surgery) were retrieved from the Histopathology Department of our institute. The clinical and histopathological details of the patients were noted from the case files maintained at the Medical Record Department of the institute.

2.3. Circulating Levels of IL-6 by Enzyme Linked Immunosorbent Assay (ELISA). The circulating levels of IL-6 were estimated from the serum samples using commercially available ELISA kit from Krishgen Biosystems following manufacturer's instructions. The unknown concentrations were interpreted from the standard curve generated in Graphpad prism 5 software.

2.4. Tumoral Protein Expression of IL-6 by Immunohistochemistry (IHC). Immunohistochemical staining was performed for detection of tumoral expression of IL-6 in primary tumours of PTC patients and in patients with benign thyroid diseases. Briefly, 3–5 μm thick sections were cut from the formalin fixed paraffin embedded tissue blocks using Leica microtome and mounted on APES coated glass slides. The immunohistochemical staining was carried out using primary mouse monoclonal IL-6 antibody from R&D Systems (MAB2061) and MACH4 Universal HRP-Polymer Detection System from Biocare Medicals, USA, as per manufacturer's protocol recommendations. Antigenicity was retrieved by heating the sections in 10 mM sodium citrate buffer (pH, 6.0) for 20 mins in a pressure cooker prior to application of the primary antibody. All the sections were scored independently by two individual observers in a blinded fashion. A semiquantitative Immunoreactive Score (IRS) method of Remmele and Stegner [26] based on staining positivity and staining intensity was implemented. Staining positivity was scored as 0 for no stained cells, 1 for staining in 1% to 10% of cells, 2 for staining in 11% to 50% of cells, 3 for staining in 50% to 80% of cells, and 4 for staining in >80% of cells. The staining intensity was scored as 0 for no staining, 1 for weak/faint staining, 2 for moderate staining, and 3 for intense/dark staining. The IRS score was then obtained by multiplying the staining positivity and the staining intensity and therefore, theoretically the scores could range from 0 to 12. For statistical evaluation, the median IRS in the two subgroups of patients was used as cut-off value to divide the patients into low (≤median IRS) and high (>median IRS) expression groups, respectively.

2.5. IL-6 mRNA Expression by Reverse Transcriptase-Polymerase Chain Reaction (RT-PCR). The total RNA was

Table 1: Clinicopathological characteristics of PTC patients.

Characteristics	N (%)	Characteristics	N (%)
Age		Bilaterality	
<45 years	41 (49)	Unilateral	61 (74)
≥45 years	42 (51)	Bilateral	22 (26)
Gender		Hemorrhagic area	
Female	56 (68)	Absent	72 (87)
Male	27 (32)	Present	11 (13)
Tumour size		Necrosis	
T1 ($N = 16$) + T2 ($N = 22$)	38 (46)	Absent	67 (81)
T3 ($N = 30$) + T4 ($N = 15$)	45 (54)	Present	16 (19)
Nodal status		Calcification	
Absent	30 (36)	Absent	32 (39)
Present	53 (64)	Present	51 (61)
Metastasis		Extrathyroidal extension	
Absent	73 (88)	Absent	52 (63)
Present	10 (12)	Present	31 (37)
Stage		Fibrosis	
Early [stage I ($N = 37$) + stage II ($N = 12$)]	49 (59)	Absent	61 (74)
Advanced [stage III ($N = 11$) + stage IV ($N = 23$)]	34 (41)	Present	22 (26)
Lymphatic permeation		Inflammation	
Absent	67 (81)	Absent	46 (55)
Present	16 (19)	Present	37 (45)
Vascular permeation		Differentiation	
Absent	74 (89)	Well	76 (92)
Present	09 (11)	Moderate/poor	07 (08)
Capsular invasion		Multifocality	
Absent	55 (66)	Absent	64 (77)
Present	28 (34)	Present	19 (23)
Encapsulation		Residual disease	
Well encapsulated	76 (92)	Absent	24 (29)
Partially/not encapsulated	07 (08)	Present	59 (71)
Treatment			
Surgery	29 (35)		
Surgery + RIA and/RT	54 (65)	Surgery + RIA	50 (60)
		Surgery + RIA + RT	04 (05)
Disease status			
Recurrence/distant metastasis ($N = 69$)		Alive/dead ($N = 76$)	
Absent	62 (90)	Alive	68 (89)
Present	07 (10)	Dead	08 (11)
Recurrence	3 (4)		
Distant metastasis	4 (6)		
Bone	1 (1.5)		
Lung	2 (3.0)		
Bone + lung	1 (1.5)		

extracted by guanidine thiocyanate-phenol-chloroform extraction method modified from that by Chomczynski and Sacchi [27] and quantitated spectrophotometrically at 260 nm and 280 nm (Helios α, Thermo Spectronic, UK). The integrity of the RNA was confirmed by on 1.4% agarose gel. RT-PCR was performed using the OneStep RT-PCR kit (Qiagen, USA) to amplify IL-6 mRNA. Primers 5′-ATG TAG CCG CCC CAC ACA GA-3′ (sense) and 5′-GCA TCC ATC TTT TTC AGC CAT C-3′ (antisense) were used to amplify a 191 bp fragment specific for IL-6. The housekeeping GAPDH mRNA was used as an internal control. Primers 5′-CGG AGT CAA CGG ATT TGG TCG TAT-3′ (sense) and 5′-AGC CTT CTC CAT GGT GGT GAA GAC-3′ (antisense) were used to amplify a 306 bp fragment specific for GAPDH.

TABLE 2: Circulating levels, tumoral protein, and mRNA expression of IL-6.

IL-6	Healthy individuals	Benign thyroid diseases		Papillary thyroid carcinoma (PTC)	
Circulating levels M ± SE (pg/mL)	4.88 ± 0.99	33.73 ± 9.93 $P = 0.004^{*}$		246.41 ± 69.41 $P = 0.002^{\dagger}$ $P = 0.007^{\ddagger}$	
Tumoral protein expression		*Low*	*High*	*Low*	*High*
N (%)		32 (71)	13 (29)	40 (48)	43 (52)
			$\chi^2 = 6.228; r = +0.221; P = 0.012^{@}$		
mRNA expression				*Primary tumour tissues*	*Adjacent normal tissues*
M ± SE (counts/mm^2)				4969.46 ± 903.77	1076.06 ± 301.70
				$P < 0.001^{\wedge}$	

*Significance of circulating IL-6 levels between benign thyroid diseases and healthy individuals.
†Significance of circulating IL-6 levels between PTC and healthy individuals.
‡Significance of circulating IL-6 levels between PTC and benign thyroid diseases.
$^{@}$Significance of tumoral protein expression of IL-6 between PTC and benign thyroid diseases.
$^{\wedge}$Significance of IL-6 mRNA expression between primary tumour tissues and adjacent normal tissues in PTC patients.

1 μg of total RNA was added per reaction. RT-PCR was performed in Mastercycler gradient (Eppendorf, Germany) using the following conditions: IL-6: 60°C for 30 minutes, 95°C for 15 minutes, followed by 36 cycles of 94°C for 45 seconds, 58.1°C for 45 seconds, and 72°C for 1 minute and final extension at 72°C for 10 minutes; and GAPDH: 60°C for 30 minutes, 95°C for 15 minutes, followed by 36 cycles of 94°C for 45 seconds, 60°C for 45 seconds, and 72°C for 1 minute and final extension at 72°C for 10 minutes. The amplified products were run on 2% agarose gels and the intensity of the products was measured as counts/mm^2 and integrated on gel documentation system (Alpha Innotech, USA) using densitometric analysis.

2.6. Statistical Analysis. The data were analyzed statistically using the Statistical Package for Social Sciences (SPSS) software version 16 (SPSS Inc., USA). Independent samples t-test was used to compare the means of circulating levels between two groups of subjects and also to assess the association of the analytes with the clinicopathological parameters of thyroid cancer patients. Receiver's operating characteristic (ROC) curve was constructed to determine the discriminating efficacy of the circulating IL-6 between healthy individuals and patients with thyroid diseases. Two-tailed χ^2 test was used to compare the tumoral protein expressions in benign and carcinoma patients and also to determine association between protein expression and clinicopathological parameters of carcinoma patients. In case of less than five patients in the cells of 2 × 2 tables, Yate's continuity correction value along with its two-tailed significance was taken into consideration. Wilcoxon signed ranks test for two-related samples was executed to compare the mRNA expressions from the malignant and corresponding adjacent normal tissues of carcinoma patients, while the correlation of mRNA expression with clinicopathological parameters was analyzed by Mann Whitney U-test. Correlation between two parameters was calculated using Spearman's correlation coefficient

(r) method. Univariate survival analysis was evaluated using Kaplan-Meier method and log rank test was used to analyze difference in survival curves and to assess the prognostic significance of DFS and OS. Multivariate survival analysis was completed using Cox forward step-wise regression model. P values ≤ 0.05 were considered to be significant.

3. Results

3.1. Circulating Levels, Tumoral Protein, and mRNA Expression of IL-6. The circulating levels were expressed as Mean ± Standard Error (M ± SE). As compared to the healthy individuals, serum IL-6 was significantly higher in both patients with benign thyroid diseases ($P = 0.004$) and PTC ($P = 0.002$). Further, its level was also significantly higher in PTC patients as compared to the patients with benign thyroid diseases ($P = 0.007$) (Table 2).

The ROC curves also confirmed that serum IL-6 exhibited a good discriminatory efficacy between healthy individuals and patients with benign thyroid diseases (AUC = 0.598, $P = 0.051$) (Figure 1(a)) and also between healthy individuals and PTC patients (AUC = 0.708, $P < 0.001$) (Figure 1(b)). Additionally, the circulating IL-6 levels could also significantly differentiate PTC patients from patients with benign thyroid diseases (AUC = 0.643, $P = 0.003$) (Figure 1(c)).

The expression of IL-6 protein was localized in cytoplasm of the thyroid follicular cells. Its expression was detectable in 87% (39/45) of the patients with benign thyroid diseases and IRS-4 was the median score, while in PTC patients it was detectable in 96% (80/83) of tumours with median IRS value as 8. Representative staining of IL-6 protein expression in benign thyroid and PTC lesions is shown in Figures 2(a) and 2(b), respectively. The incidence of immunoreactivity of IL-6 was significantly high in PTC patients as compared to the benign thyroid disease patients. It was noted that IL-6 expression was higher in 52% (43/83) of PTC patients, in comparison to only 29% (13/45) of benign thyroid disease

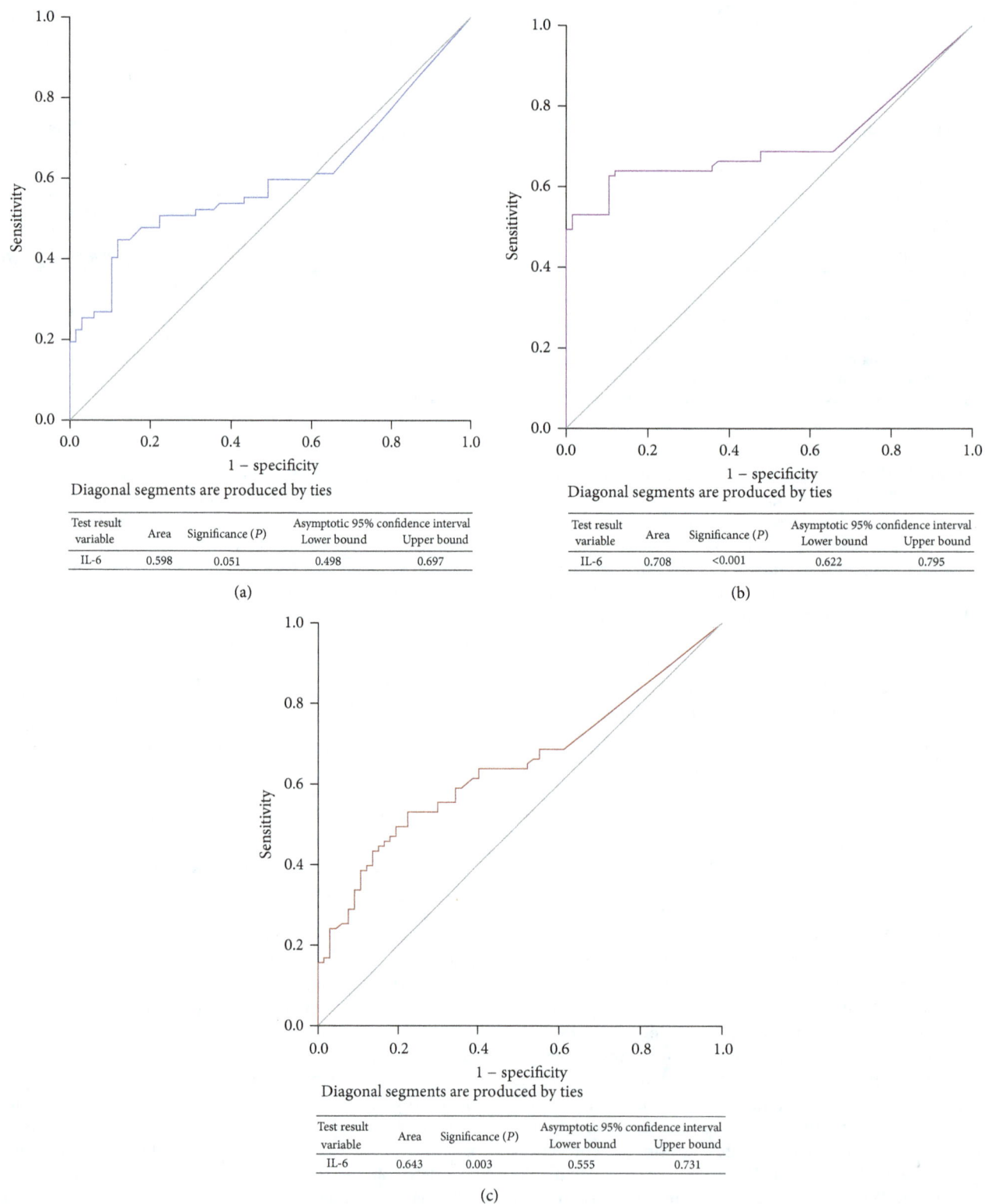

Figure 1: (a) ROC curve for IL-6 in healthy individuals versus patients with benign thyroid diseases. (b) ROC curve for IL-6 in healthy individuals versus patients with papillary thyroid carcinoma. (c) ROC curve for IL-6 in patients with benign thyroid diseases versus papillary thyroid carcinoma.

TABLE 3: Correlation of IL-6 with clinicopathological parameters in PTC patients.

Parameter	Circulating levels		Tumoral protein expression			mRNA expression (adjacent normal tissues)		
	Mean ± SE (pg/mL)	P	Low N (%)	High N (%)		Mean ± SE (counts/mm^2)	Mean rank	P
Gender								
Female	131.33 ± 36.57	0.016						
Male	485.07 ± 193.91							
Tumour size								
Small (T1 + T2)	94.08 ± 37.52	0.043	23 (61)	15 (39)	$r = +0.227$	1611.52 ± 633.60	35.52	0.037
Large (T3 + T4)	375.03 ± 121.41		17 (38)	28 (62)	$P = 0.039$	693.60 ± 240.93	26.91	
Metastasis								
Absent	157.17 ± 39.51	<0.001						
Present	897.83 ± 468.64							
Capsular invasion								
Absent			31 (56)	24 (44)	$r = +0.229$			
Present			9 (32)	19 (68)	$P = 0.037$			
Extrathyroidal extension								
Absent	121.81 ± 34.33	0.019	30 (58)	22 (42)	$r = +0.236$			
Present	455.04 ± 171.98		10 (32)	21 (68)	$P = 0.025$			
Residual disease								
Absent						1101.40 ± 785.08	24.43	0.035
Present						1113.40 ± 237.31	33.54	

r: correlation coefficient.

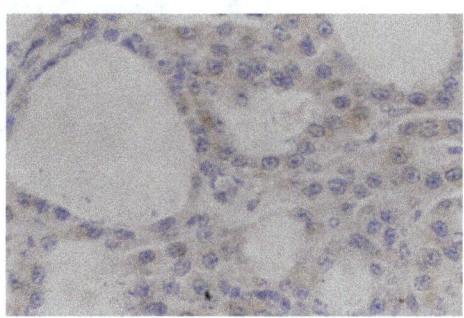
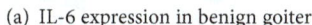

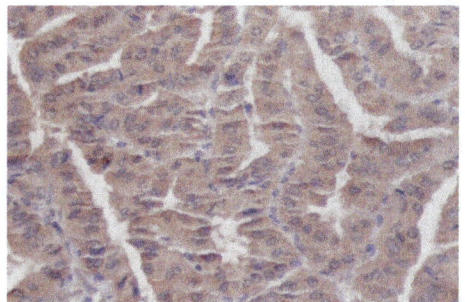

(a) IL-6 expression in benign goiter

(b) IL-6 expression in PTC

FIGURE 2: Representative staining patterns of IL-6 expression in primary tumours of patients with benign thyroid diseases and PTC.

patients exhibiting higher expressions (IL-6: $\chi^2 = 6.228$, $r = +0.221$, $P = 0.012$) (Table 2, Figure 3).

In PTC patients ($N = 60$), M ± SE of IL-6 mRNA expression in tumour and their adjacent normal tissues were 4969.46 ± 903.77 counts/mm^2 and 1076.06 ± 301.70 counts/mm^2, respectively. Using nonparametric Wilcoxon signed ranks test for two-related samples, statistical significant difference was noted in IL-6 mRNA expression between tumour and corresponding adjacent normal tissues with the primary tumour tissues showing considerably higher expression of IL-6 mRNA than the adjacent normal tissues ($P < 0.001$) (Table 2). IL-6 mRNA expression in PTC patients is depicted in Figure 4(a). GAPDH was used as housekeeping gene and Figure 4(b) is the representative picture of GAPDH mRNA expression in PTC patients.

3.2. Correlation of IL-6 with Clinicopathological Parameters in PTC Patients. As shown in Table 3, the circulating IL-6 levels were found to be significantly higher in male patients ($P = 0.016$) and in PTC patients having larger tumour size ($P = 0.043$), presence of metastasis ($P < 0.001$), and extrathyroidal extension of tumours ($P = 0.019$) when compared to their respective counterparts. Moreover, the protein expression of IL-6 was found to be significantly higher in patients with larger tumour size ($\chi^2 = 4.270$; $r = +0.227$; $P = 0.039$), in PTC patients showing capsular invasion of the tumours ($\chi^2 = 4.360$; $r = +0.229$; $P = 0.037$), and in those having extrathyroidal extension of tumours ($\chi^2 = 5.032$; $r = +0.236$; $P = 0.025$) in relation to their respective counterparts. Further, the Mann Whitney U-test revealed that IL-6 mRNA expression in primary tumours

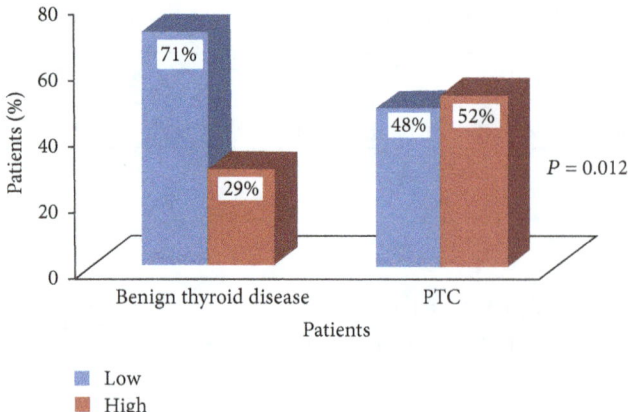

FIGURE 3: Expression of IL-6 in benign thyroid disease and PTC patients.

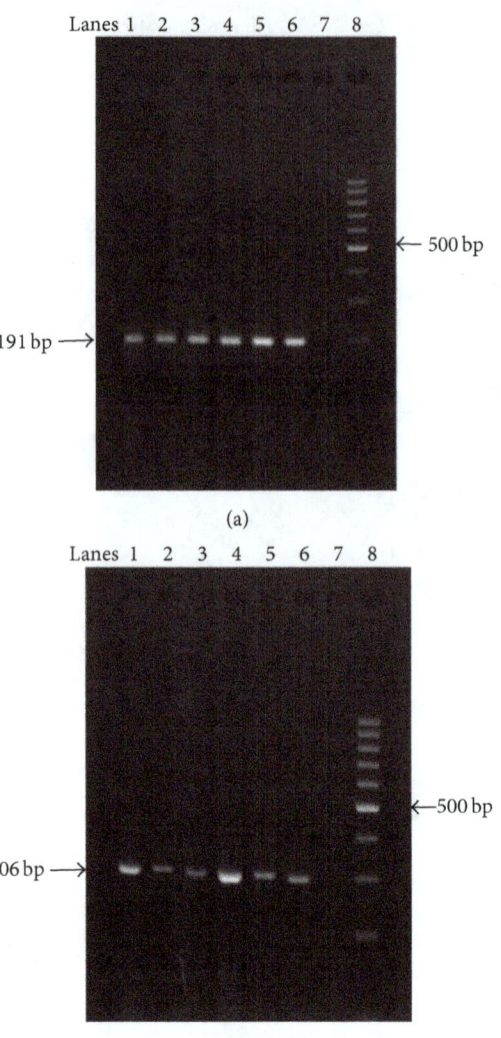

FIGURE 4: (a) Representative IL-6 mRNA expression. Lanes 1–6: presence of IL-6 mRNA in primary tumours. Lane 7: negative control. Lane 8: 100 bp ladder. (b) Representative GAPDH mRNA expression. Lanes 1–6: presence of GAPDH in primary tumours. Lane 7: negative control. Lane 8: 100 bp ladder.

did not show any significant association with any of studied clinicopathological features. On the other hand, the IL-6 mRNA expression in corresponding adjacent normal tissues was significantly higher in cases with smaller tumour size ($P = 0.037$) and in patients with presence of residual disease ($P = 0.035$) as compared to those with larger tumour size and patients showing absence of residual disease, respectively.

3.3. Association of IL-6 with Disease Free and Overall Survival in PTC Patients. Kaplan-Meier survival analysis was evaluated for DFS and OS in PTC patients. The median values of IL-6 circulating level, median IRS score for tumoral protein expression, and the median value of IL-6 mRNA expression were used as cut-off value to divide the PTC patients into low (≤median) and high (>median) expression groups, respectively. The difference in survival curves was analyzed using the log rank test. Circulating IL-6 was the significant prognosticator for OS (log rank = 4.77; df = 1; $P = 0.029$) (Table 4(b), Figure 5) while it was not able to predict DFS in the PTC patients. Further, the Kaplan-Meier survival analysis and the log rank test revealed that neither the tumoral protein expression nor the IL-6 mRNA expressions in primary tumours or the adjacent normal tissues were able to predict DFS or OS in the PTC patients (Tables 4(a) and 4(b)).

3.4. Intercorrelation between Circulating Levels of IL-6, Its Protein Expression, and mRNA Expression in PTC Patients. In PTC patients, the circulating levels of IL-6 were not significantly associated with its tumoral protein expression ($r = 0.119$, $P = 0.284$) or with the mRNA expression in primary tumour ($r = -0.130$, $P = 0.322$) or adjacent normal tissues ($r = -0.154$, $P = 0.241$). Further, nonparametric Spearman's correlation revealed a significant positive correlation of IL-6 protein expression with the IL-6 mRNA expressions in the primary tumours of PTC patients ($r = 0.333$, $P = 0.009$), while no such association was observed with the IL-6 mRNA expression in adjacent normal tissues ($r = -0.028$, $P = 0.833$) (Table 5).

4. Discussion

IL-6 is one of the most widely investigated cytokines in various diseases including cancer. As concerned with its role in thyroid, the present study demonstrated significantly higher levels of circulating IL-6 in benign as well as PTC patients as compared to the healthy individuals. This finding was further supported by the ROC curves which revealed that IL-6 could be one of the potential markers for differentiating patients with benign thyroid diseases, PTC patients from the healthy individuals. Additionally, it could also efficiently discriminate between the patients with benign thyroid diseases and PTC. Similar to present findings, Bartalena et al. reported increased serum IL-6 in multinodular goiter and they considered it as a marker of thyroid destructive inflammatory processes [28]. Recently, Provatopoulou et al. have also reported significant higher levels of serum IL-6 in

TABLE 4: (a) Univariate survival analysis of circulating IL-6, its tumoral protein expression, and mRNA in primary tumours and adjacent normal tissues for DFS in PTC patients. (b) Univariate survival analysis of circulating IL-6, its tumoral protein expression, and mRNA in primary tumours and adjacent normal tissues for OS in PTC patients.

(a)

IL-6	N	Patients relapsed N (%)	Log rank test statistics
Circulating levels	69		
Low	37	3 (8)	Log rank = 0.330, df = 1, P = 0.565
High	32	4 (12)	
Tumoral protein expression	69		
Low	35	2 (6)	Log rank = 1.480, df = 1, P = 0.224
High	34	5 (15)	
mRNA expression (primary tumour tissues)	54		
Low	25	2 (8)	Log rank = 0.119, df = 1, P = 0.730
High	29	3 (10)	
mRNA expression (adjacent normal tissues)	54		
Low	32	3 (9)	Log rank = 0.003, df = 1, P = 0.958
High	22	2 (9)	

(b)

IL-6	N	Patients died N (%)	Log rank test statistics
Circulating levels	76		
Low	37	1 (3)	Log rank = 4.772, df = 1, P = **0.029**
High	39	7 (18)	
Tumoral protein expression	76		
Low	38	4 (10)	Log rank = 0.001, df = 1, P = 0.977
High	38	4 (10)	
mRNA expression (primary tumour tissues)	60		
Low	30	5 (17)	Log rank = 1.496, df = 1, P = 0.221
High	30	2 (7)	
mRNA expression (adjacent normal tissues)	60		
Low	34	3 (9)	Log rank = 0.748, df = 1, P = 0.387
High	26	4 (15)	

TABLE 5: Intercorrelation between circulating levels of IL-6, its protein expression, and mRNA expression in PTC patients.

IL-6 mRNA expression	Circulating IL-6 levels	IL-6 protein expression
Primary tumours	$r = -0.130$ $P = 0.322$	$r = 0.333$ $P = \mathbf{0.009}$
Adjacent normal tissues	$r = -0.154$ $P = 0.241$	$r = -0.028$ $P = 0.833$
	$r = 0.119, P = 0.284$	

r: correlation coefficient.

patients with benign thyroid conditions and thyroid cancer, compared to healthy controls [29]. Also serum IL-6 levels were also found to be elevated in patients with chronic liver disease including cirrhosis and HCC [30]. Giannitrapani et al. have reported that IL-6 levels were significantly higher in HCC patients than that in patients with liver cirrhosis [31]. Similar to this and the current results, Uchiyama et al. have also shown increased levels of serum IL-6 in colorectal cancer as compared to patients with adenoma [32] while Szkarad-kiewicz et al. demonstrated that IL-6 levels were elevated in both patients with inflammatory bowel disease and colorectal cancer [33]. Multiple studies have consistently reported that, as compared to the healthy controls, the circulating levels of IL-6 were significantly higher in patients with different malignancies like colorectal cancer [33–36], breast cancer [37–40], pancreatic cancer [41], gastroesophageal cancer [42], gastric cancer [43], and non-small-cell lung carcinoma [44]. Moreover, Sun et al. have also observed that IL-6 was able to promote the proliferation of nasopharyngeal carcinoma [45].

Further, in present study, when serum IL-6 was correlated with various clinicopathological parameters of PTC patients, it was noted that levels of IL-6 showed a significant positive correlation with larger tumour size, presence of distant metastasis at the time of diagnosis, and extrathyroidal extension of tumours. Moreover, male patients had predominantly higher levels of IL-6 than the female patients. In their studies, Salgado et al., Goswami et al., Dethlefsen et al., Tripsianis et al., and Sanguinetti et al. have suggested that IL-6 assumes a role in the upregulation of malignant characteristics in breast cancer cells and that high IL-6 serum levels are associated with poor outcome in breast cancer patients [40, 46–49]. Data

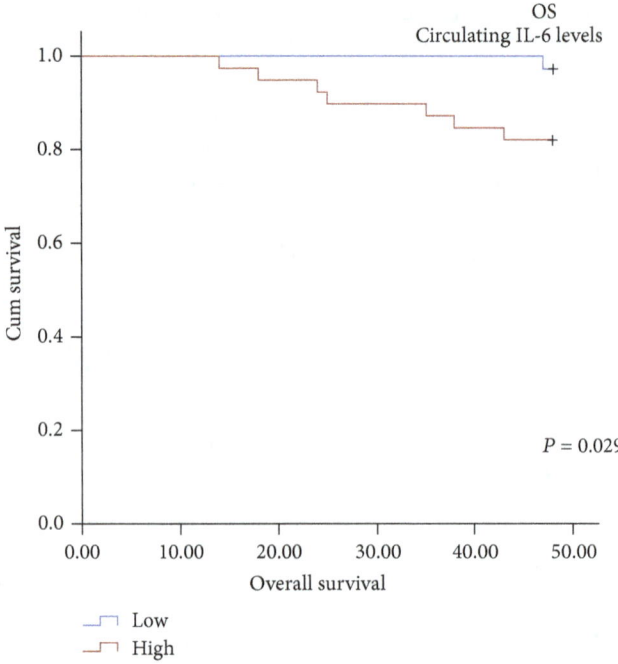

FIGURE 5: Significantly reduced OS observed in PTC patients with high levels of serum IL-6 as compared to its counterpart.

from epidemiological studies is also accruing in support of a contributory role of elevated circulating IL-6 in patients with advanced tumour stages and aggressive behaviour of various cancers, such as non-small-cell lung cancer, colorectal cancer, breast cancer, and renal cell carcinoma [11, 35, 39, 50–54]. IL-6 has been implicated as an autocrine promoter of cancer growth for various human cancers such as biliary tract epithelial cancers, multiple myeloma, and prostate cancer [55, 56]. Knüpfer and Preiss revealed that higher IL-6 levels were significantly associated with tumour size, metastasis, stage, and decreased survival in colorectal cancer patients [34] and Ahmed et al. have demonstrated its association with tumour size in breast cancer patients [37]. It can be suggested through these observations that circulating IL-6 may be partly derived from spillover of tumour produced IL-6 which hereby explains the association of high IL-6 levels with larger tumour size and presence of extrathyroidal extension of tumours.

The present study also demonstrates that higher circulating level of IL-6 was significantly associated with poor OS in PTC patients. Nakashima et al. have reported IL-6 to be independently associated with survival in prostate cancer patients [57]. Its role as an independent negative prognostic factor in patients with lymphoma has been confirmed by El Far et al. [58], and Lai et al. reported that IL-6 may be a prognostic marker in patients with Hodgkin disease or B-chronic lymphocytic leukemia [59]. Schultz et al. have demonstrated circulating IL-6 as an independent prognostic biomarker of OS in patients with locally advanced or metastatic pancreatic cancer [60]. IL-6 plays a key role as prognostic factor even in gastric cancer invasion and metastasis and its elevated level in circulation predicts shorter survival [61, 62]. Researchers

have observed that serum IL-6 concentration was associated with the progression, histological grade, and bowel wall invasion [63, 64] as well as tumour size and shorter survival periods of colorectal cancer [65]. Recently, Lu et al. have suggested the use of IL-6 concentration in the serum as an indicator of the possibility of colorectal cancer recurrence [66].

Further, the current study observed significant higher cytoplasmic expression of IL-6 protein in the primary tumours of PTC patients than in the patients with benign thyroid disease patients. The overexpression of IL-6 in PTC patients was significantly and linearly correlated with larger tumour size, presence of capsular invasion, and extrathyroidal extension of tumours. Consistent with the present finding, cytoplasmic staining pattern for IL-6 expression was also observed in ovarian cancer [67], renal cell carcinoma [68], colorectal cancer [50], and gastric cancer [61]. Expressions of IL-6 have also been observed to be higher in the primary tumour tissues than the adjacent normal tissues in prostate cancer [69], breast cancer [70], and esophageal squamous cell carcinoma [71, 72] as well as gastric cancer [62, 73]. Moreover, Depner et al. observed that IL-6 expression was strongly upregulated upon progression from benign tumours to highly malignant, metastasizing human skin squamous cell carcinoma [74]. Increased expression of IL-6 immunoreactivity in oral squamous cell carcinoma was more frequently observed in patients with advanced stage, cervical lymph node metastasis, or distant metastasis [75]. Moreover, Il-6 expression was significantly increased in advanced stage as compared to early stage of gastric cancer [73] and colorectal carcinoma [50]. However, Paule et al. found no significant difference in tumour size or grade between renal cell carcinomas with or without expression of IL-6 [68]. Moreover in the present study, IL-6 protein expression did not have a definite role in prognosis of the PTC patients. Similar to current observation, IL-6 expression in the primary tumours of patients with ovarian cancer and gall bladder cancer failed to show significant correlations with prognosis [67, 76]. Contradictory to this, IL-6 expression has been found to be significantly associated with poor prognosis in OSCC patients [75, 77], esophageal squamous cell carcinoma [72], colorectal cancer [50], and ovarian cancer [23]. In a study on colorectal cancer by Chung et al., the tissue expression of IL-6 did not correlate with the serum IL-6 levels, which is comparable to the present finding [50].

In addition to this, in the present study, the IL-6 mRNA expression was higher in the primary tumour tissues of PTC patients as compared to the corresponding adjacent normal tissues. Similar results have been reported in esophageal squamous cell carcinoma [71] and colorectal cancer [32, 66]. Moreover, Sanguinetti et al. have shown that mammospheres from node invasive breast cancer tissues express IL-6 mRNA at higher levels than the mammospheres from matched nonneoplastic mammary glands [49]. In the present study, the mRNA levels in the primary tumours were not associated with any of the clinicopathological parameters or with prognosis in PTC patients but its levels in the corresponding adjacent normal tissues were significantly higher in the PTC patients having smaller tumour size and presence of residual disease after surgery. This may be because although apparently looking normal, biologically there might be some malignant changes in the adjacent normal tissues of such patients and the concept of field cancerization may follow here. Moreover, a significant positive correlation was observed between the IL-6 protein and mRNA expression in the primary tumours of PTC patients. Data reported by Basolo et al. and Ruggeri et al. support that IL-6 tissue expression is related to aggressiveness in PTC [78, 79]. Further, Basolo et al. had shown that downregulation of IL-6 expression may represent a marker of undifferentiated thyroid carcinoma [78]. Moreover, it has also been revealed that certain polymorphisms in the genes encoding IL-6 have been associated with the risk of PTC [80]. Currently, humanized anti- IL-6 receptor monoclonal antibody tocilizumab has been adopted as a first-line biologic therapy for treatment of moderate-to-severe rheumatoid arthritis and for Castleman's disease.

5. Conclusion

From the present study, it can be evident that IL-6 has a significant role in thyroid cancer progression and targeting IL-6 signalling can be helpful in clinical management of thyroid carcinoma patients with more aggressive tumour characteristics.

Competing Interests

The authors declare that they have no competing interests.

Acknowledgments

This work was financially supported by Gujarat Cancer Society (GCS), and it was approved by the GCRI/GCS ethics committee.

References

[1] T. Nagasaki, M. Hara, H. Nakanishi, H. Takahashi, M. Sato, and H. Takeyama, "Interleukin-6 released by colon cancer-associated fibroblasts is critical for tumour angiogenesis: anti-interleukin-6 receptor antibody suppressed angiogenesis and inhibited tumour-stroma interaction," *British Journal of Cancer*, vol. 110, no. 2, pp. 469–478, 2014.

[2] T. Kishimoto, "Interleukin-6: from basic science to medicine—40 Years in immunology," *Annual Review of Immunology*, vol. 23, pp. 1–21, 2005.

[3] T. Kishimoto, "IL-6: from its discovery to clinical applications," *International Immunology*, vol. 22, no. 5, pp. 347–352, 2010.

[4] K. Tawara, J. T. Oxford, and C. L. Jorcyk, "Clinical significance of interleukin (IL)-6 in cancer metastasis to bone: potential of anti-IL-6 therapies," *Cancer Management and Research*, vol. 3, no. 1, pp. 177–189, 2011.

[5] S. Grivennikov, E. Karin, J. Terzic et al., "IL-6 and Stat3 are required for survival of intestinal epithelial cells and development of colitis-associated cancer," *Cancer Cell*, vol. 15, no. 2, pp. 103–113, 2009.

[6] T. Ara and Y. A. DeClerck, "Interleukin-6 in bone metastasis and cancer progression," *European Journal of Cancer*, vol. 46, no. 7, pp. 1223–1231, 2010.

[7] F. R. Santer, K. Malinowska, Z. Culig, and I. T. Cavarretta, "Interleukin-6 trans-signalling differentially regulates proliferation, migration, adhesion and maspin expression in human prostate cancer cells," *Endocrine-Related Cancer*, vol. 17, no. 1, pp. 241–253, 2010.

[8] H. Yi, H.-J. Cho, S.-M. Cho et al., "Blockade of interleukin-6 receptor suppresses the proliferation of H460 lung cancer stem cells," *International Journal of Oncology*, vol. 41, no. 1, pp. 310–316, 2012.

[9] G. Xie, Q. Yao, Y. Liu et al., "IL-6-induced epithelial-mesenchymal transition promotes the generation of breast cancer stem-like cells analogous to mammosphere cultures," *International Journal of Oncology*, vol. 40, no. 4, pp. 1171–1179, 2012.

[10] K.-Y. Yeh, Y.-Y. Li, L.-L. Hsieh et al., "Analysis of the effect of serum interleukin-6 (IL-6) and soluble IL-6 receptor levels on survival of patients with colorectal cancer," *Japanese Journal of Clinical Oncology*, vol. 40, no. 6, pp. 580–587, 2010.

[11] S. Mitsunaga, M. Ikeda, S. Shimizu et al., "Serum levels of IL-6 and IL-1β can predict the efficacy of gemcitabine in patients with advanced pancreatic cancer," *British Journal of Cancer*, vol. 108, no. 10, pp. 2063–2069, 2013.

[12] J. Shimazaki, Y. Goto, K. Nishida et al., "In patients with colorectal cancer, preoperative serum interleukin-6 level and granulocyte/lymphocyte ratio are clinically relevant biomarkers of long-term cancer progression," *Oncology*, vol. 84, no. 6, pp. 356–361, 2013.

[13] I. T. Cavarretta, H. Neuwirt, G. Untergasser et al., "The anti-apoptotic effect of IL-6 autocrine loop in a cellular model of advanced prostate cancer is mediated by Mcl-1," *Oncogene*, vol. 26, no. 20, pp. 2822–2832, 2007.

[14] U. H. Weidle, S. Klostermann, D. Eggle, and A. Krüger, "Interleukin 6/interleukin 6 receptor interaction and its role as a therapeutic target for treatment of cachexia and cancer," *Cancer Genomics and Proteomics*, vol. 7, no. 6, pp. 287–302, 2010.

[15] M. T. Lin, B. R. Lin, C. C. Chang et al., "IL-6 induces AGS gastric cancer cell invasion via activation of the c-Src/RhoA/ROCK signaling pathway," *International Journal of Cancer*, vol. 120, pp. 2600–2608, 2007.

[16] Z. T. Schafer and J. S. Brugge, "IL-6 involvement in epithelial cancers," *The Journal of Clinical Investigation*, vol. 117, no. 12, pp. 3660–3663, 2007.

[17] V. W. S. Wong, J. Yu, A. S. L. Cheng et al., "High serum interleukin-6 level predicts future hepatocellular carcinoma development in patients with chronic hepatitis B," *International Journal of Cancer*, vol. 124, no. 12, pp. 2766–2770, 2009.

[18] C.-C. Chen, W.-C. Chen, C.-H. Lu et al., "Significance of interleukin-6 signaling in the resistance of pharyngeal cancer to irradiation and the epidermal growth factor receptor inhibitor," *International Journal of Radiation Oncology, Biology, Physics*, vol. 76, no. 4, pp. 1214–1224, 2010.

[19] Z. Han, J. Feng, Z. Hong et al., "Silencing of the STAT3 signaling pathway reverses the inherent and induced chemoresistance of human ovarian cancer cells," *Biochemical and Biophysical Research Communications*, vol. 435, no. 2, pp. 188–194, 2013.

[20] H. Q. Yan, X. B. Huang, S. Z. Ke et al., "Interleukin 6 augments lung cancer chemotherapeutic resistance via ataxia-telangiectasia mutated/NF-kappaB pathway activation," *Cancer Science*, vol. 105, no. 9, pp. 1220–1227, 2014.

[21] M. Mihara, N. Nishimoto, and Y. Ohsugi, "The therapy of autoimmune diseases by anti-interleukin-6 receptor antibody," *Expert Opinion on Biological Therapy*, vol. 5, no. 5, pp. 683–690, 2005.

[22] M. S. Anglesio, J. George, H. Kulbe et al., "IL6-STAT3-HIF signaling and therapeutic response to the angiogenesis inhibitor sunitinib in ovarian clear cell cancer," *Clinical Cancer Research*, vol. 17, no. 8, pp. 2538–2548, 2011.

[23] J. Coward, H. Kulbe, P. Chakravarty et al., "Interleukin-6 as a therapeutic target in human ovarian cancer," *Clinical Cancer Research*, vol. 17, no. 18, pp. 6083–6096, 2011.

[24] V. Erol, Ö. Makay, G. Içöz et al., "The importance of staging systems for the determination of prognosis of well-differentiated thyroid cancer," *Turkish Journal of Surgery*, vol. 29, no. 1, pp. 7–10, 2013.

[25] T. P. Kobawala, T. I. Trivedi, K. K. Gajjar, D. H. Patel, G. H. Patel, and N. R. Ghosh, "Significance of TNF-α and the adhesion molecules: L-selectin and VCAM-1 in papillary thyroid carcinoma," *Journal of Thyroid Research*, vol. 2016, Article ID 8143695, 17 pages, 2016.

[26] W. Remmele and H. E. Stegner, "Recommendation for uniform definition of an immunoreactive score (IRS) for immunohistochemical estrogen receptor detection (ER-ICA) in breast cancer tissue," *Pathologe*, vol. 8, no. 3, pp. 138–140, 1987.

[27] P. Chomczynski and N. Sacchi, "Single-step method of RNA isolation by acid guanidinium thiocyanate-phenol-chloroform extraction," *Analytical Biochemistry*, vol. 162, no. 1, pp. 156–159, 1987.

[28] L. Bartalena, S. Brogioni, L. Grasso et al., "Interleukin-6: a marker of thyroid-destructive processes?" *The Journal of Clinical Endocrinology & Metabolism*, vol. 79, no. 5, pp. 1424–1427, 1994.

[29] X. Provatopoulou, D. Georgiadou, T. N. Sergentanis et al., "Interleukins as markers of inflammation in malignant and benign thyroid disease," *Inflammation Research*, vol. 63, no. 8, pp. 667–674, 2014.

[30] M. Trikha, R. Corringham, B. Klein, and J.-F. Rossi, "Targeted anti-interleukin-6 monoclonal antibody therapy for cancer: a review of the rationale and clinical evidence," *Clinical Cancer Research*, vol. 9, no. 13, pp. 4653–4665, 2003.

[31] L. Giannitrapani, M. Soresi, A. Giacalone et al., "IL-6-174G/C polymorphism and IL-6 serum levels in patients with liver cirrhosis and hepatocellular carcinoma," *OMICS: A Journal of Integrative Biology*, vol. 15, no. 3, pp. 183–186, 2011.

[32] T. Uchiyama, H. Takahashi, H. Endo et al., "IL-6 plays crucial roles in sporadic colorectal cancer through the cytokine networks including CXCL7," *Journal of Cancer Therapy*, vol. 3, no. 6, pp. 874–879, 2012.

[33] A. Szkaradkiewicz, R. Marciniak, I. Chudzicka-Strugała et al., "Proinflammatory cytokines and IL-10 in inflammatory bowel disease and colorectal cancer patients," *Archivum Immunologiae et Therapiae Experimentalis*, vol. 57, no. 4, pp. 291–294, 2009.

[34] H. Knüpfer and R. Preiss, "Serum interleukin-6 levels in colorectal cancer patients—a summary of published results," *International Journal of Colorectal Disease*, vol. 25, no. 2, pp. 135–140, 2010.

[35] J. Wang, K. Xu, J. Wu et al., "The changes of Th17 cells and the related cytokines in the progression of human colorectal cancers," *BMC Cancer*, vol. 12, article 418, 2012.

[36] S. Neagu, L. Lerescu, R. Costea et al., "Perioperative immunologic changes in colorectal cancer patients," *Chirurgia (Bucharest, Romania: 1990)*, vol. 107, no. 1, pp. 59–65, 2012.

[37] O. I. Ahmed, A. M. Adel, D. R. Diab, and N. S. Gobran, "Prognostic value of serum level of interleukin-6 and interleukin-8 in metastatic breast cancer patients," *The Egyptian journal of immunology/Egyptian Association of Immunologists*, vol. 13, no. 2, pp. 61–68, 2006.

[38] D. Narița, E. Seclaman, S. Ursoniu, R. Ilina, N. Cireap, and A. Anghel, "Expression of CCL18 and interleukin-6 in the plasma of breast cancer patients as compared with benign tumor patients and healthy controls," *Romanian Journal of Morphology and Embryology*, vol. 52, no. 4, pp. 1261–1267, 2011.

[39] N. Gupta, B. Goswami, and P. Mittal, "Effect of standard anthracycline based neoadjuvant chemotherapy on circulating levels of serum IL-6 in patients of locally advanced carcinoma breast—a prospective study," *International Journal of Surgery*, vol. 10, no. 10, pp. 638–640, 2012.

[40] G. Tripsianis, E. Papadopoulou, K. Anagnostopoulos et al., "Coexpression of IL-6 and TNF-α: prognostic significance on breast cancer outcome," *Neoplasma*, vol. 61, no. 2, pp. 205–212, 2014.

[41] W. Błogowski, A. Deskur, M. Budkowska et al., "Selected cytokines in patients with pancreatic cancer: a preliminary report," *PLoS ONE*, vol. 9, no. 5, Article ID e97613, 2014.

[42] M. Krzystek-Korpacka, M. Matusiewicz, D. Diakowska et al., "Impact of weight loss on circulating IL-1, IL-6, IL-8, TNF-α, VEGF-A, VEGF-C and midkine in gastroesophageal cancer patients," *Clinical Biochemistry*, vol. 40, no. 18, pp. 1353–1360, 2007.

[43] H. K. Kim, K. S. Song, Y. S. Park et al., "Elevated levels of circulating platelet microparticles, VEGF, IL-6 and RANTES in patients with gastric cancer: possible role of a metastasis predictor," *European Journal of Cancer*, vol. 39, no. 2, pp. 184–191, 2003.

[44] D. J. McKeown, D. J. F. Brown, A. Kelly, A. M. Wallace, and D. C. McMillan, "The relationship between circulating concentrations of C-reactive protein, inflammatory cytokines and cytokine receptors in patients with non-small-cell lung cancer," *British Journal of Cancer*, vol. 91, no. 12, pp. 1993–1995, 2004.

[45] W. Sun, D.-B. Liu, W.-W. Li et al., "Interleukin-6 promotes the migration and invasion of nasopharyngeal carcinoma cell lines and upregulates the expression of MMP-2 and MMP-9," *International Journal of Oncology*, vol. 44, no. 5, pp. 1551–1560, 2014.

[46] R. Salgado, S. Junius, I. Benoy et al., "Circulating interleukin-6 predicts survival in patients with metastatic breast cancer," *International Journal of Cancer*, vol. 103, no. 5, pp. 642–646, 2003.

[47] B. Goswami, P. Mittal, and N. Gupta, "Correlation of levels of IL-6 with tumor burden and receptor status in patients of locally advanced carcinoma breast," *Indian Journal of Clinical Biochemistry*, vol. 28, no. 1, pp. 90–94, 2013.

[48] C. Dethlefsen, G. Højfeldt, and P. Hojman, "The role of intratumoral and systemic IL-6 in breast cancer," *Breast Cancer Research and Treatment*, vol. 138, no. 3, pp. 657–664, 2013.

[49] A. Sanguinetti, D. Santini, M. Bonafè, M. Taffurelli, and N. Avenia, "Interleukin-6 and pro inflammatory status in the breast tumor microenvironment," *World Journal of Surgical Oncology*, vol. 13, article 129, 2015.

[50] Y.-C. Chung, Y.-L. Chaen, and C.-P. Hsu, "Clinical significance of tissue expression of interleukin-6 in colorectal carcinoma," *Anticancer Research*, vol. 26, no. 5, pp. 3905–3911, 2006.

[51] C. M. Jacobson, B. Rosenfeld, H. Pessin, and W. Breitbart, "Depression and IL-6 blood plasma concentrations in advanced cancer patients," *Psychosomatics*, vol. 49, no. 1, pp. 64–66, 2008.

[52] P. Ravishankaran and R. Karunanithi, "Clinical significance of preoperative serum interleukin-6 and C-reactive protein level in breast cancer patients," *World Journal of Surgical Oncology*, vol. 9, article 18, 2011.

[53] Y. Guo, F. Xu, T. Lu, Z. Duan, and Z. Zhang, "Interleukin-6 signaling pathway in targeted therapy for cancer," *Cancer Treatment Reviews*, vol. 38, no. 7, pp. 904–910, 2012.

[54] G. J. K. Guthrie, C. S. D. Roxburgh, C. H. Richards, P. G. Horgan, and D. C. McMillan, "Circulating IL-6 concentrations link tumour necrosis and systemic and local inflammatory responses in patients undergoing resection for colorectal cancer," *British Journal of Cancer*, vol. 109, no. 1, pp. 131–137, 2013.

[55] S. Kobayashi, N. W. Werneburg, S. F. Bronk, S. H. Kaufmann, and G. J. Gores, "Interleukin-6 contributes to Mcl-1 upregulation and TRAIL resistance via an Akt-signaling pathway in cholangiocarcinoma cells," *Gastroenterology*, vol. 128, no. 7, pp. 2054–2065, 2005.

[56] F. Meng, Y. Yamagiwa, S. Taffetani, J. Han, and T. Patel, "IL-6 activates serum and glucocorticoid kinase via p38α mitogen-activated protein kinase pathway," *The American Journal of Physiology—Cell Physiology*, vol. 289, no. 4, pp. C971–C981, 2005.

[57] J. Nakashima, M. Tachibana, Y. Horiguchi et al., "Serum interleukin 6 as a prognostic factor in patients with prostate cancer," *Clinical Cancer Research*, vol. 6, no. 7, pp. 2702–2706, 2000.

[58] M. El Far, M. Fouda, R. Yahya, and H. El Baz, "Serum IL-10 and IL-6 levels at diagnosis as independent predictors of outcome in non-Hodgkin's lymphoma," *Journal of Physiology and Biochemistry*, vol. 60, no. 4, pp. 253–258, 2004.

[59] R. Lai, S. O'Brien, T. Maushouri et al., "Prognostic value of plasma interleukin-6 levels in patients with chronic lymphocytic leukemia," *Cancer*, vol. 95, no. 5, pp. 1071–1075, 2002.

[60] N. A. Schultz, I. J. Christensen, J. Werner et al., "Diagnostic and prognostic impact of circulating YKL-40, IL-6, and CA 19.9 in patients with pancreatic cancer," *PLoS ONE*, vol. 8, no. 6, Article ID e67059, 2013.

[61] T. Ashizawa, R. Okada, Y. Suzuki et al., "Clinical significance of interleukin-6 (IL-6) in the spread of gastric cancer: role of IL-6 as a prognostic factor," *Gastric Cancer*, vol. 8, no. 2, pp. 124–131, 2005.

[62] Y. Yin, X. Si, Y. Gao, L. Gao, and J. Wang, "The nuclear factor-κB correlates with increased expression of interleukin-6 and promotes progression of gastric carcinoma," *Oncology Reports*, vol. 29, no. 1, pp. 34–38, 2013.

[63] J. Kaminska, M. P. Nowacki, M. Kowalska et al., "Clinical significance of serum cytokine measurements in untreated colorectal cancer patients: soluble tumor necrosis factor receptor type I—an independent prognostic factor," *Tumor Biology*, vol. 26, no. 4, pp. 186–194, 2005.

[64] F. Esfandi, S. M. Ghobadloo, and G. Basati, "Interleukin-6 level in patients with colorectal cancer," *Cancer Letters*, vol. 244, no. 1, pp. 76–78, 2006.

[65] N. I. Nikiteas, N. Tzanakis, M. Gazouli et al., "Serum IL-6, TNFalpha and CRP levels in Greek colorectal cancer patients: prognostic implications," *World Journal of Gastroenterology*, vol. 11, pp. 1639–1643, 2005.

[66] C.-C. Lu, H.-C. Kuo, F.-S. Wang, M.-H. Jou, K.-C. Lee, and J.-H. Chuang, "Upregulation of TLRs and IL-6 as a marker in human colorectal cancer," *International Journal of Molecular Sciences*, vol. 16, no. 1, pp. 159–177, 2015.

[67] A. Isobe, K. Sawada, Y. Kinose et al., "Interleukin 6 receptor is an independent prognostic factor and a potential therapeutic target of ovarian cancer," *PLoS ONE*, vol. 10, no. 2, Article ID e0118080, 2015.

[68] B. Paule, J. Belot, C. Rudant, C. Coulombel, and C. C. Abbou, "The importance of IL-6 protein expression in primary human renal cell carcinoma: an immunohistochemical study," *Journal of Clinical Pathology*, vol. 53, no. 5, pp. 388–390, 2000.

[69] P. F. Engelhardt, S. Seklehner, H. Brustmann, L. Lusuardi, and C. R. Riedl, "Immunohistochemical expression of interleukin-2 receptor and interleukin-6 in patients with prostate cancer and benign prostatic hyperplasia: association with asymptomatic inflammatory prostatitis NIH category IV," *Scandinavian Journal of Urology*, vol. 49, no. 2, pp. 120–126, 2014.

[70] V. Labovsky, L. M. Martinez, K. M. Davies et al., "Association between ligands and receptors related to the progression of early breast cancer in tumor epithelial and stromal cells," *Clinical Breast Cancer*, vol. 15, no. 1, pp. e13–e21, 2015.

[71] D. Chen, L. Jin, L. Zhu, X. Mou, S. Wang, and C. Mao, "Expressions and correlations of let-7a and IL-6 in esophageal squamous cell carcinoma," *Chinese Journal of Cellular and Molecular Immunology*, vol. 29, no. 11, pp. 1181–1184, 2013.

[72] M.-F. Chen, P.-T. Chen, M. S. Lu, P. Y. Lin, W.-C. Chen, and K.-D. Lee, "IL-6 expression predicts treatment response and outcome in squamous cell carcinoma of the esophagus," *Molecular Cancer*, vol. 12, article 26, 2013.

[73] Z. Wang, X. Si, A. Xu et al., "Activation of STAT3 in human gastric cancer cells via interleukin (IL)-6-type cytokine signaling correlates with clinical implications," *PLoS ONE*, vol. 8, no. 10, Article ID e75788, 2013.

[74] S. Depner, W. Lederle, C. Gutschalk, N. Linde, A. Zajonz, and M. M. Mueller, "Cell type specific interleukin-6 induced responses in tumor keratinocytes and stromal fibroblasts are essential for invasive growth," *International Journal of Cancer*, vol. 135, no. 3, pp. 551–562, 2014.

[75] T. Jinno, S. Kawano, Y. Maruse et al., "Increased expression of interleukin-6 predicts poor response to chemoradiotherapy and unfavorable prognosis in oral squamous cell carcinoma," *Oncology Reports*, vol. 33, no. 5, pp. 2161–2168, 2015.

[76] A. Chaturmohta, R. Dixit, G. Narayan et al., "Do expression profiles of cytokines VEGF, TNF- α, IL-1β, IL-6 and IL-8 correlate with gallbladder cancer?" *Journal of Cancer Science and Clinical Oncology 2*, vol. 2, no. 202, 2015.

[77] C. J. Chen, W. W. Sung, Y. M. Lin et al., "Gender difference in the prognostic role of interleukin 6 in oral squamous cell carcinoma," *PLoS ONE*, vol. 7, no. 11, Article ID e50104, 2012.

[78] F. Basolo, L. Fiore, G. Pollina, G. Fontanini, P. G. Conaldi, and A. Toniolo, "Reduced expression of interleukin 6 in undifferentiated thyroid carcinoma: in vitro and in vivo studies," *Clinical Cancer Research*, vol. 4, no. 2, pp. 381–387, 1998.

[79] R. M. Ruggeri, D. Villari, A. Simone et al., "Co-expression of interleukin-6 (IL-6) and interleukin-6 receptor (IL-6R) in thyroid nodules is associated with co-expression of CD30 ligand/CD30 receptor," *Journal of Endocrinological Investigation*, vol. 25, no. 11, pp. 959–966, 2002.

[80] A. G. Ozgen, M. Karadeniz, M. Erdogan, A. Berdeli, F. Saygili, and C. Yilmaz, "The (-174) G/C polymorphism in the interleukin-6 gene is associated with risk of papillary thyroid carcinoma in Turkish patients," *Journal of Endocrinological Investigation*, vol. 32, no. 6, pp. 491–494, 2009.

Permissions

List of Contributors

Gabriela Brenta
Department of Endocrinology, Dr. César Milstein Hospital, La Rioja 951, C1221ACI, Buenos Aires, Argentina

Nobuyuki Takasu and Mina Matsushita
Department of Endocrinology and Metabolism, Aizawa Hospital, 2-5-1 Honjo, Mtasumoto 390-8521, Japan

Pamela Bowman
Department of Paediatrics, Royal Devon and Exeter Hospital, Exeter, Devon EX25DW, UK
Department of Endocrinology, Royal Devon and Exeter Hospital, Exeter, Devon EX25DW, UK

Bijay Vaidya
Peninsula NIHR Clinical Research Facility, Level 2, Peninsula Medical School, University of Exeter, Barrack Road, Exeter, Devon EX25DW, UK

Mariella Bonzanini, LucaMorelli, Silvia Fasanella and Paolo Dalla Palma
Department of Surgical Pathology, S. Chiara Hospital, 38100 Trento, Italy

Pierluigi Amadori
Outpatient Endocrine Surgery, Local Public Health Service, 38100 Trento, Italy

Riccardo Pertile
Epidemiological Survey, Local Public Health Service, Trento, Italy

Angela Mattiuzzi and Giorgio Marini
Department of Radiology, S. Chiara Hospital, 38100 Trento, Italy

Mauro Niccolini
Department of Radiology, Villa Bianca Hospital, 38100 Trento, Italy

Giuseppe Tirone
Department of Surgery, S. Chiara Hospital, 38100 Trento, Italy

Marco Rigamonti
Department of Surgery, Cles Hospital, 38100 Trento, Italy

Amit D. Raval and Usha Sambamoorthi
Department of Pharmaceutical Systems and Policy, School of Pharmacy, West Virginia University, Morgantown, WV-26505, USA

Jonathan Chevrier, Kim G. Harley, Katherine Kogut, Nina Holland, Caroline Johnson and Brenda Eskenazi
Center for Environmental Research and Children's Health (CERCH), School of Public Health, University of California, Berkeley, CA 94704-7392, USA

Pradip K. Sarkar
Department of Basic Sciences, Parker University, 2500Walnut Hill Lane, Dallas, TX 75229, USA
Center for Computational and Integrative Biology, Rutgers University, 315 Penn Street, Camden, NJ 08102, USA
Department of Molecular Medicine, Bose Institute, P-1/12, CIT, Scheme VII-M, Calcutta 700054, India

Avijit Biswas and Joseph V. Martin
Center for Computational and Integrative Biology, Rutgers University, 315 Penn Street, Camden, NJ 08102, USA

Arun K. Ray
Department of Molecular Medicine, Bose Institute, P-1/12, CIT, Scheme VII-M, Calcutta 700054, India

Naveen Aggarwal
Department of Endocrinology, Gateshead Health NHS Foundation NHS Trust, UK

Salman Razvi
Department of Endocrinology, Gateshead Health NHS Foundation NHS Trust, UK
Institute of Genetic Medicine, Newcastle University, UK

Fabián Pitoia, Erika Abelleira, Fernanda Bueno and Hugo Niepomniszcze
Division of Endocrinology, Hospital de Clínicas, University of Buenos Aires, Córdoba 2351, 5th Floor, Buenos Aires 1424, Argentina

Robert J. Marlowe
Division of Medical Editing, Spencer-Fontayne Corporation, 33 Bentley Avenue, Jersey City, NJ 07304-1901, USA

Eduardo N. Faure and Rubén Julio Lutfi
Division of Endocrinology, Hospital Churruca Visca, Uspallata 3400, Buenos Aires 1437, Argentina

Diego Schwarzstein
Division of Endocrinology, Consultorios Integrados Rosario, Italia 424, Santa Fe, Rosario 2000, Argentina

Polyxeni Karakosta
Department of Social Medicine, Faculty of Medicine, University of Crete, 71003 Heraklion, Greece
Department of Experimental Endocrinology, Faculty of Medicine, University of Crete, 71003 Heraklion, Greece

Leda Chatzi, Emmanouil Bagkeris and Dimitris Alegakis
Department of Social Medicine, Faculty of Medicine, University of Crete, 71003 Heraklion, Greece

Marilena Kampa and Elias Castanas
Department of Experimental Endocrinology, Faculty of Medicine, University of Crete, 71003 Heraklion, Greece

Vasiliki Daraki
Department of Endocrinology, Faculty of Medicine, University of Crete, 71003 Heraklion, Greece

Manolis Kogevinas
Centre for Research in Environmental Epidemiology (CREAL), Doctor Aiguader, 88, 08003 Barcelona, Spain
National School of Public Health, Alexandras Avenue 196, 115 21 Athens, Greece

Vivek Mathew, Raiz Ahmad Misgar, Sujoy Ghosh, Pradip Mukhopadhyay, Pradip Roychowdhury, Kaushik Pandit, Satinath Mukhopadhyay and Subhankar Chowdhury
Institute of Post-Graduate Medical Education and Research, Calcutta 700020, India

Neera Sharma and Lokesh Kumar Sharma
Department of Biochemistry, Post Graduate Institute of Medical Education and Research (PGIMER) and Dr. Ram Manohar Lohia (RML) Hospital, 1 Baba Kharak Singh Marg, New Delhi 110001, India

Deep Dutta, Kumar Gaurav, Sabyasachi Mukherjee and Rahul Bansal
Department of Endocrinology, Post Graduate Institute of Medical Education and Research (PGIMER) and Dr. Ram Manohar Lohia (RML) Hospital, 1 Baba Kharak Singh Marg, New Delhi 110001, India

Adesh Kisanji Gadpayle
Post Graduate Institute of Medical Education and Research (PGIMER) and Dr. Ram Manohar Lohia (RML) Hospital, 1 Baba Kharak Singh Marg, New Delhi 110001, India

Atul Anand
Anti-Retroviral Therapy Clinic, Post Graduate Institute of Medical Education and Research (PGIMER) and Dr. Ram Manohar Lohia (RML) Hospital, 1 Baba Kharak Singh Marg, New Delhi 110001, India

Andrea Garces-Arteaga, Nataly Nieto-Garcia, Freddy Suarez-Sanchez and Héctor Reynaldo Triana-Reina
Departamento de Educación Física y Deporte, Universidad del Valle, Meléndez Cali, Colombia

Robinson Ramírez-Vélez
Grupo GICAEDS, Facultad de Cultura Física, Deporte y Recreación, Universidad Santo Tomás, Carrera 9 No 51-23, Bogotá, DC, Colombia

Michael C. Sullivan, Sanziana A. Roman and Julie A. Sosa
Department of Surgery, Yale School of Medicine, New Haven, CT 06520, USA

Osamu Tohyama and Takayuki Kimura
Biomarkers and Personalized Medicine Core Function Unit, Eisai Co., Ltd, Tsukuba, Ibaraki 300-2635, Japan

Junji Matsui, Kotaro Kodama, Naoko Hata-Sugi, Kiyoshi Okamoto, Yukinori Minoshima and Masao Iwata
Discovery Biology, Oncology Product Creation Unit, Eisai Co., Ltd, Tsukuba, Ibaraki 300-2635, Japan

Yasuhiro Funahashi
Biomarkers and Personalized Medicine Core Function Unit, Eisai Inc., 4 Corporate Drive, Andover, MA 01810, USA

Taimur Saleem
Medical College, Aga Khan University, Stadium Road, Karachi 74800, Pakistan

Aisha Sheikh and Qamar Masood
Section of Diabetes, Endocrinology, and Metabolism, Department of Medicine, Aga Khan University, Stadium Road, Karachi 74800, Pakistan

Rafal Z. Slapa, Wieslaw S. Jakubowski, Bartosz Migda and R. Krzysztof Mlosek
Department of Diagnostic Imaging, Second Faculty of Medicine, Medical University of Warsaw, ul. Kondratowicza 8, 03-242 Warsaw, Poland

Antoni Piwowonski
NZOZ Almed, 37-500 Jarosław, Poland

Jacek Bierca
Surgery Department, Solec Hospital, 00-382 Warsaw, Poland

Kazimierz T. Szopinski
Department of Dental and Maxillofacial Radiology, Institute of Stomatology, First Faculty of Medicine, Medical University of Warsaw, 02-006 Warsaw, Poland

Jadwiga Slowinska-Srzednicka
Department of Endocrinology, Centre for Postgraduate Medical Education, 01-809 Warsaw, Poland

Gustavo Vasconcelos Alves
Oncology Division, Nossa Senhora da Conceição Hospital, Porto Alegre, RS, Brazil

Ana Paula Santin
Postgraduation Program in Medicine and Medical Sciences, Universidade Federal do Rio Grande do Sul, Rua Ramiro Barcellos 2400, 90035-003 Porto Alegre, RS, Brazil

Tania Weber Furlanetto
Postgraduation Program in Medicine and Medical Sciences, Universidade Federal do Rio Grande do Sul, Rua Ramiro Barcellos 2400, 90035-003 Porto Alegre, RS, Brazil
Internal Medicine Division, Hospital de Clínicas de Porto Alegre, Universidade Federal do Rio Grande do Sul, Rua Ramiro Barcellos 2350/700, 90035-003 Porto Alegre, RS, Brazil

Jeffrey Fisher, Xiaoxia Yang and Annie Lumen
National Center for Toxicological Research, US FDA, 3900 NCTR Road, Jefferson, AR 72079, USA

Curtis Harris
College of Public Health, University of Georgia, 115 DW Brooks Dr, Barrow Hall, Room 001B, Athens, GA 30602, USA

Igor Koturbash
Department of Environmental and Occupational Health, Fay W. Boozman College of Public Health, University of Arkansas for Medical Sciences, 4301West Markham Street, Slot 820-11, Little Rock, AR 72205, USA

Emin Gurleyik
Department of Surgery, Duzce University, Medical Faculty, 81650 Duzce, Turkey

Eric T. Shinohara, Albert Attia, Matthew S. Ning, Jeffrey M. Friedman and Anthony J. Cmelak
Department of Radiation Oncology, Vanderbilt University Medical Center, Nashville, TN 37232, USA

Mark J. Stavas
Department of Radiation Oncology, Vanderbilt University Medical Center, Nashville, TN 37232, USA
Department of Radiation Oncology, Vanderbilt University School of Medicine, 1301 Medical Center Drive, B913/TVC, Nashville, TN 37232, USA

Varlık Erol, Özer Makay, Gökhan Eçöz, Mahir Akyıldız and Mustafa Yılmaz
Division of Endocrine Surgery, Department of General Surgery, School of Medicine, Ege University, Bornova, 35100 Izmir, Turkey

Yeşim Ertan
Department of Pathology, School of Medicine, Ege University, Bornova, 35100 Izmir, Turkey

Kai-PunWong and Brian Hung-Hin Lang
Division of Endocrine Surgery, Department of Surgery, The University of Hong Kong, Queen Mary Hospital, Pokfulam Road, Hong Kong, Hong Kong

Mehdi Hedayati, Marjan Zarif Yeganeh and Laleh Hoghooghi Rad
Obesity Research Center, Research Institute for Endocrine Sciences, Shahid Beheshti University of Medical Sciences, 1985717413 Tehran, Iran

Parichehr Yaghmaei and Zahra Pooyamanesh
Department of Biology, Faculty of Basic Sciences, Science Research Campus of Islamic Azad University, 1939614484 Tehran, Iran

Mario Vaisman
Endocrinology Service, Universidade Federal do Rio de Janeiro, Rio de Janiro, RJ, Brazil

Fernanda Vaisman and Rossana Corbo
Endocrinology Service, Universidade Federal do Rio de Janeiro, Rio de Janiro, RJ, Brazil
Endocrinology Service, Instituto Nacional do Cancer, Rio de Janeiro, Rio de Janiro, RJ, Brazil

Tina Toft Kristensen and Søren Jelstrup
Department of Otorhinolaryngology-Head and Neck Surgery, Koege Hospital, Region Zealand, 4600 Koege, Denmark

Jacob Larsen
Department of Clinical Pathology, Naestved Hospital, Region Zealand, 4700 Naestved, Denmark

Palle Lyngsie Pedersen and Christina Ellervik
Department of Clinical Biochemistry, Naestved Hospital, Region Zealand, 4700 Naestved, Denmark

Anne-Dorthe Feldthusen
Department of Gynecology and Obstetrics, Naestved Hospital, Region Zealand, 4700 Naestved, Denmark

Jan Kvetny
Department of Internal Medicine, Naestved Hospital, Region Zealand, 4700 Naestved, Denmark

University of Southern Denmark, 5230 Odense, Denmark

P. Torremante
Praxis für Gynäkologie und Geburtshilfe, Marktplatz 29, 88416 Ochsenhausen, Germany

F. Flock
Frauenklinik des Klinikums Memmingen, Klinikum Memmingen, Bismarckstraße 23, 87700 Memmingen, Germany

W. Kirschner
Institut Forschung, Beratung und Evaluation, FB+E Forschung, Beratung Evaluation GmbH, Postfach 10 03 35, 10563 Berlin, Germany

Mohamed Yousef, Abdelmoneim Sulieman and Alsafi Abdella
College of Medical Radiologic Science, Sudan University of Science and Technology, Baladya Street, Khartoum 11111, Sudan

Bushra Ahmed
College of Radiology and Nuclear Medicine, The National Ribat University, Nile Street, Burri, Khartoum 11111, Sudan

Khaled Eltom
Radiation and Isotope Center, Khartoum (RICK), Algaser Street, Khartoum 11111, Sudan

Indira Prabakaran, Robert Lewis, Douglas L. Fraker and Marina A. Guvakova
Department of Surgery, School of Medicine, University of Pennsylvania, Philadelphia, PA 19104, USA

Jillian R. Grau
Department of Pathology and Laboratory Medicine, School of Medicine, University of Pennsylvania, Philadelphia, PA 19104, USA

Konrad Sarosiek, Ankit V. Gandhi, Shivam Saxena, Christopher Y. Kang and Charles J. Yeo
Departments of Surgery, Jefferson Pancreatic, Biliary and Related Cancer Center, Thomas Jefferson University, Philadelphia, PA 19107, USA

Galina I. Chipitsyna and Hwyda A. Arafat
Department of Biomedical Sciences, University of New England, Biddeford, ME 04005, USA

Toral P. Kobawala, Trupti I. Trivedi, Kinjal K. Gajjar, Darshita H. Patel, Girish H. Patel and Nandita R. Ghosh
Division of Molecular Endocrinology, Cancer Biology Department, The Gujarat Cancer and Research Institute, NCH Compound, Asarwa, Ahmedabad, Gujarat 380016, India

Index

www.ingramcontent.com/pod-product-compliance
Lightning Source LLC
Chambersburg PA
CBHW080410190526
45161CB00003B/194